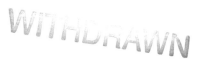

Imaging Acute Neurologic Disease

A Symptom-Based Approach

Imaging Acute Neurologic Disease

A Symptom-Based Approach

Edited by

Massimo Filippi, MD

Editor-in-Chief of *Journal of Neurology*; Professor of Neurology and Director, Neuroimaging Research Unit, Institute of Experimental Neurology, Division of Neuroscience, San Raffaele Scientific Institute, Vita-Salute San Raffaele University, Milan, Italy

Jack H. Simon, MD, PhD

Professor of Radiology and Neurology, Oregon Health and Science University (OHSU); Neuroradiologist, Portland VA Medical Center; Adjunct Scientist, Advanced Imaging Research Center, OHSU, Portland, OR, USA

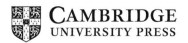
CAMBRIDGE
UNIVERSITY PRESS

CAMBRIDGE
UNIVERSITY PRESS

University Printing House, Cambridge CB2 8BS, United Kingdom

Cambridge University Press is part of the University of Cambridge.

It furthers the University's mission by disseminating knowledge in the pursuit of education, learning and research at the highest international levels of excellence.

www.cambridge.org
Information on this title: www.cambridge.org/9781107035942

© Cambridge University Press 2014

First published 2014

Printed in Spain by Grafos SA, Arte sobre papel

A catalogue record for this publication is available from the British Library

Library of Congress Cataloging in Publication data
Imaging acute neurologic disease : a symptom-based approach / edited by Massimo Filippi, Jack H. Simon.
    p. ; cm.
Includes bibliographical references and index.
ISBN 978-1-107-03594-2 (hardback)
I. Filippi, M. (Massimo), 1961– editor of compilation.   II. Simon, Jack H., editor of compilation.
[DNLM: 1. Nervous System Diseases – diagnosis.   2. Diagnostic Imaging – methods.
3. Emergency Service, Hospital. WL 141]
RC386.6.N48
616.8′0475–dc23

                                                                                    2014001848

ISBN 978-1-107-03594-2 Hardback

Contents

Contributors

Federica Agosta, MD, PhD
Neuroimaging Research Unit, Institute of
Experimental Neurology, Division of Neuroscience,
San Raffaele Scientific Institute, Vita-Salute San
Raffaele University, Milan, Italy

Alberto Albanese, MD
Istituto Neurologico Carlo Besta, Università Cattolica
del Sacro Cuore, Milan, Italy

Timothy J. Amrhein, MD
Department of Radiology, Medical University of
South Carolina, Charleston, SC, USA

A. M. Barrett, MD
Kessler Foundation, West Orange, NJ; Department of
Physical Medicine & Rehabilitation, and Department
of Neurology & Neurosciences, Rutgers – New Jersey
Medical School, Newark, NJ, USA

Walter S. Bartynski, MD
Department of Radiology, Medical University of
South Carolina, Charleston, SC, USA

Felix Benninger, MD
Department of Neurology, Rabin Medical Center,
Petach Tikva, Israel

Thomas Brandt, MD, FRCP, FANA
Clinical Neuroscience and German Center
for Vertigo and Balance Disorders – IFB,
Ludwig-Maximilians-University Munich, Germany

Andrew G. Burke, MD
Division of Neuroradiology, Oregon Health and
Science University, Portland, OR, USA

Michelle Cameron, MD, PT
Department of Neurology, Oregon Health and Science
University, Portland, OR, USA

Elisa Canu, MSc
Neuroimaging Research Unit, Institute of
Experimental Neurology, Division of Neuroscience,

San Raffaele Scientific Institute, Vita-Salute San
Raffaele University, Milan, Italy

Louis R. Caplan, MD
Department of Neurology, Beth Israel Deaconess
Medical Center, Boston, MA, USA

Christine M. Carr, MD
Division of Emergency Medicine, Medical University
of South Carolina, Charleston, SC, USA

Daniel J. A. Connolly, MRCP, FRCR
Department of Radiology, Royal Hallamshire
Hospital, Sheffield, UK

Firouz Daneshgari, MD
Department of Urology, Case Western Reserve
University, Cleveland, OH, USA

John DeLuca PhD
Kessler Foundation, West Orange, NJ; Department
of Physical Medicine & Rehabilitation, and
Department of Neurology & Neurosciences, Rutgers –
New Jersey Medical School, Newark, NJ, USA

Marianne de Visser, MD, PhD
Department of Neurology, Academic Medical Center,
University of Amsterdam, Amsterdam, The Netherlands

Marianne Dieterich, MD, FANA
Department of Neurology and German
Center for Vertigo and Balance Disorders – IFB,
Ludwig-Maximilians-University Munich, Germany

Antonio E. Elia, MD
Istituto Neurologico Carlo Besta, Università Cattolica
del Sacro Cuore, Milano, Italy

Joseph H. Feinberg, MD
Hospital for Special Surgery, New York, NY, USA

Massimo Filippi, MD
Neuroimaging Research Unit, Institute of
Experimental Neurology, Division of Neuroscience,

San Raffaele Scientific Institute, Vita-Salute San Raffaele University, Milan, Italy

Lauren C. Frey, MD
Department of Neurology, University of Colorado School of Medicine, Aurora, CO, USA

Gaëtan Garraux, MD, PhD
MOVERE Group, Cyclotron Research Center & Department of Neurology, University of Liège, Belgium

Andrea Ginestroni, MD, PhD
Department of Neuroradiology, Careggi University Hospital, Florence, Italy

Peter J. Goadsby, MD, PhD
Headache Group, Department of Neurology, University of California, San Francisco, San Francisco, CA, USA

Bronwyn E. Hamilton, MD
Division of Neuroradiology, Oregon Health and Science University, Portland, OR, USA

Simon J. Hickman, PhD, FRCP
Department of Neurology, Royal Hallamshire Hospital, Sheffield, UK

Holly E. Hinson, MD
Department of Neurology, Oregon Health and Science University, Portland, OR, USA

Jon P. Jennings, MD
Division of Emergency Medicine, Medical University of South Carolina, Charleston, SC, USA

Jan Kassubek, MD
Department of Neurology, University of Ulm, Ulm, Germany

Horacio Kaufmann, MD
Departments of Neurology, Medicine, and Pediatrics, New York University Langone Medical Center, New York, NY, USA

David M. Kaylie, MD, FACS
Division of Otolaryngology, Duke University Medical Center, Durham, NC, USA

Joanna Kitley, MBBS
Nuffield Department of Clinical Neurosciences, University of Oxford, John Radcliffe Hospital, Oxford, UK

Vladimir S. Kostic, MD, PhD
Clinic of Neurology, Faculty of Medicine, University of Belgrade, Belgrade, Serbia

C. T. Paul Krediet, MD, PhD
Department of Internal Medicine, Academic Medical Center at the University of Amsterdam, The Netherlands

Megan C. Leary, MD
Department of Neurology, Beth Israel Deaconess Medical Center, Boston, MA, USA

Farooq H. Maniyar, MD, MRCP
The Royal London Hospital, London & Basildon and Thurrock University Hospitals NHS Foundation Trust, Basildon, UK

Ken R. Maravilla, MD
Department of Radiology, University of Washington, Seattle, WA, USA

Mario Mascalchi, MD, PhD
Quantitative & Functional Neuroradiology Research Unit, Department of Experimental & Clinical Biomedical Sciences, University of Florence, Italy

Rajarshi Mazumder, MD
Oregon Health Sciences University, Portland, OR, USA

Priyesh Mehta, DO
Department of Rehabilitation Medicine, New York Presbyterian Hospital, New York, NY, USA

Jacqueline A. Palace, DM, FRCP
Nuffield Department of Clinical Neurosciences, University of Oxford, John Radcliffe Hospital, Oxford, UK

Raj M. Paspulati, MD
Department of Radiology, Case Western Reserve University, University Hospitals Case Medical Center, Cleveland, OH, USA

Christopher A. Potter, MD
Department of Radiology, University of Washington, Seattle, WA, USA

Angelo Quattrini, MD
Experimental Neuropathology Unit, Institute of Experimental Neurology, Division of Neuroscience, San Raffaele Scientific Institute, Vita-Salute San Raffaele University, Milan, Italy

Louis P. Riccelli MD
Department of Radiology, Oregon Health and Science University, Portland, OR, USA

Nilo Riva, MD, PhD
Experimental Neuropathology Unit, Division of Neuroscience, San Raffaele Scientific Institute, Vita-Salute San Raffaele University, Milan, Italy

Maria A. Rocca, MD
Neuroimaging Research Unit, Department of Neurology, San Raffaele Scientific Institute, Vita-Salute San Raffaele University, Milan, Italy

Mirabelle B. Sajisevi, MD
Division of Otolaryngology, Duke University Medical Center, Durham, NC, USA

Richard Salazar-Montero, MD
Department of Neurology, University of Maryland School of Medicine, Baltimore, MD, USA

Nicholas D. Schiff, MD, PhD
Department of Neurology, Weill Cornell Medical College, New York, NY, USA

Jack H. Simon, MD, PhD
Department of Radiology, Oregon Health and Science University; Neuroradiologist, Portland VAMC, Portland, OR, USA

Israel Steiner, MD
Department of Neurology, Rabin Medical Center, Petach Tikva, Israel

Carl D. Stevens, MD, MPH
Department of Emergency Medicine, Harbor-UCLA Medical Center, Torrance, CA, USA

Bart P. van de Warrenburg, MD, PhD
Department of Neurology, Radboud University Nijmegen Medical Centre, Donders Institute for Brain, Cognition & Behaviour, Nijmegen, The Netherlands

Judith van Gaalen, MD
Department of Neurology, Radboud University Nijmegen Medical Centre, Donders Institute for Brain, Cognition & Behaviour, Nijmegen, The Netherlands

William J. Weiner, MD (deceased)
Formerly Department of Neurology, University of Maryland School of Medicine, Baltimore, MD, USA

Jane L. Weissman, MD, FACR
Department of Radiology, Oregon Health and Science University, Portland, OR, USA

Jay Yao, MD
Department of Neurology, Oregon Health and Science University, Portland, OR, USA

G. Bryan Young, MD, FRCPC
University Hospital, London, Ontario, Canada

Preface

Acute neurologic diseases encompass a wide spectrum of medical illnesses with neurological manifestations which require rapid clinical, paraclinical, and laboratory evaluation as patients are assessed in the emergency department or acute care clinics. In the last decade, imaging has assumed far greater importance in the initial assessment of these patients, and is responsible for much of the cost and resources in the early, critical evaluation. However, the optimal approach to utilization of imaging for thorough, yet efficient and cost-responsible, care remains poorly defined for many acute neurologic presentations.

Many radiologic texts provide an invaluable overview of the many important details of the pathology of neurologic disease. But patients present to the emergency room or clinic with symptoms which typically are thoughtfully considered and guide the clinician through a decision-making process that ultimately determines the type, order, and priorities for further testing, including imaging when indicated. We have therefore prioritized a symptom-based approach to imaging in acute neurologic disease, based on the practice parameters developed by experts in the field, combining expert clinicians and imagers for each chapter. The task of developing symptom-based imaging algorithms is not always straightforward, and it is recognized that there are many potential variations in approach that are equally valid. The reader will observe that each team of authors has developed a personalized approach to the question based on their practice pattern and expertise. The approaches described in each chapter should provide a framework that we hope can be utilized by the reader to refine their approach, suggest alternative pathways, or encourage and stimulate discussion in the clinical and imaging circles that can ultimately result in more optimal clinical care. While the imaging details and differential considerations are not meant to be comprehensive, we hope that imagers will also benefit from this symptom-centric approach to disease; in the reading room evaluation always starts with consideration of history, symptoms, and signs, and imaging is an interactive process that benefits from repeated clinical input, especially in complex and unusual neurological presentations.

Currently, conventional computerized tomography (CT), magnetic resonance imaging (MRI), and nuclear medicine techniques are used to facilitate diagnosis, therapeutic decisions, to provide information regarding prognosis, and to monitor therapy response. Furthermore, the advent of quantitative CT and MRI techniques, notably diffusion and perfusion imaging, have introduced new opportunities for diagnosis of neurological diseases on the basis of objective findings. The improved and more advanced techniques offer unique anatomical as well as pathophysiological information that provides insight into neurological diseases. However, the practical value of various neuroimaging techniques in routine clinical practice in an individual patient is not as yet well defined.

The scope of this book is designed to provide a comprehensive survey of best practice for experienced clinicians and imagers as well as resident housestaff in fields such as emergency medicine, neurology, radiology and neuroradiology, neurosurgery, and critical care. The symptom-based imaging aims to guide the emergency physician in the choice of imaging tools for a correct and cost-efficient diagnosis of the common and complex neurological disorders. The integrated approach to examination algorithms includes the most common symptoms likely to be encountered in the emergency or acute care setting, ranging from global symptoms such as headache and syncope through focal neurologic symptoms such as hearing loss and paralysis. It should be emphasized that this volume is designed to provide practical algorithms and guidelines for the emergency setting. The work is not intended to discuss all possible differential diagnoses, their pathogenesis, and immediate management or treatment. For many neurologic conditions, final diagnosis is in fact not achieved in the initial or emergency department evaluation.

The organization of the book is such that the first three chapters consider evaluation of patients with altered states of consciousness: delirium, agitation, and intellectual dysfunction. The subsequent two chapters are concerned with assessment of patients with pain, a common presenting complaint for patients in an emergency department. The remaining chapters examine the frequent acute neurological complaints which are secondary to brain damage and manifest as either focal or multifocal neurological presentations. Approaches to symptoms suggestive of involvement of the spinal cord and peripheral nervous system are also considered.

Our hope is that this volume is appreciated as a comprehensive source of information and also provides an educational framework for trainees and a reference for practicing neurologists and radiologists seeking direct and authoritative answers to questions. We have encouraged authors to introduce illustrative and tabular material, including flow charts. We hope that readers will find this issue of practical relevance and a stimulus to more in-depth reading and investigation in this field.

Massimo Filippi and Jack Simon
Milan, Italy
Portland, Oregon, USA

Disorders of consciousness

G. Bryan Young and Nicholas D. Schiff

Introduction

The assessment of the patient with acute impairment of consciousness requires an organized, systematic approach, beginning with the history (the diagnosis is suspected on the history alone in over 85% of cases), the physical examination, and basic laboratory testing. It is only after these steps that well-chosen neuroimaging is performed, always with a specific question in mind. This review synthesizes clinical, laboratory, and radiological approaches with a strategy that will provide useful diagnostic and prognostic information. We also provide a special focus on the potential future role of novel neurodiagnostics in the acute care setting.

Consciousness is composed of two principal components: alertness and awareness. Alertness is a function of the ascending reticular activating system (ARAS) in the rostral brainstem tegmentum (from the midpons through the midbrain) and then the thalamus and its projections through the cerebral white matter to the cerebral cortex. This allows for an eyes-open vigilant state, including arousability and spontaneous wake and sleep cycles. (This system and its various neurotransmitters will be discussed later.)

Awareness depends on the integrity of integrated cerebral gray-matter structures and their interconnecting fibers running through the white matter. Awareness has multiple inter-related functions, including sensation, perception, memory, attention (with selectivity), emotions, judgment, motivation, and planned action, with various interconnected anatomical loci.

Thus, consciousness is not a unitary phenomenon, but has multiple components. It is best to describe impairment of consciousness in terms of the type of impairment and its degree. Note also that a patient can be fully awake and aware, but may not be responsive due to central (including psychogenic) or peripheral nervous system causes. Thus, the absence of response is not necessarily proof of a disorder of consciousness (DOC).

The approach

A patient with acutely altered consciousness is brought into the emergency room by the ambulance service. You are asked to consult on the patient to provide a diagnosis and, if necessary, a prognosis, and to recommend steps in management, including investigation and treatment.

The above is a common clinical problem and the clinician should have an approach that will maximize precision and effectiveness. Let us suppose that the initial ABC management (airway, breathing, and circulatory) has been performed and that initial blood work has been sent, so that we can concentrate on the diagnostic approach. The initial step is history-taking, followed by the neurological and relevant general examinations.

As in the clinical approach to all neurologic disorders, the initial step is to localize the problem, then to determine the etiology. In DOC, the issue of prognostic determination often follows.

A. **History**: The history can help localize the problem as well as provide a story of the tempo or course of the illness, thus addressing both where and what.

A description of the acute behavioral change is usually available from the ambulance attendants and persons living with the patient. Was the problem a disturbance in alertness or a change in behavior? Was it a sudden collapse or a gradual and progressive or fluctuating change? Were there any preceding incidents or illness, e.g., head injury, drug ingestion, fever, or headache? Were there

Imaging Acute Neurologic Disease, ed. Massimo Filippi and Jack H. Simon. Published by Cambridge University Press.
© Cambridge University Press 2014.

focal features, e.g., a hemiparesis or aphasia, which preceded the loss of consciousness? What chronic conditions were present, e.g., cancer, diabetes, epilepsy, or autoimmune diseases; or cardiac, pulmonary, hepatic, or renal impairment? What medications was the patient taking? Was there a history of drug or alcohol abuse? What were the details of the collapse – falling limply vs. like a tree? Were there convulsive movements? Did anyone feel for a pulse?

B. **The neurological examination**: The degree of obtundation, using the Glasgow Coma Scale (GCS) [1] or FOUR score if desired, is determined [2]. Observe spontaneous movements and response to stimulation. If the patient remains unresponsive one applies progressively increasing stimuli, starting with calling the patient's name then applying somatic stimulation. Cranial nerve examination can help localize the lesion to specific cranial nerves or the brainstem. Check for gaze preference or palsy (using oculocephalic or caloric testing), and pupillary reactivity and size. The corneal reflex if unilaterally absent can be localizing, but corneal reflexes being present or absent bilaterally can reflect the degree of ARAS depression from an overwhelming metabolic disorder or a drug overdose. The combination of intact pupillary and absent oculovestibular reflexes raises the possibility of Wernicke–Korsakoff's encephalopathy, but we have seen the same phenomenon with a wide variety of sedative and analgesic drugs as well as antihistamine overdoses. The presence of nystagmus with caloric testing is strongly supportive of psychogenic unresponsiveness. One should always check for vertical eye movements, as lesions of the thalamus or rostral brainstem can abolish vertical but not horizontal eye movements.

Motor tone is assessed by passively moving the patient's limbs and noting the resistance to movement. Patients with neuroleptic malignant syndrome, malignant hyperthermia, or serotonin syndrome typically have marked, persistent increased resistance to movement. Patients with other causes of encephalopathy, when comatose, may have flaccid tone, but encephalopathic patients with metabolic or septic causes often show a fluctuating, velocity-dependent increase in tone (the resistance increases with the speed of movement) known as *gegenhalten* or paratonic

rigidity. In parkinsonian rigidity (commonly produced by neuroleptic medications or metoclopramide), the resistance is present throughout the range of movement and is not as velocity-dependent as in *gegenhalten*. In spasticity, there is a velocity-dependent increase in tone and then a release as the muscle spindles fire, causing flaccidity (clasp-knife effect). It is useful to note the motor responses to stimulation. The lack of movement on one side of the body, or hemiplegia, indicates a central cause for the paralysis. Purposeful movements in which the arm moves to the stimulus, often pushing it away or crossing the midline, indicate a lighter level of consciousness and an intact motor system on the side with movement. Decerebrate (upper- and lower-limb extension) or decorticate (upper limbs flexed at the elbows) were thought to indicate lesions below or above the red nucleus in the midbrain, respectively, but in humans both can occur with deep cerebral lesions, and the type of posturing can alternate over time.

In the less obtunded patient, the presence of postural-action tremor (with the upper limbs held up against gravity and/or moving to a target), asterixis (flapping tremor caused by the loss of postural tone as the patient holds the upper limbs out and extends the wrists), and multifocal myoclonus are strongly suggestive of a toxic or metabolic encephalopathy.

C. **Routine blood and urine testing**: Routine testing of serum glucose, electrolytes, magnesium, calcium, phosphate, urea, and creatinine and arterial or capillary blood gases are usually worthwhile. Urine is commonly sent for glucose, protein, and cell counts, but bacterial culture and drug screening (usually with specific drugs in mind) are commonly indicated. Serum drug concentrations, checking for alcohol or drug intoxications or for compliance of maintenance drugs, e.g., anticonvulsants, are often performed. Blood gas determination can help narrow the differential diagnosis (e.g. a metabolic acidosis is commonly due to increased lactate (as in sepsis or hypoperfusion), ketones or uremic toxins, or some exogenous agents such as methanol or propylene glycol). Point-of-care testing often obviates the need to administer glucose intravenously; if the latter is done it is wise to give thiamine simultaneously to prevent Wernicke–Korsakoff's encephalopathy.

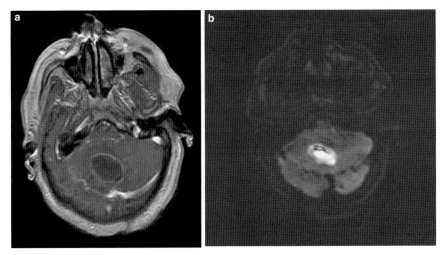

Figure 1.1 (A) Axial T1-weighted post contrast-enhanced MRI shows a ring-enhancing cerebellar abscess that occurred with purulent meningitis. There is associated compression of the fourth ventricle. (B) A diffusion-weighted MRI scan shows diffusion restriction, a feature that can help differentiate abscess from tumor.

D. **Lumbar puncture (LP)**: In the acutely comatose patient LP is used to rule out central nervous system (CNS) infection or subarachnoid hemorrhage. Less commonly, meningeal carcinomatosis can present with loss of consciousness. A computer tomography (CT) imaging of the head before LP is usually done, as unexpected mass lesions, e.g., cerebral or cerebellar abscess, can coexist with bacterial meningitis (Figure 1.1), making the LP dangerous. Subarachnoid hemorrhage can be detected by CT in over 95% of cases (Figure 1.2). Other contraindications to LP include coagulopathy and infection near or over the proposed puncture site.

E. **Neuroimaging in the acute setting**: Neuroimaging is necessary in all cases of disorders of consciousness except for those in which a non-structural cause of coma is readily identified, e.g., hypoglycemia reversed by an infusion of glucose. Even in metabolic, toxic, or infectious cases, neuroimaging is often advisable to exclude cerebral edema, associated traumatic lesions, a cerebral abscess, or empyema. CT scanning is usually available and is usually sufficient to make decisions about the safety of doing an LP.

One of the most common indications for neuroimaging in the emergency room (ER) is for stroke. Hemorrhagic stroke is readily detected on CT. However, ischemic stroke may be missed in very acute infarction. Subtle loss of gray–white differentiation can be helpful in showing ischemic damage affecting the cortex, insula, and basal ganglia. This forms the basis of the ASPECT scoring system, which has a correlation of greater than 80% between observers [3]. Recently, the American Academy of Neurology recommended diffusion-weighted MRI over CT for the assessment of acute ischemic stroke [4]. This allows for clearer delineation of the infarcted vascular territory.

A classification of DOCs

1. **Brain death**: This is the permanent cessation of all functions of the brain. Brain death is an unambiguous state when properly diagnosed but can be misidentified in situations where clinical history is unknown or the examination is limited by trauma or prior alterations of sensory-motor function. Recognition of such confounding variables is crucial for the accurate assessment of brain death [5].

2. **Coma**: An unarousable unconscious state, in which stimulation does not produce an arousal response, due to dysfunction of the ARAS. Coma can be graded dependent on motor responses. Two scales that are used to grade consciousness are the GCS [1] and the FOUR score [2]. These are listed in Tables 1.1 and 1.2. Coma is usually defined as a GCS score of 8 or less; with the FOUR score as the

3

Table 1.1 The Glasgow Coma Scale (GCS)

Best eye response	Spontaneous – open with blinking at baseline	4
	Opens to verbal command, speech or shouting	3
	Opens to pain (not applied to face)	2
	None	1
Best verbal response	Oriented	5
	Confused conversation, but able to answer questions	4
	Inappropriate responses, words discernible	3
	Incomprehensible speech	2
	None	1
Best motor response	Obeys command for movement	6
	Purposeful movement to painful stimulus	5
	Withdraws from pain	4
	Abnormal (spastic) flexion, decorticate posture	3
	Extensor (rigid) response, decerebrate posture	2
	None	1

Table 1.2 The FOUR score scale

Eye response	Eyelids open or opened, tracking, or blinking to command	4
		3
	Eyelids open but not tracking	2
	Eyelids closed but open to loud voice	1
	Eyelids remain closed to pain	0
	Eyelids closed but open to pain	4
Motor response	Thumbs up, fist or peace sign	4
	Localizing to pain	3
	Flexion response to pain	2
	Extension response to pain	1
	No response to pain or generalized myoclonus status	0
	Brainstem reflexes, pupil and corneal reflexes present	4
	One pupil wide and fixed	3
	Pupil or corneal reflexes absent	2
	Pupil and corneal reflexes absent	1
	Absent pupil, corneal, and cough reflex	0
	Respiration not intubated, regular breathing pattern	4
	Not intubated, Cheyne–Stokes breathing pattern	3
	Not intubated, irregular breathing	2
	Breathes above ventilator rate	1
	Breathes at ventilator rate or apnea	0

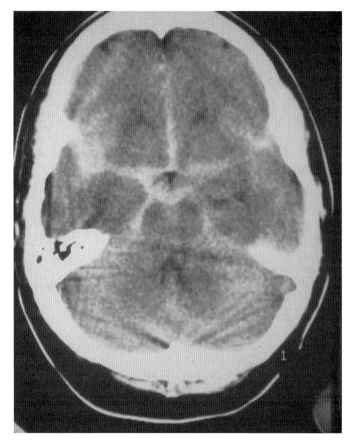

Figure 1.2 Subarachnoid hemorrhage. An axial CT scan showing severe filling of the basal cisterns with blood in a case of spontaneous subarachnoid hemorrhage due to a ruptured berry aneurysm.

failure of eye opening (0 for eye response) and a motor response of 3 or less. Coma is typically a transient state that gives way either to further recovery of brainstem function or deterioration and brain death.

3. **Stupor**: Brief arousal with eye opening or better, but the patient quickly lapses into a sleep-like state when not stimulated to waken. Stupor is, thus, also a disorder of the ARAS.

4. **Vegetative state (VS)**: VS is a behaviorally defined state in which patients show no evidence of self or environmental awareness. VS patients, like comatose patients, may have spontaneous, or stimulus-induced, stereotyped movements, and retain brainstem regulation of visceral autonomic functions. The key difference from coma is that VS patients demonstrate cyclical variation of eyes-open and eyes-closed periods across 24-hour periods. VS patients, however, do not have normal sleep–wake cycles; typically, an electroencephalogram (EEG) in VS displays a monotonous slow pattern regardless of whether the eyes are open or closed, or fragmentary components of normal electroencephalographic sleep–wake phenomenology may appear [6]. VS may represent a transitional state on the way to recovery of consciousness or could be a chronic condition in cases of more severe brain injuries. The term persistent vegetative state (PVS) has gone somewhat into desuetude and carries a temporal connotation of duration of at least one month of VS clinical features [7, 8].

VS patients typically show one of three main pathological findings if remaining in a prolonged VS following structural brain injury. Diffuse cortical and thalamic cell loss is most common and is present in the setting of global ischemia due to cardiac arrest. The second is widespread damage to axonal connections, mostly long-range fibers (as opposed to U fibers), labeled as diffuse axonal injury (DAI). The third and least-common pattern of injury is extensive damage to the upper brainstem and thalamus, which usually occurs due to basilar artery stroke [9]. The common link between these three injury types and VS is the loss of corticothalamic function, either from cell death, disconnection, or loss of brainstem activation. *In vivo* imaging studies demonstrate that VS reflects very diffuse corticothalamic dysfunction (reviewed by

Laureys and Schiff [10]). Metabolic studies reveal that VS is associated with the reduction of global metabolic rates to 50% or less of healthy control values. Comparable reductions in cerebral metabolic rate arise during generalized anesthesia and slow-wave sleep in healthy controls, both considered unconscious brain states.

5. **Minimally conscious state (MCS)**: The MCS was defined by the Aspen Workgroup as "a condition of severely altered consciousness in which there is minimal but definite behavioral evidence of conscious awareness." There is, thus, at least one aspect of awareness that is preserved [11]. Operationally, definition of MCS behaviors are often obtained from the Coma Recovery Scale Revised (CRS-R [12]) MCS patients show a wide range of behaviors from a low-level of non-reflexive behavior such as visual tracking of a mirror or localization of noxious stimuli, to high-level behavior such as consistent or inconsistent movements to command or inaccurate or inconsistent communication via gesture or even verbalization. Pathological studies indicate that MCS is typically associated with similar patterns of injury seen in VS but with considerably more preservation of cortical and particularly thalamic neuronal pools [13].

6. **Delirium (acute confusional state)**: The essential component is a disorder of sustained attention, upon which various cognitive disorders are superimposed. This has varied localization, but is often a diffuse disorder of higher cortical function (see Chapter 3).

The various DOCs will be discussed in turn.

Brain death

Illustrative case

A 70-year-old man suffered a cardiac arrest at home. He was asystole in the ER. After resuscitation and the return of spontaneous circulation (ROSC) he was treated with hypothermia (temperature 33 °C) in the intensive care unit (ICU). His pupils remained at 3 mm and were unreactive during the 24-hour period of hypothermia. His temperature remained at 33 °C for another day and he was then slowly passively rewarmed. After all sedative drugs and neuromuscular relaxants were stopped and his temperature achieved 36 °C he was neurologically reassessed. Neuromuscular blockade was excluded by a positive "train of four" response with a nerve simulator. His pupils were 3 mm and unreactive; corneal, oculovestibular, gag, and cough reflexes were absent. There was no motor response to stimulation and he made no spontaneous movements and did not breathe above the ventilator. An attempt at reducing the ventilator rate was associated with a drop in his oxygen saturation (the patient had been a very heavy smoker and suffered from emphysema). He required inotropic support to maintain his blood pressure and desmopressin (DDAVP (1-desamino-8-D-arginine vasopressin)) to treat diabetes insipidus.

Brain death was considered, but the clinical criteria could not be applied because an apnea test was not feasible. He was, therefore, transported to the radiology suite for a CT angiogram (CTA), which showed normal enhancement of the major intracranial arteries including the internal carotid arteries and the proximal middle cerebral arteries (Figure 1.3). The patient's clinical features remained the same. Although the prognosis appeared to be hopeless, the family was not willing to withdraw life-supporting therapy (LST), for religious reasons. The following day the patient had a single-photon emission computed tomographic (SPECT) scan using technetium-labeled hexamethylpropyleneamine oxime (HMPAO-Tc^{99m}). This showed no perfusion of the brain (Figure 1.4) and the patient was declared brain dead. The family was informed that the patient was declared dead and that LST would be discontinued.

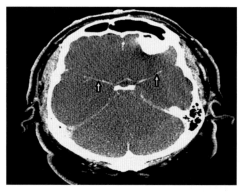

Figure 1.3 False negative CT angiogram in brain-death evaluation. The CT angiogram shows normal enhancement of the proximal portions of the major intracranial arteries, including the middle cerebral arteries (arrows).

In this scenario the patient could not be declared "brain dead" on clinical grounds alone, as the apnea test could not be performed. Therefore, an ancillary test to confirm brain death was needed (over 20% of patients being considered for the neurological determination of brain death require such ancillary testing [14]). An ancillary test for the declaration of brain death should meet the following criteria: (1) There should be no "false positives", i.e., when the test is positive for brain death there should be no patients declared who have the potential for recovery of any brain function. (2) The test should be capable of "standing alone" as proof of brain death, the test should prove that the brain is not viable. (3) The test is standardized in technique, technology, and the classification of results. (4) The test should be available in centers with ICUs. The only tests that meet these criteria are tests of intracranial circulation. In Canada, only the following tests are acceptable: (1) Standard four-vessel cerebral angiography, (2) CTA, (3) magnetic resonance angiography (MRA), and (4) nuclear medicine flow studies or SPECT [15]. A problem with most of these tests is that there can be "false negatives" as any intracranial arterial filling is regarded as negating brain death. Indeed, in some cases, as in the case illustrated above, the proximal portions of intracranial arteries can sometimes fill with contrast without the parenchyma of the brain being *perfused*. This is most commonly seen in the context of brain swelling after a neurosurgical procedure or trauma. It follows that we need a refinement of the ancillary tests that indicates *lack of perfusion of the brain*, without which the brain cannot be viable. Suitable tests include: (1) CT perfusion studies as a component of CTA, (2) radionuclide tests such as SPECT that require the agent to penetrate into the brain parenchyma from the capillary bed, (3) MRI perfusion studies, and (4) filling of the deep cerebral veins (note that superior sagittal sinus filling can occur in brain death due to contributions from diploic veins of the skull).

Coma

Two of the most common causes of acute onset coma for which outcome prediction is challenging are anoxic-ischemic encephalopathy from cardiac arrest and reperfusion and traumatic brain injury (TBI). We shall present cases of each with emphasis on prognostic determination. We shall also provide some cautionary information on acute hepatic encephalopathy.

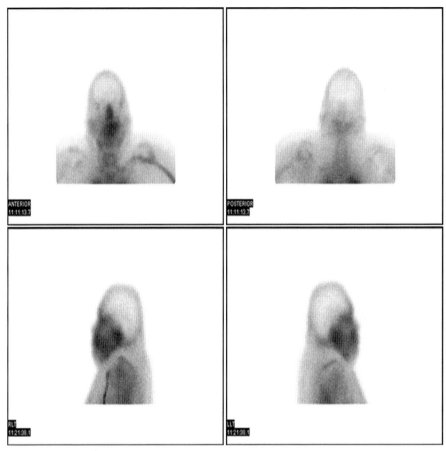

Figure 1.4 A SPECT scan using HMPAO-Tc^{99m} shows lack of brain uptake of the nucleide tracer. The other structures of the head did take up the tracer, producing the "hot nose" or "empty light bulb" sign, compatible with brain death.

Anoxic-ischemic encephalopathy

Cardiac arrest and subsequent ROSC carries a multifactorial threat to the brain's neurons.

Different brain regions and specific neuronal populations appear more susceptible to hypoxic-ischemic injury (selective vulnerability). This is likely due to being located in a vascular border zone or due to higher metabolic rates requiring increased oxygen or to density of N-methyl-D-aspartate (NMDA) or α-amino-3-hydroxy-5-methyl-4-isoxazolepropionic acid (AMPA) receptors on neuronal membranes. The CA1 neurons of the hippocampus are the most sensitive to ischemia and injury can result in memory dysfunction. The Purkinje cells of the cerebellum, the large neurons in layers 3, 5, and 6 of the neocortex, and the reticular neurons of the thalamus, are commonly affected. Brainstem nuclei are relatively more resistant. In addition, three vascular border zones are susceptible to a reduction in blood flow due to the distance from the parent vessel, and these areas become clinically important in cases of severe hypotension and incomplete cardiopulmonary arrest. The cortical border zones are the anterior border zone between the anterior cerebral artery (ACA) and the middle cerebral artery (MCA), and the posterior border zone, between the MCA and posterior cerebral artery (PCA). The internal, or subcortical, border zone is found at the junctions between the branches of the anterior, middle, and posterior cerebral arteries with the deep perforating vessels, including lenticulostriate, Heubner, and anterior choroidal arteries. Infarction of the anterior border zone results in brachial diplegia, or "man-in-a-barrel" syndrome. Infarction of the posterior border zone results in visual deficits and in severe, bilateral cases may result in cortical blindness.

Prognostic determination in patients not treated with hypothermia

In 2006, the American Academy of Neurology published practice parameters that summarized the available literature and provided an algorithm to establish a prognosis [16]. These were based on literature that antedated the use of hypothermia. The criteria appeared valid with very low false-positive rates (FPRs) for predicting an outcome no better than total dependency in a nursing home after 24 hours (Figure 1.5).

If a patient has absence of all brainstem reflexes, motor responses, and apnea, ancillary testing can be used to confirm a diagnosis of brain death. It is wise to wait at least 24 hours from the time of the arrest as some initially lost brainstem reflexes and motor responses can recover within that time. In patients who remain comatose, but have a less severe neurological insult, clinical signs and electrophysiological tests can be used to establish a poor prognosis. The clinical signs that predicted poor neurological outcome were myoclonus status epilepticus on day 1, absence of the pupillary light reflex or corneal reflex on day 3, and best motor response of extension or worse on day 3. Somatosensory evoked potentials (SSEPs) completed on day 1 to 3 that demonstrate bilateral absent N20 responses also predicted poor outcome (Figure 1.6). Serum neuronal-specific enolase (NSE) greater than 33ug/L on day 1 to 3 was also a reliable indicator of poor outcome. The practice parameters allow a physician to identify a patient who will definitely have a poor neurological outcome, but it is important to note that many patients without any of these criteria will also have poor outcomes.

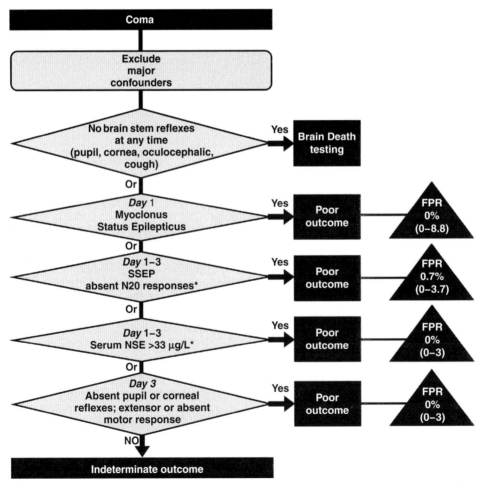

Figure 1.5 Algorithm for neurological prognostication after cardiac arrest. Note this practice parameter algorithm antedated the literature for hypothermic protocols. (From [16] Wijdicks et al., 2006, with permission.)

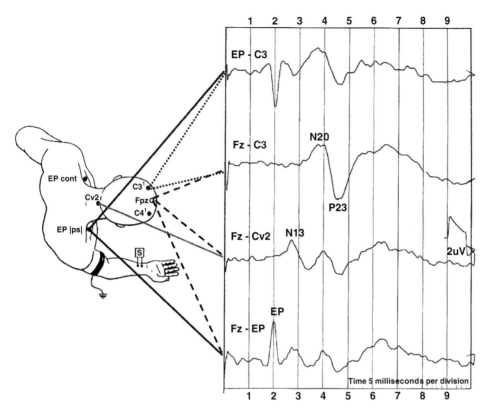

1 2 3 4 5 6 7 8 9

EP - C3

Fz - C3   N20

P23

Fz - Cv2   N13   2uV

EP
Fz - EP

Time 5 milliseconds per division

1 2 3 4 5 6 7 8 9

EP cont

C3'
Cv2   Fpz
C4'

EP |ps|

S

Figure 1.6 Setup for testing somatosensory evoked potentials. Note the potentials recorded from Erb's point over the brachial plexus, the high cervical spinal cord and the contralateral primary somatosensory area.

Although neuroimaging and EEG were not thoroughly evaluated in the 2006 AAN (American Academy of Neurology) guidelines, these tests can have great predictive value, especially when combined with other testing modalities. CT scans of the brain are often normal in the first few hours after the arrest, but at least by day 3 they show swelling and inversion of the gray–white densities (Figure 1.7) in patients with a poor prognosis [17].

The EEG may be used to prognosticate in the post-arrest period, but one must be aware of its sensitivity to multiple confounders, including sedation, hypothermia, and multi-organ failure. The presence or absence of EEG reactivity has considerable prognostic value. EEG reactivity is defined as a change in frequency and/or amplitude that occurs in response to verbal or noxious stimuli. Al Thenayan and colleagues [18] retrospectively reviewed the EEG of 29 patients post-arrest and found that 17 out of 18 patients who lacked EEG reactivity did not regain conscious awareness. In a prospective series of 34 patients conducted by Rossetti and colleagues [19], a non-reactive

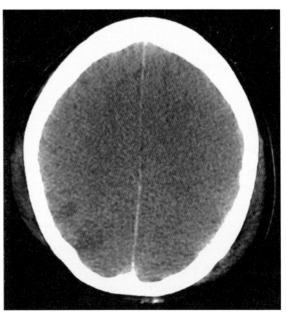

Figure 1.7 CT showing cerebral edema with generalized loss of the usual gray–white matter differentiation in a case of severe AIE.

background had a positive predictive value of 100%. In addition, all the survivors had EEG reactivity and 74% of these patients had a favorable neurological outcome. An additional series by Rossetti and colleagues [20] found that non-reactivity had an FPR of 7% for predicting mortality following cardiac arrest.

Up to 30% of post-arrest patients may develop status epilepticus. While often associated with poor outcomes [21], this same group found that epileptiform activity on the first EEG recording predicted poor outcome with an FPR of 9% [19]. Aggressive anti-epileptic treatment should be administered to these patients until other criteria suggest poor outcome. In summary, the EEG can aid in prognostication, both for favorable and unfavorable outcomes, but must be considered in context with other established prognostic indicators as the positive predictive value is insufficient to use in isolation.

Illustrative case

A 45 year-old woman with multiple comorbidities, including diabetes mellitus and chronic renal failure, suffered an asystolic cardiac arrest 2 days after an aortic valve replacement. The resuscitation was prolonged (probably more than 20 minutes) before ROSC. Because of the recent surgery she was not treated with the hypothermic protocol (see later). She remained deeply comatose with a GCS of 3. On day 3, while off all sedation for more than 24 hours, her pupils showed slight reactivity, the corneal reflexes were bilaterally absent and there was no motor response to noxious stimuli. The CT scan (also done on day 3) showed marked swelling of the hemispheres

with loss of sulci, basal cisterns, and loss of gray–white differentiation (Figure 1.7).

The EEG, also on day 3, was iso-electric (flat) without reactivity (Figure 1.8).

Since the 2006 AAN guidelines could be applied (no hypothermia), her clinical findings (absent corneal reflexes and no motor response on day 3) and the unfavorable CT scan and EEG indicated a poor prognosis. On discussion with the family, LST was withdrawn and she suffered a terminal cardiac arrest within 1 hour.

Prognosis of cardiac-arrest patients treated with hypothermia

In 2002, two landmark studies published in the *New England Journal of Medicine* showed that therapeutic hypothermia (TH) (32–34 °C) significantly improved the mortality and morbidity post-arrest [22, 23].

Studies done on cardiac-arrest patients treated with hypothermia have shown that many of the 2006 AAN guideline features have reduced prognostic accuracy. Rossetti and colleagues [20] found higher FPRs for predicting mortality for absence of pupillary reactivity (FPR 4%), presence of axial myoclonus (FPR 3%), and best motor response of extensor or worse (FPR 24%). Al Thenayan and colleagues [24] found that motor response, specifically extension or worse, was not prognostically reliable at day 3 following TH. In their prospective review 14 patients had delayed return of the motor response as late as day 6 post-arrest and two of these patients had favorable

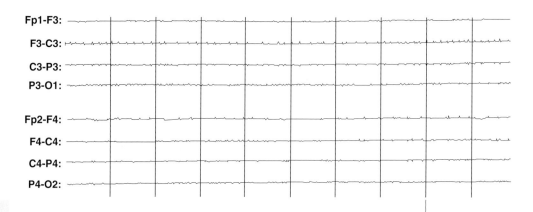

Figure 1.8 Flat or iso-electric EEG.

outcomes [24]. We have encountered an anoxic-ischemic encephalopathy (AIE) patient treated with TH who lacked motor response until day 21 post-arrest (unpublished data).

Axial myoclonus may be cortical in origin, having an EEG correlation, or reticular, meaning originating from the brainstem, and having a variable EEG correlation. Until recently (i.e. in the pre-hypothermic era), the presence of axial myoclonus was considered uniformly fatal. Several recently published cases of good outcome despite axial myoclonus suggest that TH may modify the outcome of a small but significant number of patients who develop status myoclonus after resuscitation from cardiac arrest [25, 26, 27].

Illustrative case

A 68 year-old man suffered an out-of-hospital cardiac arrest, but was given cardiopulmonary resuscitation (CPR) promptly by a physician who witnessed his collapse. The patient had pulseless electrical activity on arrival in ER, but ROSC was achieved within another 10 minutes. Before the patient was cooled in the ICU he exhibited bilaterally synchronous myoclonus of the proximal limbs. His pupils retained their reactivity. After achieving normal temperature a day later his cranial nerve reflexes were intact. The EEG did not show epileptiform activity but did reveal reactivity to stimulation and his MRI was unremarkable. He was part of a project on assessing the default-mode network on functional MRI (fMRI), and this was found to be intact (Figure 1.9).

The patient made a complete recovery and returned to his previous occupation. The case illustrates that axial myoclonus alone does not reliably predict a poor outcome. It also shows the positive implications of a reactive EEG and the preservation of the default-mode network on fMRI [28].

Several other investigative procedures have been utilized to help determine prognosis. Thus far, these have been tested in small research projects, but they offer further insights and may prove practical when technological advances become more widespread.

Hyperacute hepatic failure: a special prognostic trap

Hyperacute hepatic failure is defined by the appearance of encephalopathy within 7 days of the onset of liver dysfunction. Mortality is high and is commonly due to cerebral edema and herniation. In contrast to the clinical, EEG, and MRI prognostic features described above for AIEs, patients with absent cranial nerve reflexes, flat EEGs, and diffuse cytotoxic edema can recover awareness and some can make a complete neurological recovery [29].

Illustrative case

A 62-year-old-man with viral hepatitis presented in deep coma (GCS of 3 and FOUR score of 0). Despite a liver transplant he remained comatose. On neurological examination there was loss of all brainstem reflexes. His EEG was isoelectric and his MRI scan showed severe cytotoxic edema (Figure 1.10). He was treated with mannitol and hypothermia. After 24 hours his EEG showed low-voltage delta activity and the brain swelling on MRI had improved. The patient ultimately recovered his cranial nerve reflexes and opened his eyes to stimulation. He ultimately recovered to answer questions. Unfortunately, he died several days later of sepsis.

Traumatic brain injury

TBI can result from direct head impact, from rapid acceleration–deceleration, or from a penetrating object. The resulting pathology may be diffuse, such as diffuse axonal or diffuse vascular injury, or focal. Focal lesions include subdural hematomas, epidural hematomas, intracerebral contusions or hematomas, and skull fractures [30]. This variability in mechanism and resulting pathology complicates the formulation of uniform guidelines for prognosis.

The most widely used classification of head trauma utilizes the GCS. Severe TBI is defined as GCS scores of 3 to 8, moderate as 9 to 13, and mild at 14 or 15. An initial GCS has been frequently reported as an important prognosticator, although more recent research suggests the isolated motor score may be more valuable. One study found that 77% of patients with extensor posturing as the best motor response on admission had unfavorable outcomes [31]. Herniation from supratentorial lesions often results in pupillary asymmetry and loss of pupillary reactivity and also carries a poor prognosis (77% with bilateral fixed pupils and 54% with unilateral fixed pupils) [31]. Other features associated with poor outcome include increasing age, hypoxia, hypotension, traumatic subarachnoid hemorrhage, and pathology other than epidural hematoma [32].

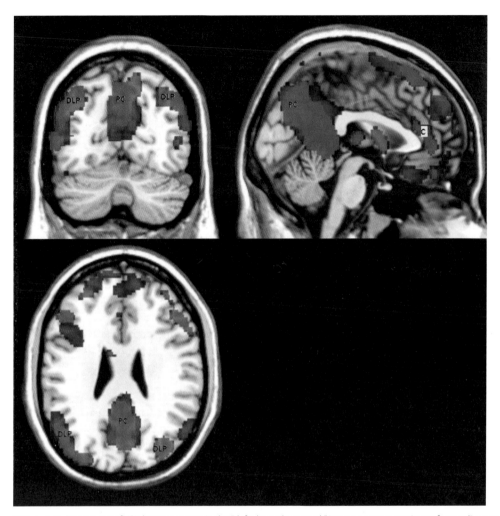

Figure 1.9 Resting-state fMRI showing activity in the "default-mode network" in two comatose patients after cardiac arrest. Blue is one patient's activation, red the other coma patient and the purple are areas of overlap between the two patterns. There is activation of the dorsolateral parietal regions (DLP), the precuneus (PC), and the cingulate gyrus (C).

The diagnosis of traumatic axonal injury (TAI), characterized by axonal swelling and secondary axotomy, is grossly underestimated by CT, and plays a crucial role in prognostication for severe head trauma. MRI has greater spatial resolution as well as better sensitivity for posterior fossa and brainstem lesions. Gradient echo sequences are sensitive to hemoglobin breakdown products and depict hemorrhagic TAI lesions. Fluid-attenuated inversion recovery (FLAIR) sequences are useful for depicting non-hemorrhagic (edematous) TAI lesions as well as periventricular lesions. There has been increasing interest in diffusion-tensor (DT) MRI, which looks at the direction of water-associated proton diffusion and can be used to generate three-dimensional images of white-matter tracts.

MRI is routinely ordered in head-trauma patients for prognostication and in situations where the neurological examination cannot be explained by the findings on CT. A recent study found that with FLAIR and T2-weighted imaging, the median number of lesions detected, median total volume of lesions, and median volume per lesion could discriminate between good and poor outcome [33]. Skandsen and colleagues [34] found that bilateral brainstem lesions on MRI, done within 4 weeks of severe head injury, predicted poor neurological outcome at 1-year follow-up with a sensitivity of 75% and specificity of 94%. The timing

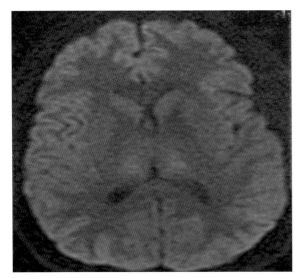

Figure 1.10 A diffusion-weighted MRI showing cytotoxic edema of the cortex, thalami, and basal ganglia in a patient with acute hepatic encephalopathy.

possible for clinically unresponsive patients to provide yes/no type answers to questions [39]. This approach requires further exploration, but clearly has important implications for exploring issues such as patient comfort/pain and determining wishes. Such insights are also of great importance to families who benefit from knowing that the patient is aware.

EEG testing, including long-term monitoring, evoked potentials, and event-related potentials, also has a role in prognostic assessment and in detecting seizures and monitoring the effect of treatment.

A systematic review of 25 studies of high-grade TBI patients showed that SSEPs provide a more reliable prediction of poor outcome than the GCS, EEG, CT scan, or clinical examination. The bilateral absence of the cortical component of the SSEP was associated with an outcome no better than VS. Unilateral absence and contralateral delay were still associated with significant impairment [40]. Combining the SSEP results with GCS, pupillary, and motor responses enhanced the predictive value for intermediate degrees of SSEP abnormalities [40, 41]. In applying SSEPs for prognosis it is best to record along the sensory pathway, as shown in Figure 1.6, to ensure that the problem lies intracranially. Although SSEPs are not affected as much by sedation as EEGs are, it is wise to minimize anesthetic drugs when applying this test.

Vegetative and minimally conscious states

The VS is described as wakefulness without awareness [7], which implies that the arousal system is able to function, allowing for arousability and wake and sleep cycles. However, integrated corticothalamic function, responsible for conscious awareness, is severely dysfunctional. Jennett and Plum [7] chose the term "vegetative" to denote vegetative functions. These include the preservation of homeostatic temperature regulation, hormonal secretion, adequate blood pressure and tissue perfusion, digestion, and respirations. The term PVS was introduced to classify VS lasting for 1 month or more. Some patients spontaneously emerge from the vegetative state and regain cognitive responses, indicative of comprehension and at least some degree of awareness. Others then were thought to remain in a *permanent* VS.

Diagnostic criteria for VS were published in 1994 [8] and were entirely based on observed behaviors. The essential features included: (1) no evidence of awareness of the self or the environment (no interaction with other individuals); (2) no response to verbal,

of MRI may also affect its utility. Moen and colleagues [35] found that at 3-month follow-up, MRI demonstrated fewer hemispheric, central, and brainstem lesions on FLAIR and DT sequences. Most notably, 31% of patients had brainstem lesions on initial imaging and this decreased to 17% at 3 months. Further discussion of brain trauma can be found in Chapter 15.

Advanced imaging techniques, especially fMRI, are beginning to provide some diagnostic and prognostic clues. This began with the seminal work of Owen and colleagues, who studied a TBI patient who was considered to be vegetative [36]. There was activation of the supplementary motor area when the patient was asked to pretend she was playing tennis. Similarly, several areas in the posterior cerebrum were activated when she was asked to imagine she was walking through rooms of her house. In one study of 41 VS and MCS patients, predominantly TBI, a strong association was observed between the fMRI results and the Coma Recovery Scale-Revised (CRS-R) score 6 months after scanning. Importantly, no such association was evident between the fMRI results and the CRS-R at the time of the scan [37]. A review of the available literature from 15 separate fMRI studies, involving 48 published cases, also concluded that atypical activity (e.g. on the fMRI scan) patterns appear to predict recovery from VS with 93% specificity and 69% sensitivity [38]. Using the above binary responses it is auditory, tactile, or noxious stimuli; (3) lack of evidence of language comprehension or expression; (4) sufficient vegetative (hypothalamic and autonomic) function to sustain life; (5) incontinence of bowel and bladder; and (6) variable preservation of cranial nerve and spinal reflexes.

The findings issued by the Task Force, derived from careful analysis of the literature and clinical experience, formulated timeline criteria for declaring that the VS was, in fact, permanent. For non-traumatic brain injury (non-TBI), this was set to be 3 months for both children and adults. For TBI, most patients plateaued at about 6 months to 1 year from the time of injury. The diagnostic timeline for the transition from "persistent" to "permanent" VS was set accordingly.

The minimally conscious state (MCS) was defined by the Aspen Workgroup [11] and allowed for minimal/markedly limited but definite behavioral evidence of conscious awareness. The essential aspect was that there was evidence of some, very limited, awareness of self or the environment as evidenced by one of the following: (1) simple following of commands; (2) "yes/no" responses (regardless of accuracy); (3) limited intelligible verbalization; (4) purposeful behavior or movements, e.g., smiling or laughing, response to the content of questions by a verbal utterance or gesture, reaching for an object, touching or manipulating an object, or sustained visual fixation or tracking. As with VS criteria, these are based on clinical observations.

As neurological improvement from and beyond the MCS could sometimes occur, the Aspen group proposed that *emergence from* MCS would require a consistent demonstration of volitional behavior, e.g., yes/no or binary responses to questions [11].

Prognostic errors

Although establishing working definitions of VS and MCS was valuable for clinical practice, it became apparent, from careful clinical and neuropsychological studies, that the diagnosis of VS was inaccurate in up to 30–40% of cases [42–44]. Furthermore, recent studies suggest up to 17% of patients accurately diagnosed in VS on clinical grounds have exhibited volitional cognitive responses with fMRI, ERPs, and EEG testing [45].

The diagnosis of MCS has somewhat different implications, in that MCS is primarily based on positive findings indicative of at least some degree of awareness. There can be a wide range of severity and possibly, partial recovery. There is clearly room for

better precision in establishing prognosis in MCS patients.

Novel diagnostic tests and their potential role in the acute care setting

Recent work utilizing fMRI and electrophysiological methods has led to a new, but currently incompletely defined, category of patients with DOCs or highly preserved cognition and the false appearance of such a DOC [36, 39, 46–49]. In some patients who show bedside behavioral examinations consistent with VS or MCS, signals extracted by fMRI or quantitative measures of EEG activity (qEEG) may provide evidence of high-level cognitive processes, including command following or even communication.

Illustrative case

A 23-year-old man suffered a severe traumatic brain injury from a motor-vehicle accident. The initial diagnosis was VS with no evidence of response to external stimulation or spontaneous purposeful movement. Four months after the injury, the first evidence of brief visual fixation was noted with visual tracking appearing by 6 months. The patient's condition slowly continued to improve and at 1 year a single caregiver identified that the patient was able to effectively communicate using head movements and eventually he became communication-capable through the use of a letter board. Using these methods of communication the patient completed an independent evaluation of cognitive function which indicated normal intelligence.

Figure 1.11 shows the results of fMRI studies [46] and qEEG studies [49] on this man used to assess changes in cortical activity when he was asked to imagine swimming. As seen in the left-hand image in Figure 1.11a, a statistically significant activation of the supplementary motor area is present consistent with normal control patterns of activation. Similar methods have identified a subset of patients fulfilling VS or MCS behavioral features on bedside examination who can generate similar fMRI responses for motor imagery [36, 39]. The severity of structural injury following DAI in this subject as assessed by structural MRI is comparable with patients remaining clinically in VS over long time periods [50], although he demonstrated bedside evidence of consciousness. Of note,

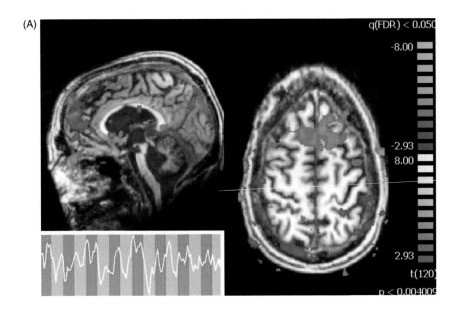

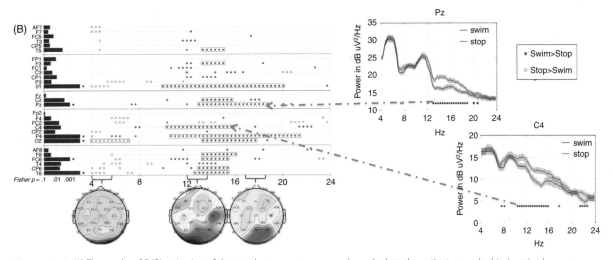

Figure 1.11 (A) The results of fMRI activation of the supplementary motor area (arrow) when the patient was asked to imagine he was swimming compared with time periods of fMRI signal acquisition after a "stop imagining swimming command" (graph on lower left shows time series for voxel within the supplementary motor area). (B) The results of a power spectral analysis of EEG signals acquired in separate experimental studies utilizing the same task structure and timing of signal acquisition. The power spectra show the significant differences between the swimming task and post-stop signal period in the bar histogram and raster display (left of the figure), the spectral plot of the EEG (to the right), and the topographic map (bottom). Increases in signal power for swimming compared with post-stop baseline are shown in red (decreases in blue).

despite the clear activation of the supplementary motor area to the mental imagery, this subject could not use this fMRI-based method to establish a non-gestural communication channel as has been demonstrated in other severely brain-injured subjects using fMRI [39, 46, 47]. Figure 1.11b shows an independent measurement of the same command following a task carried out while the EEG was recorded. A quantitative analysis of the EEG signal examining changes in power at different frequencies revealed a robust and clear task-related response. Collectively, the results of the two studies and the bedside communication skills (utilizing head movements and a letterhead) indicate that the failure to demonstrate fMRI-based communication may hint at major challenges for the wide translation of these tools in either the chronic or acute settings.

The importance of diagnostic precision in use of available nosological distinctions

A diagnosis of VS should be questioned when evidence for covert cognitive capacities is established in an individual who appears unresponsive. By definition, a diagnosis of VS should be considered inconsistent with any evidence of response to the environment or self-awareness.

It is important that as knowledge evolves to better predict the risk of such a broad dissociation of motor and cognitive function in patients who remain behaviorally non-responsive (either at the level of VS or only low-level non-reflexive responses consistent with MCS such as fixation, visual tracking, or auditory localization [11] yet carry out fMRI- or qEEG-based cognitive tasks, those who do should not be described as in VS and able to carry out the tasks. At present, the broader clinical implications of these and related findings in the published literature for assessments in the acute care setting are not yet very clear. However, once these measurements are successfully obtained, it is clear that the patients have interacted with their environment, thereby placing them in an ill-defined category somewhere between a high-level MCS and locked-in state. In principle, neuroimaging tools provide unambiguous methods for excluding false-positive VS diagnoses although clinical guidelines for introducing such methods as ancillary assessments and their operational requirements have not been established.

At a minimum, clinicians need to be aware that such confounds exist and need to be considered in formulating diagnostic assessments in the acute care (or any other) setting. Recent work by Forgacs et al. [51] suggests that straightforward assessments with clinically available tools will potentially improve the clinician's capacity to adjudicate the risk of misidentifying such patients. In a study of 38 patients ranging in function from VS to partially LIS, Forgac et al. identified four subjects capable of fMRI-based command following, all of whom preserved most features of a normal wakeful EEG architecture used by clinical neurophysiologists to identify cerebral dysfunction; all subjects capable of the fMRI tasks showed only mild or moderate cerebral dysfunction and preserved global metabolic rates (dissociating their basic profile from the known pathophysiologic features of VS reviewed above).

References

1. Teasdale G, Jennett B (1974). Assessment of coma and impaired consciousness. A practical scale. *Lancet* **2**: 81–84.

2. Wijdicks EF, Bamlet WR, Maramattom BV, Manno EM, McClelland RL (2005). Validation of a new coma scale: the FOUR score. *Ann Neurol* **58**: 585–593.

3. Finlayson O, John V, Yeung R, *et al.* (2013). Interobserver agreement of ASPECT score distribution for noncontrast CT, CT angiography, and CT perfusion in acute stroke. *Stroke* **44**: 234–246.

4. Schellinger PD, Bryan RN, Caplan LR (2010). Evidence-based guideline: the role of diffusion and perfusion MRI for the diagnosis of acute ischemic stroke. *Report of the Therapeutics and Technology Assessment Subcommittee of the American Academy of Neurology* **75**: 177–185.

5. Wijdicks EF (2001). The diagnosis of brain death. *N Engl J Med* **344**:1215–1221.

6. Kobylarz EJ, Schiff ND (2004). Functional imaging of severely brain-injured patients: progress, challenges, and limitations. *Arch Neurol* **61**: 1357–1360.

7. Jennett B, Plum F (1972). Persistent vegetative state after brain damage: a syndrome in search of a name. *Lancet* **1**: 734–737.

8. The Multi-Society Task Force on PVS (1994). Medical aspects of the vegetative state. The Multi-Society Task Force on PVS. *N Engl J Med* **330**: 1499–1508.

9. Ingvar DH, Sourander P (1970). Destruction of the reticular core of the brainstem. *Arch Neurol* **23**: 1–8.

10. Laureys S, Schiff ND (2012). Coma and consciousness: paradigms (re)framed by neuroimaging. *Neuroimage* **61**: 478–491.

11. Giacino JT, Ashwal S, Childs N, *et al.* (2002). The minimally conscious state: definition and diagnostic criteria. *Neurology* **58**: 349–353.

12. Giacino J, Kalmar K, Whyte J (2004). The JFK Coma Recovery Scale-Revised: measurement characteristics and diagnostic utility. *Arch Phys Med Rehabil* **85**: 2020–2029.

13. Jennett B, Adams JH, Murray LS, *et al.* (2001). Neuropathology in vegetative and severely disabled patients after head injury. *Neurology* **56**: 486–490.

14. Savard M, Turgeon AF, Gariepy J-L, Trottier T, Langevin S (2010). Selective 4-vessel angiography in brain death: a retrospective study. *Can J Neurol Sci* **37**: 492–497.

15. Young GB, Shemie SD, Doig CJ, Teitelbaum J (2006). Brief review of the role of ancillary tests in the neurological determination of death. *Can J Anaesth* **53**: 620–627.

16. Wijdicks EFM, Hijdra A, Young GB, *et al.* (2006). Practice parameter: prediction of outcome in comatose survivors after cardiopulmonary resuscitation (an evidence-based review): report of the Quality Standards Subcommittee of the American Academy of Neurology. *Neurology* **67**: 203–210.

17. Zingler VC, Krumm B, Bertsch T, Fassbender K, Pohlmann-Eden B (2003). Early prediction of outcome after cardiopulmonary resuscitation: a multi-modal approach combining neurobiochemical and electrophysiological investigations may provide higher prognostic certainty in patients after cardiac arrest. *Eur Neurol* **49**: 79–84.

18. Al Thenayan E, Savard M, Sharpe MD, *et al.* (2010). Electroencephalogram for prognosis after cardiac arrest. *J Crit Care* **25**: 300–304.

19. Rossetti AO, Urbano LA, Delodder F, *et al.* (2010a). Prognostic value of continuous EEG monitoring during therapeutic hypothermia after cardiac arrest. *Crit Care* **14**(5): R173.

20. Rossetti AO, Oddo M, Logroscino G, *et al.* (2010b) Prognostication after cardiac arrest and hypothermia: A prospective study. *Ann Neurol* **67**: 301–307.

21. Rossetti AO, Lorgoscino G, Liaudet L, *et al.* (2007). Status epilepticus. An independent outcome after cerebral anoxia. *Neurology* **69**: 255–260.

22. Bernard SA, Gray TW, Buist MD, *et al.* (2002). Treatment of comatose survivors of out-of-hopsital cardiac arrest with induced hypothermia. *N Engl J Med* **346**: 557–563.

23. Hypothermia after Cardiac Arrest Study Group (2002). Mild therapeutic hypothermia to improve the neurologic outcome after cardiac arrest. *N Engl J Med* **346**: 549–556.

24. Al Thenayan EA, Savard M, Sharpe M, *et al.* (2008). Predictors of poor neurologic outcome after induced mild hypothermia following cardiac arrest. *Neurology* **71**: 1535–1537.

25. Chen CJ, Coyne PJ, Lyckhom LJ, *et al.* (2012). A case of inaccurate prognostication after the ARCTIC protocol. *J Pain Symptom Manage* **43**: 1120–1125.

26. Lucas JM, Cocchi MN, Salciccioli J, *et al.* (2012). Neurologic recovery after hypothermia in patients with post-cardiac arrest myoclonus. *Resuscitation* **83**: 265–269.

27. Rossetti AO, Oddo M, Liaudet L, *et al.* (2009). Predictors of awakening from postanoxic status epilepticus after therapeutic hypothermia. *Neurology* **72**: 744–749.

28. Norton L, Hutchison RM, Young GB, *et al.* (2012). Distributions of functional connectivity in the default network of comatose patients. *Neurology* **78**: 175–181.

29. Hunter GRW, Young GB (2010). Recovery of awareness after hyperacute hepatic encephalopathy with "flat" EEG, severe cerebral edema and deep coma. *Neurocrit Care* **13**: 247–251.

30. Posner JB, Saper CB, Schiff ND, Plum F (2007). *Plum and Posner's Diagnosis of Stupor and Coma*, 4th edn. New York: Oxford University Press.

31. Steyerberg EW, Mushkudiani N, Perel P, *et al.* (2008). Predicting outcome after traumatic brain injury: development and international validation of prognostic scores based on admission characteristics. *PLOS Med* **5**: e165.

32. Roozenbeek B, Lingsma HF, Lecky FE, *et al.* (2012). Prediction of outcome after moderate and severe traumatic brain injury: external validation of the International Mission on Prognosis and Analysis of Clinical Trials (IMPACT) and Corticoid Randomisation After Significant Head injury (CRASH) prognostic models. *Crit Care Med* **40**: 1609–1617.

33. Chastain CA, Oyoyo UE, Zipperman M, *et al.* (2009). Predicting outcomes of traumatic brain injury by imaging modality and injury distribution. *J Neurotrauma* **26**: 1183–1196.

34. Skandsen T, Kvistad KA, Solheim O, *et al.* (2011). Prognostic value of magnetic resonance imaging in moderate and severe head injury: a prospective study of early MRI findings and one-year outcome. *J Neurotrauma* **28**: 691–9.

35. Moen KG, Skandsen T, Folvik M, *et al.* (2012). A longitudinal MRI study of traumatic axonal injury in patients with moderate and severe traumatic brain injury. *J Neurol Neurosurg Psychiatry* **83**: 1193–1200.

36. Owen AM, Coleman MR, Boly M, *et al.* (2006) Detecting awareness in the vegetative state. *Science* **313**: 1402.

37. Coleman MR, Davis MH, Rodd JM, *et al.* (2009). Towards the routine use of brain imaging to aid the clinical diagnosis of disorders of consciousness. *Brain* **32**: 2541–2552.

38. Di H, Boly M, Weng X, Ledoux D, Laureys S (2008). Neuroimaging activation studies in the vegetative state: predictors of recovery? *Clin Med* **8**: 502–507.

39. Monti MM, Vanhaudenhuyse A, Coleman MR, *et al.* (2010). Willful modulation of brain activity and communication in disorders of consciousness. *N Engl J Med* **362**: 579–589.

40. Houlden DA, Chen RAK, Schwartz MI, Katic M (1990). Median nerve somatosensory evoked potentials and the Glasgow Coma Scale as predictors of outcome in comatose patients with head injuries. *Neurosurgery* **27**: 701–708.

41. Carter BG, Butt W (2005). Are somatosensory evoked potentials the best predictor of outcome after severe

brain injury? A systematic review. *Intensive Care Med* **31**: 765–775.

42. Andrews K, Murphy L, Munday R, *et al.* (1996). Misdiagnosis of the vegetative state: retrospective study in a rehabilitation unit. *BMJ* **7048**:13–16.

43. Childs NL, Mercer WN, Childs HW (1993). Accuracy of diagnosis of persistent vegetative state. *Neurology* **43**: 1465–1467.

44. Schnakers C, Ledoux D, Majerus S, *et al.* (2008). Diagnostic and prognostic use of bispectral index in coma, vegetative state and related disorders. *Brain Inj* **22**: 926–931.

45. Naci L, Monti MM, Cruse D, *et al.* (2012). Brain–computer interfaces for communication with nonresponsive patients. *Ann Neurol* **72**: 312–323.

46. Bardin JC, Fins JJ, Katz DI, *et al.* (2011). Dissociations between behavioural and functional magnetic resonance imaging-based evaluations of cognitive function after brain injury. *Brain* **134**: 769–782. doi: 10.1093/brain/awr005.

47. Bardin JC, Schiff ND, Voss HU (2012). Pattern classification of volitional functional magnetic resonance imaging responses in patients with severe brain injury. *Arch Neurol* **69**: 176–181.

48. Cruse D, Chennu S, Fernandez-Espejo D, *et al.* (2012). Detecting awareness in the vegetative state: electroencephalographic evidence for attempted movements to command. *PLoS One* **7**(11): e49933-e40040.

49. Goldfine AM, Victor JD, Conte MM, Bardin JC, Schiff ND (2011). Determination of awareness in patients with severe brain injury using EEG power spectral analysis. *Clin Neurophsiol* **122**: 2157–2168.

50. Kampfl A, Schmutzhard E, Franz G, *et al.* (1998). Prediction of recovery from post-traumatic vegetative state with cerebral magnetic-resonance imaging. *Lancet* **351**:1763–1767.

51. Forgacs PB, Conte MM, Schiff ND (2013). Reframing the big picture: characterization of patients with disorders of consciousness and evidence of covert high-level cognitive functions. Society for Neuroscience Meeting, Abstract 442.25

Chapter 2

Delirium and confusion

Jay Yao, Holly E. Hinson, and Jack H. Simon

Introduction

Delirium and confusional states are among the most common disorders affecting adults admitted to a hospital. Delirious patients may present dramatically, exhibiting agitated, combative behavior. Or, signs of delirium might be more subtle, remaining undetected by an unsuspecting clinician. The spectrum of delirium poses significant challenges for hospital staff and family alike. Moreover, delirium is also strongly associated with negative outcomes and adds significantly to the cost of healthcare.

The recognition of confusion and delirium may, on the surface, seem simple, but the available evidence suggests otherwise [1, 2]. These are not disease diagnoses in their own right, but rather symptoms of an underlying disorder. Delirium and confusional states are clinical syndromes with many potential causes. The greater diagnostic challenge often lies in identifying the underlying disease or disturbances. Obtaining a useful history and examination can be difficult, if not impossible. Since delirium and confusional states can be seen in such a wide range of diseases, no one diagnostic test is reliably informative in their evaluation. Therefore, the clinician must take a systematic approach to the delirious patient.

Despite being a daily occurrence in nearly every hospital, our understanding of delirium and confusional states remains limited. The heterogeneous nature of the condition makes studying delirium difficult, which is a barrier to both clinical management and research. Practice guidelines based on expert opinion must still rely heavily on the results of small and/or observational rather than prospective studies [3].

This chapter reviews the current definition of delirium and confusional states, highlighting its key features. A systematic approach is key to identifying the underlying cause or causes of delirium so that the appropriate treatment can then be applied.

Delirium vs. confusional state

There is no consensus as to whether or not delirium and confusional states are the same entity. Additional related or synonymous terms include "acute confusional state," "encephalopathy," "organic brain syndrome," "symptomatic psychosis," and even simply "confusion." Many experts use delirium and confusional states interchangeably [1, 4] while others attribute specific additional features to delirium [5]. In this latter schema, delirium is a special form of confusional state characterized by agitation, prominent perceptual disturbances such as hallucinations, delusions, lack of sleep, emotional lability, tremulousness, and hyperactivity. There is no clear data to settle the debate. In this chapter, delirium and confusional states are taken to be synonymous and refer to the condition as defined above.

Epidemiology

Delirium is common. Prevalence has been found to be as high as 70% in the intensive care unit (ICU), 10% in emergency departments, 42% in inpatient hospices, and 16% in post-acute care settings [6–9]. The risk increases for older patients, ranging from 10% to 50% in the hospitalized elderly, and patients with medical comorbidities, especially dementia and polypharmacy [10–13].

Patients who develop delirium have increased 6- and 12-month mortality as well as less favorable functional outcome [14, 15]. Length of hospitalization is longer, functional and cognitive status is worse, and likelihood of institutionalization is greater in patients with delirium [11, 16, 17].

Imaging Acute Neurologic Disease, ed. Massimo Filippi and Jack H. Simon. Published by Cambridge University Press.
© Cambridge University Press 2014.

Treatment

Treatment of delirium is included only briefly here to highlight the importance of recognizing delirium and identifying its underlying cause or causes. There is a significant body of literature on the prevention of delirium [18–20]. This focuses on providing a stable, safe environment and preventing physiologic disturbances that can lead to delirium. The current armamentarium for the treatment of delirium itself, however, is fairly limited. There are no specific treatments [5–21]. The key measures are the correction of the underlying cause and supportive care, including reorientation and the prevention of additional factors that can worsen the delirium. It is therefore critically important to identify patients at risk of delirium, so that the appropriate supportive and preventive measures can be applied, and to identify the underlying disease or diseases causing the delirium, so that the root cause may be corrected.

Definition and clinical characteristics

Delirium is a clinical syndrome that can result from a wide variety of diseases, ranging from stroke to simple constipation. The clinical presentation of delirium extends over a wide spectrum with many possible features, some of which are even contradictory (see below). Our current understanding characterizes delirium by several key features [4, 5, 21, 22].

Core features

1. Inattention

    This feature is often termed disturbance of consciousness. It is being referred to as inattention here to highlight the fact that this does not refer to a depressed level of consciousness. Patients with delirium may be somnolent, but may also be agitated and hyperactive. The key feature for delirium is the inability to focus, sustain, and shift attention. One way this can be seen is that the patient is easily distracted and quickly loses his/her train of thought.

    As a consequence of impaired attention, there is decreased awareness of the environment. The patient is often unaware of what is happening around and to him/her. Similarly, because the patient is not able to pay attention to and register events, there is impaired memory.

2. Impairment of cognition

    There is global impairment and slowing of executive functions. Problems include perceptual disturbances, poor memory, difficulty with language, and disorientation, among other things. Patients who are multilingual often revert to only using their native tongue. There is usually a lack of insight. Normal inhibition is lost, manifesting as inappropriate behavior and perseveration. Changes in perception can include illusions and hallucinations. These can involve any of the senses and can be crude or well formed.

    With inattention, testing of cognitive functions is difficult, if not impossible. Interpretation of the results of cognitive testing is also problematic as it is impossible to determine if an incorrect response reflects a deficit in a particular cognitive domain or is the result of inattention. However, as inattention is a core feature of delirium, the inability to perform the testing is often the important finding.

3. Acuity

    Delirium is an acute process that results in a change from a pre-existing baseline. The symptoms develop over hours to days, but may persist for days to months. Acuity is the key differentiating feature between delirium and dementia. Dementia is a chronic condition that develops over months to years, but otherwise may overlap with delirium in cognitive deficits. A patient with dementia, with impaired baseline cognitive function, can (and often does) develop acute worsening from that baseline, becoming acutely confused or delirious. Good collateral information can be essential in this differentiation, as the patient is often unable to provide the critical information.

4. Fluctuation

    Temporal variability is often considered a hallmark of delirium. Symptoms can vary from normal (or baseline) cognitive function to severely abnormal over the course of hours. Often there is a diurnal variation with symptom improvement or even resolution in the morning and daylight hours and worsening at night. This pattern can also be seen in dementia, where patients can settle into a consistent pattern of agitation at night. However, as this pattern is their baseline status, this would not be considered delirium in a patient with dementia. Of course, a demented patient can develop delirium and become even more symptomatic at night. The term "sundowning" has been used inconsistently to refer to either phenomenon [23].

This variation over time in symptoms of delirium can present a pitfall for diagnosis. If a patient is seen by a provider only once or infrequently, the patient may be normal or only subtly symptomatic at the time of evaluation and the condition may be unrecognized. Variation over time increases the importance of serial examinations and collateral information in suspected or at-risk patients.

Additional symptoms

There are a wide array of additional features that may be seen in delirium. If present, the severity of any symptom can also vary greatly. They include, but are not limited to, lethargy and somnolence, agitation, tremulousness, hyperactivity, irritability, fear and anxiety, emotional lability, delusions, paranoia, disturbance of sleep-wake cycle, and hypersensitivity to light and sound.

Psychiatric conditions

Delirium is considered a consequence of organic disease or physiologic stressors. While psychiatric disease can manifest symptoms very similar to those seen in delirium, they are, by definition, not considered delirium. However, delirium can develop on top of an existing psychiatric illness and present a considerable diagnostic challenge.

Pathogenesis

1. Neurobiology

The brain remains a poorly understood organ. This is particularly true for cognitive functions. To date, no single or definitive mechanism has been implicated in the pathogenesis of delirium [5, 21]. Taking into account the wide array of potential causes of delirium and the wide spectrum of symptoms, it is very possible that what is classified as delirium today is a variety of pathologic processes, as delirium is a clinical syndrome, not an etiology.

While focal lesions in the brain can cause delirium, it is also clear that delirium can result without any structural abnormality in the brain. The range of cognitive processes affected suggests a diffuse process. This is supported by electroencephalogram (EEG) studies showing

generalized slowing in delirium [24]. Evidence also exists for subcortical involvement.

The role of neurotransmitters has also been studied. Acetylcholine has been implicated in a number of studies and has implications for diagnosis and management [25, 26]. Anticholinergic medication is a common cause of delirium. Also, many common medications have anticholinergic activity (Table 2.1) and can precipitate delirium, especially in at-risk populations, including the elderly.

2. Causes

Delirium can result from essentially any form of physiologic stress (Table 2.2). This can be as simple as disruption of the normal sleep routine or sleep deprivation. In a patient who is at high risk (e.g. elderly with dementia), simply being awakened regularly for vital checks and examinations throughout the night can be sufficient to precipitate a delirium. On the other end of the spectrum, subarachnoid hemorrhage can cause a delirium, and confound the presentation with additional focal deficits related to the associated brain injury.

Table 2.1 Medications with anticholinergic effects

Antidepressants	**Urinary antispasmodics**
tricyclic antidepressants	oxybutynin
paroxetine	flavoxate
	tolteradine
Antiemetics	**Gli antispasmodics**
promethazine	dicyclomine
prochlorperazine	hyoscyamine
trimethobenzamide	belladonna alkaloids
meclizine	clindinium
scopolamine	propantheline
Antihistamines	**Antiarrhythmics**
any non-selective antihistamine	disopyramide
	procainamide
	quinidine
Muscle relaxants	**Antipsychotics**
metazalone	chlorpromazine
cyclobenzaprine	thioridazine
orphenadrine	clozapine
methocarbamol	thiothixene
carisoprodol	fluphenazine
Cardiovascular medications	
furosemide	
digoxin	
nifedipine	
disopyramide	

Table 2.2 Potential causes of delirium. This list is not comprehensive, but serves to highlight the wide range of conditions that can contribute to delirium. From Francis J Jr, Young GB. Diagnosis of delirium and confusional states. Aug, 2012. Uptodate.com; with permission.

Drugs and toxins
prescription medications
oct medications
drugs of abuse
withdrawal states
medication side effects
poisons (e.g. methanol, carbon monoxide, cyanide, hydrogen sulfide, alvia)

Infections
UTI
pneumonia
meningitis
encephalitis
any other infection

Metabolic derangements
electrolyte disturbance
endocrine disturbance
hypercarbia
hypoxia
hyper- or hypoglycemia
hyper- or hypoosmolar states
inborn errors of metabolism
nutritional (e.g. thiamine, niacin, B12, folate)

Neurologic disorders
stroke
epidural hematoma
subdural hematoma
subarachnoid hemorrhage
intraparenchymal hemorrhage
seizure
hypertensive encephalopathy
pain

Systemic organ failure
cardiac failure
liver failure
renal failure
pulmonary disease
hematologic (e.g. blast cell crisis)

Physical disorders
trauma
burns
electrocution
hyperthermia
hypothermia

Furthermore, multiple underlying conditions are often present in delirium [27]. The most common conditions include:

a. fluid and electrolyte disturbances;
b. infections;
c. drug side effect (see Table 2.3)
d. metabolic disorders;
e. low perfusion states;
f. withdrawl from alcohol and sedatives.

Pain alone can be a cause of delirium. In many instances, pain is a marker of pathology. But when other conditions have been ruled out, uncontrolled pain is a potential etiology that should not be overlooked. In fact, adequate pain control is essential in recommendations for preventing delirium [18, 19].

Table 2.3 Some of the medications that have been implicated in causing or worsening delirium. This list is by no means comprehensive. If another cause is not readily apparent, all medications should be reviewed and considered. From Francis J Jr, Young GB. Diagnosis of delirium and confusional states. Aug, 2012. Uptodate.com; with permission.

Analgesics
opioids
Antibiotics and antivirals
acyclovir
aminoglycosides
amphotericin b
antimalarials
cephalosporins
fluroquinolones

isoniazid
interferon
linezolid
macrolides
metronidazole
nalidixic acid
penicillins
rifampin
sulfonamides
Anticholinergics
Antiepileptics
carbamazepine
levetiracetam

phenytoin
valproate
vigabatrin
Antidepressants
mirtazapine
SSRIs
TCAs
Other CNS acting agents
lithium
phenothiazines
disulfiram
cholinesterase inhibitors
IL-2

Cardiovascular drugs
antiarrhythmics
beta blockers
clonidine
digoxin
diuretics
methyldopa
Corticosteroids
Anti-parkinsonian agents
amantadine
bromocriptine
levodopa
pergolide
dopamine agonists
benztropine
GI drugs
antiemetics
antispasmodics
h2 blockers
loperamide
Antihistamines
Hypoglycemic agents
Sedatives
barbiturates
benzodiazepines
Muscle relaxants
baclofen
cyclobenzaprine
Herbal supplements
atropa belladonna extract
henbane
mandrake
jimson weed
St. John's wort
valerian

Differential diagnosis

The evaluation of delirium is difficult for many reasons. Attention should be paid to conditions that can present similarly to delirium, but are distinct. The fact that delirious patients typically are unable to provide any useful history or cooperate fully with an examination poses significant challenges. As such, great attention should be paid to the details of the presentation to help clarify the differential. Collateral information, when available, can also be especially helpful.

Key features of delirium can help set it apart from other similar conditions and in determining the underlying cause. Delirium is an acute process that represents a change from baseline. It is a diffuse process affecting multiple cognitive domains. There is always impairment of attention.

1. Dementia

    Dementia is a chronic condition that involves impairment of memory as well as other cognitive functions. There are multiple dementing diseases and they differ in the set of cognitive functions affected. However, all are slow processes. Even the so-called rapidly progressive dementias develop over months – as opposed to the hours and days over which delirium develops. An acute decline in mental function in a patient with dementia should, however, prompt a work-up for acute illness that could cause delirium. A dementia patient who becomes more confused in the evening hours or at night without a prior established pattern of "sundowning" [23] may warrant a work-up for delirium due to the change in baseline.

2. Non-convulsive status epilepticus (NCSE)

    NCSE is a condition that is difficult to detect and can cause persistent altered mental status or confusion. The only symptom can be persistently depressed mental status, potentially mistaken for hypoactive delirium. Additional symptoms, if present, may be subtle. There can be slight rhythmic movements such as twitching of an extremity or the face. Rhythmic nystagmoid eye movements or hippus may also be seen. NCSE can also cause a focal deficit, such as aphasia, in the absence of a structural lesion.

    NCSE is likely under-recognized in the critically ill. As it is easily missed, there must be a high level of suspicion in patients at risk of seizures. NCSE, although rare in the general population, can affect up to one third of the patients in a neurological ICU and up to 10% of patients in a general medical ICU [28, 29]. The incidence of convulsive and non-convulsive status epilepticus is 100,000 to 200,000 annually in the United States [30], most of which have convulsive features at presentation. Risk factors for status epilepticus include a prior history of seizures, any structural lesion (e.g. infarct, hemorrhage, tumor) that affects the cortex, central nervous system (CNS) infection, neurodegenerative process that affects the cortex (e.g. Creutzfeldt–Jakob disease), sedative withdrawal, metabolic abnormalities (e.g. hypoglycemia, hyponatremia), and use of medications that lower seizure threshold (Table 2.4). NCSE should be considered for any persistently depressed mental status that remains unexplained, especially in the context of risk factors. Work-up for non-convulsive status epilepticus requires continuous EEG monitoring.

3. Encephalitis

    Encephalitis is an acute process that can cause depressed consciousness, inattention, confusion,

Table 2.4 Medications that can lower seizure threshold. *Italics* – tramadol and bupropion have been reported to precipitate seizures in otherwise healthy individuals with no seizure history. From Bromfield EB. Epilepsy and the elderly. In: Schachter SC, Schomer DL, eds. *The Comprehensive Evaluation and Treatment of Epilepsy*. San Diego, CA: Academic Press; 1997; with permission.

Antiasthmatics
aminophylline
theophylline

Antibiotics
isoniazid
lindane
metronidazole
nalidixic acid
penicillins

Antidepressants
tricyclic antidepressants
bupropion

General anesthetics
enflurane
ketamine

Hormones
estrogens

Immunosuppressants
chlorambucil
cyclosporine A

Local anesthetics
lidocaine
bupivacaine
procaine

Narcotics
tramadol
meperidine
pentazocine
propoxyphene

Antipsychotics
clozapine
phenothiazines
butyrophenones

and global cognitive dysfunction. Work-up for any acute confusion should involve evaluation for infection (as discussed below) and encephalitis or meningitis should be included in the differential.

4. Focal cognitive deficits

Focal deficits in cognitive function can appear like delirium. It is important to remember that delirium is a diffuse process that affects attention and all cognitive functions. If one cognitive domain is disproportionately affected, a focal lesion is suggested, but the distinction can be difficult to make.

A patient with aphasia may not answer or follow commands and may therefore appear confused. The deficit, however, is limited to language, and the patient may be able to mimic and maintain attention on the examiner.

An amnestic syndrome can have the appearance of confusion, with the patient repeating (the same) questions. However, within the time limits of working memory – a few minutes – the patient would appear normal, demonstrating normal attention and other cognitive faculties. Working memory requires focal attention to a task, such as silently repeating a telephone number while writing that number down.

Cortical lesions in the parietal lobe can cause a neglect syndrome, especially right-sided lesions. The laterality of the deficits distinguishes these from a global process such as delirium.

Frontal lesions may be the most difficult to distinguish from delirium. There can be perseveration, lack of motivation, disinhibition, and poor judgment and insight. Again, if one cognitive domain is more affected than others, this can help distinguish the process from delirium. In the end, any suggestion of focality should prompt additional work-up for a structural brain lesion.

5. Psychiatric illness

Mild delirium may be similar to depression, with decreased concentration, lethargy, and irritability. More severe delirium may be similar to acute psychosis, with disorganized thinking, hallucinations, paranoia, and agitation. Generally, there is less variability in psychiatric illness, especially over short time courses such as hours. The ability to sustain attention may not be affected in psychiatric illness and there may not be disorientation. A prior history of psychiatric illness can be helpful. However, when the distinction is

not clear, a work-up for medical illness may be necessary to rule out delirium.

Evaluation

Recognizing delirium

The first task in the evaluation of delirium is recognition of the condition. While this may seem easy and obvious – for example an elderly patient calling out to imagined characters in an empty hospital room – often it is not so straightforward [1, 2]. Delirium may be subtle. In the ICU, where patients are routinely in and out of consciousness, mild lethargy and disorientation are easily missed unless specific questions are asked. Patients may retain the ability to interact socially in the midst of delirium. The fluctuating course of delirium can also be misleading. The patient can be normal during morning rounds, only to become quite delirious later in the day.

Determining baseline status is an essential first set in assessing delirium. Unfortunately, it is often a difficult task. A poor understanding of the patient's baseline can lead to both over-diagnosis (mistaking baseline dementia for delirium) and under-diagnosis (attributing confusion to known dementia when it is actually new). The patient may not be able to provide a useful history. Therefore, collateral history is vital. If no information is available, then the evaluation must proceed on the assumption of delirium until proven otherwise.

For patients already in the hospital, a considerable body of evidence exists for the use of a formalized method to detect delirium [18, 31, 32]. Several screening tools have been developed for this purpose, such as the Confusion Assessment Method for the ICU (CAM-ICU) [33] (Figure 2.1) and the Intensive Care Delirium Screening Checklist (ICDSC) [34] (Figure 2.2). As the names suggest, they are designed to be used in the ICU, where patients are at high risk of delirium. Both are designed to be short examinationss focused on the core features of delirium. The CAM-ICU includes onset, inattention, level of consciousness, and disorganized thought. The ICDSC is slightly longer and assesses level of time course, inattention, level of consciousness, disorganized thought, hallucinations or delusions, psychomotor agitation or retardation, appropriateness of speech and mood, and sleep/wake cycle. Recommendations are that every patient be checked at least daily in the ICU [32].

CAM-ICU Worksheet

Feature 1: Acute Onset or Fluctuating Course	Score	Check here if Present
Is the pt different than his/her baseline mental status? OR Has the patient had any fluctuation in mental status in the past 24 hours as evidenced by fluctuation on a sedation scale (i.e., RASS), GCS, or previous delirium assessment?	Either question Yes →	☐
Feature 2: Inattention		
Letters Attention Test (See training manual for alternate **Pictures**) Directions: Say to the patient, *"I am going to read you a series of 10 letters. Whenever you hear the letter 'A,' indicate by squeezing my hand."* Read letters from the following letter list in a normal tone 3 seconds apart. **S A V E A H A A R T** **Errors are counted when patient fails to squeeze on the letter "A" and when the patient squeezes on any letter other than "A."**	Number of Errors >2 →	☐
Feature 3: Altered Level of Consciousness		
Present if the Actual RASS score is anything other than alert and calm (zero)	RASS anything other than zero →	☐
Feature 4:Disorganized Thinking		
Yes/No Questions (See training manual for alternate set of questions) 1. Will a stone float on water? 2. Are there fish in the sea? 3. Does one pound weigh more than two pounds? 4. Can you use a hammer to pound a nail? **Errors are counted when the patient incorrectly answers a question.** **Command** Say to patient: "Hold up this many fingers" (Hold 2 fingers in front of patient) "Now do the same thing with the other hand" (Do not repeat number of fingers) *If pt is unable to move both arms, for 2nd part of command ask patient to "Add one more finger" **An error is counted if patient is unable to complete the entire command.**	Combined number of errors >1→	☐

Overall CAM-ICU	Criteria Met →	☐ **CAM-ICU Positive** (Delirium Present)
Feature 1 **plus** 2 **and** either 3 **or** 4 present = CAM-ICU positive	Criteria Not Met →	☐ **CAM-ICU Negative** (No Delirium)

Figure 2.1 Confusion Assessment Method for the ICU (CAM-ICU) Worksheet. Copyright © 2002, E. Wesley Ely, MD, MPH and Vanderbilt University, all rights reserved; with permission.

History and examination

Once it is established that the patient is delirious, the evaluation turns to uncovering the underlying cause or causes of delirium. The history, if one can be obtained, should include a general review of systems to look for any evidence of active disease or ingestion of medication, recreational drug, or other harmful substance. Since the list of potential causes of delirium is so large and varied, it is important to cast a wide net. It is also important to keep in mind the possibility of atypical presentations of common conditions. For example, a myocardial infarction could cause delirium in a patient who may be unable then to report the usual symptoms of chest pain.

Similarly, the physical examination should be comprehensive, to the degree that patient cooperation allows. Even dehydration can cause delirium in the elderly or other at-risk populations. As such, simple findings such as skin turgor can be informative. Mild facial or scalp injuries suggest the possibility of head trauma. In the elderly or patients on anticoagulation, even mild trauma can cause intracranial hemorrhage or expanding chronic subdural hemorrhage

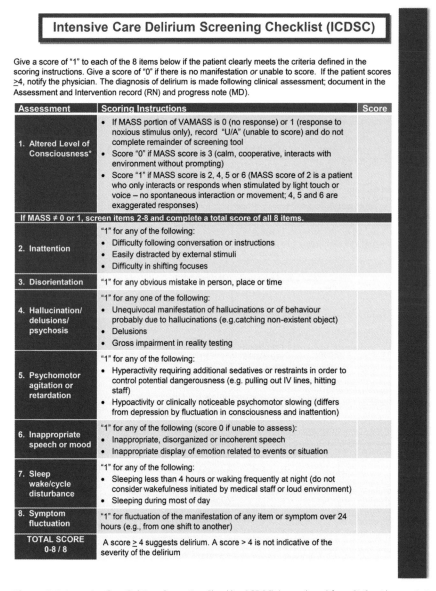

Intensive Care Delirium Screening Checklist (ICDSC)

Give a score of "1" to each of the 8 items below if the patient clearly meets the criteria defined in the scoring instructions. Give a score of "0" if there is no manifestation *or* unable to score. If the patient scores ≥4, notify the physician. The diagnosis of delirium is made following clinical assessment; document in the Assessment and Intervention record (RN) and progress note (MD).

Assessment	Scoring Instructions	Score
1. Altered Level of Consciousness*	• If MASS portion of VAMASS is 0 (no response) or 1 (response to noxious stimulus only), record "U/A" (unable to score) and do not complete remainder of screening tool • Score "0" if MASS score is 3 (calm, cooperative, interacts with environment without prompting) • Score "1" if MASS score is 2, 4, 5 or 6 (MASS score of 2 is a patient who only interacts or responds when stimulated by light touch or voice – no spontaneous interaction or movement; 4, 5 and 6 are exaggerated responses)	
If MASS ≠ 0 or 1, screen items 2-8 and complete a total score of all 8 items.		
2. Inattention	"1" for any of the following: • Difficulty following conversation or instructions • Easily distracted by external stimuli • Difficulty in shifting focuses	
3. Disorientation	"1" for any obvious mistake in person, place or time	
4. Hallucination/ delusions/ psychosis	"1" for any one of the following: • Unequivocal manifestation of hallucinations or of behaviour probably due to hallucinations (e.g.catching non-existent object) • Delusions • Gross impairment in reality testing	
5. Psychomotor agitation or retardation	"1" for any of the following: • Hyperactivity requiring additional sedatives or restraints in order to control potential dangerousness (e.g. pulling out IV lines, hitting staff) • Hypoactivity or clinically noticeable psychomotor slowing (differs from depression by fluctuation in consciousness and inattention)	
6. Inappropriate speech or mood	"1" for any of the following (score 0 if unable to assess): • Inappropriate, disorganized or incoherent speech • Inappropriate display of emotion related to events or situation	
7. Sleep wake/cycle disturbance	"1" for any of the following: • Sleeping less than 4 hours or waking frequently at night (do not consider wakefulness initiated by medical staff or loud environment) • Sleeping during most of day	
8. Symptom fluctuation	"1" for fluctuation of the manifestation of any item or symptom over 24 hours (e.g., from one shift to another)	
TOTAL SCORE 0-8 / 8	A score ≥ 4 suggests delirium. A score > 4 is not indicative of the severity of the delirium	

Figure 2.2 Intensive Care Delirium Screening Checklist (ICDSC) (reproduced from [34]; with permission).

presenting as delirium. Oral trauma, on the sides of the tongue or cheeks, could be the result of a seizure and delirium may be part of the post-ictal state or ongoing seizure activity, as in NCSE.

The neurologic examination is often difficult in the setting of limited patient cooperation. However, an examination can provide valuable information regarding potential etiologies of delirium. Any focal findings should prompt neuroimaging for a structural lesion. Deficits may be apparent upon observation of the patient, including hemiplegia, hemisensory loss, or neglect. Others can be subtle and elicited only with difficulty, such as visual deficits. Testing for blink response to visual threat can be useful in such instances. Findings, including myoclonus or asterixis, may suggest metabolic disturbances.

Medications

Medications should be carefully reviewed. Drug toxicity is a common cause of delirium [35], including many common medications. New medications or medications whose dose has been adjusted should be suspect even if not usually associated with delirium. If the medication history is uncertain, non-critical medications can be held and any medications with high potential to cause delirium should be avoided. (Table 2.3).

Investigational studies

Diagnostic testing should be guided by the history and physical examination to evaluate for the most likely causes of delirium in a given situation. Nonetheless, despite best efforts, it is not uncommon for the history and physical examination to be uninformative. In such instances, empiric application of basic tests may be required to search for the most common causes of delirium.

Laboratory studies

"Basic" laboratory studies are appropriate for most patients when no cause for delirium is immediately apparent. Serum electrolytes, blood urea nitrogen (BUN) and creatinine, liver function tests, glucose, complete blood count, and urine analysis can inform regarding the most common metabolic disturbances as well as common infectious etiologies. A urine drug screen and serum alcohol level may also be warranted. However, it should be kept in mind that many recreational drugs are not detected by a standard urine drug screen. Additionally, many prescribed medications can cause delirium. Therapeutic drug levels should be tested when appropriate. If there is evidence of respiratory distress or respiratory disease (such as chronic obstructive pulmonary disease) arterial blood gas can also be useful to rule out CO_2 narcosis. Finally, with any suggestion of infection, blood, urine, and sputum cultures and chest X-ray may be informative.

Lumbar puncture

If there is evidence of infection and no other source of infection is apparent, then lumbar puncture (LP) should be considered to evaluate for CNS infection. If there is evidence of meningeal irritation such as meningismus, LP should be performed even if there is evidence of other infection. It should be remembered that in the elderly or immunosuppressed the usual signs of infection may be absent. Hypothermia and leukopenia can also be signs of infections just as fever and leukocytosis. If no other cause of delirium is

apparent, LP should considered, as should screening neuroimaging.

EEG testing

As noted previously, NCSE can be a cause of depressed mental status and present with no other signs of seizure activity. If no other cause of delirium is evident, EEG testing should be considered to rule out seizures. While there is no prospective evidence for the evaluation of occult seizure in delirium, two case series of patients with unexplained altered consciousness for whom an EEG was ordered showed seizures in 19% and 37% [36, 37]. If any evidence of seizure activity is present, then EEG testing is a must. If used to evaluate for NCSE, then 24-hour monitoring should be used as the yield of a spot EEG is not sufficient [36, 38].

Neuroimaging

Delirium is somewhat unique compared to most of the symptoms discussed in this imaging text. As alluded to above, the vast majority of patients with delirium in an ICU setting, or those presenting acutely to an emergency department can be expected to have a non-contributory brain-imaging study, apart from those incidental findings that may be related to the medical or surgical conditions responsible for the state of health that led to the admission. For example, patients in a cardiovascular ICU are more likely to have non-specific white-matter lesions from chronic ischemia or pre-existent lacunar or lobar infarctions (Figure 2.3A). Brain volume loss may reflect baseline alcoholism, seizure history, or treatment (e.g. cerebellar volume loss) (Figure 2.3B). Although many forms of brain pathology may, or may not contribute to a patient's delirium, the relationship is often difficult to predict (Figure 2.4).

As there is no known unifying pathophysiology of delirium, and no specific abnormal structural finding that is pathognomonic, suggestive of, or highly associated with delirium, it is not surprising that the one highly correlated brain-imaging finding for delirium is an essentially unremarkable brain, or a brain with relatively non-specific findings (atrophy or white-matter changes) that do not necessarily imply that they are causal in delirium, but may simply indicate a more generally vulnerable brain [39]. The frequent associations with delirium such as systemic infection, fluid and electrolyte disturbances, dehydration, or

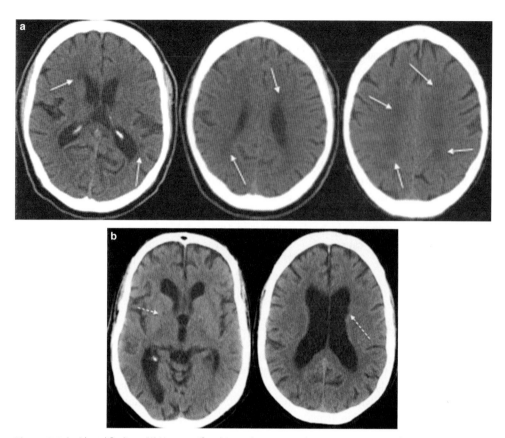

Figure 2.3 Incidental findings: (A) Non-specific white and gray matter lesions are common, often incidental findings on CT or MRI in patients with delirium, related to age and particularly vascular-disease risk factors. Arrows indicate typical non-specific white-matter hypodensities on non-contrast CT. (B) Parenchymal atrophy with secondarily enlarged ventricles and sulci is also not uncommon in the hospitalized patient related to age, and/or pre-existing medical conditions, and is not specifically associated with delirium. Dashed arrows indicate gray-matter hypodensities, most likely from remote lacunar infarctions.

drug effects are not typically associated with positive brain-imaging findings.

The literature for imaging in delirium is remarkably small, despite the prevalence of delirium, but not surprising given the consistent experiences and results of the few series that seem to be in agreement that there are no specific features relating the syndrome and brain structure. Not surprisingly, several studies suggest that patients with pre-existing findings on imaging are more likely to develop delirium. Pre-existing white-matter and thalamic pathology has been implicated in post-operative delirium particularly in an elderly population [40], in electro-convulsive-therapy-induced delirium [41], and several studies suggest an association with brain atrophy [42]. Others suggest that serious medical disease is a better predictor of the development of delirium than the presence of abnormal brain imaging [43].

A possible exception to the rule that imaging studies are generally normal or show unrelated pathology is the literature linking delirium to abnormal brain perfusion; a number of reports suggest a possible association between delirium and focal (reduced) brain perfusion [44]. In one series [45] of 22 patients studied by technetium-labeled hexamethylpropylene-amine oxime (HMPAO-Tc99m) single photon emission computed tomography (SPECT), frontal and parietal perfusion abnormality was observed by visual criteria in half of them, and there was a more widespread abnormality by regional measurements. Of the six patients who had serial measures, three did not have visually apparent perfusion change with change in their level of delirium. Unfortunately, most of these studies cannot account for the many potential confounding factors [44] including pre-existing pathology in the study population, which is

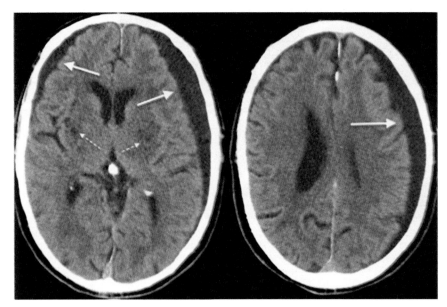

Figure 2.4 Major structural findings in the brain may be unrelated to delirium. A 92-year-old patient was evaluated in the emergency department for altered mental status. CT showed chronic, bilateral hypodense subdural hematomas (arrows), and non-specific hypodensities in the basal ganglia (dashed arrow), the latter most likely remote lacunar infarctions. After hospitalization, treatment was initiated for urinary-tract and gall-bladder infections, with rapid improvement in mental status to baseline (pre-admission) levels. Subsequently, there were intermittent periods of confusion, inattention, disorientation, typical of mild delirium, which also resolved prior to discharge, and were apparently unrelated to the major imaging findings.

typically elderly, and ill with a variety of comorbidities. Currently, perfusion imaging by computed tomography (CT), magnetic resonance imaging (MRI), or nuclear medicine would not be considered a clinical standard of care, as these require and deserve further investigation in controlled studies [44].

There are very few conventional imaging studies that are generally applicable to most populations, either those with delirium in an ICU setting or presenting to an emergency room (ER), and enrollment bias reflects the specifics of each study. However, the findings of one large retrospective study of patients admitted to a neurology service for acute confusion (delirium) are informative. Hufschmidt *et al.* [46] reported imaging findings by CT and/or MRI in 14% of the patients, overall. When patients with focal signs were excluded, the risk of positive imaging decreased to 7%. And the probability of abnormal imaging decreased even further in the group with no focal signs but with either fever or dehydration. Including patients with dementia also reduces the likelihood of abnormal imaging. Consistent with several small series and case reports, when imaging was positive, there was a wide range in pathology, including stroke presenting with the clinical manifestation of confusion, thalamic infarction, intracranial hemorrhage, metastatic and primary brain tumor, and infectious processes, including herpes simplex encephalitis.

When no focal deficits are evident, provided that a neurologic examination can be performed, the yield of neuroimaging is low [46, 47]. If a cause of delirium is otherwise evident, then neuroimaging may not be necessary. However, if the patient fails to improve with appropriate treatment of the presumed cause, then the diagnosis needs to be reconsidered and imaging may be considered. Also, if no cause of delirium is readily evident, even if there are no focal deficits, screening neuroimaging may still be prudent to rule out unlikely, but highly morbid, intracranial pathology. Similarly, if the delirious patient is so impaired as to prevent any useful history or examination, imaging is also warranted.

Irrespective of the high probability of a negative imaging study in the population of patients with delirium, the likelihood, as indicated above, of an important positive finding increases in patients with focal deficits, or signs of elevated intracranial pressure, and/or concerning history (Figure 2.5). Any evidence of trauma should prompt immediate

29

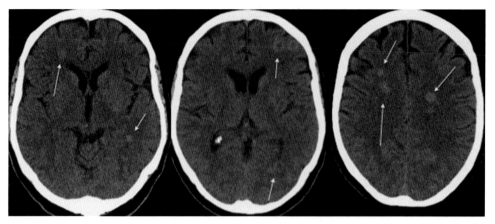

Figure 2.5 Positive non-contrast CT scan in a patient with small cell lung carcinoma and confusion. Arrows indicate some of the multiple dense mass lesions. Imaging evaluation of unexplained confusion/delirium in the absence of focal findings will only rarely reveal significant findings, although the likelihood of significant findings by imaging is greater in patients with specific risk factors including neoplasm. Note that most small mass lesions will be inapparent without intravenous contrast enhancement, and MRI would provide even greater sensitivity for cases that remain diagnostic dilemmas after CT.

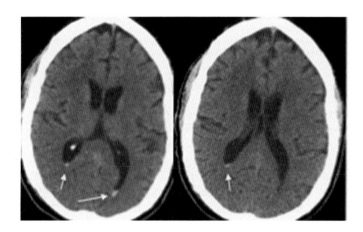

Figure 2.6 Critical finding of intraventricular hemorrhage but considered unrelated to delirium. Patient with acute lymphocytic leukemia, under treatment and with an Omaya reservoir, who developed neutropenia and fever. The reservoir and drain were removed. A non-contrast CT for altered mental status and delirium showed new intraventricular hemorrhages (arrows), but in this case, these were considered to be unrelated to the symptoms.

neuroimaging, and typically CT in this patient population. CT requires only minutes of actual scan time, which is especially important in the uncooperative and/or disoriented patient. Screening requirements are minimal for CT compared to MRI, and the technique is available 24/7 with in-house technologist staff at most hospitals.

Non-contrast CT imaging will detect most of the actionable acute pathology, including hemorrhage with mass effect, large mass lesions, large or subacute cerebral infarction, and hydrocephalus. Contrast-enhanced CT would provide additional sensitivity to infectious etiologies, notably abscess, subdural empyema, ventriculitis, and some cases of meningitis, cerebritis, and encephalitis. However, a negative CT does not exclude acute or small, yet critically located infarctions, many posterior fossa lesions, small mass lesions, and will miss most early findings in herpes and other types of encephalitis (Figure 2.6).

MRI is generally more sensitive but is also more time intensive, and requires greater care in prescreening and monitoring. Non-sedated, delirious patients do not do well in the confined environment of the MRI magnet bore, and inability to control motion is a contraindication to MRI. Moreover, it is not certain that the additional pathology that can be identified on MRI provides information that changes the acute management of delirious patients [48]. However in problematic cases, and when patients are deteriorating without explanation, the relatively small risk and gain of MRI may be justified (Figure 2.7).

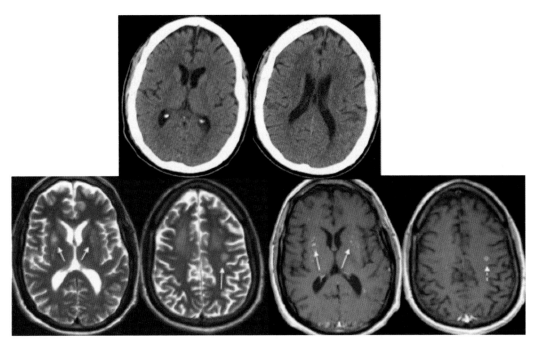

Figure 2.7 Negative CT followed by MRI for unexplained findings. Same patient as Fig 2.6. Top panel. After treatment for infection with clinical improvement, the patient was discharged home, but returned to the emergency department 11 days later, with fever, nausea, and confusion. A repeat CT showed resolution of the hemorrhages; the CT was otherwise unremarkable. Bottom panel. In view of concern for unexplained findings, an MRI was acquired the same day as the CT and showed multiple foci of T2-hyperintensity on the T2-weighted images (arrows, two bottom-left panels) and enhancement on the T1-weighted images (arrows, two bottom-right panels) in the basal ganglia and white matter, typical of micro-abscesses. With few exceptions (e.g. some acute hemorrhages, including subarachnoid hemorrhage), MRI will most often provide greater sensitivity to intracranial pathology compared to CT, and will have a higher yield for critical findings in patients with specific risk factors (infection, neoplasm, focal findings) when CT is negative.

Conclusion

Delirium is not a singular clinical entity, but rather a clinical syndrome. It is not a unifying diagnosis, but rather a range of symptoms that reflect brain dysfunction caused by physiologic stress that can be from almost any cause. It is, unfortunately, an imperfect classification based on imperfect understanding of how the brain works. When confronted with delirium, the clinician's task is to maintain a broad differential while searching for evidence that will inform on the underlying disease process and to select judiciously the tests and studies that will lead to the diagnosis of what is actually ailing the patient.

References

1. Cole MG (2004). Delirium in elderly patients. *Am J Geriatr Psychiatry* **12**: 7–21.

2. Marcantonio E, Ta T, Duthie E, Resnick NM (2002). Delirium severity and psychomotor types: their relationship with outcomes after hip fracture repair. *J Am Geriatr Soc* **50**: 850–857.

3. Inouye, SK (1994). The dilemma of delirium: clinical and research controversies regarding diagnosis and evaluation of delirium in hospitalized elderly medical patients. *Am J Med* **97**: 278–288.

4. American Psychiatric Association (2000). *Diagnostic and Statistical Manual of Mental Disorders, Fourth Edition: DSM-IV-TR®*. Arlington, VA: American Psychiatric Publishing.

5. Ropper A, Adams RD, Victor M, Samuels M (2009). *Adams and Victor's Principles of Neurology*, 9th edn. New York: McGraw Hill Professional.

6. McNicoll L, Pisani MA, Zhang Y, *et al.* (2003). Delirium in the intensive care unit: occurrence and clinical course in older patients. *J Am Geriatr Soc* **51**: 591–598.

7. Elie M, Rousseau F, Cole M, *et al.* (2000). Prevalence and detection of delirium in elderly emergency department patients. *Can Med Assoc J* **163**: 977–981.

8. Lawlor PG, Gagnon B, Mancini I L, *et al.* (2000). Occurrence, causes, and outcome of delirium in

patients with advanced cancer: a prospective study. *Arch Intern Med* **160**: 786–794.

9. Kiely DK, Bergmann MA, Murphy KM, *et al.* (2003). Delirium among newly admitted postacute facility patients: prevalence, symptoms, and severity. *J Gerontol A Biol Sci Med Sci* **58**: M441–445.

10. Francis J (1992). Delirium in older patients. *J Am Geriatr Soc* **40**: 829–838.

11. Inouye SK, Rushing JT, Foreman MD, Palmer RM, Pompei P (1998). Does delirium contribute to poor hospital outcomes? A three-site epidemiologic study. *J Gen Intern Med* **13**: 234–242.

12. Dyer CB, Ashton CM, Teasdale TA (1995). Postoperative delirium. A review of 80 primary data-collection studies. *Arch Intern Med* **155**: 461–465.

13. Pisani MA, Murphy TE, Van Ness PH, Araujo KLB, & Inouye SK (2007). Characteristics associated with delirium in older patients in a medical intensive care unit. *Arch Intern Med* **167**: 1629–1634.

14. Cole MG, Primeau FJ (1993). Prognosis of delirium in elderly hospital patients. *Can Med Assoc J* **149**: 41–46.

15. Ely EW, Shintani A, Truman B, *et al.* (2004). Delirium as a predictor of mortality in mechanically ventilated patients in the intensive care unit. *JAMA* **291**: 1753–1762.

16. Witlox J, Eurelings LSM, de Jonghe JFM, *et al.* (2010). Delirium in elderly patients and the risk of postdischarge mortality, institutionalization, and dementia: a meta-analysis. *JAMA* **304**: 443–451.

17. Girard TD, Jackson JC, Pandharipande PP, *et al.* (2010). Delirium as a predictor of long-term cognitive impairment in survivors of critical illness. *Crit Care Med* **38**: 1513–1520.

18. O'Mahony R, Murthy L, Akunne A, Young J, Guideline Development Group (2011). Synopsis of the National Institute for Health and Clinical Excellence guideline for prevention of delirium. *Ann Intern Med* **154**: 746–751.

19. Brown TM, Boyle MF (2002). Delirium. *BMJ* **325**: 644–647.

20. Inouye SK, Bogardus ST Jr, Charpentier PA, *et al.* (1999). A multicomponent intervention to prevent delirium in hospitalized older patients. *N Engl J Med* **340**: 669–676.

21. Inouye SK (2006). Delirium in older persons. *N Engl J Med* **354**: 1157–1165.

22. American Psychiatric Association (1999). Practice guideline for the treatment of patients with delirium. *Am J Psychiatry* **156**: 1–20.

23. Bliwise DL (1994). What is sundowning? *J Am Geriatr Soc* **42**: 1009–1011.

24. Romano J, Engel G (1944). Delirium: I. Electroencephalographic data. *Arch Neurol Psychiatry* **51**: 356–377.

25. Mach JR Jr, Dysken MW, Kuskowski M, *et al.* (1995). Serum anticholinergic activity in hospitalized older persons with delirium: a preliminary study. *J Am Geriatr Soc* **43**: 491–495.

26. Campbell N, Boustani M, Limbil T, *et al.* (2009). The cognitive impact of anticholinergics: a clinical review. *Clin Interv Aging* **4**: 225–233.

27. Francis J, Martin D, Kapoor WN (1990). A prospective study of delirium in hospitalized elderly. *JAMA* **263**: 1097–1101.

28. Jordan KG (1994). Status epilepticus. A perspective from the neuroscience intensive care unit. *Neurosurg Clin N Am* **5**: 671–686.

29. Towne AR, Waterhouse EJ, Boggs JG, *et al.* (2000). Prevalence of nonconvulsive status epilepticus in comatose patients. *Neurology* **54**: 340–345.

30. DeLorenzo RJ, Pellock JM, Towne AR, Boggs JG (1995). Epidemiology of status epilepticus. *J Clin Neurophysiol* **12**: 316–325.

31. Neto AS, Nassar AP Jr, Cardoso SO, *et al.* (2012). Delirium screening in critically ill patients: a systematic review and meta-analysis. *Crit Care Med* **40**: 1946–1951.

32. Jacobi J, Fraser GL, Coursin DB, *et al.* (2002). Clinical practice guidelines for the sustained use of sedatives and analgesics in the critically ill adult. *Crit Care Med* **30**: 119–141.

33. Ely EW, Inouye SK, Bernard GR, *et al.* (2001). Delirium in mechanically ventilated patients: validity and reliability of the confusion assessment method for the intensive care unit (CAM-ICU). *JAMA* **286**: 2703–2710.

34. Bergeron N, Dubois MJ, Dumont M, Dial S, Skrobik Y (2001). Intensive Care Delirium Screening Checklist: evaluation of a new screening tool. *Intensive Care Med* **27**: 859–864.

35. Francis J Jr (1996). Drug-induced delirium. *CNS Drugs* **5**: 103–114.

36. Claassen J, Mayer SA, Kowalski RG, Emerson RG, Hirsch LJ (2004). Detection of electrographic seizures with continuous EEG monitoring in critically ill patients. *Neurology* **62**: 1743–1748.

37. Privitera M, Hoffman M, Moore JL, Jester D (1994). EEG detection of nontonic-clonic status epilepticus in patients with altered consciousness. *Epilepsy Res* **18**: 155–166.

38. Claassen J, Hirsch LH (2009). Status epilepticus. In Frontera JA, ed. *Decision Making in Neurocritical Care.* New York: Thieme, pp. 63–75.

39. Soiza RL, Sharma V, Ferguson K, *et al.* (2008). Neuroimaging studies of delirium: a systematic review. *J Psychosom Res* **65**: 239–248.

40. Shioiri A, Kurumaji A, Takeuchi T, *et al.* (2010). White matter abnormalities as a risk factor for postoperative delirium revealed by diffusion tensor imaging. *Am J Geriatr Psychiatry* **18**: 743–753.

41. Figiel GS, Coffey CE, Djang WT, Hoffman G Jr, Doraiswamy PM (1990). Brain magnetic resonance imaging findings in ECT-induced delirium. *J Neuropsychiatry Clin Neurosci* **2**: 53–58.

42. Koponen H, Hurri L, Stenback U, *et al.* (1989). Computed tomography findings in delirium. *J Nerv Ment Dis* **177**: 226–231.

43. Kishi Y, Iwasaki Y, Takezawa K, Kurosawa H, Endo S (1995). Delirium in critical care unit patients admitted through an emergency room. *Gen Hosp Psychiatry* **17**: 371–379.

44. Alsop DC, Fearing MA, Johnson K, *et al.* (2006). The role of neuroimaging in elucidating delirium pathophysiology. *J Gerontol A Biol Sci Med Sci* **61**: 1287–1293.

45. Fong TG, Bogardus ST Jr, Daftary A, *et al.* (2006). Cerebral perfusion changes in older delirious patients using 99mTc HMPAO SPECT. *J Gerontol A Biol Sci Med Sci* **61**: 1294–1299.

46. Hufschmidt A, Shabarin V (2008). Diagnostic yield of cerebral imaging in patients with acute confusion. *Acta Neurol Scand* **118**: 245–250.

47. Inouye SK (1998). Delirium in hospitalized older patients. *Clin Geriatr Med* **14**: 745–764.

48. Morandi A, Gunther, ML, Vasilevskis EE, *et al.* (2010). Neuroimaging in delirious intensive care unit patients: a preliminary case series report. *Psychiatry Edgmont Pa Townsh* **7**: 28–33.

Intellectual dysfunction

Massimo Filippi, Federica Agosta, and Elisa Canu

Introduction

Cognitive impairment is very common and is associated with many neurological and systemic disorders. Cognitive impairment is an umbrella term that comprises a number of conditions ranging from confusional state (or delirium) to severe dementia in patients with Alzheimer's disease (AD). Neurologists together with primary care physicians play an important role in the assessment, interpretation, and treatment of symptoms, disability, and needs of patients with cognitive deficits. Delirium is discussed in Chapter 2. The present chapter is focused on clinical disorders associated with cognitive impairment leading to dementia (Table 3.1) and comprises three sections. In the first, the main cognitive functions are reviewed along with their anatomical correlates, and the most important (and common) cognitive deficits are defined. In the second, basic clinical, cognitive, and laboratory investigations recommended in the assessment of patients with cognitive impairment are described, with a particular focus on neuroimaging techniques. In the last section, clinical and cognitive findings and diagnostic work-up of the principal treatable, vascular, and neurodegenerative causes of cognitive impairment are discussed.

Cognitive functions and impairment

Memory

"LEONARD SHELBY: Burt. I'm not sure, I think I may have asked you to hold my calls.

BURT: You don't know?

LEONARD SHELBY: Well, I think I may have. I'm not too good on the phone.

BURT: Right, you said you like to look people in the eye when you talk to them.

LEONARD SHELBY: Yeah, yeah.

BURT: You don't remember saying that.

LEONARD SHELBY: Well, that's the thing. I have this condition.

BURT: A condition?

LEONARD SHELBY: It's my memory [...]. I have no short-term memory. I know who I am, I know all about myself. I just... since my injury I can't make new memories. Everything fades. If we talk for too long I'll forget how we started and next time I see you I'm not gonna remember this conversation. I don't even know if I've met you before. So if I seem a little strange or rude, or something, uh...

[He notices Burt is staring at him strangely]

LEONARD SHELBY: I've told you this before, haven't I?

BURT: Yeah ... I don't mean to mess with you but it's so weird. You don't remember me at all?

LEONARD SHELBY: No.

BURT: We've talked a bunch of times.

LEONARD SHELBY: I'm sure we have."

From "Memento", a Christopher Nolan movie.

Definitions

Human memory is a collection of mental abilities that serve the brain for registering incoming information (storage), processing the information to be consolidated, and making it accessible to use seconds, minutes, days, and even years later [1]. Memory is subserved by several different brain networks, which

---

Imaging Acute Neurologic Disease, ed. Massimo Filippi and Jack H. Simon. Published by Cambridge University Press.

Table 3.1 Common clinical causes of cognitive impairment

Category of disease	Most common causes
Metabolic/endocrine disorders	Respiratory/cardiac failure, hepatic/uremic encephalopathy, pancreatic encephalopathy, hypoglycemia, pellagra, hypoxia, acute intermittent porphyria, Wilson disease, hypothyroidism, hypopituitarism, hypo- or hyperparathyroidism, adrenocortical insufficiency
Intoxication	Drugs, alcohol, carbon monoxide, substance abuse, heavy-metal poisoning, organic toxins
Malnutrition	Thiamine, vitamin B12, nicotin acid, multiple vitamin deficiencies
Infections	HIV and other viral encephalitis, neurosyphilis, tuberculosis, Whipple's disease, Lyme disease, cryptococcal/fungal meningitis, neurocysticercosis, JC virus infection (progressive multifocal encephalopathy), measles (subacute sclerosing panencephalitis)
Inflammatory/autoimmune diseases	Multiple sclerosis, cerebral vasculitis, neurosarcoidosis, Behçet disease, VGKC channelopathy, anti-basal ganglia antibody syndrome, Hashimoto's encephalopathy, celiac disease
Head trauma	Chronic subdural hematoma, post-traumatic phenomenon, punchdrunk syndrome (dementia pugilistica)
Tumors	Brain tumors, CNS lymphoma, carcinomatous meningitis, paraneoplastic syndromes (e.g. limbic encephalitis), post-radiotherapy syndrome
Epileptic disorders	Non-convulsive status, transient epileptic amnesia
Other treatable causes	Normal-pressure hydrocephalus, obstructive hydrocephalus, side effects of medication,
Vascular	Multiple cortical and subcortical infarcts, strategic infarcts (e.g. thalamus), subcortical ischemic vascular disease, lacunae
Neurodegenerative	CJD, AD, FTLD syndromes, PD, atypical parkinsonisms, motor neuron disease
Psychiatric diseases	Depression
Genetic diseases	Leucodystrophies, familial neurodegenerative diseases (e.g. Huntington's disease)

Abbreviations: AD, Alzheimer's disease; CJD, Creutzfeldt–Jakob disease; CNS, central nervous system; FTLD, frontotemporal lobar degeneration; HIV, human immunodeficiency virus; VGKC, voltage-gated potassium channels.

rely on a dissociable neuroanatomy. These networks have a variable sensitivity to different disease processes and, thus, allow localizing the site of impairment which has important diagnostic implications. Some networks are associated with conscious awareness (explicit) and can be consciously recalled (declarative), whereas others are expressed by a change in behavior (implicit) and are typically unconscious (nondeclarative) [1]. Memory can also be categorized in many other ways, such as by the nature of the material to be remembered (e.g. verbal or visuospatial) [1].

Explicit memory has short-term and long-term components [1]. The **short-term memory** is the ability to retain a small amount of information for a brief period of time without consolidation if the data are not refreshed. The registration, i.e., the sensorial memory, selects and records the incoming information through the sensorial system for immediate repetition or reproduction. This first storage has a low ability to record information and, if the information is not converted to a more stable memory trace, it will disappear without learning records. The **long-term memory** is

the ability to retain a large amount of information for extensive periods (days, weeks, years) depending on the information salience. It is a consolidated memory with learning (encoding) and retrieval (a mechanism which allows us to restore memories) as the key processes. The retrieval can occur in two ways: through recall or, much more easily, through recognition. During the retrieval process, explicit memory requires a conscious access to information related to events (episodic) or knowledge (semantic) [1].

Episodic memory is the memory system that allows us to remember past experiences and episodes of our lives [1]. Episodic memory can be divided into item and associative memory. Item memories are for individual items without context, while associative memories involve multiple aspects of the same event. The medial temporal lobe (MTL), including the hippocampus and the entorhinal and perirhinal cortices, is the anatomical storage of the episodic memory [2]. Other critical structures involved in the episodic memory system are the forebrain, retrosplenial cortex, presubiculum, fornix, mammillary bodies, mammillothalamic tract, and anterior nucleus of the thalamus, which are all part of the circuit described by Papez in 1937 [3]. The episodic memory system also includes the prefrontal cortex [4], which is involved in different aspects of cognitive control mechanisms that enhance memory encoding and retrieval rather than supporting the retention of information.

Semantic memory defines what you know about the world, including general information about objects, people, events, and word meaning [1]. It is different from episodic memory because such a knowledge is not associated with a sense of self-experience or linked to a particular spatial or temporal context. For instance, remembering the day spent in Rome with friends is different from remembering that Rome is the capital city of Italy. While semantic memory is likely represented in a distributed network throughout much of the neocortex, the inferolateral and anterior temporal lobes (particularly the left) are considered critical for semantic knowledge (for further details see the language section).

Implicit (or procedural) memory refers to the ability to learn cognitive and behavioral skills and algorithms and use them without access to declarative consciousness [1], i.e., it works at an automatic, unconscious level. Examples are learning to ride a bicycle or play the piano. Brain regions involved in the procedural memory are the basal ganglia, cerebellum, and supplementary motor area.

Related cognitive deficits

When registration or storage processes are impaired by disease or accident, acquisition of new information is difficult or impossible (**amnesia**) [1]. Lesions involving the Papez circuit cause amnesia. An important distinction of episodic memory deficits is between anterograde and retrograde amnesia. Relative to the time of the brain injury, **anterograde amnesia** is the inability to form new memories, whereas **retrograde amnesia** is the loss of previously acquired memories. The extent of the loss of old memories could be in terms of days, years, sometimes decades. These disturbances may co-occur. Usually, a severe retrograde memory deficit is also accompanied by an anterograde amnesia. On the contrary, impairment of anterograde memory can occur in the absence of a frank retrograde amnesia. Consistent with Ribot's law, [5] subjects are more likely to lose recent memories that are closer to the injury onset than more

remote memories. This occurs because the most consolidated (oldest) memories are stored in the neocortical regions connected to the MTL; thus, an isolated lesion to the MTL is not likely to affect old memories [6]. Damage to the prefrontal cortex can contribute to the amnestic syndrome making collection and consolidation of information difficult. Disorders of episodic memory can be transient, such as those attributable to concussion, seizures, or transient global amnesia [1]. Furthermore, episodic memory deficits due to medications, hypoglycemia, tumors, and Korsakoff's syndrome can have a variable time course and be transient and non-progressive [1]. Episodic memory impairment following traumatic brain injury, hypoxic or ischemic injury, surgical lesions, and viral and limbic encephalitis, is more severe at onset (or for several days), improves (sometimes over periods of two years or more), and then stabilizes [1]. In the context of a neurodegenerative condition, such as AD, memory impairment begins insidiously and progresses gradually [1]. In disorders affecting multiple brain regions, such as vascular dementia (VaD) and multiple sclerosis, memory deficits usually progress in a stepwise manner [1].

Semantic memory impairment is most frequently manifested by naming deficits (see language section). In addition, patients with semantic memory impairment can display evidence of non-verbal impairment, such as matching pictures of items into different semantic categories [1]. Causes of semantic memory impairment include almost any disorder that disrupts the inferolateral temporal lobes, such as brain trauma, stroke, surgical lesions, encephalitis (typically herpes simplex virus (HSV) encephalitis), and tumors. AD is the most common neurodegenerative disorder disrupting semantic memory. A selective and progressive deterioration of semantic knowledge is the cardinal feature of the semantic variant of primary progressive aphasia (PPA), which is characterized by anatomical damage to anterior and inferior temporal regions [7].

Disruption of procedural memory includes either the loss of previously learned skills or substantial difficulties in learning new skills [1]. Tumors, strokes, hemorrhages, and other causes of injury to the basal ganglia, cerebellum, or supplementary motor area may disrupt procedural memory. Patients with Parkinson's disease (PD) show impaired procedural memory [8]. Other, less-common, neurodegenerative causes that affect procedural memory are Huntington's disease and olivopontocerebellar degeneration [8].

Language

"With an inked brush he marked everything with its name: table, chair, clock, door, wall, bed, pan. He went to the corral and marked the animals and plants: cow, goat, pig, hen, cassava, caladium, banana. [. . .] He realized that the day might come when things would be recognized by their inscriptions but that no one would remember their use."

From *One Hundred Years of Solitude*,
G.G. Márquez, 1970 [9].

Definitions

Language refers to the capacity for communication through productive combination of symbolic representations. In formulating a general definition of this kind, however, it is critical to keep in mind that language is not a unitary process, but rather a collection of processes operating at distinct levels and on distinct types of information [10, 11]. The complex operations of language can be broadly classified as comprehension, retrieval, and production. Each of these operations can refer to single words or sentences.

Comprehension of speech begins with the interpretation of acoustic–phonetic input as word forms in the surround of the auditory cortex located in the posterior superior temporal lobe [12]. Then, the concepts to which the word forms are semantically associated must be retrieved (semantic memory), in parallel with interpretation of word order and grammatical marking, to achieve comprehension of a discourse [12]. Comprehension can be facilitated by auditory cues from prosody and visual cues from concurrent hand gestures, lip movements, and facial expressions, and writing.

Naming (word retrieval) requires many distinct cognitive processes [13]. First, the item to be named needs to be recognized as a familiar entity by the subject (e.g. **visual recognition**) [13]. Then, it is essential to access the item meaning (semantics) [13]. Semantics includes two levels of knowledge: **conceptual knowledge** (information shared by a culture about an item) and **lexical semantics** (the defining features of the item). The meaning of the item is used to select a lexical representation or **lemma** that is independent of output modality (oral vs. written), and then the lemma is used to select a **modality-specific lexical representation**, i.e., the phonologic (spoken) representation or the orthographic (written) representation [13]. Once a spoken word form has been accessed, it must be spoken aloud. This process is based on two aspects: one requires maintaining the correct sequence of speech sounds that comprise the pronunciation while the sounds are produced, and the second is the motor output (**articulation**) [13]. Articulation of the word requires motor planning of complex movements of the lips, tongue, palate, vocal folds, and respiratory muscles, followed by implementation of these movements. Due to its complex entity, the process of naming is subtended by several brain regions, such as the anterior and inferior temporal lobes bilaterally for the conceptual knowledge; by the posterior superior temporal gyrus or Wernicke area for the lexical semantics; and by the superior and inferior division of the left middle cerebral artery, and by the left angular gyrus, for access to the lemma [13].

According to the Garrett model [14], **sentence production** starts with a concept to be conveyed (the message level). Then, a particular syntactic structure and particular lemmas are selected at the functional level. Next, a sentence planning frame is created that specifies the word order and the grammatical morphemes (positional-level representation). Specific words are then selected to fill the "slots" in the sentence planning frame [13]. The sentence production system involves the left posterior and inferior frontal cortex (including the Broca area) [13].

Related cognitive deficits

Since language is a complex task different aspects of it can be selectively impaired by focal or widespread brain damage, usually located in the left hemisphere [10]. It has been reported that language deficits (dysphasia or **aphasia**) are one of the most common consequences of stroke in both the acute and chronic phases [13]. Language impairment can also occur in head injury, brain tumors, and neurodegenerative dementias. The types of errors made by the patient and the pattern of performance across tasks can provide clues regarding the location of the lesion [13].

Impaired speech comprehension can be the result of a number of causes such as failure in discriminating speech sounds, word recognition, auditory working memory, or syntactic structure building. In strokes, impaired speech comprehension is generally associated with damage to the left posterior superior temporal region (Wernicke area). Typically caused by an insult to the inferior division of the middle cerebral artery, **Wernicke's aphasia** is marked by severe impairment in comprehension of both speech and written language [15]. Speech can be hyperfluent but dominated by low-information content [12]. Verbatim repetition and naming are also impaired, while prosody, articulation, and fluency remain intact [12]. **Transcortical sensory aphasia** is a condition in which spoken and written language comprehension is impaired but word-form processing is spared, in contrast to Wernicke's aphasia. Transcortical sensory aphasia differs from Wernicke's aphasia in that patients still have intact repetition [12]. Fluency and articulation are also spared [12]. Transcortical sensory aphasia is associated with damage of a region that is behind the Wernicke area, near the temporoparieto-occipital junction, usually caused by infarcts in territory of the left posterior cerebral artery. Impaired speech comprehension also occurs in the semantic (impaired single-word comprehension) and non-fluent (impaired syntactic comprehension) variants of PPA [7].

Naming failure can be attributed to a number of distinct phenomena [13]. Impaired visual recognition (apperceptive visual agnosia) and impaired access to lexical semantics from vision (associative visual agnosia) are discussed in the perception section. Patients with **impaired conceptual knowledge** often use objects, particularly less familiar ones, inappropriately [13]. Impaired access to conceptual knowledge is associated with a bilateral damage to the anterior and inferior temporal lobes. The most common disease affecting the bilateral anterior temporal lobes is the semantic variant of PPA [7]. HSV encephalitis also can affect this area bilaterally. **Deficits in lexical semantics** are associated with lesions in the Wernicke area [13]. Stroke in this region causes impaired word comprehension (see above). Impaired access to the lemma is known as **anomia** (or impaired word retrieval) [13]. Anomia can manifest as the inability to retrieve either spoken or written names. Anomia is associated with word-finding pauses and circumlocutions in everyday conversation. Patients with anomia can retrieve some partial information such as the first letter or sound (leading to the familiar tip-of-the-tongue state). This partial information often activates phonologically similar words, i.e., **phonemic paraphasias**, or semantically related words, i.e., **semantic paraphasias**, for output. Anomia can result from strokes in the territory of the superior (Broca aphasia) or inferior (Wernicke's aphasia) divisions of the left middle cerebral artery, and isolated infarcts of the left angular gyrus, thalamus, or posterior inferior

and middle temporal gyri. Anomia is a common deficit in patients with AD [16], and is frequently the onset symptom of PPA (mainly the logopenic variant) [7]. Patients with impaired access to phonologic or orthographic lexical representations (**modality-specific naming deficits**) can write names even when they cannot retrieve the pronunciation of the names, or vice versa [13]. These deficits are uncommon and can be observed in strokes affecting the left posterior inferior frontal cortex or in the non-fluent/agrammatic variant of PPA [7]. Failure to maintain activation of the complete phonological representation results in phonemic paraphasia. Impairment of motor planning of speech articulation is known as **apraxia of speech** and can also be associated with errors of insertion, deletion, transposition, substitution, or distortions of speech sounds [17]. However, patients with apraxia of speech are aware of their errors and try to correct them, while those who make phonemic paraphasias are generally unaware of them.

In sentence production, impairment at the message level manifests with strings of words that do not make sense together, or neologisms, or both, and is associated with left temporal lesions [13], as in posterior strokes and in patients with the semantic variant of PPA. A problem at the functional level results in **agrammatism**, with uncorrected or missing verbs or nouns [13]. This is usually caused by damage to the left inferior frontal (Broca area) and inferior temporoparietal regions. Agrammatism is also characterized by an impairment at the positional level with correct words in an incorrect order and omission of grammar functors (prepositions, auxiliary verbs, etc.) [13]. In this latter case, the lesion typically involves the left inferior frontal region and posterior insula, as in strokes in the territory of the superior division of the middle cerebral artery (**Broca aphasia**), and in patients with the non-fluent variant of PPA. Broca aphasia is the most common variety of aphasia following stroke [15]. Patients with Broca aphasia have a slow, incomplete, and laboured production of language, with a major breakdown of grammatical output. The ability to repeat phrases is lost. Comprehension is relatively preserved but complex multiple commands usually reveal a partial lack of understanding since the grammatical deficit is not confined to production but also involves speech comprehension (e.g. they do poorly at interpreting reversible passive sentences). Lesions of the left anterior superior frontal region typically cause a **transcortical motor aphasia** [12, 15]. Patients with transcortical motor aphasia have a halting and effortful speech, with phrases typically of only one or two words. However, repetition of words and sentences is spared. Comprehension is reasonably normal.

Perception

I tried one final test. It was still a cold day, in early spring, and I had thrown my coat and gloves on the sofa. 'What is this?' I asked, holding up a glove. 'May I examine it?' he asked, and, taking it from me, he proceeded to examine it as he had examined the geometrical shapes. 'A continuous surface,' he announced at last, 'infolded on itself. It appears to have' – he hesitated – 'five outpouchings, if this is the word'. 'Yes,' I said cautiously. 'You have given me a description. Now tell me what it is.' 'A container of some sort?' 'Yes,' I said, 'and what would it contain?' 'It would contain its contents!' said Dr P., with a laugh".

From *The Man Who Mistook His Wife For a Hat*,
O. Sacks, 1985 [18].

Definitions

Perception is the organization, identification, and interpretation of sensory information in order to represent and understand the environment. Commonly recognized sensory systems are those for vision, hearing, somatic sensation (touch), taste, and olfaction. Visual processing is the most widely studied modality and in general the most clinically relevant. Numerous regions of the brain are involved in visual processing, and are thought to belong to two main processing streams: a ventral medial occipitotemporal stream (the "what" pathway), which is critical for the processing of form and color for object recognition; and a dorsolateral occipitoparietal stream (the "where" pathway), which is involved in motion and spatial processing, including attention and localization.

Related cognitive deficits

Agnosia is the loss of the ability to interpret sensory stimuli, such as sounds or images. Although the sensorial system is preserved, the ability to recognize a stimulus or know its meaning is lost. Teuber defined agnosia as *"a normal percept stripped of its meaning"* [19]. Patients with agnosia cannot understand or recognize what they see, hear, or feel. It is a very rare condition, occurring in less than 1% of all neurological patients [20]. Examination involves assessing what the patient sees, hears, or feels when presented with objects, pictures, or sounds using a combination of clinical procedures and neuropsychological tests.

Agnosia can present in different ways depending on the nature and extent of brain lesion and the modality involved. Disorders of higher visual processing can be grouped into two broad categories [21]: the ventral and the dorsal groups. In the ventral group, there is damage to the medial occipitotemporal structures that participate in object identification and recognition [21]. This can result in a variety of syndromes, including general visual agnosia, achromatopsia, or more selective object recognition deficits such as prosopagnosia, and certain forms of topographagnosia. In the second, dorsal group, there is damage to lateral occipitoparietal structures that participate in visuospatial processing and localization [21]. Patients with such a damage may experience akinetopsia, neglect (the patient is unaware of, and as a consequence ignores, the contralesional half of space), various components of the Bálint syndrome, or astereopsis. Dorsal syndromes are discussed in the visuospatial processing section. **Visual agnosia** is the inability to recognize or identify objects visually, despite an intact primary visual function [21]. Patients are usually able to recognize the same objects using other sensorial modalities, such as touch or sound thanks to the intact dorsal stream. There are two main types of visual agnosia: apperceptive and associative [21]. In the **apperceptive visual agnosia**, the patient is unable to access the structure or spatial properties of a visual stimulus and the object is not seen as a whole or in a meaningful way. In **associative visual agnosia**, patients are unable to name visually presented objects but have no difficulty in naming those objects on tactile or verbal presentation and can copy or match simple figures, indicating that they can perceive objects correctly. Associative visual agnosia is thought to be the result of a disconnection between the perceptual representation of the object and the relative semantic knowledge. Apperceptive agnosia is typically associated with large temporal and occipital lesions, most typically due to hypoxic-ischemic injury in the posterior cerebral or vertebrobasilar territories, HSV encephalitis, or posterior cortical atrophy (PCA). Associative agnosia is typically associated with left temporo-occipital damage involving the parahippocampal, fusiform, and lingual gyri and the splenium of the corpus callosum, and is frequently caused by a stroke in the distribution territory of the posterior cerebral artery. **Achromatopsia** is the loss of color vision [21]. Patients with achromatopsia report that everything appears in shades of gray. Hemiachromatopsia is loss of color limited to the contralateral hemifield. Bilateral lesions of the lingual and fusiform gyri, most often secondary to strokes in the territory of the posterior cerebral artery, cause achromatopsia, while unilateral lesions in the same territory cause hemiachromatopsia. **Prosopagnosia** is the impaired ability to recognize familiar faces and to learn new faces [21]. Patients with prosopagnosia can identify facial parts, recognize a face as a face but with no recognition of the person. In severe cases, patients cannot recognize their own face. It is important to exclude alternatively a problem in retrograde memory (in the case of failure to recognize old faces) or anterograde memory (in cases of failure to recognize new faces) [22]. In order to compensate, patients often identify people through their voices or gestures, facial expressions, or particular hairstyles. The context usually helps them in recognizing a person at work for instance, but not across the street. Lesions causing prosopagnosia usually involve the lingual and fusiform gyri bilaterally and the subjacent white matter. Unilateral right occipitotemporal lesions (involving the right fusiform gyrus) and bilateral or right anterior temporal lesions have also been described [23, 24]. The most common causes of prosopagnosia are posterior cerebral artery infarctions, head trauma, and viral encephalitis. Progressive forms occur in patients with the semantic variant of PPA [7]. **Topographagnosia** (or topographic disorientation) is the loss of ability to make a correct representation of the surrounding environment [21]. Patients with this disturbance get lost in familiar places. Several types of topographagnosia have been described, including among others: landmark agnosia, the failure to recognize buildings and scenes, which is associated with lesions in the right medial occipitotemporal region; impaired cognitive map formation, the inability to form a mental layout of scenes, which is associated with hippocampal and retrosplenial lesions; and heading disorientation, the failure in discerning the relationship between objects in the environment, which is typically related to posterior cingulate involvement.

In addition to visual agnosia, other types of agnosia involving different sensory modalities can occur. Despite relatively preserved primary and discriminative somesthetic perception, patients can have a selective impairment of object recognition by touch. The ability to recognize basic features such as size, weight,

and texture may be dissociated from the ability to name or recognize the object. This is usually an unilateral disorder resulting from lesions to the contralateral inferior parietal cortex. In this framework, **finger agnosia** is defined as the loss of the ability "to distinguish, name, or recognize the fingers," not only when the patient's own fingers are involved, but also with the fingers of others, when drawing and in case of other representations of fingers [25]. Usually, lesions of the left angular gyrus and posterior parietal areas can be the cause of this disturbance.

Attention

On any given day, something claims our attention. Anything at all, inconsequential things. A rosebud, a misplaced hat, that sweater we liked as a child, an old Gene Pitney record. A parade of trivia with no place to go. Things that bump around in our consciousness for two or three days then go back to wherever they came from . . . to darkness. We've got all these wells dug in our hearts. While above the wells, birds flit back and forth.
From *Pinball, 1973*, H. Murakami, 1980 [26].

Definitions

Attention refers to the preferential allocation of neuronal resources to events that become relevant in a specific period of time [27, 28]. Attention can be distributed globally or focally, can work in parallel or in serial, and can be directed to external stimuli or to internal mental states [29]. The attentional abilities vary not only from one individual to another, but also from a moment to another in the same subject. Attention can be described in terms of the task contexts in which it operates as sustained attention, selective attention, divided attention, and attention switching [28]. **Sustained attention** (vigilance) is the ability to maintain a consistent behavioral response over prolonged periods of time. **Selective attention** is the ability to focus on just one source of information for processing it in the face of distracting or competing stimuli. Thus, selective attention is accomplished not only by an active processing of target information, but also by an active inhibition or suppression of distracting information [30]. **Divided attention** is the highest level of attention and it refers to the ability to process more than one source of information at a time or perform more than one task at a time. Attention switching describes the task context in which a person alternates the focus of attention between two different tasks or sources of information.

Attentional functions are a set of complex cognitive processes, and are distributed throughout the human brain as postulated by both the Posner's attentional network and Mesulam's attentional matrix. Posner and colleagues have proposed three separate functions for attention [31, 32]: alerting, orienting, and executive control. **Alerting** is the ability to stay focused in anticipation of an expected event, is subserved by the thalamus and frontal and parietal cortices, and is regulated by norepinephrine from the locus coeruleus. The **orienting** function allows the selection of one source of information for processing among many possible sources; it has been linked to the superior parietal lobe, temporal parietal junction, and frontal eye fields, and is thought to be modulated mainly by cholinergic inputs from the basal forebrain. Finally, **executive control attention** plays a role when more complex behavioral responses are necessary, such as doing two things at once, performing a novel task, or assessing all aspects of a situation before making a response; it has been associated with the anterior cingulate cortex, lateral prefrontal cortex, and dopaminergic system. According to Mesulam's **attentional matrix** [28], attention can be driven by specific domains (e.g. visual neurons mediate domain-specific attentional responses to visual stimuli) or be domain-independent. Domain-independent modulations are exerted through the bottom-up influence of the ascending reticular activating system (ARAS), which projects to the thalamus and cortex, and the top-down influence of the association and limbic cortices [29]. While the ARAS responds mainly to arousal, the prefrontal, parietal, and limbic cerebral areas are more closely involved in the modulation of the cognitive state, past experience, and expectation [29].

Related cognitive deficits

Given the importance of attention to sensory and cognitive processing, it is not surprising that attentional disorders are among the most common and devastating neurological deficits. The main attentional disorders are confusional states, hemispatial neglect, and partial (domain-specific) attentional syndromes [27]. The syndrome of acute confusional state (or delirium) reflects an impairment of the attention system as a whole and has been reviewed in Chapter 2. The syndrome of hemispatial neglect is a disorder of spatial attention and is discussed in the visuospatial

processing section. Attentional impairment can also present more focally as domain-specific or "partial" attentional syndromes [27]. These syndromes are not well defined because partial attentional impairment does not tend to present as a set of separately definable syndromes, but it rather manifests as reduced performances in one or more cognitive domains. For example, changes in visual-based attention could result in reduced detection of stimuli in the environment, while changes in language-based attention could present as a reduced verbal fluency. The most striking deficits of attention occur with focal lesions, such as strokes, involving the non-dominant parietal lobe. In addition, impaired or inefficient attention is a feature of many types of neurodegenerative dementia and neuropsychiatric conditions.

Visuospatial processing

Buttoning the length of my shirt with left neglect and one right hand takes the same kind of singular, intricate, held-breath concentration that I imagine someone trying to dismantle a bomb would need to have.

From *Left Neglected*, L. Genova, 2011 [33].

Definitions

Spatial attention is the ability to focus on specific stimuli in the external environment [28]. Spatial attention is oriented endogenously to stimuli that are relevant for the task at hand, either because the observer has expectancy of where the relevant stimuli would appear, or given certain incentives for responding efficiently to specific attributes of the stimuli regardless of their spatial features. Additionally, spatial attention can be exogenously captured by salient stimuli (such as luminance changes or moving stimuli) even if the observer has no intention of orienting his/her attention to that object or location. During the last decades, numerous neuroimaging studies have demonstrated that spatial attention is implemented in a bilateral network with core regions in parietal and frontal brain areas [34].

Related cognitive deficits

Disorders of visuospatial processing usually result from frontoparietal damage, whether induced by focal (mainly vascular) lesions or degenerative conditions. The major disorders of visuospatial processing are the hemineglect syndrome, simultanagnosia, and optic ataxia [35]. Visuospatial deficits are frequently associated with dementia affecting the posterior brain regions, such as AD, PCA, dementia with Lewy bodies (DLB), and corticobasal syndrome (CBS). Patients with AD might present with spatial attentional impairment before experiencing memory deficits.

Hemineglect is a disorder of spatial attention characterized by a domain-specific impairment in distributing attention across the extrapersonal space [28]. In neglect, spatial attention is biased so that patients preferentially process stimuli in ipsilesional space over those in contralesional space. These patients may be inattentive or even deny the existence of parts of their own body. For instance, patients may be aware of their contralesional limb but not that it is paralyzed (anosognosia for hemiplegia) [36]. Neglect is a multimodal deficit and may affect any or all sensory modalities, motor behavior, or even the internal representations of memories and thoughts. Lesions causing neglect have been found throughout the network of cortical and subcortical areas responsible for attention. These regions include the posterior parietal cortex/temporoparietal junction, frontal eye fields, cingulate and supplementary motor cortex, basal ganglia, thalamus, midbrain, and superior colliculus. Typically, the lesions affect the right hemisphere [37, 38]. **Simultanagnosia** is the inability to perceive more than one aspect of a visual stimulus at the same time and to integrate visual details into a coherent whole [39]. The deficit is more evident when the patient is questioned in front of a complex stimulus, and more with unfamiliar than with familiar stimuli. Simultanagnosia is still a debated phenomenon in which visual, semantic, and attentive aspects seem to play a relevant role. This deficit is associated with bilateral damage to the posterior parietal lobes with a limited occipital lobe involvement [40]. Simultanagnosia has also been reported in patients with unilateral left occipital lesions, but the disturbance is less severe. Patients with **optic ataxia** fail to reach accurately for objects, particularly when they are presented in peripheral vision [41]. Patients can describe an object within arm's reach but, when attempting to pick up the object, miss the target. Optic ataxia is typically associated with lesions of the posterior parietal lobe. Simultanagnosia, optic ataxia, and "psychic paralysis of gaze" (also known as oculomotor apraxia, i.e., the inability to voluntarily guide eye movements, changing to a new location of visual fixation) are the three classic features of the **Bálint syndrome** [42].

Praxis

Every morning he struggles trying to tie his shoes. "I know how to do it, Mary", he keeps saying, "but I can't do it". Then, sadly, I stare at his hands attempting dozens of times. Finally, I show him (hopelessly, I have to say!) how to do it. "Tomorrow I'll do it by myself, Mary, I promise".

A caregiver report during a clinical visit at the San Raffaele Hospital, Milan, Italy (July 2013)

Definitions

Praxis refers to the ability to perform learned gestures, that is, to generate, coordinate, and execute an acquired intentional motor program. The network of structures underlying praxis involves the frontal and parietal cortex, basal ganglia, and white-matter tracts connecting these areas [43–45].

Related cognitive deficits

Apraxia is the inability to perform learned, skilled motor acts, despite preserved motor and sensory systems, coordination, comprehension, and cooperation [43–45]. There are two major forms of forelimb apraxia: task specific and general. **Task-specific apraxias** are disorders that are limited to one form of activity, e.g., dressing apraxia, constructional apraxia, apraxia of speech, and apraxic agraphia [44]. The four principal types of **general apraxia** are: ideomotor, ideational, conceptual, and limb-kinetic [44]. Ideally, any neurologic disease that impairs the brain networks responsible for programming forelimb movements can induce apraxia. Apraxia is often observed in patients with hemispheric (especially left) strokes, subcortical vascular dementia, and neurodegenerative diseases like AD. Apraxia is also seen in patients with movement disorders, including CBS, PD, progressive supranuclear palsy (PSP), and Huntington's disease.

Ideomotor apraxia, the most common and recognized form of apraxia, can be defined as the inability to perform a gesture with a limb when the subject is asked verbally to carry out the movement [43–45]. The gestures may appear awkward with incorrect timing, sequencing, and spatial position of the limb. For some authors, the ideomotor apraxia also includes the inability to imitate a gesture (meaningful or meaningless), to perform an action in response to a visually presented object, or to demonstrate the object use (patients usually use their limb as an object rather than demonstrating how to use the object) [46]. The same gestures can be performed normally by the patients in their daily life, a phenomenon which is called "voluntary-automatic dissociation" [46]. Limb ideomotor apraxia is associated with injury to several structures, including the inferior parietal lobe, premotor cortex, and anterior corpus callosum. Subcortical lesions that involve the basal ganglia, thalamus, and white-matter tracts connecting these areas with the cortex can also be associated with limb ideomotor apraxia. Orofacial apraxia, which is characterized by an impairment of skilled movements involving the face, mouth, tongue, larynx, and pharynx, can be considered a subtype of ideomotor apraxia [43]. Orofacial apraxia is associated with lesions in the inferior frontal gyrus, deep frontal white matter, insula, and basal ganglia lesions [47]. Automatic movements of the same muscles are often preserved [47]. Orofacial apraxia can coexist with limb apraxia; however, orofacial and limb apraxia can also be dissociated, suggesting that the neural systems underlying these disorders are at least partially different [47].

Patients with **ideational apraxia** have difficulty in correctly sequencing a series of acts that lead to a goal [43–45]. Ideational apraxia is often seen in patients with extensive left hemisphere damage or dementia. Lesions that induce such a disorder have been located in the left occipitoparietal region [45], although damage to the left prefrontal lobe is also associated with sequencing deficits [44]. Some authors have made a distinction between ideational and conceptual apraxia [44]. **Conceptual apraxia** is the loss of mechanical knowledge [44]. Patients with conceptual apraxia may misuse objects, have difficulty matching objects and actions, be unaware of the mechanical advantage afforded by tools, or be unable to judge whether a gesture is well formed [44]. In right-handed people, this mechanical knowledge is stored in the left hemisphere [44]. Therefore, conceptual deficits can be seen in patients with a callosal disconnection as well as in those with diseases affecting the (posterior) left hemisphere [44, 48, 49].

The term **limb-kinetic apraxia** refers to a loss of dexterity, including the ability to make precise independent but coordinated finger movements [44]. Limb-kinetic apraxia tends to be independent of modality (e.g. verbal command vs. imitation), with no voluntary-automatic dissociation [50]. Inaccurate distal limb movements are often seen in the limb contralateral to the affected hemisphere [44, 50]. This disorder has been associated with frontal (motor and premotor) lesions and can be difficult to differentiate from limb weakness [50]. Limb-kinetic apraxia is frequently observed in patients with movement disorders such as CBS [51], PSP [52], and PD [53], although it can be challenging to differentiate limb-kinetic apraxia from the extrapyramidal features of these disorders [54].

Executive functions

We leaf through a book but we tap a computer keyboard [as I am doing right now]. Does this mean that we grab a knife, lift a cup, leaf through a book, or tap a keyboard every time we encounter one in our environment [like young children often do]? Not at all – we do it only when a larger context warrants it: when we need to cut a steak, when we are thirsty and the cup is filled and clean, when we want to extract some information from a book, or send an e-mail to a friend. In fact, most of the time we encounter any of these objects we simply ignore them. A mere encounter with an object does not automatically trigger the object-associated behavior. But in patients [. . .] it often does.

From *The New Executive Brain: Frontal Lobes in a Complex World*, E. Goldberg, 2009 [55].

Definitions

Executive functions are defined as high-order processes involved in the top-down control of cognition and goal-directed behavior. Intact executive functioning supports a multitude of behaviors, such as planning a complex task, solving a problem, and being flexible and adaptive to the environment and to specific circumstances when complex tasks are presented [56]. Although the frontal areas, in particular the prefrontal cortex, are the most recognized brain regions subserving executive functions, growing evidence demonstrates that frontal structures are part of larger cortico-cortical and cortico-subcortical networks associated with this cognitive domain [57, 58].

Executive functions are not a unitary phenomenon and are composed of related, but separable, components which could be affected independently, including working memory, planning and organization, and inhibitory control [59].

With the term **working memory**, we refer to the ability to temporarily maintain and manipulate information that one needs to keep in mind during a high-order operation, such as planning and organizing, decision-making, and problem solving [60]. Most models of working memory separate two components of working memory: temporary stores of information, in the form of "buffers" or "slave systems," that are usually modality-specific, and a central "executive" or set of processes that manipulate the information [60]. Baddeley proposed a model of memory that has influenced virtually all subsequent research in the area [60]. The model is composed of a three-component system: (1) the "phonological loop," comprising a limited-capacity phonological store in which verbal information is stored temporarily and maintained by subvocal rehearsal (e.g. repeated subvocal articulation when trying to keep a phone number in mind); (2) the "visuospatial sketchpad," a storage buffer for non-verbal material, such as the visual representations of objects; and (3) the "central executive," which is responsible for strategic manipulation and execution of the above-mentioned "slave" systems. The original model has recently been updated [61] to include an "episodic buffer" that provides an interface between the subsystems of working memory and long-term memory. The phonological loop has been localized in the left perisylvian regions, including the left inferior parietal area and the dorsal part of the Broca area, while the visuospatial sketchpad is localized in the right inferior parietal and prefrontal structures [62, 63]. The central executive is located in the prefrontal lobe [62, 63], with the ventrolateral part more involved in online maintenance of information and the dorsolateral one in monitoring and manipulating the information [64]. Frontal areas are very likely to be important for the episodic buffer [61].

Planning and organizing is the ability to identify and organize the many elements required in order to achieve a goal while performing complex tasks, and is associated with the dorsolateral frontal lobe [65]. Planning and organizing also play a crucial role in language, since words and phrases must be organized into sentences and story events, as does the theory of mind, i.e., the ability to perceive subtle, nuanced behavior in a social interaction and modify one's behavior accordingly.

Inhibitory control can be defined as a range of mechanisms that allow the suppression of previously activated cognitions and inappropriate actions and resistance to interference from irrelevant stimuli [66]. In brief, inhibitory control is the ability to suppress the processing or expression of information that would disrupt the efficient completion of the goal at hand. Inhibition can be applied to control of behavioral responses in both motor and cognitive domain. On the other hand, the **control behavior** is the ability to maintain the focus on the relevant information to achieve a goal, and to shift the attention when necessary. Inhibitory control is mediated by the prefrontal cortex together with the parietal lobe and basal ganglia [67]. The network involved in the control behavior includes the anterior cingulate cortex [68], anterior insula [69], and areas of the prefrontal cortex [68, 70].

Related cognitive deficits

Various aspects of executive functions can be damaged independently in patients with diseases affecting different brain regions [56]. Because executive functioning depends on a brain network that includes frontal and parietal cortical cortices as well as subcortical regions, any disease that disrupts the frontal lobes or their connections with posterior cortical and subcortical regions can interfere with executive resources, e.g., stroke, tumors, brain trauma, multiple sclerosis, and hydrocephalus. Several neurodegenerative diseases are characterized by executive dysfunction, including AD, PD, and frontotemporal dementia (FTD), and less common disorders such as PSP. Executive dysfunction is also increasingly being recognized as an important component of a number of neuropsychiatric disorders.

Executive impairment can have an enormous impact on patient independence and quality of life [56]. A patient with working memory deficit can experience an inability to concentrate or pay attention and difficulties in performing new tasks involving multistep instructions. Patients losing planning ability may be not able to start an action, sequence the steps to be performed in a correct order, or be flexible to change strategy with another one more appropriate for the circumstances. A patient with deficits in planning may become defective in organizing sentences and phrases in speech (see the language section). Due to a deficit of the theory of mind, patients can have difficulty in determining the intentions of others, a lack of understanding of how their behavior may affect others, and they can have a difficult time with social reciprocity. Failure to inhibit and to shift the focus may lead to perseverative and stimulus-bound behaviors, e.g., echolalia, echopraxia, and utilization behavior [67].

Basic evaluation of the patient with cognitive deficits

Clinical and neuropsychological examinations

Clinical history, which needs to be supplemented by an informant, should focus on the affected cognitive domains, the course of the illness, and the impact on activity of daily living, together with any associated non-cognitive symptoms [71]. Past medical history, comorbidities, and family and education history are all important [71]. A general and neurological physical examination should be performed in all patients with cognitive impairment [71]. It is also important to evaluate hearing and vision because sensory deficits can influence the mental status and neurological examination.

Neuropsychological assessment is central to diagnosis and management of disorders associated with cognitive impairment and should be performed in all patients [71]. Preferably, the neuropsychological evaluation should be performed at an early stage of the disease when the cognitive impairment is likely to reflect the disruption of selective brain structures [71]. Neuropsychological assessment should include a global cognitive measure and more detailed testing of the main cognitive domains. The most frequently used cognitive screening test is the Mini-Mental State Examination. However, it is important to highlight that, in most cases, the neuropsychological assessment itself is not enough to perform a diagnosis. For instance, an impairment of episodic memory is not enough for diagnosing AD. It needs to be associated with other clinical and cognitive disturbances, progressive onset of the disease, suggestive laboratory findings, and so on (see below). In addition, during the neuropsychological assessment, one of the important things to understand is whether or not the patient is performing at the same level of his/her cognitive abilities prior to lesion/disease. To do so, it is important to have an indirect measure of the premorbid functions. Various methods can be used to test the premorbid intelligence quotient. One of the most common is the reading of irregular words, which requires the patient having a previous knowledge of them [72, 73]. The accuracy of these tests is limited in subjects with a low education level.

Laboratory investigations

Clinical and neuropsychological examinations should be supported by a number of laboratory investigations.

Initial investigations should be minimally invasive and aimed at the identification of reversible conditions, such as metabolic, infectious, inflammatory, or other systemic processes (Table 3.1) [71]. A basic initial battery should include the following:

- blood tests: full blood count, erythrocyte sedimentation rate, renal and liver functions, electrolytes, glucose, C-reactive protein, coagulation profile, thyroid function, B12 and folate, syphilis serology; ammonia and amylase are recommended in case of rapid onset cognitive impairment;
- urine test;
- electrocardiogram;
- chest X-ray;
- computed tomography (CT) or, preferably, magnetic resonance imaging (MRI) of the brain.

Electroencephalogram testing (EEG) is recommended in rapid dementia, and when Creutzfeldt–Jakob disease (CJD) or transient epileptic amnesia are suspected. International guidelines do not support the use of EEG testing for the initial assessment of any patients with cognitive impairment [71].

In selected patients, additional investigations may be useful, such as cerebrospinal fluid (CSF) examination, autoimmune screening, human immunodeficiency virus (HIV) serology, echocardiography, drug/toxicological and nutritional screenings, sleep study, psychiatric evaluation, and genetic testing [71]. Routine analysis of CSF (cell count, protein level, glucose, oligoclonal bands, cytology, cultures, and viral polymerase chain reactions (PCRs)) should be performed if there is a suspicion of inflammatory diseases, infections, syphilis, HIV encephalitis, and paraneoplastic disease. Assessment of CSF total tau and 14-3-3 protein is recommended in rapidly progressive cases when CJD is suspected. CSF assessment of amyloid β ($A\beta_{1-42}$), and total- and phosphor-tau levels may help in the diagnosis of AD.

Neuroimaging examination of the patient with cognitive impairment: the general approach (sequences to be used)

Structural brain imaging should be performed at least once in the diagnostic work-up of patients with cognitive impairment [68, 69]. Exclusion of a potentially (surgically) treatable cause of dementia (e.g., tumor, subdural hematoma, brain abscess, or normal-pressure hydrocephalus (NPH)) and evaluation of the presence and extent of cerebrovascular disease can be ascertained using CT [74]. However, MRI offers benefits over CT for the detection of abnormalities suggestive of specific diseases, particularly cerebral atrophy patterns (e.g. hippocampal atrophy for AD; focal temporal and/or frontal atrophy for FTD; and midbrain atrophy for PSP) and subtle, small-vessel vascular changes [74]. Therefore, MRI should be considered the "preferred modality to assist with early diagnosis" in a subject suspected of having dementia [68, 70, 71].

The essential MRI sequences that provide the important minimum set of information required to be addressed in a subject with cognitive impairment are: three-dimensional (3D) T1-weighted gradient echo; turbo/fast spin echo T2-weighted and fluid attenuated inversion recovery (FLAIR), and T2*-gradient echo [68, 69]. If 3D T1-weighted techniques are unavailable, coronal-oblique two-dimensional (2D) images can be the alternative. Multiplanar reformatting can be applied to 3D T1-weighted images in order to assess specific brain regions (e.g. to reslice the data on the anterior/posterior commissure line or perpendicularly to the long axis of the hippocampus). Two other MRI sequences that are frequently used in the clinical setting include diffusion-weighted imaging (DWI) and post-contrast 2D T1-weighted spin echo images [68, 69]. DWI can be useful to identify recent infarcts, even in patients with vascular dementia or in the context of vasculitis, and neocortical or striatal abnormalities in patients with CJD. Post-contrast T1-weighted images are recommended in those patients, typically in the young age range, where there is a suspicion of infectious (e.g. HSV encephalitis) or inflammatory disorders (e.g. vasculitis, sarcoid, or multiple sclerosis).

Although typical cases of dementia may not benefit from routine functional imaging, these tools are recommended in those cases where diagnosis remains in doubt after clinical evaluation and structural imaging and in particular clinical settings [74]. Single-photon emission computed tomography (SPECT) and positron emission tomography (PET) both rely on the detection of radioactive signals from a labeled compound that selectively binds in the brain. The most commonly used tracer to examine cerebral blood flow (CBF) using SPECT is 99m-technetium-labeled hexamethylpropylene. ^{18}F-Fluorodeoxyglucose (FDG) serves as a marker of cerebral glucose metabolism for

PET. SPECT is technically less demanding and more widely available, while PET is more sensitive, mainly due to its higher resolution [75], but comes at the cost of a more complex detector system and tracer-production facilities. In general, the magnitude of hypometabolism seen with FDG PET is greater than the amplitude of hypoperfusion seen with CBF SPECT [75].

Specific clinical and laboratory findings in the most common clinical disorders associated with cognitive impairment

Major reversible causes of dementia

Normal-pressure hydrocephalus

(a) Clinical findings

Normal-pressure hydrocephalus (NPH) occurs when there is an increase in intracranial pressure due to an abnormal accumulation of CSF in the ventricles of the brain causing ventriculomegaly [76]. Although the exact mechanism is unknown, NPH is thought to be a form of communicating hydrocephalus with impaired CSF reabsorption at the arachnoid granulations. NPH can follow arachnoiditis, subarachnoid hemorrhage, or head trauma (secondary NPH). In a high proportion of cases, however, NPH has an unknown (idiopathic) cause. Clinically, NPH is characterized by a classic symptom triad: gait apraxia, urinary incontinence, and cognitive decline; but the clinical picture can be incomplete. Cognitive dysfunction in NPH is characterized by frontal and subcortical deficits (psychomotor slowing and impaired attention, executive deficits, and visuospatial dysfunction). "Pure cortical deficits" such as apraxia, agnosia, and aphasia are rare [77]. It has been shown that frontal lobe dysfunction accounts for 50% of the whole cognitive deficit in NPH. The most common behavioral abnormality is apathy [75] that, together with inattentiveness, agitation, and poverty of thought, may mimic a depressive illness delaying the diagnosis and treatment of the underlying structural injury [78]. NPH patients may respond to shunting procedures (i.e. surgically implanting a ventriculoperitoneal shunt to drain excess CSF to the abdomen where it is absorbed) with amelioration of their clinical symptoms, though the rate of clinical improvement after shunting is only

50%. Clinical improvement after removal of a diagnostic aliquot of CSF (30 mL or more) has a high predictive value for subsequent success with shunting. The most likely patients to show improvement are those that show only gait disturbance, mild or no incontinence, and mild dementia.

(b) Investigative findings

CT and MRI are helpful to exclude mass lesions, obstructions or primary neurodegenerative diseases, and to show ventriculomegaly, with particular enlargement of the temporal horns, that is disproportionate to the degree of gyral atrophy [79] (Figure 3.1). The corpus callosum may be bowed upward [79]. No signs of increased CSF pressure should be present, although there can be evidence of subtle transependymal CSF leakage on T2-weighted and FLAIR images (i.e. relatively thin, slightly blurry zone of increased signal, extending homogeneously around the whole ventricular system) [79]. Pressure bands should not be confused with periventricular white-matter changes that may occur with normal aging. In NPH, MRI often shows the accentuation of the cerebral aqueduct flow void [79] (Figure 3.1). CSF flow can be quantified using phase-contrast MRI; however, its diagnostic/predictive role in NPH remains uncertain.

Nuclear medicine studies in NPH patients usually reveal a reduction of cortico-subcortical cerebral blood flow [81, 82] and metabolism [83, 84].

Limbic encephalitis

(a) Clinical findings

Limbic encephalitis (LE) is a subacute encephalopathy characterized by the acute or subacute onset of short-term memory loss and disorientation [76]. Patients may show psychosis including visual or auditory hallucinations, or paranoid obsession. Confusion, depression, and anxiety are also common. Generalized or partial complex seizures are seen in about 50% of these patients. LE can be caused by a variety of conditions, including paraneoplastic syndromes (paraneoplastic LE (PLE)), autoimmune encephalitis with voltage-gated potassium channels (VGKC) antibodies, and inflammatory vasculitides. Inflammatory vasculitides are described in Chapter 13.

PLE is preferentially associated with small-cell lung cancer (40%), germ cell tumors of the testis (20%), breast cancer (8%), Hodgkin's lymphoma, thymoma, and immature teratoma [85]. The neurological presentation of PLE antedates the diagnosis of cancer in approximately 60% of the cases. Early detection and treatment of the underlying tumor is the approach that

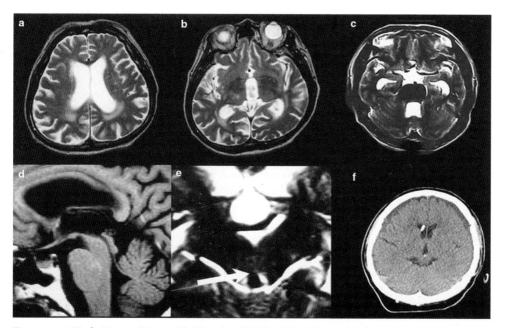

Figure 3.1 MRI of a 72-year-old man with idiopathic NPH. (A to C) Axial T2-weighted images reveal disproportionately enlarged lateral, third, and fourth ventricle and T2 hyperintensity in the subependymal area. The sagittal T1 (D) and coronal T2-weighted images (E) show an apparently normal cerebral aqueduct with no stenosis. (F) Follow-up brain CT (after ventriculoperitoneal shunt) shows a reduction of third ventricle size. Reproduced with permission from reference [80].

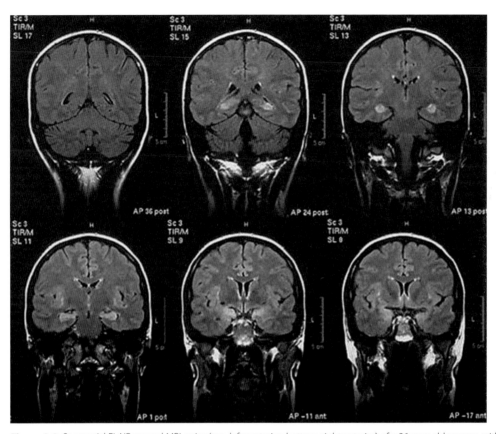

Figure 3.2 Sequential FLAIR coronal MRI series (top, left posterior, bottom, right anterior) of a 36-year-old woman with limbic encephalitis of presumed autoimmune origin. There are bilateral symmetric hyperintensities of the hippocampus (posteriorly) and amygdala (anteriorly). Reproduced with permission from reference [87].

offers the greatest chance for neurological improvement or symptom stabilization of PLE patients, but there is often a considerable residual cognitive impairment and seizures may persist. The increasing evidence that PLE is immune-mediated has prompted the use of immunomodulating therapies. In VGKC-LE, persistent hyponatremia, resistant to treatment, is often present, and appears to be a strong indicator of the diagnosis. VGKC-LE may respond to corticosteroids, plasma exchange, or intravenous immunoglobulin.

(b) Investigative findings

In PLE, CSF examination shows inflammatory signs (i.e. pleocytosis, oligoclonal bands) in about 80% of the cases. Antineuronal antibodies are found in the serum and CSF of about 60% of the patients with histologically proven PLE. VGKC antibodies can be associated with PLE and small-cell lung cancer and thymoma, although the great majority of patients with these antibodies present with non-paraneoplastic LE [86]. The EEG reveals diffuse slowing with epileptic foci in the temporal lobe(s).

In LE, T2 and FLAIR MRI alterations are seen in about 70–80% of patients (Figure 3.2) [79]. The MRI appearance simulates an HSV encephalitis (see below), consisting of a usually bilateral (though it may be unilateral in 40% of the cases), extensive, high-signal-intensity alteration on T2-weighted and FLAIR images in the temporal lobes [88]. On T1-weighted sequences, this temporal lesion can appear as hypointense and rarely enhance after contrast injection. Atrophy of the temporal lobe may coexist [79]. Hemorrhage is uncommon [79]. Abnormal signal intensity in the brainstem and/or hypothalamus can be seen in about 10 to 20% of the cases. Subcortical white-matter abnormalities and DWI abnormalities, including a bright cortical ribbon or altered basal ganglia similar to those seen in CJD have also been reported [89]. Meningeal enhancement following gadolinium administration is found in ~ 7% of patients [79]. In the absence of MRI abnormalities, FDG PET may offer useful hints when showing an increased metabolism in the medial temporal lobe, which may reflect an acute inflammatory process.

HSV encephalitis

(a) Clinical findings

HSV is the causative organism in approximately 10% of patients with encephalitis due to an identified organism [90]. The majority of cases of HSV encephalitis in immune-competent adults are caused by HSV-1. Ten percent are caused by HSV-2, usually associated with immune compromise or occurring in neonates. HSV-1 encephalitis is thought to be a result of either acute primary infection or reactivation of latent viral infection of the dorsal root ganglia [90], although the exact pathophysiology is unknown.

Patients are usually below 20 or above 50 years old and present with fever, headache, and alteration of consciousness, which may develop gradually or rapidly over a matter of hours [76]. The most common manifestations are behavioral, speech, and gait disturbances and occasionally psychotic features. Focal or generalized seizures are often associated with olfactory or gustatory hallucinations. Those patients with left-temporal disease become symptomatic earlier because of their language impairment. Death follows in up to 70% of untreated cases and prompt administration of acyclovir is strongly correlated with a better outcome. Of treated survivors, 30% suffer chronic neurological deficits, including memory and personality problems, and empirical antiviral treatment is therefore administered when encephalitis is suspected [90]. In patients with impaired immunity, HHV-6 encephalitis should be considered in the differential diagnosis because it is unresponsive to acyclovir and carries a poor prognosis [90].

(b) Investigative findings

Routine CSF analysis should be performed and may show a mild to moderate lymphocytic pleocytosis and elevation of proteins, and a normal or mildly decreased glucose level. PCR examination of the CSF is sensitive and specific for the detection of HSV DNA. However, PCR can be negative especially in patients who have received empirical antiviral medication. The EEG is characterized by spikes and slow-wave activity and periodic lateralized epileptiform discharges, which arise from the temporal lobe [91, 92]. The sensitivity of EEG testing is high (approximately 80%), but the specificity is low (only 30%).

Within the first 5 days of the disease, MRI shows hyperintense lesions on T2-weighted and FLAIR images in the medial and inferior temporal lobes extending into the insular cortex and frontal lobe, diffusion restriction on DWI, and progressive mass effect including the cingulate region. At this stage CT findings are subtle [79]. Imaging abnormalities can be uni- or bilateral. The lesions may appear necrotic, and are frequently hemorrhagic (hyperintense on T1-weighted images) [79]. Basal ganglia are rarely involved. Negative DWI may indicate an increased likelihood of lesion recovery [79]. The earliest CT abnormalities are hypodense areas in the temporal lobe and insular cortex, and cerebral swelling with local sulcal effacement [79]. Later, gyriform and leptomeningeal enhancement on post-contrast MRI can be seen. Residual abnormalities on MRI include areas of hyperintensity and parenchymal loss at the site of involvement.

Alcohol-dementia

(a) Clinical findings

Intake of alcohol has several effects on the brain, which are only partially reversible. Alcohol abuse is associated with Wernicke–Korsakoff's encephalopathy (WE) and chronic alcohol-dementia [76]. WE results from an alcoholism-related deficiency of thiamine (vitamin B1) [93]. Other main causes of thiamine deficiency are a poor diet or gastrointestinal disturbances including diarrhoea and vomiting. In WE, pathology involves the periaqueductal gray matter, thalamus, superior cerebellar vermis, and mamillary bodies. The classical clinical presentation of WE syndrome is characterized by an acute onset of oculomotor symptoms, altered consciousness, and ataxia. Mental status changes occur in the vast majority of WE patients including confusion, apathy, concentration deficits, hallucinations, progressing to coma and death over days or weeks. Some patients develop a Korsakoff's syndrome, which is an amnestic syndrome characterized by a profound involvement of both anterograde and retrograde memory, loss of working memory, and disorientation [93]. Other cognitive domains are relatively spared. Alcohol-dementia patients display a more global cognitive decline. Memory deficits can be associated with aphasia, apraxia, agnosia, and disturbances in executive functioning [94].

49

(b) Investigative findings

WE should be differentiated from acute delirium secondary to hypoxia, CNS infections, and seizures (Chapter 2). Ataxic and ocular disorders can result from cerebral infarction. Laboratory investigations in patients suspected of having WE include routine blood examinations and serum thiamine-level tests [93]. CSF may be normal or characterized by mildly elevated proteins without pleocytosis [93]. Hyperintense T2 and FLAIR lesions in the periaqueductal gray matter of the midbrain, thalamic regions, mamillothalamic tract, and tissue surrounding the third ventricle are frequently seen in patients with WE (Figure 3.3) [79]. DWI shows high signal intensity of the corresponding T2 hyperintense regions [79]. Lesions may or may not enhance (Figure 3.3), and may be associated with mamillary body atrophy. These abnormalities can be reversible after thiamine administration.

In chronic alcohol-induced dementia, MRI may show atrophy, with a particular involvement of the brainstem, cerebellum, hippocampus, thalamus and frontal lobes, and ventricular enlargement [79].

Vascular cognitive impairment

The clinical findings and neuroimaging protocol in a patient with focal, acute symptoms (including cognitive disturbances) thought to be due to suspected stroke have been extensively discussed in Chapter 12. Here, we focus on VaD.

(a) Clinical findings

Recently, the concept of VaD caused by small or large brain infarcts has been extended from only multi-infarct (multi-stroke) dementia to a whole spectrum of vascular causes of cognitive impairment and dementia, subsumed under the term vascular cognitive impairment (VCI) [96]. The main subtypes of VCI included in current classifications are large-vessel VCI (also referred to as cortical VCI), multi-infarct VCI or post-stroke VCI, small-vessel VCI, subcortical ischemic vascular disease and dementia, strategic infarct dementia, and hypoperfusion VCI resulting from global cerebrovascular insufficiency. Further subtypes include hemorrhagic dementia, hereditary vascular causes, and AD with cerebrovascular disease [96].

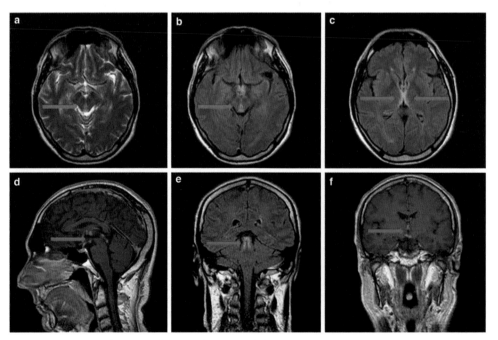

Figure 3.3 MRI scans of a 51-year-old man with WK encephalopathy associated with pyloric stenosis. Axial T2-weighted (A) and FLAIR (B, C) images show marked hyperintensity of the mammillary bodies, tectal region, and periaqueductal area. Post-contrast sagittal and coronal T1-weighted images (D and E, F, respectively) show abnormal enhancement of the mammillary bodies. The coronal FLAIR series confirms hyperintensity with respect to the pons of the periaqueductal area and tectal plate, with involvement of inferior quadrigeminal tubercula. Reproduced with permission from reference [95].

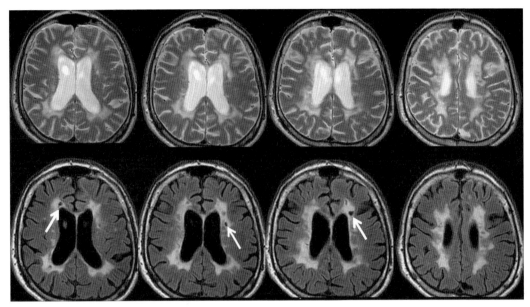

Figure 3.4 Extensive and diffuse white-matter hyperintensities (WMH) in a 60-year-old man with vascular dementia. Axial T2-weighted (top panel) and FLAIR images (bottom panel) show WMH predominantly involving the deep and periventricular white matter. U-fibers are relatively spared. Scattered, fluid-like lacunar infarcts (arrows) are also identified in the white matter. There is moderate ex vacuo dilatation of the lateral ventricles.

VCI can give rise to any form of cognitive decline from mild deficits in one or more cognitive domains to a broad dementia-like syndrome [96]. Executive and attentional impairment, behavioral changes (disinhibiton or abulia), and cognitive slowing with relative sparing of memory are clinical features common to many forms of vascular damage. Frequently, VCI is the result of a diffuse involvement of the brain white matter and subcortical nuclei caused by small-vessel disease. These patients typically present with an indolent cognitive decline and lack a history of clinical vascular episodes. Clinical features often include fluctuating deficits, bradyphrenia, and prominent dysexecutive disturbances. Memory impairment is generally due to attentional deficits. On neurological examination, patients may show brisk facial and limb reflexes, pseudobulbar palsy, apraxic gate, extrapyramidal signs, and urinary incontinence.

(b) Investigative findings

Cerebrovascular disease can be detected by CT and structural MRI [74, 97]. Although both modalities perform relatively well in depicting large-vessel infarcts, MRI is more sensitive to subtle small-vessel vascular abnormalities than CT. T2-weighted and FLAIR sequences are highly sensitive for detecting major strokes as well as small strategic infarcts and small-vessel ischemic white-matter damage (Figure 3.4). Compared to T2, FLAIR sequences have, however, a reduced sensitivity for lesions in the infratentorial region as well as in the diencephalon (including the thalamus) [98]. On T2-weighted sequences, all these lesions are seen as bright areas; on FLAIR images fluid cavities can be seen as dark areas (Figure 3.4). This facilitates the differentiation of enlarged perivascular spaces from white-matter hyperintensities. T2* sequences are used to detect microbleeds, hemorrhages, and calcifications. T1-weighted sequences are used for regional atrophy assessment.

The most widely used clinical diagnostic criteria for VaD are the National Institute for Neurological Disorders and Stroke–Association pour la Recherche et l'Enseignement en Neurosciences (NINDS–AIREN) criteria [99]. NINDS–AIREN criteria require the demonstration of cerebrovascular disease using structural brain imaging, and a link between such a finding and the onset of cognitive impairment [99]. In addition, the operational radiological definitions for the NINDS–AIREN criteria provided guidelines on the topography and severity of vascular lesions [100]. Bilateral infarcts in the territory of the anterior cerebral artery, and infarcts in the territory of the posterior cerebral artery, association areas, or in watershed regions are thought to be causative of large vessel VaD [100]. Extensive white-matter lesions involving at least 25% of the white matter, multiple basal ganglia, thalamic, and frontal-white-matter lacunar infarcts, or bilateral thalamic lesions are considered typical radiological findings associated with small-vessel VaD [100].

Criteria to diagnose subcortical ischemic VaD have also been proposed [86, 101]: these require demonstration of extensive periventricular and deep-white-matter lesions and lacunar infarcts in the deep gray matter, or multiple lacunae in the deep gray matter, and at least moderate white-matter lesions, in the absence of cortical and/or cortical-subcortical (non-lacunar) territorial infarcts, watershed infarcts, hemorrhages, and other specific causes of white-matter lesions.

Neurodegenerative dementia

DLB, PD, CBS, and PSP are discussed in Chapters 17 and 19.

Creutzfeldt-Jakob disease

(a) Clinical findings

Sporadic Creutzfeldt–Jakob disease (sCJD), which is the most common prion disease (85% of cases), is a neurodegenerative, uniformly fatal disease characterized pathologically by spongiform abnormalities of the brain [76]. The cause is unknown. Genetic forms (e.g. familial CJD) occur in 10–15% of the cases and are caused by prion protein gene mutations. In addition, CJDs have been related to corneal graft transplantation, contaminated human pituitary-derived growth hormone, or gonadotropin and dura mater grafts (iatrogenic CJD). The very rare new variant CJD (vCJD) was first reported in the UK in March 1996 and has been related to bovine spongiform encephalopathy.

The characteristic clinical picture of sCJD is one of rapidly progressive dementia with associated neurological features, particularly cerebellar ataxia, pyramidal signs, and myoclonus [76]. Visual disturbances, ocular movement disorders, extrapyramidal signs, and hallucinations are also well recognized. The clinical progression is typically over weeks, and ends with an akinetic mute state and death often in 2–3 months (usually less than 6). The illness may be preceded by a non-specific prodrome, including fatigue, low mood, weight loss, and headache for a few months. Although the most common sCJD presentation is a subacute encephalopathy, patients can also present with a pure cerebellar ataxia (10% of the cases, so-called ataxic CJD), and visual, psychiatric, and stroke-like syndromes [76]. vCJD is characterized by atypical features including a predominantly psychiatric presentation, some cases with sensory disturbances, and a relatively extended duration of illness (median = 14 months) [76].

(b) Investigative findings

Diagnostic criteria for sCJD are based on clinical signs, 14-3-3 protein in the CSF, EEG, and MRI findings [102]. The classical diagnostic triad is a rapidly progressive dementia, myoclonus, and a characteristic EEG pattern [103]. Myoclonus is an important manifestation, but is seen often only in late stages of the disease. The CSF is usually unremarkable with normal glucose levels and no cells although proteins may be modestly elevated. The most valuable CSF test is the analysis of the neuronal protein 14-3-3, which has a sensitivity of 85–95% in patients with suspected sCJD [104]. However, CSF 14-3-3 protein can be positive in recent cerebral strokes, viral encephalitis, and rapidly progressive AD. EEG examination is a useful investigation in sCJD, classically showing periodic, triphasic sharp wave complexes at a frequency of 1 per second (70% of the cases), usually generalized throughout the trace. In vCJD, the EEG is abnormal showing generalized slow wave activity, but without the pseudoperiodic pattern seen in most cases of sCJD. Brain biopsy may be considered in highly selected cases to exclude alternative, treatable diagnoses.

MRI has emerged as an increasingly valuable tool in identifying sCJD, both by excluding other disorders and demonstrating typical features. In sCJD, T2-weighted and especially FLAIR sequences can show a very characteristic pattern of hyperintense signal in the striatum and/or cortex (Figure 3.5) [102, 105]. DWI can detect focal abnormalities in patients with sCJD not yet apparent on FLAIR images (up to 20% of the cases) [102, 105, 106]. In sCJD, involvement of either the striatum or neocortex or both is usually found (Figure 3.5) [105]. Both sensitivity and specificity based on either bilateral basal ganglia changes or cortical hyperintensity in at least two areas is up to 80% [102]. In vCJD, there is a selective involvement of the medial and dorsal (pulvinar) thalamic nuclei, leading

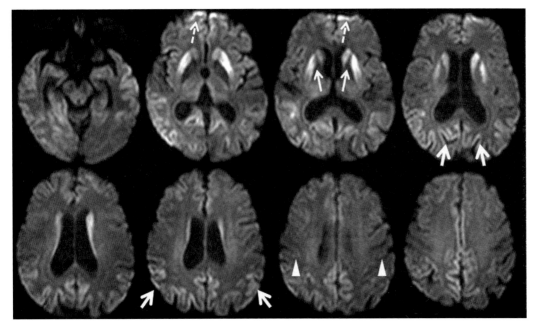

Figure 3.5 Axial DWI scans in a 65-year-old woman with sCJD. Images show extensive, abnormal symmetric hyperintensity of the caudate nucleus and putamen (arrows) and pathologic hyperintensity in the bilateral parietal and temporo-occipital neocortex (wide arrows). Note the sparing of cortex of the precentral and postcentral gyri (arrowheads). Dashed arrows show typical severe magnetic susceptibility artifacts in the frontal regions bilaterally. Courtesy of Professor Andrea Falini.

to the so-called hockey-stick sign [107]. However, this sign appears as a late feature of vCJD and is not specific; similar MRI appearances have been described in sCJD and PLE. Cerebral and cerebellar atrophy can occur in patients with longer disease duration. FDG PET may show marked hypometabolism in early CJD, even when no brain abnormalities are visible on MRI scans.

The most common sCJD mimics are neurodegenerative diseases, including AD, DLB, and FTD syndromes [103]. In addition, psychiatric disorders, immune-mediated encephalopathies, metabolic derangements, toxins, and infections are generally considered in the differential work-up of patients suspected of having a prion disorder [103]. A large number of potential causes can be confirmed or excluded fairly quickly with a detailed history, including the search for drug and alcohol use, and some investigations such as routine blood, CSF proteins, and brain imaging (e.g. drug/toxic encephalopathy, brain metastases, systemic and common CNS infections, and many metabolic causes). However, the difficulty in diagnosis remains in atypical presentations, or in those cases with negative investigations [103].

Alzheimer's disease

(a) Clinical findings

AD is the most common neurodegenerative disorder leading to dementia. AD is a slowly progressive disorder with a broad spectrum of symptoms, reflecting the wide array of cortical regions that may be involved [108]. Typically, AD presents with an insidious onset of cognitive decline, starting with deficits of episodic memory [108]. For example, patients and their family complain of forgetting recent personal or family events, seldom-used names of persons and objects, losing items around the house, repetitive questioning. These complaints reflect early involvement of the neuroanatomically vulnerable basal forebrain and MTL, including the hippocampus and the adjacent areas [109]. Remote memories are usually preserved. As the disease pathology spreads to other cortical areas, primarily the posterior cingulate gyrus and the temporoparietal cortices, additional deficits arise [109]. Visuospatial deficits are often present, with patients getting lost or disoriented while navigating. Misplacement of personal objects may also reveal a visual memory deficit. In the language domain, reduced spontaneous verbal output often accompanies early memory symptoms. The patient's speech is frequently interrupted because of anomias, with recurrent use of circumlocutions. The same difficulty interrupts writing. Vocabulary becomes restricted and expressive language stereotyped. Grammar and syntax may also become progressively less complex. Many patients undergo a phase when comprehension is impaired, but repetition is normal (transcortical sensory aphasia). This disturbance further progresses to Wernicke's aphasia with poor comprehension and repetition. Finally, after many years of illness, patients develop global aphasia or mutism. The language dysfunctions observed in AD correlate with the severity of left-posterior parietal and temporal-lobe disease.

Other cognitive symptoms occur with variable frequency in patients with AD, most often in the moderate to late stages of the illness. Apraxia leads to difficulties in using utensils or dressing. Agnosia often arises later in the disease course and manifests as a failure to recognize objects and family members. Executive dysfunction, as a result of prefrontal cortex involvement, leads to deficits in focusing attention, problem-solving, abstraction, reasoning, decision-making, and judgment. Psychiatric and behavioral symptoms occur more frequently as the disease advances.

The general neurologic examination is typically unremarkable in mild to moderate AD [108]. In the late stages of the disease, sphincteric continence fails and difficulty in locomotion emerges gradually. Ultimately, the patient loses their ability to stand and walk. Convulsions are rare until late in the illness. Dysphagia is an important symptom that occurs in the last stages. Eventually, with the patient in a bedridden state, an intercurrent infection such as aspiration pneumonia or some other disease terminates life. The average survival of AD patients is typically about 8–13 years from the onset of symptoms.

In addition to the typical presentation of AD characterized by early anterograde memory deficits, there is evidence from clinico-pathological studies that AD patients may present with different neuropsychological profiles [110]. In atypical forms, patients may experience language or visuospatial deficits or executive dysfunction as the first symptoms with a relatively spared memory. PCA is a rare and atypical AD presentation with early-onset (usually before 65 years), characterized by an initially isolated, progressive impairment of high-order visual and visuospatial

skills, which usually manifest as visual agnosia, prosopagnosia, environmental disorientation, elements of Balint syndrome, visual neglect, and alexia [111]. The logopenic variant of PPA is considered an atypical, early-onset presentation of AD pathology [7]. Patients usually come to the neurologist's attention for impaired single-word retrieval in spontaneous speech and naming, and impaired repetition of sentences; phonologic errors are frequent in the absence of frank agrammatism; whilst single-word comprehension, object knowledge, and motor speech are preserved.

(b) Investigative findings

There is general consensus that $A\beta_{1-42}$, an important constituent of the neuritic plaques, is significantly reduced in the CSF of AD patients compared with normal elderly adult controls [102, 112, 113]. On the contrary, CSF tau, an important component of the neurofibrillary tangles, is significantly increased in patients with AD compared with normal controls [112, 113]. The combined reduction of the CSF $A\beta_{1-42}$ and elevation of the CSF tau protein yields a sensitivity and specificity of approximately 80–90% in comparing AD patients and controls, but this is not the case when other dementing syndromes, such as FTD or DLB, are considered.

Coronal T1-weighted MRI imaging should be acquired to assess MTL atrophy to support a clinical diagnosis of AD (Figure 3.6) [74]. Although MRI is superior to conventional CT in the evaluation of MTL atrophy, high-resolution CT with coronal reformatted images should be used when MRI is not utilized [114]. Prediction of subsequent evolution of AD in individuals with amnestic mild cognitive impairment (MCI) can also be obtained with MRI volumetric measures of the MTL [74]. At present, however, accepted standards for quantitative MTL volume measurement are lacking. Therefore, quantification must rely on local specific standards. Combining MTL measures with other potentially informative markers, such as posterior cingulate cortex and precuneus volumetric measures (Figure 3.6), is likely to improve diagnostic confidence, mainly in young AD cases [74].

In cases of atypical AD presentations, the involvement of the MTL is reported less consistently than that of lateral temporal and medial parietal regions. Structural MRI scans of patients with PCA show atrophy of parieto-occipital and posterior temporal cortices [115, 116]. Compared with typical AD cases, PCA

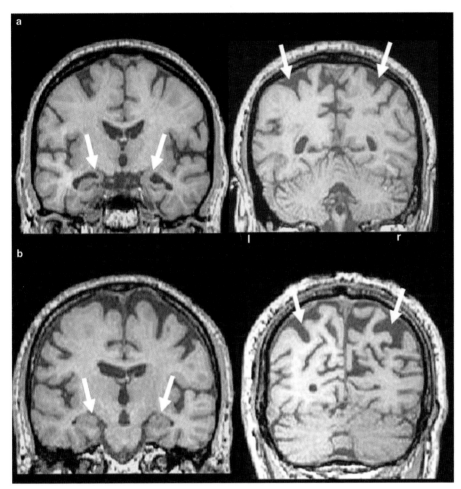

Figure 3.6 MRI of (A) a typical case of AD and (B) a patient with PCA. Coronal T1-weighted images show prominent bilateral hippocampal and parietal atrophy in AD (arrows), and the relatively asymmetric (right greater than left) parieto-occipital atrophy with relative preservation of the medial temporal lobe in PCA (arrows).

patients have a more-severe right parietal and a less-pronounced left MTL atrophy (Figure 3.6) [115]. Data from functional imaging studies demonstrate a comparable involvement of temporoparietal cortex and precuneus in PCA and typical AD, with extension of hypoperfusion or hypometabolism into occipital and posterior temporal lobes in PCA patients [117, 118]. In the logopenic variant of PPA, the pattern of atrophy and hypometabolism primarily affects the left temporoparietal junction, including the left posterior superior and middle temporal gyri, as well as the inferior parietal lobule [119, 120].

Functional imaging using CBF SPECT or FDG PET can be of value to diagnose (or exclude) a neurodegenerative dementia in those subjects with cognitive impairment presenting with severe psychiatric disturbances (including depression and agitation), and in cases where proper cognitive testing is difficult, e.g., when the patients and the examiner do not speak the same language [74]. The overall regional pattern of metabolic impairment of the posterior cingulate/precuneus and lateral temporoparietal cortices, more accentuated than frontal-cortex abnormalities, together with the relative preservation of the primary sensorimotor and visual cortices, basal ganglia, and cerebellum defines the metabolic phenotype of AD (Figure 3.7) [74]. AD-like metabolic patterns in patients with MCI are predictive of conversion to AD within several years [74].

PET amyloid imaging has very high (90% or greater) sensitivity for AD pathology [122]. Amyloid-tracer binding is diffuse and symmetric, with high

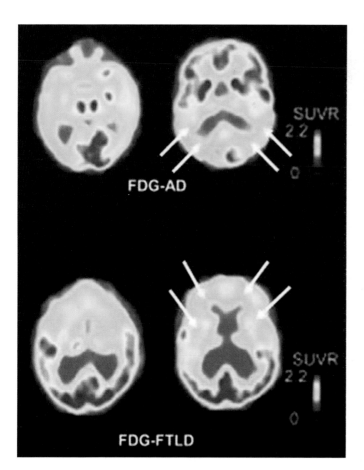

FDG-AD

SUVR
2 2

0

FDG-FTLD

SUVR
2 2

0

Figure 3.7 FDG PET scans of AD and FTLD. In AD, note the reduced glucose metabolism in the superior/posterior temporal and parietal regions (arrows). In FTLD, hypometabolism is seen in the frontal and anterior temporal regions, with a relative sparing of the posterior brain regions (arrows). Reproduced with permission from reference [121].

uptake consistently found in the prefrontal cortex, precuneus, and posterior cingulate cortex, followed by the lateral parietal and lateral temporal cortices, and the striatum (Figure 3.8). This pattern closely mirrors the distribution of plaques found at autopsy [124]. However, some healthy elderly controls show high binding, with the frequency of increased cortical binding increasing rapidly from 10% below the age of 70 to 30–40% at the age of 80 years [125]. Thus, although negative amyloid scans indicate the absence of AD pathology with a high level of accuracy, in the other cases the predictive value of the amyloid scan per se is not clear. According to the EFNS guidelines, amyloid imaging is not yet recommended for routine use in the clinical setting, especially in the diagnostic work-up of patients with straightforward clinical AD as these patients are very likely to have positive scans [74]. On the other hand, amyloid imaging is likely to find clinical utility in the following fields: (a) the stratification of MCI patients into those with and without underlying AD; (b) the evaluation of early-onset AD

patients, as these patients often present with atypical symptoms, or patients with atypical clinical presentations (e.g. PPA), as these are pathologically heterogeneous syndromes that are variably associated with AD pathology; and (c) the differential diagnosis between AD and FTD, since amyloid plaques are not part of the FTLD pathologic spectrum [74].

The US National Institute on Aging (NIA) and the Alzheimer's Association (AA) have recently developed new diagnostic guidelines for AD [126, 127]. These recommendations emphasize the evolving recognition that AD represents a continuum, starting from a pre-clinical stage in which the pathophysiological process begins, through an early symptomatic phase referred to as prodromal AD or MCI due to AD, and ending with a dementia phase that represents a fairly late stage in the illness. The NIA–AA guidelines include a specific framework for biomarkers across the continuum of the disease, dividing them into two categories [128]: (a) markers of $A\beta$ accumulation, i.e. low CSF $A\beta_{1\text{-}42}$ concentrations or positive PET amyloid imaging; and

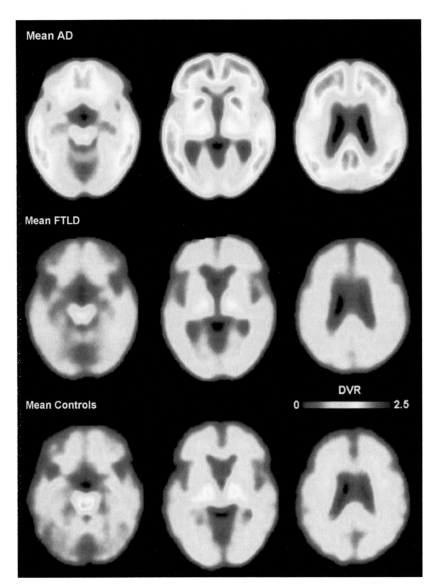

Mean AD

Mean FTLD

Mean Controls

DVR
0 ▬▬▬▬▬▬▬ 2.5

Figure 3.8 Axial slices of mean ^{11}C-labeled Pittsburgh compound B images (normalized to cerebellum) in patients clinically diagnosed with AD (top row, N = 27, mean age 67.1±9.9), FTLD (middle row, N = 31, mean age 64.5±7.5), and cognitively normal controls (bottom row, N = 12, mean age 73.9±6.1). Patients with AD show tracer uptake throughout the frontal, parietal, and lateral temporal cortex, and the striatum, while most patients with FTLD and controls show only mild non-specific tracer binding in white matter. Reproduced with permission from reference [123].

(b) markers of neuronal injury, i.e. elevated CSF tau, decreased FDG uptake on PET in temporoparietal cortex, and disproportionate atrophy on structural MRI in the medial, basal, and lateral temporal lobe, and the medial parietal cortex. In individuals who meet the core clinical criteria for probable AD dementia, biomarker abnormalities increase the certainty that AD pathology is the basis of the clinical dementia syndrome. Similar considerations can be made for the diagnosis of prodromal (MCI) stages of the disease. In terms of core clinical criteria, the NIA–AA guidelines do not require an amnestic presentation, recognizing that the disorder can present as deficits in other cognitive and behavioral domains [126].

Frontotemporal lobar degeneration

(a) Clinical findings

The most frequent presentations of frontotemporal lobal degeneration (FTLD) are the behavioral and the language variants. The behavioral variant (bvFTD) is a clinical syndrome characterized by a progressive deterioration of personality, social behavior, and cognition [129]. These patients typically present with an early behavioral disinhibition, loss of sympathy or empathy (~ 70%), apathy, impairment in personal care, and emotional blunting (~ 80%), perseverative stereotyped or compulsive behavior (~ 65%), hyperorality and dietary changes (~ 60%), and loss of insight (~ 85%).

At the neuropsychological assessment patients may manifest with an executive impairment (mainly deficits of executive control, planning, and organization) and relatively spared memory and visuospatial functions [129].

The language variants are also known as PPAs. In PPA, language deficits are the core cognitive features at onset [130]. There are three variants of PPA: non-fluent/agrammatic, semantic, and logopenic [7]. The non-fluent variant is characterized by agrammatism in language production, effortful, halting speech with inconsistent speech sound errors and distortions (apraxia of speech); patients with the non-fluent variant may present with disturbances in comprehension of syntactically complex sentences; however, they have spared single-word comprehension and object knowledge. The semantic variant is characterized by impaired confrontation naming, single-word comprehension, and object knowledge; repetition and speech production are spared. The logopenic variant has been discussed as an atypical presentation of AD.

Neurological examination in patients suspected of having FTLD syndromes is usually normal, although a subgroup of cases have or may develop later additional signs of weakness in bulbar and/or limb muscles, in a pattern indistinguishable from that of amyotrophic lateral sclerosis. In all stages, primitive reflexes may also become prominent. Parkinsonism can occur in some cases.

(b) Investigative findings

CSF is usually normal or shows elevated tau levels. In the majority of FTLD cases, the distinctive anatomical distribution of damage can be appreciated on structural MRI and functional imaging. According to recent criteria [7, 129], in patients clinically diagnosed with either bvFTD or PPA, an "imaging-supported" diagnosis can be made with structural MRI scans or functional SPECT and FDG PET.

Structural MRI studies showed that classical bvFTD presents with a combination of medial frontal, orbital-insular, and anterior temporal cortical atrophy (Figure 3.9) [131, 132]. Such an atrophy pattern can be readily appreciated on coronal T1-weighted MRI scans. The MTL is affected more anteriorly than in AD cases, i.e., the amygdala is more affected than the hippocampus, and the posterior hippocampus often appears normal. According to the recent EFNS recommendations for the diagnosis of degenerative dementia, the whole pattern of atrophy is more useful than

atrophy of single regions in the differential diagnosis of bvFTD compared with AD: knife-edge, severe frontotemporal atrophy combined with dilatation of the frontal horn and an anterior greater than posterior gradient is suggestive of a diagnosis of bvFTD [74]. Nevertheless, the typical pattern is not necessarily present in all cases [133, 134]. A large structural MRI study suggested that bvFTD may be divided into four anatomically different subtypes, two of which are associated with a prominent frontal atrophy (i.e. frontal-dominant and frontotemporal variants) and two with prominent temporal-lobe atrophy (i.e. temporal-dominant and temporofrontoparietal subtypes) [135]. Brain atrophy in bvFTD also involves several subcortical structures, such as the striatum [131, 135, 136]. Although an overlap of PET and SPECT functional abnormalities between bvFTD and AD has been shown to occur, the presence of posterior temporal and parietal brain hypoperfusion or hypometabolism is predictive of AD pathology, whereas a disproportionate reduction of frontal perfusion/metabolism is more common in FTLD cases (Figure 3.7) [74].

Generally speaking, the presence of knife-edge frontal and/or temporal-lobe atrophy in patients with PPA is predictive of FTLD pathology, while the presence of temporoparietal atrophy is highly associated with AD [74]. More specifically, the non-fluent PPA variant is associated with a characteristic pattern of left anterior perisylvian atrophy involving inferior, opercular, and insular portions of the frontal lobe (Figure 3.9) [119]. Motor and premotor regions and Broca's area are also involved [119]. The semantic variant PPA is associated with temporal-lobe atrophy, which is maximal at the ventral and lateral portions of the anterior temporal lobe (Figure 3.9) [137].

In a previous study [138], we observed that white-matter damage is related to gray-matter atrophy in these conditions; however, we could not exclude a primary white-matter degeneration. Furthermore, using diffusion tensor (DT) MRI measures, we ran a random forest analysis in order to provide information on the predictive value of white-matter-tract measures [138]. We found that the uncinate fasciculus was able to distinguish all FTLD variants compared with controls, while the genu of the corpus callosum (CC), left superior longitudinal fasciculus (SLF), and left inferior longitudinal fasciculus (ILF) were able to specifically distinguish respectively bvFTD, non-fluent, and semantic variants from controls. When we compared these syndromes to each other, the left

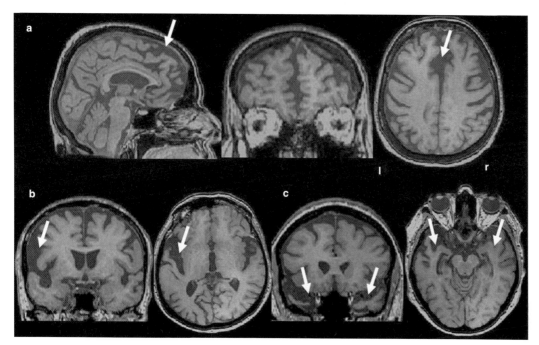

Figure 3.9 MRI of patients with frontotemporal lobar degeneration syndromes. (A) Sagittal, coronal, and axial T1-weighted images show a pattern of knife-edge frontal atrophy (arrows) in a patient with the behavioral variant of frontotemporal dementia (bvFTD). (B) Coronal and axial T1-weighted images show a marked left frontal atrophy (arrows) in a patient with the non-fluent variant of PPA. Major involvement of the anterior temporal lobes, with left predominance (arrows), is shown in (C) in a patient with the semantic variant of PPA. Furthermore, the white matter needs to be considered when investigating FTLD syndromes, since it seems to play a crucial role in defining the neuropsychological profile and provides information for monitoring the progression of the disease.

SLF and the genu of the CC DT MRI measures provided the highest accuracy in distinguishing bvFTD from non-fluent cases (more severe left SLF damage in non-fluent and more severe genu of CC damage in bvFTD). When bvFTD patients were compared with the semantic group, the most important predictors were DT MRI variables of the left ILF and uncinate fasciculus (more severe left ILF damage in semantic, and more severe left uncinate fasciculus damage in bvFTD). Finally, for non-fluent vs. semantic patients, left uncinate fasciculus and ILF DT MRI measures resulted in the highest patient classification accuracy. White-matter DT MRI measures are promising for FTLD diagnosis and for their utility in the differential diagnosis with AD.

Finally, the study of resting state (RS) activity using functional MRI has been found to be useful in differential diagnosis between AD and bvFTD patients, by detecting specific disconnections between regions of the most relevant cerebral networks [139, 140]. Furthermore, RS functional connectivity combined with advanced methodological approaches, such as the graph theory [141], are promising imaging markers of the disease.

Conclusions

This chapter has provided a guide for evaluating neurological cases presenting with cognitive disturbances, potentially leading to dementia. It is based on awareness and understanding of the multiple acquired cognitive deficits and combines a neuropsychological and anatomical approach. When the neuropsychological assessment is not fully informative in providing a diagnosis, there are a number of appropriate laboratory investigations that can be helpful. Neuroimaging tools, mainly MRI, are useful not only for the exclusion of potentially treatable causes of dementia, such as tumor and subdural hematoma, but also for the detection of abnormalities suggesting specific disorders. These biomarkers are increasingly relevant to assess individual clinical cases.

References

1. Budson AE, Price BH (2005). Memory dysfunction. *N Engl J Med* **352**: 692–699.
2. Bayley PJ, Hopkins RO, Squire LR (2006). The fate of old memories after medial temporal lobe damage. *J Neurosci* **26**: 13311–13317.

59

3. Papez JW (1937). A proposed mechanism of emotion. *Arch Neurol Psychiatry* **38**: 725–743.

4. Nolde SF, Johnson MK, D'Esposito M (1998). Left prefrontal activation during episodic remembering: an event-related fMRI study. *Neuroreport* **9**: 3509–3514.

5. Ribot T (1882). *Diseases of Memory: An Essay in the Positive Psychology*. Smith WH, trans. New York: Appleton.

6. Moscovitch M, Nadel L, Winocur G, Gilboa A, Rosenbaum RS (2006). The cognitive neuroscience of remote episodic, semantic and spatial memory. *Curr Opin Neurobiol* **16**: 179–190.

7. Gorno-Tempini ML, Hillis AE, Weintraub S, *et al.* (2011). Classification of primary progressive aphasia and its variants. *Neurology* **76**: 1006–1014.

8. Heindel WC, Salmon DP, Shults CW, Walicke PA, Butters N (1989). Neuropsychological evidence for multiple implicit memory systems: a comparison of Alzheimer's, Huntington's, and Parkinson's disease patients. *J Neurosci* **9**: 582–587.

9. Marquez GG (1970). *One Hundred Years of Solitude*, Rabassa G, trans. London: Harper Collins.

10. Damasio AR, Geschwind N (1984). The neural basis of language. *Annu Rev Neurosci* **7**: 127–147.

11. Price CJ (2010). The anatomy of language: a review of 100 fMRI studies published in 2009. *Ann NY Acad Sci* **1191**: 62–88.

12. Shim H, Grabowski TJ (2010). Comprehension. *Continuum (Minneap Minn)* **16**: 45–58.

13. Hillis AE (2010). Naming and language production. *Continuum (Minneap Minn)* **16**: 29–44.

14. Garrett MF. Levels of processing in sentence production (1980). In Butterworth B, ed. *Language Production: Speech and Talk*. New York: Academic Press, pp. 177–220.

15. Damasio AR (1992). Aphasia. *N Engl J Med* **326**: 531–539.

16. Taler V, Phillips NA (2008). Language performance in Alzheimer's disease and mild cognitive impairment: a comparative review. *J Clin Exp Neuropsychol* **30**: 501–556.

17. Ogar J, Slama H, Dronkers N, Amici S, Gorno-Tempini ML (2005). Apraxia of speech: an overview. *Neurocase* **11**: 427–432.

18. Sacks O (1985). *The Man Who Mistook His Wife For a Hat*. New York: Summit Books.

19. Teuber HL (1968). Alteration of perception and memory in man. In Weiskrantz L, ed. *Analysis of Behavioral Change*. New York: Harper & Row, pp. 268–375.

20. Burns MS (2004). Clinical management of agnosia. *Top Stroke Rehabil* **11**: 1–9.

21. Barton JJ (2011). Disorders of higher visual processing. *Hand Clin Neurol* **102**: 223–261.

22. Barton JJ, Cherkasova M, O'Connor M (2001). Covert recognition in acquired and developmental prosopagnosia. *Neurology* **57**: 1161–1168.

23. Barton JJ (2008). Structure and function in acquired prosopagnosia: lessons from a series of 10 patients with brain damage. *J Neuropsychol* **2**: 197–225.

24. Haxby JV, Gobbini MI, Furey ML, *et al.* (2001). Distributed and overlapping representations of faces and objects in ventral temporal cortex. *Science* **293**: 2425–2430.

25. Della Sala S, Spinnler H (1994). Finger agnosia: fiction or reality? *Arch Neurol* **51**: 448–450.

26. Murakami H (1980). *Pinball, 1973*. Tokyo: Kodansha International Ltd.

27. McDowd JM (2007). An overview of attention: behavior and brain. *J Neurol Phys Ther* **31**: 98–103.

28. Mesulam MM (2000). *Principles of Behavioral and Cognitive Neurology*. New York: Oxford University Press.

29. Mesulam MM (2010). Attentional and confusional States. *Continuum (Minneap Minn)* **16**: 128–139.

30. Kok A (1999). Varieties of inhibition: manifestations in cognition, event-related potentials and aging. *Acta Psychol (Amst)* **101**: 129–158.

31. Fan J, McCandliss BD, Fossella J, Flombaum JI, Posner MI (2005). The activation of attentional networks. *Neuroimage* **26**: 471–479.

32. Fan J, Posner M (2004). Human attentional networks. *Psychiatr Prax* **31** (suppl 2): S210–214.

33. Genova L (2011). *Left Neglected*. New York: Gallery Books.

34. Ikkai A, Curtis CE (2011). Common neural mechanisms supporting spatial working memory, attention and motor intention. *Neuropsychologia* **49**: 1428–1434.

35. Chatterjee A, Coslett HB (2010). Disorders of visuospatial processing. *Continuum (Minneap Minn)* **16**: 99–110.

36. Chatterjee A (1996). Anosognosia for hemiplegia: patient retrospections. *Cogn Neuropsychiatry* **1**: 221–237.

37. Heilman KM, Watson RT, Valenstein E (1979). Neglect and related disorders. In Heilman KM, Valenstein E, eds. *Clinical Neuropsychology*. New York: Oxford University Press, pp. 268–307.

38. Mesulam MM (1981). A cortical network for directed attention and unilateral neglect. *Ann Neurol* **10**: 309–325.

39. Coslett HB, Saffran E (1991). Simultanagnosia. To see but not two see. *Brain* **114**: 1523–1545.

40. Coslett HB, Chatterjee A (2003). Balint syndrome and related disorders. In Feinberg TE, Farah MJ, eds. *Behavioral Neurology and Neuropsychology*. New York: McGraw-Hill, pp. 325–335.

41. Jax SA, Buxbaum LJ, Lie E, Coslett HB (2009). More than (where the target) meets the eyes: disrupted visuomotor transformations in optic ataxia. *Neuropsychologia* **47**: 230–238.

42. Harvey M, Milner AD (1995). Bálint's patient. *Cogn Neuropsychol* **12**: 261–265.

43. Gross RG, Grossman M (2008). Update on apraxia. *Curr Neurol Neurosci Rep* **8**: 490–496.

44. Heilman KM, Rothi LJG (2003). Apraxia. In Heilman KM, Valenstein E, eds. *Clinical Neuropsychology*. New York: Oxford University Press, pp. 215–235.

45. Liepmann H (1920). Apraxia. *Erbgn der ges Med* **1**: 516–543.

46. Schnider A, Hanlon RE, Alexander DN, Benson DF (1997). Ideomotor apraxia: behavioral dimensions and neuroanatomical basis. *Brain Lang* **58**: 125–136.

47. Ozsancak C, Auzou P, Dujardin K, Quinn N, Destee A (2004). Orofacial apraxia in corticobasal degeneration, progressive supranuclear palsy, multiple system atrophy and Parkinson's disease. *J Neurol* **251**: 1317–1323.

48. Heilman KM, Rothi LJ, Valenstein E (1982). Two forms of ideomotor apraxia. *Neurology* **32**: 342–346.

49. Ochipa C, Rothi LJ, Heilman KM (1992). Conceptual apraxia in Alzheimer's disease. *Brain* **115**: 1061–1071.

50. Leiguarda RC, Marsden CD (2000). Limb apraxias: higher-order disorders of sensorimotor integration. *Brain* **123**: 860–879.

51. Leiguarda RC, Merello M, Nouzeilles MI, *et al.* (2003). Limb-kinetic apraxia in corticobasal degeneration: clinical and kinematic features. *Mov Disord* **18**: 49–59.

52. Leiguarda RC, Pramstaller PP, Merello M, *et al.* (1997). Apraxia in Parkinson's disease, progressive supranuclear palsy, multiple system atrophy and neuroleptic-induced parkinsonism. *Brain* **120**: 75–90.

53. Quencer K, Okun MS, Crucian G, *et al.* (2007). Limb-kinetic apraxia in Parkinson disease. *Neurology* **68**: 150–151.

54. Graham NL, Zeman A, Young AW, Patterson K, Hodges JR (1999). Dyspraxia in a patient with corticobasal degeneration: the role of visual and tactile inputs to action. *J Neurol Neurosurg Psychiatry* **67**: 334–344.

55. Goldberg E (2009). *The New Executive Brain: Frontal Lobes in a Complex World*. Oxford: Oxford University Press.

56. Gross RG, Grossman M (2010). Executive resources. *Continuum (Minneap Minn)* **16**: 140–152.

57. Carpenter PA, Just MA, Reichle ED (2000). Working memory and executive function: evidence from neuroimaging. *Curr Opin Neurobiol* **10**: 195–199.

58. Morris RG (1994). Working memory in Alzheimer-type dementia. *Neuropsychology* **8**: 544–554.

59. Godefroy O, Cabaret M, Petit-Chenal V, Pruvo JP, Rousseaux M (1999). Control functions of the frontal lobes. Modularity of the central-supervisory system? *Cortex* **35**: 1–20.

60. Baddeley AD (1986). *Working Memory*. Oxford: Psychology Press.

61. Baddeley A (2000). The episodic buffer: a new component of working memory? *Trends Cogn Sci* **4**: 417–423.

62. Smith EE, Jonides J (1999). Storage and executive processes in the frontal lobes. *Science* **283**: 1657–1661.

63. D'Esposito M, Postle BR, Ballard D, Lease J (1999). Maintenance versus manipulation of information held in working memory: an event-related fMRI study. *Brain Cogn* **41**: 66–86.

64. Owen AM, Doyon J, Petrides M, Evans AC (1996). Planning and spatial working memory: a positron emission tomography study in humans. *Eur J Neurosci* **8**: 353–364.

65. Shallice T, Burgess PW (1991). Deficits in strategy application following frontal lobe damage in man. *Brain* **114**: 727–741.

66. Friedman NP, Miyake A (2004). The relations among inhibition and interference control functions: a latent-variable analysis. *J Exp Psychol Gen* **133**: 101–135.

67. Dillon DG, Pizzagalli DA (2007). Inhibition of action, thought, and emotion: a selective neurobiological review. *Appl Prev Psychol* **12**: 99–114.

68. Bush G, Luu P, Posner MI (2000). Cognitive and emotional influences in anterior cingulate cortex. *Trends Cogn Sci* **4**: 215–222.

69. Dosenbach NU, Fair DA, Miezin FM, *et al.* (2007). Distinct brain networks for adaptive and stable task control in humans. *Proc Natl Acad Sci USA* **104**: 11073–11078.

70. Fan J, Flombaum JI, McCandliss BD, Thomas KM, Posner MI (2003). Cognitive and brain consequences of conflict. *Neuroimage* **18**: 42–57.

71. Sorbi S, Hort J, Erkinjuntti T, *et al.* (2012). EFNS–ENS guidelines on the diagnosis and management of disorders associated with dementia. *Eur J Neurol* **19**: 1159–1179.

72. Grober E, Sliwinski M. (1991). Development and validation of a model for estimating premorbid verbal intelligence in the elderly. *J Clin Exp Neuropsychol* **13**: 933–949.

73. Nelson HE (1991). *The National Adult Reading Test*. Windsor: NFER-Nelson.

74. Filippi M, Agosta F, Barkhof F, *et al.* (2012) EFNS task force: the use of neuroimaging in the diagnosis of dementia. *Eur J Neurol* **19**: e131–140, 1487–1501.

75. Herholz K, Schopphoff H, Schmidt M, *et al.* (2002) Direct comparison of spatially normalized PET and SPECT scans in Alzheimer's disease. *J Nucl Med* **43**: 21–26.

76. Ropper AH, Samuels MA (2009). *Adams and Victor's Principles of Neurology*. New York: McGraw-Hill.

77. Saito M, Nishio Y, Kanno S, *et al.* (2011). Cognitive profile of idiopathic normal pressure hydrocephalus. *Dementia Ger Cogn Disord Extra* **1**: 202–211.

78. Rosen H, Swigar ME (1976). Depression and normal pressure hydrocephalus. A dilemma in neuropsychiatric differential diagnosis. *J Nerv Ment Dis* **163**: 35–40.

79. Yousem DM, Grossman RI (2010). *Neuroradiology: The Requisites*. Philadelphia, PA: Mosby Elsevier.

80. Jung KH, Chu K, Jeong SW, *et al.* (2003). Idiopathic normal pressure hydrocephalus predominantly with prolonged fever and hyponatremia. *Neurology* **61**: 554–556.

81. Kristensen B, Malm J, Fagerland M, *et al.* (1996). Regional cerebral blood flow, white matter abnormalities, and cerebrospinal fluid hydrodynamics in patients with idiopathic adult hydrocephalus syndrome. *J Neurol Neurosurg Psychiatry* **60**: 282–288.

82. Waldemar G, Schmidt JF, Delecluse F, *et al.* (1993). High resolution SPECT with [99mTc]-d,l-HMPAO in normal pressure hydrocephalus before and after shunt operation. *J Neurol Neurosurg Psychiatry* **56**: 655–664.

83. Klinge P, Berding G, Brinker T, *et al.* (2002). Regional cerebral blood flow profiles of shunt-responder in idiopathic chronic hydrocephalus – a 15-O–water PET-study. *Acta Neurochir Supplement* **81**: 47–49.

84. Momjian S, Owler BK, Czosnyka Z, *et al.* (2004). Pattern of white matter regional cerebral blood flow and autoregulation in normal pressure hydrocephalus. *Brain* **127**: 965–972.

85. Gultekin SH, Rosenfeld MR, Voltz R, *et al.* (2000). Paraneoplastic limbic encephalitis: neurological symptoms, immunological findings and tumour association in 50 patients. *Brain* **123**: 1481–1494.

86. Vincent A, Buckley C, Schott JM, *et al.* (2004). Potassium channel antibody-associated encephalopathy: a potentially immunotherapy-responsive form of limbic encephalitis. *Brain* **127**: 701–712.

87. Chinnery PF, Cottrell DA, Birchall D, Griffiths TD (2004). Limbic encephalitis: not a picture to forget. *Neurology* **62**: 1019.

88. Dirr LY, Elster AD, Donofrio PD, Smith M (1990). Evolution of brain MRI abnormalities in limbic encephalitis. *Neurology* **40**: 1304–1306.

89. Geschwind MD, Tan KM, Lennon VA, *et al.* (2008). Voltage-gated potassium channel autoimmunity mimicking Creutzfeldt–Jakob disease. *Arch Neurol* **65**: 1341–1346.

90. Steiner I (2011). Herpes simplex virus encephalitis: new infection or reactivation? *Curr Opin Neurol* **24**: 268–274.

91. Ch'ien LT, Boehm RM, Robinson H, Liu C, Frenkel LD (1977). Characteristic early electroencephalographic changes in herpes simplex encephalitis. *Arch Neurol* **34**: 361–364.

92. Upton A, Gumpert J (1970). Electroencephalography in diagnosis of herpes-simplex encephalitis. *Lancet* **1**: 650–652.

93. Sechi G, Serra A (2007). Wernicke's encephalopathy: new clinical settings and recent advances in diagnosis and management. *Lancet Neurol* **6**: 442–455.

94. American Psychiatric Association (1994). *Diagnostic and Statistical Manual of Mental Disorders (DSM-IV)*. Washington, DC: American Psychiatric Press.

95. Caso F, Fiorino A, Falautano M, *et al.* (2010). Treatment of Wernicke's encephalopathy with high dose of thiamine in a patient with pyloric sub-stenosis: description of a case. *Neurol Sci* **31**: 859–861.

96. Erkinjuntti T, Gauthier S (2009). The concept of vascular cognitive impairment. *Front Neurol Neurosci* **24**: 79–85.

97. Barkhof F, Fox NC, Bastos Leite AJ, Scheltens P (2011). *Neuroimaging in Dementia*. Berlin: Springer.

98. Bastos Leite AJ, van Straaten EC, Scheltens P, Lycklama G, Barkhof F (2004). Thalamic lesions in vascular dementia: low sensitivity of fluid-attenuated inversion recovery (FLAIR) imaging. *Stroke* **35**: 415–419.

99. Roman GC, Tatemichi TK, Erkinjuntti T, *et al.* (1993) Vascular dementia: diagnostic criteria for research studies. Report of the NINDS-AIREN International Workshop. *Neurology* **43**: 250–260.

100. van Straaten EC, Scheltens P, Knol DL, *et al.* (2003). Operational definitions for the NINDS–AIREN criteria for vascular dementia: an interobserver study. *Stroke* **34**: 1907–1912.

101. Erkinjuntti T, Inzitari D, Pantoni L, *et al.* (2000). Research criteria for subcortical vascular dementia in clinical trials. *J Neural Transm Suppl* **59**: 23–30.

102. Zerr I, Kallenberg K, Summers DM, *et al.* (2009). Updated clinical diagnostic criteria for sporadic Creutzfeldt-Jakob disease. *Brain* **132**: 2659–2668.

103. Paterson RW, Takada LT, Geschwind MD (2012). Diagnosis and treatment of rapidly progressive dementias. *Neurol Clin Pract* **2**: 187–200.

104. Collins SJ, Sanchez-Juan P, Masters CL, *et al.* (2006). Determinants of diagnostic investigation sensitivities across the clinical spectrum of sporadic Creutzfeldt-Jakob disease. *Brain* **129**: 2278–2287.

105. Young GS, Geschwind MD, Fischbein NJ, *et al.* (2005). Diffusion-weighted and fluid-attenuated inversion recovery imaging in Creutzfeldt–Jakob disease: high sensitivity and specificity for diagnosis. *AJNR* **26**: 1551–1562.

106. Vitali P, Maccagnano E, Caverzasi E, *et al.* (2011). Diffusion-weighted MRI hyperintensity patterns differentiate CJD from other rapid dementias. *Neurology* **76**: 1711–1719.

107. Collie DA, Summers DM, Sellar RJ, *et al.* (2003). Diagnosing variant Creutzfeldt–Jakob disease with the pulvinar sign: MR imaging findings in 86 neuropathologically confirmed cases. *AJNR* **24**: 1560–1569.

108. Cummings JL (2004). Alzheimer's disease. *N Engl J Med* **351**: 56–67.

109. Thompson PM, Hayashi KM, de Zubicaray G, *et al.* (2003). Dynamics of gray matter loss in Alzheimer's disease. *J Neurosci* **23**: 994–1005.

110. Alladi S, Xuereb J, Bak T, *et al.* (2007). Focal cortical presentations of Alzheimer's disease. *Brain* **130**: 2636–2645.

111. Crutch SJ, Lehmann M, Schott JM, *et al.* (2012). Posterior cortical atrophy. *Lancet Neurol* **11**: 170–178.

112. Andreasen N, Minthon L, Davidsson P, *et al.* (2001). Evaluation of CSF-tau and CSF-Abeta42 as diagnostic markers for Alzheimer disease in clinical practice. *Arch Neurol* **58**: 373–379.

113. Sunderland T, Linker G, Mirza N, *et al.* (2003). Decreased beta-amyloid1–42 and increased tau levels in cerebrospinal fluid of patients with Alzheimer disease. *JAMA* **289**: 2094–2103.

114. Wattjes MP, Henneman WJ, van der Flier WM, *et al.* (2009). Diagnostic imaging of patients in a memory clinic: comparison of MR imaging and 64-detector row CT. *Radiology* **253**: 174–183.

115. Migliaccio R, Agosta F, Rascovsky K, *et al.* (2009). Clinical syndromes associated with posterior atrophy: early age at onset AD spectrum. *Neurology* **73**: 1571–1578.

116. Whitwell JL, Jack CR, Jr., Kantarci K, *et al.* (2007). Imaging correlates of posterior cortical atrophy. *Neurobiol Aging* **28**: 1051–1061.

117. Kas A, de Souza LC, Samri D, *et al.* (2011). Neural correlates of cognitive impairment in posterior cortical atrophy. *Brain* **134**: 1464–1478.

118. Nestor PJ, Caine D, Fryer TD, Clarke J, Hodges JR (2003). The topography of metabolic deficits in posterior cortical atrophy (the visual variant of Alzheimer's disease) with FDG-PET. *J Neurol Neurosurg Psychiatry* **74**: 1521–1529.

119. Gorno-Tempini ML, Dronkers NF, Rankin KP, *et al.* (2004). Cognition and anatomy in three variants of primary progressive aphasia. *Ann Neurol* **55**: 335–346.

120. Rohrer JD, Ridgway GR, Crutch SJ, *et al.* (2010). Progressive logopenic/phonological aphasia: erosion of the language network. *Neuroimage* **49**: 984–993.

121. Rabinovici GD, Rosen HJ, Alkalay A, *et al.* (2011). Amyloid vs FDG PET in the differential diagnosis of AD and FTLD. *Neurology* **77**: 2034–2042.

122. Herholz K, Ebmeier K (2011). Clinical amyloid imaging in Alzheimer's disease. *Lancet Neurol* **10**: 667–670.

123. Tartaglia MC, Vitali P, Migliaccio R, Agosta F, Rosen H (2010). Neuroimaging in dementia. *Continuum (Minneap Minn)* **16**: 153–175.

124. Braskie MN, Klunder AD, Hayashi KM, *et al.* (2008). Plaque and tangle imaging and cognition in normal aging and Alzheimer's disease. *Neurobiol Aging* **31**: 1669–1678.

125. Rowe CC, Ng S, Ackermann U, *et al.* (2007). Imaging beta-amyloid burden in aging and dementia. *Neurology* **68**: 1718–1725.

126. McKhann GM, Knopman DS, Chertkow H, *et al.* (2011). The diagnosis of dementia due to Alzheimer's disease: recommendations from the National Institute on Aging–Alzheimer's Association workgroups on diagnostic guidelines for Alzheimer's disease. *Alzheimers Dement* **7**: 263–269.

127. Albert MS, DeKosky ST, Dickson D, *et al.* (2011). The diagnosis of mild cognitive impairment due to Alzheimer's disease: recommendations from the National Institute on Aging–Alzheimer's Association workgroups on diagnostic guidelines for Alzheimer's disease. *Alzheimers Dement* **7**: 270–279.

128. Jack CR, Jr., Knopman DS, Jagust WJ, *et al.* (2010). Hypothetical model of dynamic biomarkers of the Alzheimer's pathological cascade. *Lancet Neurol* **9**: 119–128.

129. Rascovsky K, Hodges JR, Knopman D, *et al.* (2011). Sensitivity of revised diagnostic criteria for the behavioural variant of frontotemporal dementia. *Brain* **134**: 2456–2477.

130. Mesulam MM (2001). Primary progressive aphasia. *Ann Neurol* **49**: 425–432.

131. Boccardi M, Sabattoli F, Laakso MP, *et al.* (2005). Frontotemporal dementia as a neural system disease. *Neurobiol Aging* **26**: 37–44.

132. Rosen HJ, Gorno-Tempini ML, Goldman WP, *et al.* (2002). Patterns of brain atrophy in frontotemporal dementia and semantic dementia. *Neurology* **58**: 198–208.

133. Knopman DS, Boeve BF, Parisi JE, *et al.* (2005). Antemortem diagnosis of frontotemporal lobar degeneration. *Ann Neurol* **57**: 480–488.

134. Pijnenburg YA, Mulder JL, van Swieten JC, *et al.* (2008). Diagnostic accuracy of consensus diagnostic criteria for frontotemporal dementia in a memory clinic population. *Dement Geriatr Cogn Disord* **25**: 157–164.

135. Whitwell JL, Przybelski SA, Weigand SD, *et al.* (2009). Distinct anatomical subtypes of the behavioural variant of frontotemporal dementia: a cluster analysis study. *Brain* **132**: 2932–2946.

136. Seeley WW, Crawford R, Rascovsky K, *et al.* (2008). Frontal paralimbic network atrophy in very mild behavioral variant frontotemporal dementia. *Arch Neurol* **65**: 249–255.

137. Hodges JR, Patterson K (2007). Semantic dementia: a unique clinicopathological syndrome. *Lancet Neurol* **6**: 1004–1014.

138. Agosta F, Scola E, Canu E, *et al.* (2012). White matter damage in frontotemporal lobar degeneration spectrum. *Cerebral Cortex* **22**: 2705–2714.

139. Filippi M, Agosta F, Scola E, *et al.* (2012). Functional network connectivity in the behavioral variant of frontotemporal dementia. *Cortex* **49**: 2389–2401.

140. Seeley WW, Allman JM, Carlin DA, *et al.* (2007). Divergent social functioning in behavioral variant frontotemporal dementia and Alzheimer disease: reciprocal networks and neuronal evolution. *Alz Dis Assoc Disord* **21**: S50–57.

141. Agosta F, Sala S, Valsasina P, *et al.* (2013). Brain network connectivity assessed using graph theory in frontotemporal dementia. *Neurology* **81**: 134–143.

Headache

Farooq H. Maniyar and Peter J. Goadsby

Introduction

A significant proportion of patients admitted to the emergency medical wards have headache as a presenting symptom. Usually patients mention an acute, new headache or acute worsening of an existing headache. Headache, or pain in the head as some patients may express it, is one of the most important and common presenting symptoms in neurology. While headache is common and most often benign in presentation, its emergent presentation can signal life-threatening disorders that need immediate attention and pivotally involve neuroimaging. Here we address the major clinical presentations of this crucial acute neurological symptom.

Perhaps the key question in this presentation for clinicians to always ask is the following: "is this thunderclap headache (TCH)?" TCH is defined by the *International Classification of Headache Disorders*, second edition (ICHD-II) as an acute headache reaching maximum intensity within 1 minute [1]. Many patients considered to have or referred to neurology as "thunderclap headache" do not fulfill this diagnostic criteria. It is not enough to ask patients, "is this the worst headache of your life?", rather to enquire about the rapidity of the onset. Thunderclap headache can present as the sole complaint or may be associated with several symptoms including but not limited to nausea, vomiting, photophobia, phonophobia, neck stiffness, altered vision, altered level of consciousness, seizures, and focal neurological symptoms. Here, we discuss the various causes of TCH that an emergency doctor may encounter with particular emphasis on imaging modalities that can be useful in its diagnosis. It should be pointed out right at the outset that the conditions discussed below may present with a more gradual headache not fitting in with the diagnosis of TCH. Therefore, patients may still need a thorough work-up if clinically indicated.

Subarachnoid hemorrhage (SAH)

Up to one-quarter of patients presenting with TCH have SAH; approximately half, including out-of-hospital deaths, die [2]. Therefore, all patients presenting with TCH need a thorough work-up for SAH. The most common cause of SAH is saccular aneurysms (85%). Less common causes include non-aneurysmal perimesencephalic SAH, arterial dissection, arteriovenous malformation, dural arteriovenous fistula, reversible segmental vasoconstriction syndrome, substance abuse, mycotic aneurysms, bleeding disorders, vasculitis, and spinal cord vascular lesions [3, 4].

An unenhanced computer tomography (CT) scan of the brain is the most appropriate first investigation in patients presenting with TCH. The sensitivity of CT to detect SAH depends on several factors – the time of scan after onset of symptoms, the scanner details, and the skill of the reporting professional [5, 6]. Almost all patients can be expected to be diagnosed if scanned within 12 hours of onset on a third-generation scanner and reported by a skilled reader [5]. CT becomes less reliable as time elapses after onset – for example, the sensitivity was 86% on day 2, 76% after 2 days, and 58% after 5 days [5]. Because of these factors, all patients presenting with TCH with a negative CT should be considered for a lumbar puncture to look for the presence of blood products.

CT may show the presence of blood in the subarachnoid space (Figure 4.1). In addition, intracerebral extension is present in 20% to 40% of patients and intraventricular and subdural blood may be seen in 15% to 35% and 2% to 5%, respectively [7]. As well as the presence of subarachnoid blood, CT may help to localize the source and hence the location of the aneurysm if the subarachnoid collections are most dense at one of the classical aneurysm sites. Examples are the anterior interhemispheric cistern (aneurysm of the anterior

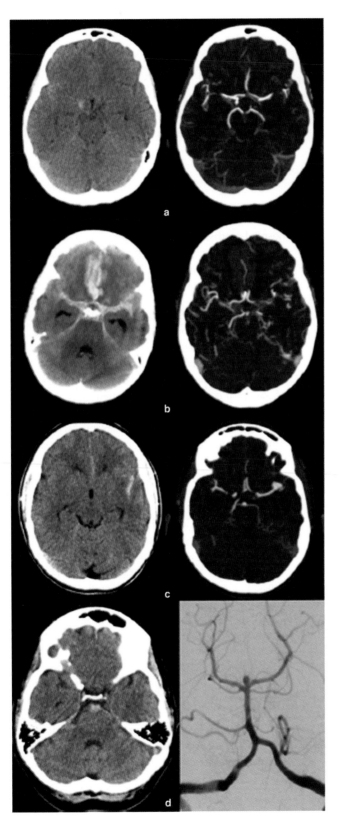

Figure 4.1 Patterns of aneurysmal SAH on unenhanced CT (left) with CT angiography or digital subtraction angiography (DSA) (right) demonstrating the site of aneurysm: (a) posterior communicating artery; (b) anterior communicating artery; (c) middle cerebral artery; (d) terminal basilar artery. Beware a subtle focus of hyperdensity from basilar tip aneurysm mimicking a perimesencephalic hemorrhage (d). Reprinted from Mortimer AM, Bradley MD, Stoodley NG, Renowden SA (2013). Thunderclap headache: diagnostic considerations and neuroimaging features. *Clin Radiol* 68(3): e101–13. Copyright (2013), with permission from Elsevier.

cerebral artery), the suprasellar cistern on one side (aneurysm of the internal carotid artery usually at the origin of the posterior communicating artery), or the most lateral part of the Sylvian fissure (aneurysm of the middle cerebral artery). However, in practice, localization of the source is often difficult, reliable only in the case of a ruptured anterior cerebral artery or anterior communicating artery aneurysm or when SAH is associated with intraparenchymal hematoma [8].

Bleeding from more unusual sites may be more difficult to recognize, for example SAH from rupture of a posterior inferior cerebellar artery aneurysm may be missed on CT [9]. The head CT should be performed with thin cuts through the base of the brain to increase sensitivity for small amounts of blood [10, 11]. Despite this, small SAHs are missed in about half the patients who can be diagnosed by lumbar puncture (LP) [12].

Not all hemorrhages in the basal cisterns are of aneurysmal origin, particularly if the blood is restricted to the interpeduncular, ambient, or the quadrigeminal cisterns. In these cases, this may represent a perimesencephalic SAH, the source of which is usually a venous bleed. The clinical presentation may be different from a typical aneurysmal SAH. The headache may be more gradual and less often associated with loss of consciousness. This type of SAH accounts for 10% of all SAH cases and generally carries a good prognosis. However, with this presentation, a basilar artery aneurysm bleed needs to be ruled out with an angiogram, although basilar artery aneurysms are rare amongst ruptured aneurysms and usually present with more widespread blood in the basal cisterns [13].

If the patient presents a few days after the onset of the TCH, CT may not detect SAH. Magnetic resonance imaging (MRI) can be useful in these cases. T2*-weighted (T2*) and fluid-attenuated inversion recovery (FLAIR) sequences can detect SAH in a high proportion of cases and a practical advantage is that the sensitivity increases after the first 4 days. In one study, T2* MRI detected 94% of cases in the first 4 days and 100% of cases after the first 4 days [14].

Thus, in the acute setting, an unenhanced CT with or without LP, and, where indicated, an MRI scan, will detect the majority of patients with SAH. If diagnostic uncertainty still remains on the basis of a strong history suggestive of SAH, one should proceed to an angiographic study. Once the diagnosis of SAH is made, conventional cerebral angiography with digital subtraction angiography (DSA) is thought to be the gold standard with the highest sensitivity for detection

of cerebral aneurysms [15]. If the initial angiogram is negative, it should be repeated in 4–14 days as the ruptured aneurysm is not always detected on first examination, especially in the presence of large collections of blood in the cisterns. CT angiography (CTA) and magnetic resonance angiography (MRA) are alternatives that can detect aneurysms 3 to 5 mm or larger with a high degree of certainty but they are not as sensitive as conventional angiography.

Unruptured cerebral aneurysm

In retrospective studies, between 10% and 43% of patients with SAH who are cognitively well are able to recall TCH days to weeks prior to SAH [16]. A majority of these headaches occur within 2 weeks of SAH, most of these within 24 hours [17]. This headache is called "sentinel headache," which is not associated with the demonstration of SAH by available diagnostic means. The cause of this headache is not clear but may include SAH in very small amounts or stretching or other physical changes to the wall of the aneurysm. Sentinel headache can potentially warn of impending SAH and hence timely treatment can prevent SAH. However, the prevalence of sentinel headache is based on retrospective recollection by those who have had SAH and is hence open to recall bias. Also, cerebral aneurysms occur in 3.2% of the population and hence some of these aneurysms will be incidental [18]. Therefore, if the initial work-up for SAH is negative, the question remains: "is this a sentinel headache warning of impending SAH, such that the patient needs an angiogram?" Although there is no clear evidence, we think that if the history is typical for TCH, a CT angiogram or MRI angiogram is advisable given the morbidity and mortality of SAH.

Cerebral venous sinus thrombosis (CVST)

CVST usually presents with gradually worsening headache associated with focal neurological symptoms or signs: papilledema, an altered level of consciousness, and seizures in varying combinations. Usually patients have risk factors including pregnancy, dehydration, thrombophilia, cancer, oral contraceptives, and head trauma [19]. However, about one-quarter of patients with CVST may present with headache only as the presenting symptom [19]. Some 2–10% of patients may present with TCH [20, 21]. Hence, CVST should be in the differential diagnosis of TCH, particularly if risk factors are present. If LP is done for the work-up of TCH, a raised cerebrospinal fluid (CSF) opening pressure may be a hint towards the possibility of CVST and hence the opening pressure should always be measured [20].

An unenhanced CT is likely to be normal in CVST without focal neurological signs but can be abnormal when such signs are present. In one study, up to two-thirds of patients had abnormal unenhanced CT in the acute setting. The changes may include hyperdensities suggestive of thrombosed cortical veins or dural sinuses [22]. A more subtle finding is a low-density signal in the dural sinus representative of a subacute thrombus. Absence of signal void and changes in signal intensity are characteristic changes of sinus thrombosis in MRI but these signs are variable depending on the age of the thrombus. T2* sequences may be more useful when T1 and T2 changes are equivocal by T1- or T2-weighted imaging. Blood breakdown products can produce blooming artifacts in the thrombosed sinuses detected on T2*. Finally MRI and CT venography has similar sensitivity for detecting CVST [23] (Figure 4.2).

It is useful to remember that patients with CVST may also have SAH detected on LP. In one series this occurred in half the cases [24]. Therefore, positive LP for SAH should prompt investigations for CVST if risk factors are present or in the setting where investigations are negative for a cerebral aneurysm.

Reversible cerebral vasoconstriction syndrome (RCVS)

RCVS is a group of conditions presenting with a single or multiple episodes of thunderclap headache with or without other neurological symptoms. RCVS is associated with reversible narrowing of intracerebral arteries [25]. Various names are in use, which probably include the same syndrome, such as post-partum angiopathy, benign angiopathy of the central nervous system (CNS), Call–Fleming syndrome, and drug-induced vasospasm. Various drugs have been implicated including cocaine, cannabis, selective serotonin reuptake inhibitors (SSRIs), nasal decongestants, and nicotine patches [26, 27]. RCVS is also noted to occur in the setting of a catecholamine-secreting tumor, and also without a readily identifiable cause [25].

The initial CT or MRI may not show any abnormality in more than half the patients presenting with this condition [26]. However, the majority develop one or more of ischemic infarctions, convexity SAH, lobar intracerebral hemorrhage (ICH), or brain edema (Figure 4.3). Isolated ischemic infarction is the most common lesion seen followed by isolated convexity SAH and isolated ICH. Rarely, ICH may coexist with SAH or infarction. The infarction or hemorrhages are typically seen in the watershed areas and edematous regions. These lesions are more common in the posterior supratentorial brain in a pattern consistent with posterior reversible encephalopathy syndrome (PRES) with which it can overlap in 10% of cases [26, 27]. Angiographic studies typically show smooth or tapered narrowing followed by normal-caliber or dilated intracerebral arteries; the findings can be bilateral and multifocal. The extracranial arteries are usually not affected. The angiographic study (DSA, CTA, or MRA) may be normal in the first 4–5 days. Therefore, if strong clinical suspicion remains, imaging should be repeated. The abnormalities usually normalize within 3 months. CSF studies are usually normal [25].

In the acute setting it may be difficult to differentiate RCVS from cerebral vasculitis. The CSF is more likely to be abnormal in cerebral vasculitis. Recent work suggests high-resolution, contrast-enhanced vessel wall MRI with flow compensation and fat saturation may be useful to differentiate between the two [28].

Therefore, if the initial CT and LP are negative for SAH, one should consider RCVS if risk factors are present or if TCH has been recurrent. An angiographic study, CTA or MRA, is indicated in such cases with a repeat in due course if normal.

Spontaneous intracranial hypotension (SIH)

SIH classically presents with a postural or orthostatic headache, i.e., worse in the upright position and better in supine position, although the postural element may become less distinct with time. Usually, the postural headache is associated with other symptoms like neck stiffness, hypacusis, and tinnitus. In patients with a personal or family history of migraine, migrainous features such as photophobia or phonophobia may be present. The mechanism is thought to be a dural tear leading to CSF leak. Although the term SIH suggests reduction in intracranial pressure, the CSF pressure may be normal on repeated measures [29] and the pathogenic mechanism may well be related to reduction in volume rather than pressure. In one series, 14% of patients with SIH presented with TCH [30].

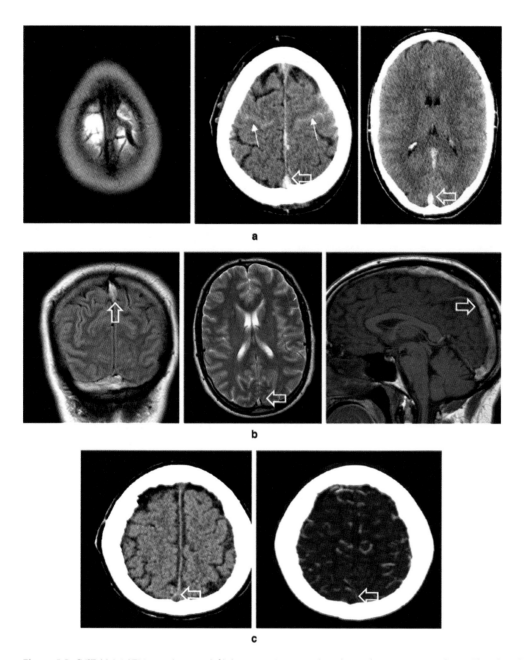

Figure 4.2 CVST. (a) Axial T2 image (top row, left) demonstrating acute thrombus in the superior sagittal sinus. The relatively low signal of acute thrombus mimics flow void and can be difficult to appreciate. Unenhanced CT images (center and right) in another patient demonstrating bilateral hyperdensity in the subarachnoid space suggestive of secondary SAH (arrows) with hyperdensity noted in the superior sagittal sinus representative of acute thrombus (open arrows). (b) Coronal FLAIR (left), axial T2 (middle), and sagittal T1 (right) images demonstrating subacute thrombus in the superior sagittal sinus (arrows). (c) Axial unenhanced CT (left) and CT venogram (right) demonstrating the low density of subacute thrombus in the superior sagittal sinus, difficult to distinguish from normal appearances if not alert to this possibility (arrows). Reprinted from Mortimer AM, Bradley MD, Stoodley NG, Renowden SA (2013). Thunderclap headache: diagnostic considerations and neuroimaging features. *Clin Radiol* 68(3): e101–13. Copyright (2013), with permission from Elsevier.

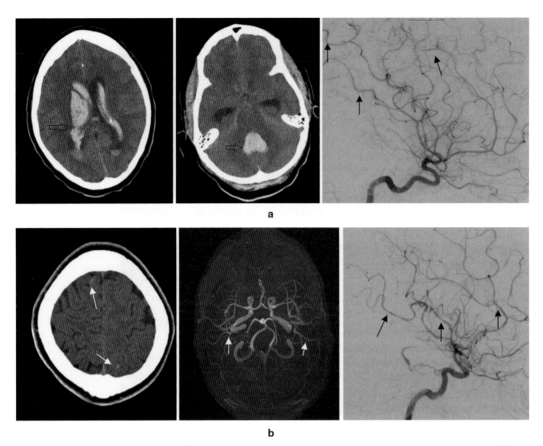

a

b

Figure 4.3 RCVS. (a) Post-partum headache and subsequent collapse in a 30-year-old woman. Axial unenhanced CT (left and center) demonstrates parenchymal hemorrhage (arrows) dissecting into the ventricles with secondary obstructive hydrocephalus. DSA (right) demonstrating areas of narrowing with subsequent vessel dilatation. (b) Acute headache following recreational use of cocaine. Axial unenhanced CT (left) demonstrates small areas of convexity SAH (arrows). Time-of-flight MRA (center) shows subtle vessel irregularity and DSA (right) confirms this, demonstrating multiple areas of vessel narrowing and dilatation. Reprinted from Mortimer, AM, Bradley, MD, Stoodley, NG, Renowden, SA (2012). Thunderclap headache: diagnostic considerations and neuroimaging features. *Clin Radiol* 68(3): e101–13. Copyright (2013), with permission from Elsevier.

Following a normal CT, a low opening pressure during LP may be a hint towards SIH. The ideal investigation is MRI with contrast. The typical finding is diffuse dural enhancement with gadolinium seen on a T1-weighted MRI scan [31] (Figure 4.4). This is thought to reflect the compensatory increase in venous blood volume secondary to reduction to CSF volume in keeping with the Monroe–Kellie doctrine. Pituitary enlargement due to hyperemia may also be seen for the same reason. However, up to 20% may not have dural enhancement on MRI [32]. Other changes on MRI include sagging of the brain, flattening of the anterior portion of the pons, reduction in ventricle size, and downward displacement of the optic chiasm [31]. Subdural collections may occur in 17–60% of patients [33].

The majority of patients improve conservatively, or with intravenous caffeine, while 36–57% respond to a "blind" lumbar epidural patch [34, 35]. Therefore, investigations for demonstrations of CSF leak and the site of the leak may be reserved for patients who do not respond to conservative measures, or one or more lumbar epidural blood patches. A spinal MRI scan may show signs suggestive of a CSF leak including extra-arachnoid fluid collections (often extending across several levels), extra-dural extravasations of fluid (extending to paraspinal soft tissues), meningeal diverticula, CSF leaks around nerve roots, spinal pachymeningeal enhancement, and engorgement of the spinal epidural venous plexus. The level of the leak may also be identified [36]. Short tau inversion recovery (STIR) may be better than T2-weighted

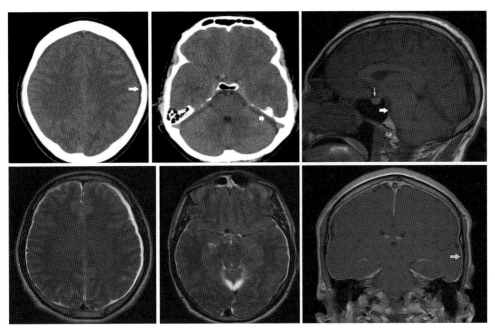

Figure 4.4 SIH. Axial CT and sagittal T1 (top row) plus axial T2, and contrast-enhanced coronal T1 images (bottom row) in a patient with SIH. Note the subdural collections on CT with effacement of the suprasellar cistern in keeping with brain sagging. This is confirmed on the sagittal images, with loss of the prepontine cistern. Note also mild pituitary enlargement. Subdural hygromas are confirmed on T2 images, and dural enhancement is demonstrated on the contrast-enhanced T1 images. Reprinted from Mortimer, AM, Bradley, MD, Stoodley, NG, Renowden, SA (2012). Thunderclap headache: diagnostic considerations and neuroimaging features. *Clin Radiol* 68(3): e101–13. Copyright (2013), with permission from Elsevier.

imaging in demonstrating the extra-dural extravasations of CSF. Sensitivity of spinal MRI in diagnosing low CSF volume states may be as high as 94% [37].

Various methods have been used to demonstrate the exact site of the CSF leak. CT myelography has been widely used and considered by some as the diagnostic test of choice [38, 39]. However, the dural puncture required for the procedure can potentially aggravate the symptoms of SIH and may be challenging to do in the presence of a collapsed dural sac. Also, ionizing X-irradiation and exposure to iodinated contrast medium may be concerns. CT myelography is not ideal for follow-up scans if required. One may also need to do a delayed scan for slow flow or intermittent leaks. A non-invasive alternative is heavily T2-weighted MRI myelography using a single-shot fast spin-echo (SSFSE) sequence and prolonged echo time or equivalent. A study comparing MRI and CT myelography showed comparable results for the detection of spinal CSF leaks along nerve roots, high-spinal retro-spinal CSF collections, and epidural CSF collections [40]. Evaluation of axial views can give information regarding both the level and the specific site of the CSF leak. Multiple spontaneous CSF leaks are common. Another

option is radioisotope cisternography, which involves LP to introduce a radioisotope in the CSF space. A study comparing radioisotope cisternography and MRI myelography in 15 patients with clinical symptoms of SIH showed comparable results for the two methods. Sensitivity was 86.7% for MRI myelography and 93% for radioisotope cisternography. In another study using MRI with intrathecal gadolinium the site of the leak was identified in nine out of fourteen patients [41]. It should be noted that the intrathecal use of gadolinium-based MRI contrast is not Food and Drug Administration (FDA)-approved and would be an off-label use in the United States [42].

We therefore feel in patients not responding to conservative measures and one or more "blind" lumbar epidural blood patches, one should undertake investigations to locate the exact site of CSF leak to facilitate targeted blood-patch or surgical repair. We feel MRI myelography should be tried first since it is non-invasive yet effective. If this fails to detect the site of the leak, CT myelography, MRI with intrathecal gadolinium, or radioisotope cisternography may be considered, although in our experience the latter has not often been very useful.

Pituitary apoplexy

Pituitary apoplexy occurs due to hemorrhage or infarction in the pituitary gland. Pituitary apoplexy can present with TCH with or without SAH [43]. Symptom scan be mild to severe including coma and death. This can occur in the setting of a pituitary adenoma but commonly occurs in patients with no known pituitary disease [44]. Common circumstances in which pituitary apoplexy is known to occur include pregnancy, bromocriptine therapy, general anesthesia, and pituitary irradiation. An acute CT frequently shows hyperintensity in the pituitary fossa and MRI shows an altered signal, the nature of which depends on the age of the hemorrhage.

Colloid cyst of the third ventricle

Headache is the most common symptom of a colloid cyst of the third ventricle, reported by 68–100 % of patients [45]. Typically the headache is abrupt in onset, endures for seconds to a day, and resolves quickly [46]. Often the pain is relieved by recumbency.

Associated features include nausea, vomiting, loss of consciousness, seizures, coma, and death.

Both CT and MRI may be used for diagnosis. Most colloid cysts are oval or rounded and located at the foramen of Monro. Typically, they are hyperdense on CT (Figure 4.5) but may be isodense or hypodense. On MRI, most are hyperintense on T1-weighted images (from methemoglobin) but may be isointense or hypointense. On T2-weighted images most are hypointense.

Cervical artery dissection

Headache is the most common symptom of cervical artery dissection. Headache is reported by 60–95% of patients with carotid artery dissection and 70% of patients with vertebral artery dissection [47]. In around 20% the headache can be TCH [48]. Headache is commonly associated with focal neurological symptoms of a stroke but may precede these symptoms or occur in isolation. The CT and LP are usually normal when headache is not accompanied by other neurological symptoms. Diagnosis can be based

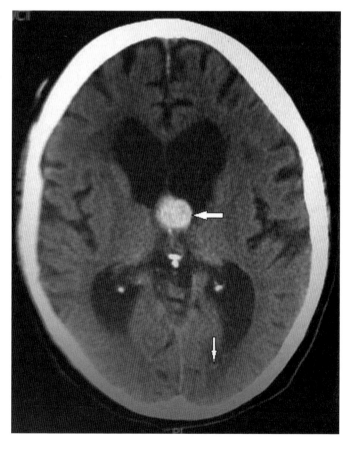

Figure 4.5 Non-contrast brain CT demonstrating a hyperdense colloid cyst (horizontal arrow) with evidence of intraventricular hemorrhage (hyperdensity in the dependent portion of the occipital horns of lateral ventricles, vertical arrow). Reproduced from Ogbodo E, Kaliaperumal C, Bermingham N, O'Sullivan M (2012). Spontaneous haemorrhage and rupture of third ventricular colloid cyst. *BMJ Case Rep*: Sep 3. With permission from BMJ Publishing Group Ltd.

on ultrasound, although ultrasound may be inadequate due to its limited coverage, CTA, or MRA. MRI of the neck with a fat-saturation protocol may show the characteristic partial circumferential appearance of methemoglobin in the wall of the vessel in the subacute stages of dissection.

Acute hypertensive crisis

There are a few case reports of TCH being the main presenting symptom of hypertensive crisis or PRES [49, 50]. Usually, PRES presents with a reduced level of consciousness, visual symptoms, and seizures. The pathophysiology of PRES is thought to be the failure of cerebral autoregulation leading to vasogenic edema, secondary to endothelial damage in the setting of acute rise in blood pressure. The posterior circulation is more commonly involved. The initial CT scan may be abnormal in about half the patients ultimately showing hypodensity in the posterior areas [51]. The typical MRI changes are hyperintense lesions on T2-weighted imaging seen over the parieto-occipital and posterior frontal cortex, and the subcortical white matter. Rarely, the brainstem, basal ganglia, and the cerebellum may be involved. Hemorrhage, contrast enhancement, and restricted diffusion are atypical but noted [52]. PRES may be associated with angiographic changes seen in RCVS.

Retroclival hematoma

Retroclival hematoma (RCH) may present with TCH. RCH may rarely occur in neck injuries causing atlanto-axial dislocations [53]. Spontaneous RCH may occur in the setting of dural-based meningeal tumors or arteriovenous fistula [54]. MRI with gadolinium contrast and cerebral angiography with selective external carotid artery injection have been recommended for diagnosis [55].

Acute ischemic stroke

One-quarter of patients with acute stroke have headache, half of which develop before other manifestations of stroke [56]. Although most patients with stroke-related headache do not present with TCH, this may occur rarely. There is a case report of a patient with bilateral cerebellar infarcts presenting with TCH as the main complaint [57]. CT is often normal. MRI with diffusion-weighted sequences is recommended for the diagnosis.

Other causes of acute headache

Conditions like meningitis, brain abscess, brain tumors, adult aqueductal stenosis, intracerebral hemorrhage and subdural hematoma can also present with an acute headache which may or may not be TCH [58–61]. These conditions are usually associated with other neurological symptoms and signs, including fever, rash, focal neurological symptoms/signs, reduced level of consciousness, and seizures. Both CT and MRI may detect the abnormality.

Lastly, one should also keep in mind that the cause for the acute headache presentation may be a primary headache disorder, most often migraine. Indications for imaging in migraine include a change in quality of headache including TCH, unresponsiveness to therapy, and development of other neurological symptoms atypical for migraine aura, which are suggestive of focal parenchymal brain involvement. Migraine is a common disorder and therefore, from time to time, one can expect to encounter other pathology in migraine patients presenting with headache.

To conclude, in an emergency setting, assessing the rapidity of headache onset, i.e. if the headache is a TCH, is a useful way to plan investigations and manage patients. However, patients exhibiting the conditions we have discussed above may present with a headache that may not peak in 1 or several minutes, i.e. not truly TCH. If other clinical pointers are present a thorough work-up is still required.

References

1. Headache Classification Committee of the International Headache Society (2004). The international classification of headache disorders. *Cephalalgia* **24**(supp 1): 1–151.

2. Hop JW, Rinkel GJE, Algra A, van Gijn J (1997). Case–fatality rates and functional outcome after subarachnoid hemorrhage: a systematic review. *Stroke* **28**: 660–664.

3. Rinkel GJ, van Gijn J, Wijdicks EF (1993). Subarachnoid haemorrhage without detectable aneurysm. A review of the causes. *Stroke* **24**: 1403–1409.

4. van Gijn J, Rinkel GJE (2001). Subarachnoid haemorrhage: diagnosis, causes and management. *Brain* **124**: 249–278.

5. van Gijn J, van Dongen KJ (1982). The time course of aneurysmal haemorrhage on computed tomograms. *Neuroradiology* **23**: 153–156.

6. Hutchinson PJ, Kirkpatrick PJ (2012). Diagnosing subarachnoid hemorrhage: are CT scans enough? *Nat Rev Neurol* **10**: 126–127.

7. Latchaw RE (1997). The role of CT following aneurysmal rupture. *Neuroimaging Clin N Am* **7**: 693–708.

8. VanderJagt M (1999). Validity of prediction of the site of ruptured intracranial aneurysms with CT. *Neurology* **52**: 34–39.

9. Ruelle A, Cavazzani P, Andrioli G (1988). Extracranial posterior inferior cerebellar artery aneurysm causing isolated intraventricular hemorrhage: a case report. *Neurosurgery* **23**: 774–777.

10. Schmid UD, Steiger HJ, Huber P (1987). Accuracy of high resolution computed tomography in direct diagnosis of cerebral aneurysms. *Neuroradiology* **29**: 152–159.

11. Latchaw RE (1997). The role of CT following aneurysmal rupture. *Neuroimaging Clin N Am* **7**: 693–708.

12. Leblanc R (1987). The minor leak preceding subarachnoid hemorrhage. *J Neurosurg* **66**: 35–39.

13. VanGijn J, VanDongen KJ, Vermeulen M, Hijdra A (1985). Perimesencephalic hemorrhage: a nonaneurysmal and benign form of subarachnoid hemorrhage. *Neurology* **35**: 493–497.

14. Mitchell P, Wilkinson ID, Hoggard N, *et al* (2001). Detection of subarachnoid haemorrhage with magnetic resonance imaging. *J Neurol Neurosurg Psychiatry* **70**: 205–211.

15. Bederson JB, Connolly ES Jr, Batjer HH, *et al.* (2009). Guidelines for the management of aneurysmal subarachnoid hemorrhage: a statement for healthcare professionals from a special writing group of the Stroke Council, American Heart Association. *Stroke* **40**: 994–1025.

16. Polmear A (2003). Sentinel headaches in aneurysmal subarachnoid hemorrhage: what is the true incidence? A systematic review. *Cephalalgia* **23**: 935–941.

17. de Falco FA (2004). Sentinel headache. *Neurol Sci* **25**(suppl 3): S215–S217.

18. Vlak MHM, Algra A, Brandenburg R, Rinkel GJE (2011). Prevalence of unruptured intracranial aneurysms, with emphasis on sex, age, comorbidity, country, and time period: a systematic review and meta-analysis. *Lancet Neurol* **10**: 626–636.

19. Saposnik G, Barinagarrementeria F, Brown RD, *et al.* (2011). Diagnosis and management of cerebral venous thrombosis: a statement for healthcare professionals from the American Heart Association/American Stroke Association. *Stroke* **42**: 1158–1192.

20. de Bruijn SF, Stam J, Kappelle LJ, for the CVST study group (1996). Thunderclap headache as the first symptom of cerebral venous sinus thrombosis. *Lancet* **348**: 1623–1625.

21. Cumurcic R, Crassard I, Sarov M, *et al.* (2005). Headache as the only neurological sign of cerebral venous thrombosis: a series of 17 cases. *J Neurol Neurosurg Psychiatry* **76**: 1084–1087.

22. Roland T, Jacobs J, Rappaport A, *et al.* (2010). Unenhanced brain CT is useful to decide on further imaging in suspected venous sinus thrombosis. *Clin Radiol* **65**: 34–39.

23. Leach JL, Fortuna RB, Jones BV, *et al.* (2006). Imaging of cerebral venous thrombosis: current techniques, spectrum of findings, and diagnostic pitfalls. *RadioGraphics* **26**: S19–43.

24. Oppenheim C, Domigo V, Gauvrit JY, *et al.* (2005). Subarachnoid hemorrhage as the initial presentation of dural sinus thrombosis. *AJNR* **26**: 614–617.

25. Calabrese LH, Dodick DW, Schwedt TJ, Singhal AB (2007). Narrative review: reversible cerebral vasoconstriction syndromes. *Ann Intern Med* **146**: 34–44.

26. Shinghal AB, Hajj-Ali RA, Topcuoglu MA, *et al.* (2011). Reversible cerebral vasoconstriction syndromes: analysis of 139 cases. *Arch Neurol* **68**: 1005–1012.

27. Ducros A, Boukobza M, Porcher R, *et al.* (2007). The clinical and radiological spectrum of reversible cerebral vasoconstriction syndrome. A prospective series of 67 patients. *Brain* **130**: 3091–3101.

28. Mandell DM, Matouk CC;, Farb RI, *et al.* (2012). Vessel wall MRI to differentiate between reversible cerebral vasoconstriction syndrome and central nervous system vasculitis: preliminary results. *Stroke* **43**: 860–862.

29. Mokri B (2000). Cerebrospinal fluid volume depletion and its emerging clinical/imaging syndromes. *Neurosurg Focus* **9**: e6.

30. Schievink WI, Wijdicks EF, Meyer FB, *et al.* (2001). Spontaneous intracranial hypotension mimicking aneurysmal subarachnoid hemorrhage. *Neurosurgery* **48**: 513–516.

31. Spelle L, Boulin A, Tainturier C, *et al.* (2001). Neuroimaging features of spontaneous intracranial hypotension. *Neuroradiology* **43**: 622–627.

32. Mokri B (1999). Spontaneous cerebrospinal fluid leaks: from intracranial hypotension to cerebrospinal fluid hypovolemia – evolution of a concept *Mayo Clin Proc* **74**: 1113–1123.

33. McKinney AM, Short J, Truwit CL, *et al.* (2007). Posterior reversible encephalopathy syndrome: incidence of atypical regions of involvement and imaging findings. *AJR* **189**: 904–912.

34. Sencakova D, Mokri B, McClelland RL (2001). The efficacy of epidural blood patch in spontaneous CSF leaks. *Neurology* **57**: 1921–1923.

35. Berroir S, Loisel B, Ducros A, *et al.* (2004). Early epidural blood patch in spontaneous intracranial hypotension. *Neurology* **63**: 1950–1951.

36. Tomoda Y, Korogi Y, Aoki T, *et al.* (2008). Detection of cerebrospinal fluid leakage: initial experience with three-dimensional fast spin-echo magnetic resonance myelography. *Acta Radiol* **49**: 197–203.

37. Watanabe A, Horikoshi T, Uchida M, *et al.* (2009). Diagnostic value of spinal MR imaging in spontaneous intracranial hypotension syndrome. *AJNR* **30**: 147–151.

38. Schievink WI (2006). Spontaneous spinal CSF leaks and intracranial hypotension. *JAMA* **295**: 2286–2296.

39. Mokri B (2003). Headaches caused by decreased intracranial pressure: diagnosis and management. *Curr Opin Neurol* **16**: 319–326.

40. Wang YF, Lirng JF, Fuh JL, Hseu SS, Wang SJ (2009). Heavily T2-weighted MR myelography vs. CT myelography in spontaneous intracranial hypotension. *Neurology* **73**: 1892–1898.

41. Vanopdenbosch LJ, Dedeken P, Casselman JW, Vlaminc SA (2011). MRI with intrathecal gadolinium to detect a CSF leak: a prospective open-label cohort study. *J Neurol Neurosurg Psychiatry* **82**: 456–458.

42. Dillon WP (2008). Intrathecal gadolinium: its time has come? *AJNR* **29**: 3–4

43. van Gijn J, Rinkel GJ (2001). Subarachnoid haemorrhage: diagnosis, causes and management. *Brain* **124**: 249–278.

44. Schwedt TJ, Matharu MS, Dodick DW (2006). Thunderclap headache. *LancetNeurol* **5**: 621–631.

45. Young WB, Silberstein SD (1997). Paroxysmal headache caused by colloid cyst of the third ventricle: case report and review of the literature. *Headache* **37**: 15–20.

46. Kelly R (1951). Colloid cysts of the third ventricle: analysis of twenty-nine cases. *Brain* **74**: 23–65.

47. Silbert PL, Mokri B, Schievink WI (1995). Headache and neck pain in spontaneous internal carotid and vertebral artery dissections. *Neurology* **45**: 1517–1522.

48. Mitsias P, Ramadan NM (1992). Headache in ischemic cerebrovascular disease. Part I:clinical features. *Cephalalgia* **12**: 269–274.

49. Tang-Wai DF, Phan TG, Wijdicks EF (2001). Hypertensive encephalopathy presenting with thunderclap headache. *Headache* **41**: 198–200.

50. Dodick DW, Eross EJ, Drazkowski JF, *et al* (2003). Thunderclap headache associated with reversible vasospasm and posterior leukoencephalopathy syndrome. *Cephalalgia* **23**: 994–997.

51. McKinney AM, Short J, Truwit CL, *et al.* (2007). Posterior reversible encephalopathy syndrome: incidence of atypical regions of involvement and imaging findings. *AJR* **189**: 904–912.

52. Hefzya HM, Bartynskib WS, Boardmanb JF, *et al.* (2009). Hemorrhage in posterior reversible encephalopathy syndrome: imaging and clinical features. *AJNR* **30**: 1371–1379.

53. Kurosu A, Amano K, Kubo O, *et al.* (1990). Clivus epidural hematoma. *J Neurosurg* **72**: 660–662.

54. Tomaras C, Horowitz BL, Harper RL (1995). Spontaneous clivus hematoma: case report and literature review. *Neurosurgery* **37**: 123–124.

55. Schievink WI, Thompson RC, Loh CT, Maya MM (2001). Spontaneous retroclival hematoma presenting as thunderclap headache. *J Neurosurg* **95**: 522524.

56. Ferro JM, Melo TP, Oliveira V, *et al.* (1995). A multivariate study of headache associated with ischemic stroke. *Headache* **35**: 315–319.

57. Schwedt TJ, Dodick DW (2006). Thunderclap stroke: embolic cerebellar infarcts presenting as thunderclap headache. *Headache* **46**: 520–522.

58. Lamonte M, Silberstein SD, Marcelis JF (1995). Headache associated withaseptic meningitis. *Headache* **35**: 520–526.

59. Evans RW (2007). Thunderclap headache associated with a nonhemorrhagic anaplastic oligodendroglioma. *MedGenMed* **9**: 26.

60. Mucchiut M, Valentinis L, Tuniz F, *et al.* (2007). Adult aqueductal stenosis presenting as thunderclap headache: a case report. *Cephalalgia* **27**: 1171–1173.

61. Kotwica Z, Brezinski J (1985). Chronic subdural hematoma presenting as spontaneous subarachnoid hemorrhage. Report of six cases. *J Neurosurg* **63**: 691–692.

Back pain

Timothy J. Amrhein, Jon P. Jennings, Christine M. Carr, and Walter S. Bartynski

Introduction

Low-back pain (LBP) is a common presenting complaint to the primary care physician and in the emergency department. In the majority of cases, symptoms arise from benign conditions that do not merit emergent imaging studies. There are several causes, however, which may lead to disability or death if not promptly identified and treated including epidural abscess, discitis/osteomyelitis, unstable spinal fracture, cord-compressive metastasis, and expanding/leaking abdominal aortic aneurysm (AAA). It is important for physicians to maintain a high index of suspicion for these potentially devastating pathologies and to be able to discern these from more benign causes of back pain. It is also important that primary care and emergency department physicians do not over-utilize diagnostic imaging in patients without appropriate clinical indications, as this leads to increased costs, unnecessary radiation exposure, and can potentially result in unnecessary interventions or undue psychological distress. Satisfying these obligations requires a systematic approach that relies on historical and clinical features to guide appropriate use of imaging resources.

In this chapter, we will outline a clinical paradigm approach to the patient who presents with acute LBP. This will include identifying relevant factors in the clinical history, examination, and laboratory features that are important in the diagnosis of a patient with acute LBP all of which enable the physician to establish an initial differential diagnosis. We will also review an approach to imaging in these patients and emphasize how individual imaging tests can help to refine the diagnosis, and result in a specific diagnosis, in most patients.

Clinical approach/algorithm

Most new-onset or acute LBP resolves spontaneously. In work-related acute LBP, improvement with return to work is seen in 50% of patients in the first 12 days, 85% at 6 weeks, and 95% at 12 weeks with approximately 5% continuing with pain and not returning to work after 3 months [1, 2]. Strict, conservative management including a short course of bed rest is effective in early control of acute LBP [3]. These clinical trends are important to consider when assessing the patient with new-onset significant LBP and deciding on a course of evaluation and management.

The lower spine is made up of five lumbar segments containing the intervertebral disk spaces, bilateral facet joints, and the sacrum. With the addition of the sacroiliac joints (SIJs) there are 17 joints and eight distinct bones (five vertebrae, the sacrum, and two iliac bones) to assess in the average patient. In addition, a complex arrangement of muscles (spinal erectae, multifidis) span and cross between the transverse processes, facet joints, lamina, and the sacroiliac region, any of which could develop primary injury or secondary spasm. These anatomic structures lie in close proximity to each other, work together to facilitate spine motion, and may develop pathological change in isolation or together as a group. Even without the added challenge of a larger body habitus, the lower back is not a simple system to physically examine or evaluate.

With age, progressive spine degenerative changes occur [4, 5] and can be identified on routine radiographs, computed tomographic (CT) imaging and magnetic resonance imaging (MRI) [6–8]. These common degenerative changes are typically asymptomatic and therefore may be an underlying presence in patients who develop superimposed causes of urgent

Chapter 5

Imaging Acute Neurologic Disease, ed. Massimo Filippi and Jack H. Simon. Published by Cambridge University Press.

acute LBP (i.e. infection, fracture, and tumor). However, these degenerative changes may also, themselves, be the cause of new, acute LBP. An acute or repetitive biomechanical stress, challenge, or injury to pre-existing degenerative spine structures can lead to new onset and therefore perceived "acute" LBP.

The choice of imaging modality is dependent upon the particular clinical question posed as well as patient-dependent factors. Routine radiographs may be conveniently available, but are less sensitive to bone loss and subtle fracture compared with CT. MRI may be preferred for cord compression/injury or cauda equina compression, but the presence of a contraindicated device (pacemaker, certain metallic implants) or

condition (orbital metallic foreign body) might prevent the examination.

In systematically assessing back pain the medical provider must consider the nature of the pain, duration, relevant history and risk factors, and, in particular, noted "red flags" [9–11]. Generally, patients presenting with acute back pain are first risk stratified into one of two broad categories: traumatic (traumatic fracture, osteoporotic vertebral compression fracture (VCF)), or atraumatic (Figure 5.1).

In addition to the standard physical examination, all LBP patients should undergo focused neurologic testing of lower extremity strength, reflexes, and sensation. Further, efforts should be taken to

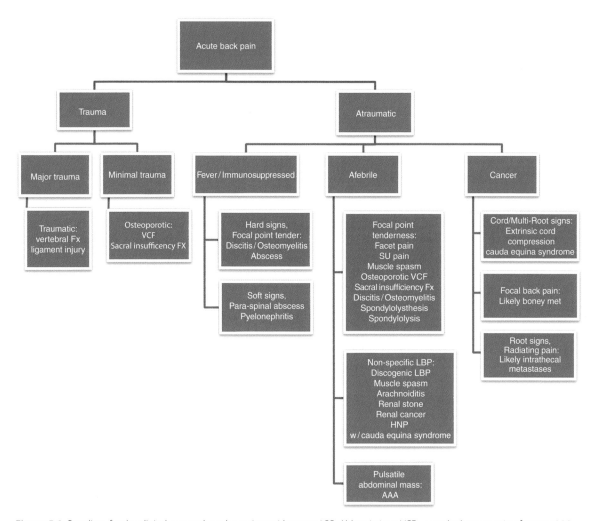

Figure 5.1 Paradigm for the clinical approach to the patient with severe LBP. Abbreviations: VCF – vertebral compression fracture; AAA – abdominal aortic aneurysm; HNP – herniated nucleus pulposus; Fx – fracture; SIJ – sacroiliac joint

characterize the LBP as low risk or high risk (pain secondary to trauma, symptoms of cord compression or cauda equina syndrome, history of cancer, osteoporosis or prolonged corticosteroid use, systemic illness or immune-suppression, or risk factors for AAA).

Patients who present with LBP secondary to trauma must be assessed for point tenderness, deformity, and neurological signs and symptoms. In the obtunded trauma patient with concern for spinal injury, a digital rectal examination must be performed to assess for sphincter laxity. In the absence of neurological findings, patients with suspected fractures are evaluated preferentially with CT or with plain radiographs if CT cannot be immediately obtained. In contradistinction, trauma patients with new neurologic symptoms will require emergent MRI for evaluation of the soft-tissue structures of the spine. While many patients with significant trauma and neurologic symptoms will first undergo emergent CT scanning, MRI should be subsequently obtained – even in the absence of identifiable spinal pathology on CT.

All patients with LBP should be screened for symptoms of cauda equina syndrome. The cauda equina is sensitive to rapidly compressive insult. Early surgical decompression is required to prevent progression of symptoms and reduce the risk of permanent disability. Therefore, regardless of other risk factors, all LBP patients must be specifically questioned about urinary retention with or without overflow incontinence, stool incontinence, and saddle anesthesia. If any of these are present, a digital rectal examination should be performed to test for sphincter laxity. Of these signs, urinary retention (bladder distension > 500 cc; post-void residual volume > 100 cc) is the most sensitive and is usually evaluated with bedside sonography in the emergency department. Plain radiographs have little utility in the assessment of cauda equina syndrome. Emergent systemic corticosteroids should be administered to these patients prior to MRI, with concomitant intravenous (IV) antibiotics if an infectious cause is of clinical concern.

Risk factors for osteoporotic VCFs, which may occur even after relatively minor trauma, include age greater than 50, a known history of osteoporosis, and prolonged corticosteroid use. Patients with these demographic features should be evaluated for point tenderness and deformity on physical examination. Those with new onset neurologic findings and clinical suspicion for fracture should undergo imaging, preferably MRI.

In patients presenting with LBP without trauma, alternative etiologies must be considered including infectious causes, non-infectious causes, and malignancy. Infectious processes include discitis/osteomyelitis, and paraspinal or epidural abscess. These infections are not common and, unfortunately, may not be initially detected unless a high index of suspicion is maintained. Ill-appearing patients with LBP and systemic signs such as fever, rigors, or unexplained weight loss must be assessed for infection. Unfortunately, fever, the classic sign used to stratify patients into this category, is relatively insensitive, being present in a little over half of cases. Therefore, physicians must assess for concerning elements of the patient history to risk-stratify patients into this category (i.e. history of pneumonia, skin infection, urinary-tract infection, IV drug use, tuberculosis, immunosuppression, recent spinal fracture, or spinal surgery). Other risk factors, such as uncontrolled diabetes, alcoholism, and chronic renal failure are lower yield and must be interpreted in light of the clinical picture.

Patients with spine infections typically report prolonged, unrelenting back pain, which may be excruciating in severity. The spine should be specifically assessed for point tenderness. While not commonly present, the skin overlying the spine should be examined for warmth, erythema, induration, or fluctuance. Appropriate laboratory tests include a complete blood count, erythrocyte sedimentation rate (ESR), and C-reactive protein (CRP). While these patients may not have a leukocytosis, most will have an elevated ESR. Urinalysis and culture should be performed to exclude a possible source of infection. There is little to no role for plain films in the evaluation of LBP patients suspected of having spinal infection, as radiographic abnormalities will not be present in the absence of significant osseous destruction. MRI is helpful for adequate visualization of the soft tissues involved and should be ordered emergently.

In cancer patients presenting with LBP, spinal or epidural metastasis is always a concern. Spine metastasis is typical of solid tumors including breast, prostate, lung, renal, thyroid, and gastrointestinal carcinomas. Historical features are, of course, of paramount importance in identifying these patients. In patients without a known history of underlying malignancy, unexplained weight loss and pain lasting greater than 6 months may raise the clinician's concern. Additionally, benign back pain typically improves with rest, while patients with spinal metastasis often experience unrelenting discomfort that is present in the recumbent position. LBP patients with a history of cancer and new-onset neurologic symptoms warrant emergent MRI. In patients presenting with new-onset LBP without neurologic signs, one potential strategy is to obtain enhanced lumbosacral MRI and proceed with CT only if necessary to confirm subtle lesions, which demonstrate trabecular bone destruction.

Patients with AAA may present with LBP alone or in association with abdominal pain, lower extremity pallor or mottling, diaphoresis, nausea, or other signs of distress. AAA should be considered in patients older than 50 presenting with LBP. Atherosclerotic disease, history of tobacco use, or a family history of AAA are also risk factors. The nature of pain has wide variability. The classical physical examination finding of a pulsatile abdominal mass has limited sensitivity. Although sensitivity of palpation increases with increasing aneurysm size, physical examination alone is insufficient to rule out AAA in the high-risk patient. In addition to abdominal examination, the lower extremities should be evaluated for signs of embolism. The flanks should be evaluated for ecchymosis, as patients with AAAs that have ruptured posteriorly may present with relative hemodynamic stability.

Properly performed emergent bedside ultrasound has excellent sensitivity and should be utilized as a screening tool in patients who are good sonographic candidates. Large body habitus or bowel gas can significantly impair sonographic evaluation of the aorta. For this reason, contrast-enhanced CT remains the gold standard and should be obtained in patients when ultrasound is indeterminate or unavailable. All patients with symptomatic AAA require stabilization and emergent evaluation by a surgeon.

Patients who do not fall into one of these categories most likely have a benign cause of pain. Conservative management with outpatient follow-up is the standard of care. Emergency-department imaging plays little role in these patients. Ideally, these patients should be followed by a primary care provider, who may then utilize imaging if it becomes appropriate in their clinical course.

Imaging in acute LBP

Trauma

Major trauma

Back pain in the setting of major trauma (i.e. motor-vehicle collision, fall) is not a diagnostic dilemma.

While an all-inclusive description of the types of traumatic spinal injury and vertebral fracture is beyond the scope of this text, several general principles apply when considering imaging evaluation of the spine in the acute trauma patient. CT is the first-line imaging examination of choice secondary to its widespread availability, rapid examination time, reduced sensitivity to patient motion artifacts, and increased sensitivity for fracture. CT is best for detecting and characterizing fractures [12]. MRI excels in the evaluation of the spinal canal, spinal cord, and spine soft tissues, including detecting injury to the spinal ligaments and paraspinal soft tissues, which are all poorly evaluated with CT. MRI of the spine in the setting of trauma should include a sagittal short tau inversion recovery (STIR) sequence as the fat suppression markedly increases the conspicuity of edema within injured paraspinal soft tissues, the spinal cord, and in fractured vertebral bodies. Intravascular contrast is of minimal utility in trauma imaging. MRI can be complementary to CT, but is often performed in the subacute or non-acute setting given the longer imaging acquisition times and more limited availability.

Evaluating traumatic injury of the spine on imaging requires an understanding of the three-column model, which is used to assess spinal stability [13]. The anterior column extends from the anterior aspect of the vertebral column to the midaspect of the vertebral body and disk interspace. The middle column extends from the mid-aspect of the vertebral body and disk interspace to the posterior aspect of the vertebral body and posterior longitudinal ligament. Finally, the posterior column includes the neural arch and posterior elements.

A burst fracture occurs in the setting of significant axial loading forces and results in comminution and fragmentation of the affected vertebral body commonly resulting in both anterior and posterior translocation of the osseous fragments (Figure 5.2).

Burst fractures may involve the anterior column alone, both the anterior and middle columns, or all three columns of the spine, the latter two considered unstable. Retropulsion of osseous fragments can result in compression and injury to the neural structures. Cord compression is best assessed with MRI, which demonstrates mass effect upon a narrowed spinal cord often containing internal T2 hyperintense edema. In patients with spinal injury and concern for cord compression that have an absolute contraindication to MRI (i.e. MRI-non-compatible pacemaker), myelography may be performed followed by CT to confirm compressive sequelae.

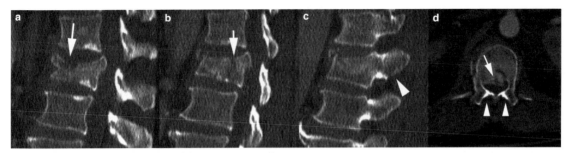

Figure 5.2 Patient with recent motor-vehicle collision with severe LBP. CT scan obtained in the emergency department demonstrates fracture of the L1 vertebral body. (a)–(c) Sagittal reconstructed images demonstrate that the fracture subtends two columns with fracture through the anterior L1 vertebral body (anterior column, (a): long arrow) and posterior L1 vertebral body (middle column, (b): short arrow) but sparing of the posterior elements including the pedicles, facet joints, and lamina (posterior column, (c): arrowhead). (d) Axial image demonstrates the burst fracture through L1 with two-column involvement, retropulsion of posterior fracture elements (arrow) and sparing of the posterior elements (arrowheads).

Chance fractures occur most commonly secondary to lap-seat-belt injuries in motor-vehicle collisions and are diagnosed by identifying a horizontally oriented fracture extending through the midaspect of the affected vertebral body, most commonly L2 or L3. Typically a chance fracture involves all three columns of the spine and has a high probability of associated ligamentous injury. It is important to note that the extreme forces required to cause these fractures may result in injury to ligaments and soft tissues of the spine that are not apparent with CT. For this reason, patients with concerning clinical findings and fracture findings on CT will commonly undergo an MRI to exclude soft-tissue and spinal cord injury.

Osteoporotic VCFs

Patients with osteoporosis can present with nonspecific focal back pain in the absence of significant trauma secondary to vertebral body insufficiency fractures [14]. Osteoporotic VCFs are common and predisposing risk factors include female gender, advancing age, and long-term corticosteroid use. Physical examination often reveals considerable pain on palpation over the spinous process of the fractured vertebral body.

Imaging findings include a wedge deformity or flattening of the fractured vertebral body and marrow edema best demonstrated with a sagittal STIR MRI sequence (Figure 5.3).

Plain radiography can be helpful in establishing the diagnosis if recent prior examinations are available for comparison to assess for interval change. Establishing fracture acuity requires a recent MRI revealing marrow edema or a bone scan documenting increased radiotracer uptake in the fractured vertebra.

As with other fractures in the spine, spinal stenosis, lateral recess stenosis, and neuroforaminal narrowing can occur and may lead to neurologic symptoms. Complicating the pain presentation, VCF commonly results in accelerated degenerative changes of the adjacent facet joints and disk secondary to altered biomechanics creating several additional potential sources of pain.

Sacral insufficiency fractures occur in the same patient population as VCF and can be subtle on imaging [15, 16]. Plain radiography and CT demonstrate linear sclerosis along the fracture, typically running parallel to the SIJ within the lateral sacral alae. MRI may demonstrate marrow edema (Figure 5.4).

A bone scan can be helpful in uncertain cases, classically revealing increased radiotracer uptake in the regions of fracture (the "Honda sign").

Non-traumatic conditions

Infectious/febrile conditions

Patients presenting with acute back pain in the absence of an inciting traumatic event should be assessed for the possibility of an underlying causative infection [17]. This is typically determined through a combination of physical examination findings, vital signs, clinical history, and laboratory tests. Spinal infection is notoriously insidious and clinical presentation can be both variable and non-specific. Patients are often afebrile and the absence of an elevated white-blood-cell count is not reliable for excluding spinal infection. Elevated ESR and CRP are considered the most reliable laboratory abnormalities [18]. Given the protean manifestations of spinal infection, imaging often plays a critical role in either its confirmation or exclusion.

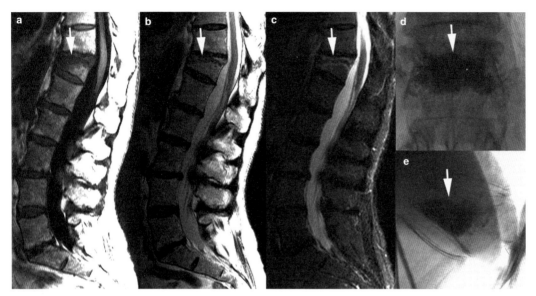

Figure 5.3 The patient is a 68-year-old female with a 6-week history of relentless severe thoraco-lumbar pain. MRI demonstrated an osteoporotic vertebral compression fracture at T12. (a) – (c) Sagittal MRI demonstrates the vertebral compression fracture. Marrow edema is seen as a low signal on the sagittal T1 weighted image (a, arrow), a cleft-like area seen on the T2-weighted image (b, arrow) and edema with a bright signal on the sagittal STIR image (c, arrow) signifying the fracture has acute to subacute features. Edema can remain for an extended period of time in a fracture likely due to persistent motion and failed union within the fracture. (d), (e) Vertebral augmentation was performed with balloon-assisted kyphoplasty and injection of polymethylmethacrylate (PMMA, arrows) cement resulting in near-complete elimination of the patient's pain.

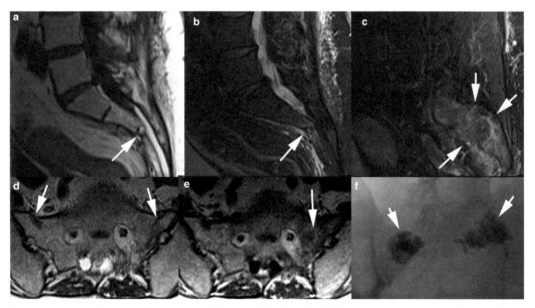

Figure 5.4 Patient with recent fall with severe LBP and radiating leg pain, initially thought to be related to disk protrusion and radiculopathy. MRI is challenging in patients with sacral fractures as the features are often subtle and seen only when looked for in the lateral sacral alar regions on the sagittal images. (a) Sagittal T1-weighted image demonstrates the subtle angulation of the sacrum at the S2–3 segment junction (arrow), but the fracture is difficult to perceive. (b) Sagittal fat-saturated T2-weighted image demonstrates pre-sacral edema, the fracture of the sacral body with slight angulation and edema in the sacral marrow (arrow). (c) Sagittal fat-saturated T2-weighted image more lateral in position through the sacral ala demonstrates edema in the lateral sacral ala (arrows), consistent with the osteoporotic fracture in this area. (d) Axial T2-weighted image demonstrates the subtle fractures bilaterally (arrows). (e) Axial T1-weighted image through the mid body of the sacral ala demonstrate the low signal from the marrow edema (arrow), similar to the bright signal seen on the sagittal T2 image (c). (f) Fluoroscopic image with slight pelvic obliquity demonstrates bilateral sacroplasty performed with PMMA (arrows) using fluoroscopy and CT guidance with excellent pain relief and marked improvement in patient mobility.

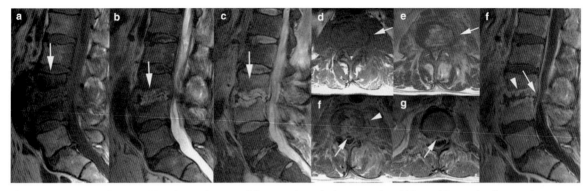

Figure 5.5 Patient with severe LBP and a combination of discitis and vertebral osteomyelitis. (a) Sagittal T1-weighted image demonstrates marrow edema at L3 and L4 (arrow) as well as disk abnormality with endplate irregularity. (b) Sagittal T2-weighted image demonstrates abnormal signal in the L3–4 disk space with irregular endplates (arrow). (c) Sagittal STIR image demonstrates the bright signal in the L3 and L4 marrow from edema along with the abnormal signal in the L3–4 disk space. (d) Axial T1- and (e) T2-weighted images demonstrate disk space and paravertebral signal abnormality from peri-discal and peri- vertebral edema (arrows). Distinction between the disk margin and surrounding fat is lost. (f), (g) Axial post-contrast T1-weighted images demonstrate extensive enhancement within the disk space and surrounding tissues. A focal epidural abscess cavity is present (arrow) along with small paraspinal abscess cavities adjacent to the psoas muscle (arrowhead). (h) Sagittal post-contrast T1-weighted image demonstrates abnormal enhancement in the L3–4 disk space (arrowhead) along with the small epidural abscess cavity in the spinal canal adjacent to the disk margin (arrow).

Contrast-enhanced MRI is the most sensitive imaging test to evaluate for the presence of spinal infection with a negative predictive value approaching 100%. It is therefore the radiologic examination of choice. Standard spinal imaging for infection should include the acquisition of a sagittal STIR sequence given its markedly increased sensitivity for marrow edema (Figure 5.5).

Contrast should be administered, in the absence of a known contraindication (i.e. renal insufficiency), as it aids in visualizing areas of infection and adjacent inflammation and is particularly helpful in differentiating abscesses from phlegmon. Alternative imaging modalities such as CT have reduced sensitivity in the evaluation of infection and are typically only employed if MRI is contraindicated.

Infectious causes of back pain include discitis/osteomyelitis, epidural abscess, and paraspinal abscess.

Discitis/osteomyelitis

The MRI findings in discitis/osteomyelitis are the result of the infectious process and the associated adjacent inflammation with accompanying marrow edema (Figure 5.5) [19]. In adults, infections typically begin in the vertebral body metaphysis and subsequently extend into the adjacent avascular disk. There is considerable edema within the affected marrow space manifesting as STIR hyperintensity with a concomitant reduction in signal on T1-weighted images (obliteration of the normal fatty marrow). Typically,

there is associated endplate destruction and enhancement progressing to involvement of the adjacent disk, termed discitis, which exhibits STIR hyperintensity and enhancement. CT is insensitive to the marrow signal changes identified on MRI. Signs of discitis and osteomyelitis on CT primarily involve endplate destruction surrounding the affected disk. Additionally, infection can originate within the facet joint with analogous imaging features [20].

Epidural abscess

Spinal infection may be confined to the endplate/disk or may extend into adjacent structures [21–23]. Posterior extension into the ventral epidural space can take the form of phlegmonous inflammation identified as heterogeneous soft-tissue enhancement on post-contrast T1-weighted MRI (Figure 5.5). Eventually, the infectious process can lead to the formation of an abscess. On MRI an epidural abscess is diagnosed via identification of a centrally non-enhancing and T2-hyperintense (fluid-signal) structure demonstrating peripheral rim-like enhancement that is often heterogeneous and irregular. Abscesses in the ventral epidural space can become large enough to cause compressive sequelae on the neural structures, an emergency that may require neurosurgical intervention.

Paraspinal abscess

Anterior or lateral extension of a spinal infection may result in a paraspinal abscess, commonly located within the paraspinal musculature (iliopsoas muscle in the lumbar spine) [21–23]. MRI features of a paraspinal abscess mirror those of an epidural abscess: near fluid-bright T2 hyperintensity and peripheral rim-like enhancement (Figure 5.5). Not uncommonly, contiguity can be demonstrated between the abscess and the disk interspace from which it originated. If MRI is contraindicated, CT with contrast may be used to demonstrate endplate destruction and collections of fluid-density material within the paraspinal soft tissues concerning for abscess. These collections may demonstrate rim enhancement, increasing the specificity for an infectious process.

Non-infectious/afebrile conditions

There are multiple possible etiologies for non-infectious acute back pain. Clinical presentation, past medical history, and imaging findings are used in combination to arrive at a diagnosis.

Degenerative changes

Degenerative changes of the spine develop early in life. In studies of children, disk degeneration noted at one or more levels by MRI is seen in approximately 30% of individuals at 13 years of age, 19–42% of children 14 years of age, 26–38% of children 15 years of age, and in approximately 50% of people by 20–22 years of age [24–27]. The frequency increases in young elite athletes [28]. Disk degeneration is known to further increase with advancing adult age and is nearly ubiquitous in the elderly [6–8]. The degenerative disk includes areas of radial annular tears and annular lamellar fragmentation resulting in disk height loss, disk bulge and protrusion, end-plate spur formation, and reactive vertebral body changes (often called Modic changes) that include vertebral marrow edema/fibrosis and end-plate degenerative erosions [29, 30]. These degenerative disk and vertebral body changes can certainly be the source of primary LBP.

Facet degenerative changes are also known to develop and progress with advancing age. This includes areas of facet cartilage loss, facet subchondral erosions, facet hypertrophy and ligamentum flavum hypertrophy. Similar SIJ degenerative changes also develop with age. These facet and SIJ degenerative features may be related to the source of acute LBP or "referred" radiating leg pain mimicking true radiculopathy, but facet and SIJ pain is often present in the absence of an imaging abnormality. Therefore, these degenerative changes do not specifically correlate with LBP in and of themselves. In addition, disk and facet degenerative changes (disk bulge, protrusion, facet hypertrophy) may lead to secondary compression of neural structures resulting in true radiculopathy or neurogenic claudication.

Therefore, when evaluating a patient with acute LBP, it is important to recognize that acute pain might be related to older, previously degenerative spine structures.

The intervertebral disk

The intervertebral disk as a direct cause of LBP has been long debated. A growing body of literature has provided considerable evidence of a patho-anatomic correlate for discogenic pain, helping to establish its validity with documented ingrowth of pain fibers deep in the annulus and nucleus. Complicating matters, it is well known that asymptomatic individuals of all ages will exhibit abnormalities of the disk on imaging studies. Therefore, determining the source of a patient's back pain requires the integration of physical examination, clinical history, imaging findings, and, on occasion, diagnostic anesthetic injections.

Most discogenic LBP develops as a chronic process. At times, acute disk herniation develops with acute-onset radiculopathy/LBP, likely related to ongoing disk extrusion, with the potential for acute cauda equina compression and the development of cauda equina syndrome (Figure 5.6).

The pathological and imaging findings in disk degenerative change have been well established [31–33]. The normal intervertebral disk consists of a central gelatinous nucleus pulposus contained by a surrounding annulus fibrosus. The disk has a density similar to soft tissue on CT with features of degeneration limited to disk height loss, disk bulge, disk protrusion, and adjacent bony sclerosis/erosions. MRI is more sensitive for the detection of disk degenerative changes and for the evaluation of the disk margins. In selected patients, the disk may be evaluated under fluoroscopy via direct-contrast injection, a discogram, and subsequent CT.

On MRI, the water and proteoglycans within the nucleus pulposus of a normal intervertebral disk results in T2 hyperintensity and an intermediate-to-low signal on non-contrast T1-weighted images similar in intensity to that of muscle. Degeneration and aging results in decreased water and proteoglycan content within the nucleus pulposus reducing the T2 signal within the disk [34, 35]. Anatomically, the

83

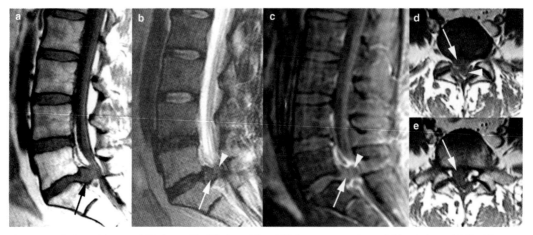

Figure 5.6 Patient with severe LBP along with difficulty voiding. MRI demonstrates a large disk herniation at L5 S1 with severe compression of the distal cauda equina. Sagittal T1-weighted (a), T2-weighted (b), and post-contrast T1-weighted (c) images demonstrate a large disk protrusion at L5 S1 (arrows) with what likely represents an extruded fragment (arrowhead) with significant compression of the distal cauda equina. (d), (e) Axial T1-weighted images demonstrate the large disk protrusion (arrow, d) and extruded fragment (arrow, e) with significant compression of the distal thecal sac and nerve roots (arrowheads).

degenerated disk may lose height and may extend beyond the cortical margin of the adjacent vertebral bodies, characteristics not typically seen in healthy discs. Marrow signal abnormalities may be identified within the endplates of the adjacent vertebral bodies in reaction to the degenerated disk. These signal abnormalities typically take the form of edema (T2 hyperintensity with T1 hypointensity), fat replacement (relative T2 hypointensity with T1 hyperintensity), or fibrosis (T1 and T2 hypointensity).

Painful disk degeneration typically presents with complaints of deep or dull aching lower-back pain or sharp, stabbing, knife-like pain. This pain may be exacerbated by certain movements and can be provoked with discography. Acute discogenic pain may develop in chronically degenerative discs with areas of annular degeneration or radial annular tear. Disk pain provoked at discography has been shown to correlate with a peripheral radial annular fissure, or "high-intensity zone" along the posterior annular margin seen on sagittal T2-weighted MRI.

Acute disk pain can also be seen in the setting of acute disk herniation. A large protrusion or extrusion of disk material can cause rapid and significant compression of the cauda equina with potential for the development of cauda equina syndrome.

A focal disk "herniation" is defined as extension of disk material beyond the expected limits of the intervertebral disk space that is less than 90° of the periphery of the disk [36]. Extension of disk material greater than 90° is considered a disk "bulge" and may

be circumferential (360° of disk margin) or asymmetric (to the left or right). Focal disk herniations are further subdivided into "protrusions," so termed when the greatest diameter of herniated disk material does not exceed the distance between the edges of the base of the herniated disk at the margin of the parent disk, and "extrusions," when the greatest diameter of herniated disk material *exceeds* the distance between the edges of the base of the herniated disk at the margin of the parent disk. Finally, a disk sequestration is defined as a fragment of disk within the spinal canal that has lost connection with the parent disk.

The facet
The facet joint and surrounding ligaments, tendons, and muscles can be a source of acute or longstanding LBP. Degenerative changes of the facet may be present, but it is common to identify facet pain in the absence of significant facet degeneration [37]. On physical examination, facet origin pain is typically elicited by direct palpation over the joint and may be exacerbated with flexion, extension, or rotation of the spine (motion of the joint). Facet pain can radiate to the lower extremities overlapping with radiculopathy from nerve-root compression, thereby complicating the diagnosis [38].

Facet degeneration includes joint-space narrowing, cartilage breakdown, osteophytosis, subchondral geode formation, peri-facet inflammatory change, and sclerosis [39, 40]. Both MRI and CT are adept at demonstrating these findings, although the osseous overgrowth is somewhat better depicted with CT. Facet-joint effusions, which appear as fluid T2 hyperintensity within the joint on MRI, may be present and can occasionally lead to expansion of the synovial lined facet-joint capsule to produce synovial cysts. These synovial cysts may extend either anteriorly or posteriorly from the joint space; when anterior, they extend into the spinal canal and cause mass effect on neural structures [41]. Inflammatory changes of the facet joint can result in edema (T2 hyperintensity) within the marrow spaces of the adjacent pedicle. Spondylolisthesis is commonly seen in association with facet degeneration and can lead to nerve compression including central spinal canal stenosis, lateral recess stenosis, and foraminal stenosis. The tissues that are compressed by the facet hypertrophy are identified to better advantage with MRI, making it the first-line imaging modality.

Sacroiliac joint
Similar degenerative processes can occur at the SIJs. Patients with SIJ pain present with back pain located at the SIJs with or without radiating lower extremity pain and often exhibit exquisite point tenderness with directed palpation of the affected joint [42]. SIJ degenerative changes can be identified on both CT and MRI as joint-space narrowing, osseous proliferation, and adjacent subchondral sclerosis.

Spondylolisthesis and spondylolysis
Spondylolisthesis, or translocation of one adjacent vertebral body in relation to another, may occur secondary to proliferative degenerative changes (typically of the facets) or secondary to spondylolysis, also known as pars defects (Figure 5.7).

Other less-common causes include acute trauma, tumor with bone destruction, and congenital facet anomalies. Degenerative spondylolisthesis is typically accompanied by hypertrophic facet changes, which results in narrowing of the lateral recesses and the spinal canal. This is well depicted with both CT and MRI, the latter being particularly useful for evaluating the integrity of neural structures. Spondylolysis typically results in anterior translocation of the affected vertebral body independent of the detached posterior elements, which acts to *widen* the spinal canal and lateral recesses [43]. Pars defects are usually bilateral (85–90%) and are most commonly found in the lower lumbar spine (80% at L5). Pars defects themselves can be a source of pain or may generate pain via compression of adjacent nerves.

While MRI is excellent at demonstrating these compressive sequelae, directly identifying the pars defects can be challenging. Often, the radiologist is dependent upon secondary findings of the defect (such as spinal canal widening) to arrive at the diagnosis. CT best depicts the fractures, confirming the diagnosis. Bone scan is also very sensitive for the diagnosis, exhibiting increased radiotracer uptake in the region of the fracture.

Arachnoiditis
Arachnoiditis is an inflammatory process involving all three meningeal layers as well as the nerve roots and is an uncommon cause of LBP in the modern era. In the past, oil-based myelographic contrast (i.e. Pantopaque) was considered a cause of arachnoiditis, especially when mixed with blood. Today, these agents are no longer in use. Arachnoiditis can be seen in the setting of spine infection, intrathecal steroid

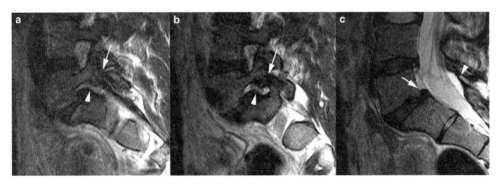

Figure 5.7 Patient with persistent LBP in spite of bed rest and several weeks of anti-inflammatory medications. MRI was used for further evaluation. (a), (b) Sagittal T2-weighted images demonstrate a pars defect, or spondylolysis (arrows), along with significant compression of the L5 nerve root in the foramen (arrowheads) due to anterolisthesis of L5 relative to S1 along with disk height loss. (c) The central canal is widened in a pars defect since the L5 vertebral body slips forward (arrow) but the L5 lamina remains posterior (arrowhead), enlarging the canal.

injections, trauma, spine surgery, and subarachnoid hemorrhage. It often presents as non-specific LBP or radiating leg pain, dysethesias, or spastic paraparesis.

T2-weighted MRI images are the most sensitive examination for the detection of suspected arachnoiditis. Findings reflect the underlying inflammation and resultant root-to-root and root-to-dural adhesions, which manifest as clumping of nerve roots and the "empty-sac sign," respectively [44]. Contrast is not necessary or helpful in diagnosing arachnoiditis. If MRI is contraindicated, a CT myelogram can be performed demonstrating similar findings.

Seronegative arthropathies

The serogenative spondyloarthropathies (ankylosing spondylitis (AS), Reiter's syndrome, psoriatic arthritis, and arthritis of inflammatory bowel disease) are a group of multisystem inflammatory disorders that affect various joints throughout the body, including the spine and SIJ. Sacroiliitis manifests as joint-space narrowing, subchondral sclerosis, and erosion, which can be identified by plain radiography, CT, or MRI [45]. Severe cases may result in fusion across the joint. Classically, SIJ involvement is asymmetric with Reiter's syndrome and psoriatic arthritis, while AS and arthritis of inflammatory bowel disease result in bilaterally symmetric sacroiliitis.

Ossification of the anterior spinal ligament and ankylosis of the facet joints in AS in combination with osteopenia lead to a markedly increased proclivity to spinal fracture, even in the setting of minor trauma. Therefore, AS patients with acute back pain should be evaluated with a high level of suspicion for fracture and clinicians should have a low threshold for obtaining imaging. CT should be performed in these patients, as subtle fractures may not be visible on plain radiographs. MRI is complementary to CT and can demonstrate marrow edema or injury to soft tissues, ligaments, and the spinal cord.

Spontaneous epidural hemorrhage

An uncommon cause of LBP, spontaneous epidural hemorrhage typically presents as knife-like, lancinating pain with or without radicular symptoms [46]. The patient often has an underlying coagulopathy. While more commonly found within the cervicothoracic spine, spontaneous epidural hemorrhage can occasionally occur within the lumbar spine. Imaging demonstrates hemorrhage in the epidural space, which, in the acute phase, will be hyperdense on CT.

Spinal epidural hemorrhage has a variable appearance on MRI depending on its age, similar to intracranial hemorrhage. In the acute phase, epidural hematomas will be T1 isointense and T2 hypointense. In the subacute phase, they exhibit T1 hyperintensity secondary to methemoglobin. Gradient-echo sequences may be acquired, which may exhibit magnetic susceptibility artifact in the region of hemorrhage, increasing the sensitivity and specificity for the diagnosis.

LBP after prior surgical intervention

Causes of LBP after surgical intervention can be multifactorial, providing a diagnostic challenge. Postoperative infections are uncommon, but should always be considered in evaluating these patients. More commonly, recurrent disk herniation and post-operative scarring are the underlying etiology, both presenting in a manner analogous to a virgin disk herniation (typically LBP and radiculopathy). MRI is the imaging method of choice and the administration of contrast is imperative as it helps to distinguish between enhancing scar tissue and non-enhancing residual/recurrent disk material. This distinction is of increased utility greater than 6 months after surgical intervention, as scar tissue may not enhance centrally in the first few months.

In patients with prior fusion, new-onset back pain may arise from hardware loosening or accelerated degenerative changes at levels immediately above or below the fusion, which now experience increased stresses and altered biomechanics. On imaging, these levels may demonstrate disk degeneration and protrusions, facet arthropathy, and resultant neuroforaminal and spinal-canal stenoses.

Retroperitoneal abnormalities

Astute clinicians and radiologists should be mindful of the fact that LBP is not always spinal in origin. Mimickers include referred pain from abdominal and pelvic pathologies. Common examples include nephrogenic pain (i.e. renal stones or pyelonephritis), pancreatitis, and an abdominal aortic aneurysm, as described in the clinical approach/algorithm (Figure 5.8).

Cancer
Osseous metastatic disease

Neoplastic involvement of the spine is more commonly the result of metastatic disease rather than a primary spinal malignancy. Patients often have a known history of cancer and may present with central axial back pain, radiating leg pain, or some

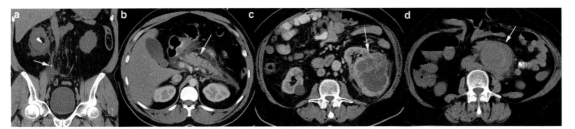

Figure 5.8 Retroperitoneal causes of LBP. (Images courtesy of Stephen Schabel, MD.) (a) Coronal abdominal CT reconstruction demonstrates a stone in the right mid to distal ureter (arrow) with peri-ureteral fluid suggesting collecting-system rupture and proximal ureteral dilatation indicating obstruction. Other stones are still noted in the renal parenchyma (arrowhead) and some peri-renal fluid is also noted. (b) Axial abdominal CT image demonstrates pancreatitis with pancreatic and peri-pancreatic edema (arrow). (c) Axial abdominal CT image demonstrates a large renal mass (arrow) with some peri-nephric stranding. (d) Axial abdominal CT image demonstrates aortic enlargement along with peri-aortic edema and fluid (arrow) from a leaking abdominal aortic aneurysm.

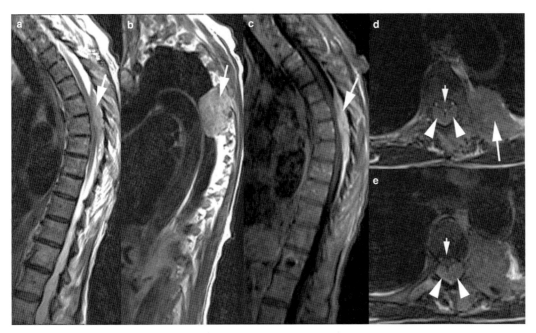

Figure 5.9 Patient with cancer who presents with mid-thoracic back pain along with bilateral lower-extremity weakness, paresthesias, and a sensory level to pin in the mid chest. MRI was used for further neurologic evaluation. (a), (b) Sagittal T2-weighted images demonstrate a large mass infiltrating the spinal canal posteriorly with extensive compression of the thoracic cord (a, arrow) along with a paraspinal component on the left overlying the chest wall and ribs (b, arrow). (c) Sagittal post-contrast T1-weighted image demonstrates the enhancing mass in the posterior spinal canal with extensive compression of the spinal cord (arrow). (d), (e) Axial T2-weighted images demonstrate the large paraspinal mass with extensive involvement of the ribs and chest wall (larger arrows), extensive infiltration of the tumor into the posterior spinal canal (arrowheads), and significant compression of the spinal cord (smaller arrows).

combination therein, depending upon the structures involved. Involvement of the cortical surface of the vertebral body can result in central axial back pain secondary to irritation of the innervated periosteum. Aggressive osseous destruction with extension beyond the confines of the vertebral body can cause compression of adjacent neural structures leading to symptoms of cord compression and/or radiculopathy (Figure 5.9).

Metastatic disease is usually focal and multiple. MRI is most useful in demonstrating the location of the lesions, which replace the normally hyperintense fatty marrow on sagittal T1-weighted images (Figure 5.9) [47, 48]. Most metastases also exhibit T2 hyperintensity (best identified on sagittal STIR sequences) and enhance after the administration of contrast. However, sclerotic lesions (such as in prostate and breast cancer) are dark on all sequences.

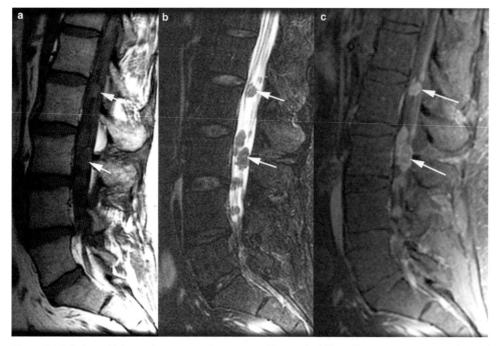

Figure 5.10 Patient with known lung cancer who presents with complex LBP and lower extremity pain and paresthesias in a non-specific distribution. MRI was used to assess for neurologic status. (a) Sagittal T1-weighted image demonstrates faint visualization of large masses in the spinal canal (arrows). (b) Sagittal T2-weighted image more clearly demonstrates the large lesions in the spinal canal, consistent with lung carcinoma drop metastasis. (c) Sagittal post-contrast T1-weighted image demonstrates faint enhancement in the drop metastasis.

Plain radiography or CT can be complementary in the evaluation of metastatic disease, particularly when of the sclerotic variety or when cortical destruction is suspected [47, 48]. MRI remains most sensitive for the evaluation of effects upon adjacent soft-tissue structures and, in particular, the neural structures within the spinal canal. Further, epidural extension of malignancy is best evaluated with post-contrast MRI, which often shows enhancing soft tissue extending into the epidural space and causing a mass effect (Figure 5.9).

Intrathecal: spinal cord and drop metastasis

Intrathecal metastatic disease can be subdivided into intramedullary (within the cord) and extramedullary (external to the cord: carcinomatous meningitis and drop metastasis). Both types of intrathecal metastasis can result in non-specific back pain, radiating leg pain, or focal neurologic deficits, depending on the affected structures [49, 50]. Intramedullary metastatic disease is exceedingly rare, occurring in only 0.9–2.1% of autopsied cancer patients. When present, they enlarge the cord, enhance, and are associated with considerable adjacent edema (T2 hyperintensity).

Most intrathecal metastatic disease is extramedullary with deposits on the dura and in the pia-arachnoid including the cord surface and nerves of the cauda equina (Figure 5.10).

Many different types of primary malignancies, both from within the central nervous system (CNS) and external to the CNS, can cause intrathecal metastases including breast or lung cancer, leukemia/lymphoma, glioblastoma multiforme, ependymoma, and medulloblastoma. Thin-section post-contrast axial MRI is most sensitive for the detection of these sometimes subtle metastatic lesions, demonstrating enhancing nodules of variable size along the cord surface or the cauda equina with associated surface irregularity. Cerebral spinal-fluid cytology also plays an important role in diagnosis and is positive in the vast majority of cases when serial lumbar punctures are performed.

Conclusion

The evaluation of patients with acute LBP is complex. Clinical direction is critical in guiding optimal imaging approaches. A paradigm approach to patient assessment and optimal imaging can be helpful in guiding patient work-up, choice of imaging, assessment, and definitive clinical management.

References

1. Frymoyer JW, Pope MH, Costanza MC, *et al.* (1980). Epidemiologic studies of low-back pain. *Spine* **5**: 419–423.

2. Andersson GB, Svensson HO, Oden A (1983). The intensity of work recovery in low back pain. *Spine (Phila Pa 1976)* **8**: 880–884.

3. Wiesel SW, Cuckler JM, Deluca F, *et al.* (1980). Acute low-back pain. An objective analysis of conservative therapy. *Spine (Phila Pa 1976)* **5**: 324–330.

4. Miller JA, Schmatz C, Schultz AB (1988). Lumbar disc degeneration: correlation with age, sex, and spine level in 600 autopsy specimens. *Spine (Phila Pa 1976)* **13**: 173–178.

5. Eubanks JD, Lee MJ, Cassinelli E, Ahn NU (2007). Prevalence of lumbar facet arthrosis and its relationship to age, sex, and race: an anatomic study of cadaveric specimens. *Spine (Phila Pa 1976)* **32**: 2058–2062.

6. Stadnik TW, Lee RR, Coen HL, *et al.* (1998). Annular tears and disc herniation: prevalence and contrast enhancement on MR images in the absence of low back pain or sciatica. *Radiology* **206**: 49–55.

7. Weishaupt D, Zanetti M, Hodler J, Boos N (1998). MR imaging of the lumbar spine: prevalence of intervertebral disk extrusion and sequestration, nerve root compression, end plate abnormalities, and osteoarthritis of the facet joints in asymptomatic volunteers. *Radiology* **209**: 661–666.

8. Jarvik JJ, Hollingworth W, Heagerty P, Haynor DR, Deyo RA (2001). The Longitudinal Assessment of Imaging and Disability of the Back (LAIDBack) Study: baseline data. *Spine (Phila Pa 1976)* **26**: 1158–1166.

9. Chou R, Qaseem A, Snow V, *et al.* (2007). Diagnosis and treatment of low back pain: a joint clinical practice guideline from the American College of Physicians and the American Pain Society. *Ann Internal Med* **147**: 478–491.

10. Dagenais S, Tricco AC, Haldeman S (2010). Synthesis of recommendations for the assessment and management of low back pain from recent clinical practice guidelines. *Spine J* **10**: 514–529.

11. Jarvik JG, Deyo RA (2002). Diagnostic evaluation of low back pain with emphasis on imaging. *Ann Internal Med* **137**: 586–597.

12. McAfee PC, Yuan HA, Fredrickson BE, Lubicky JP (1983). The value of computed tomography in thoracolumbar fractures. An analysis of one hundred consecutive cases and a new classification. *J Bone Joint Surg Am* **65**: 461–473.

13. Denis F (1983). The three-column spine and its significance in the classification of acute thoracolumbar spinal injuries. *Spine* **8**: 817–831.

14. Jensen ME, McGraw JK, Cardella JF, Hirsch JA (2007). Position statement on percutaneous vertebral augmentation: a consensus statement developed by the American Society of Interventional and Therapeutic Neuroradiology, Society of Interventional Radiology, American Association of Neurological Surgeons/ Congress of Neurological Surgeons, and American Society of Spine Radiology. *J Vasc Interv Radiol* **18**: 325–330.

15. Dasgupta B, Shah N, Brown H, *et al.* (1998). Sacral insufficiency fractures: an unsuspected cause of low back pain. *Br J Rheumatol* **37**: 789–793.

16. Blake SP, Connors AM (2004). Sacral insufficiency fracture. *Br J Radiol* **77**: 891–896.

17. Mylona E, Samarkos M, Kakalou E, Fanourgiakis P, Skoutelis A (2009). Pyogenic vertebral osteomyelitis: a systematic review of clinical characteristics. *Semin Arthritis Rheum* **39**: 10–17.

18. Cahill DW, Abshire BB (2003). Pyogenic vertebral osteomyelitis. In Barjer HH, Loftus CM, eds. *Textbook of Neurological Surgery*. Philadelphia, PA: Lippincott Williams & Wilkins, pp. 3239–3247.

19. Ledermann HP, Schweitzer ME, Morrison WB, Carrino JA (2003). MR imaging findings in spinal infections: rules or myths? *Radiology* **228**: 506–514.

20. Michel-Batot C, Dintinger H, Blum A, *et al.* (2008). A particular form of septic arthritis: septic arthritis of facet joint. *Joint Bone Spine* **75**: 78–83.

21. Nussbaum ES, Rigamonti D, Standiford H, *et al.* (1992). Spinal epidural abscess: a report of 40 cases and review. *Surg Neurol* **38**: 225–231.

22. Varma R, Lander P, Assaf A (2001). Imaging of pyogenic infectious spondylodiskitis. *Radiol Clin N Am* **39**: 203–213.

23. Huang PY, Chen SF, Chang WN, *et al.* (2012). Spinal epidural abscess in adults caused by *Staphylococcus aureus*: clinical characteristics and prognostic factors. *Clin Neurol Neurosurg* **114**: 572–576.

24. Kjaer P, Leboeuf-Yde C, Sorensen JS, Bendix T (2005). An epidemiologic study of MRI and low back pain in 13-year-old children. *Spine* **30**: 798–806.

25. Tertti MO, Salminen JJ, Paajanen HE, Terho PH, Kormano MJ (1991). Low-back pain and disk degeneration in children: a case–control MR imaging study. *Radiology* **180**: 503–507.

26. Erkintalo MO, Salminen JJ, Alanen AM, Paajanen HE, Kormano MJ (1995). Development of degenerative changes in the lumbar intervertebral disk: results of a prospective MR imaging study in adolescents with and without low-back pain. *Radiology* **196**: 529–533.

27. Takatalo J, Karppinen J, Niinimaki J, *et al.* (2009). Prevalence of degenerative imaging findings in lumbar magnetic resonance imaging among young adults. *Spine (Phila Pa 1976)* **34**: 1716–1721.

28. Sward L, Hellstrom M, Jacobsson B, Nyman R, Peterson L (1991). Disc degeneration and associated abnormalities of the spine in elite gymnasts. A magnetic resonance imaging study. *Spine (Phila Pa 1976)* **16**: 437–443.

29. Bartynski WS, Rothfus WE, Kurs-Lasky M (2008). Postdiskogram CT features of lidocaine-sensitive and lidocaine-insensitive severely painful disks at provocation lumbar diskography. *AJNR* **29**: 1455–1460.

30. Bartynski WS, Rothfus WE (2012). Peripheral disc margin shape and internal disc derangement: imaging correlation in significantly painful discs indentified at provocation lumbar discography. *Interventional Neuroradiology* **18**: 227–241.

31. Videman T, Malmivaara A, Mooney V (1987). The value of the axial view in assessing discograms. An experimental study with cadavers. *Spine* **12**: 299–304.

32. Thompson JP, Pearce RH, Schechter MT, *et al.* (1990). Preliminary evaluation of a scheme for grading the gross morphology of the human intervertebral disc. *Spine (Phila Pa 1976)* **15**: 411–415.

33. Pfirrmann CW, Metzdorf A, Zanetti M, Hodler J, Boos N (2001). Magnetic resonance classification of lumbar intervertebral disc degeneration. *Spine* **26**: 1873–1878.

34. Adams MA, Roughley PJ (2006). What is intervertebral disc degeneration, and what causes it? *Spine.* **31**: 2151–2161.

35. Urban J (2002). The physiology of the intervertebral disk. In Grunzburg R, Szpalski M, eds. *Lumbar Disk Herniation*. Philadelphia, PA: Lippincott Williams and Wilkins, pp. 22–30.

36. Fardon DF, Williams AL (in press). Nomenclature and classification of lumbar disc pathology. Version 2.0. *AJNR*.

37. Kalichman L, Li L, Kim DH, *et al.* (2008). Facet joint osteoarthritis and low back pain in the community-based population. *Spine (Phila Pa 1976)* **33** : 2560–2565.

38. Mooney V, Robertson J (1976). The facet syndrome. *Clin Orthop Relat Res* **115**: 149–156.

39. Czervionke LF, Fenton DS (2008). Fat-saturated MR imaging in the detection of inflammatory facet arthropathy (facet synovitis) in the lumbar spine. *Pain Med (Malden Mass)* **9**: 400–406.

40. Pneumaticos SG, Chatziioannou SN, Hipp JA, Moore WH, Esses SI (2006). Low back pain: prediction of short-term outcome of facet joint injection with bone scintigraphy. *Radiology* **238**: 693–698.

41. Metellus P, Fuentes S, Adetchessi T, *et al.* (2006). Retrospective study of 77 patients harbouring lumbar synovial cysts: functional and neurological outcome. *Acta neurochirurgica* **148**: 47–54.

42. Slipman CW, Jackson HB, Lipetz JS, *et al.* (2000). Sacroiliac joint pain referral zones. *Arch Phys Med Rehabil* **81**: 334–338.

43. Ulmer JL, Elster AD, Mathews VP, King JC (1994). Distinction between degenerative and isthmic spondylolisthesis on sagittal MR images: importance of increased anteroposterior diameter of the spinal canal ("wide canal sign"). *AJR* **163**: 411–416.

44. Ross JS (1999). MR imaging of the postoperative lumbar spine. *MRI Clin N Am* **7**: 513–524.

45. Amrami KK (2012). Imaging of the seronegative spondyloarthopathies. *Radiol Clin N Am* **50**: 841–854.

46. Groen RJ (2004). Non-operative treatment of spontaneous spinal epidural hematomas: a review of the literature and a comparison with operative cases. *Acta neurochirurgica* **146**: 103–110.

47. Shah LM, Salzman KL (2011). Imaging of spinal metastatic disease. *Int J Surg Oncol* Nov 3. doi: 10.1155/2011/769753.

48. Roberts CC, Daffner RH, Weissman BN, *et al.* (2010). ACR appropriateness criteria on metastatic bone disease. *J Am Coll Radiol* **7**: 400–409.

49. Entin g RH (2005). Leptomeningeal neoplasia: epidemiology, clinical presentation, CSF analysis and diagnostic imaging. *Cancer Treat Res* **125**: 17–30.

50. Clarke JL, Perez HR, Jacks LM, Panageas KS, Deangelis LM (2010). Leptomeningeal metastases in the MRI era. *Neurology* **74**: 1449–1454.

Acute vision loss

Simon J. Hickman and Daniel J. A. Connolly

Introduction

When approaching a patient who complains of acute vision loss it is important to consider what the cause might be and the anatomical location before proceeding to further investigations and imaging, as vision loss can occur due to lesions anywhere from the front of the eye to the association visual cortices. Ocular causes of acute loss of vision should be apparent from the history and ocular examination, backed up by optical coherence tomography (OCT) and electrophysiology. They will not be considered further, unless neuro- or vascular imaging is required in management. In neurologic causes of acute loss of vision, the ocular examination may be unremarkable and therefore the pattern of vision loss, the history of onset, and other associated features are important in working out the diagnosis.

The pattern of vision loss will give some clues. Uniocular vision loss will be due to pathology in the eye or the ipsilateral optic nerve. Bitemporal vision loss will be due to pathology affecting the central optic chiasm, whereas hemianopic loss arises from the post-chiasmatic visual pathways. Bilateral vision loss can be harder to localize. It can occur due to bilateral simultaneous ocular or optic nerve disease, more extensive optic chiasm disease, or bilateral simultaneous disease in the posterior visual pathways (termed cerebral vision loss). The history of onset, pattern of vision loss, and other features of the examination can help in localization, as will be discussed.

The history of the onset and progression of vision loss can give important clues as to the etiology. A sudden onset with fast recovery within seconds usually occurs due to a transient failure of arterial perfusion to the eye or brain, such as in pre-syncope. A sudden onset with fast recovery within minutes suggests either a transient ischemic attack or a migrainous visual aura. Loss of vision to its maximal extent, either suddenly or within seconds, without recovery, suggests that the cause is vascular, either due to ischemia or hemorrhage, or due to trauma. Progression of vision loss over hours to days is more indicative of an inflammatory or infectious cause. Neoplastic or degenerative causes of loss of vision usually progress more indolently although there are cases of optic nerve compression and posterior cortical atrophy that have presented with acute loss of vision.

It is important to find out if there are other associated symptoms that can also help in finding the etiology. Fever might suggest an infective cause, retro-ocular pain and pain on eye movement occurs in inflammatory optic neuropathies, and headaches can occur in cerebral hemorrhage and migraine.

The examination should include a formal measure of visual acuity with a retro-illuminated chart at the appropriate viewing distance as this will gauge the severity of vision loss as well as providing a baseline against which to assess progression or recovery. Color vision should also be assessed with an appropriate screening test, such as the Ishihara charts, Hardy–Rand–Rittler plates, or the desaturated D15 test. A color vision deficit in excess of what would be expected from the visual acuity is often a very sensitive and specific clue as to the presence of an optic neuropathy. The visual field should be assessed in each eye, ideally by formal perimetry, but if this is unavailable then the most accurate confrontation test is with a kinetic red target [1]. The pattern of loss should be charted with the left-eye visual field on the left side of the page and the right-eye visual field on the right, which corresponds to how the visual fields are presented using formal perimetry. The pupillary responses need to be examined in each eye. This should be done in a dark room with a very bright light. In terms of assessing

Imaging Acute Neurologic Disease, ed. Massimo Filippi and Jack H. Simon. Published by Cambridge University Press.
© Cambridge University Press 2014.

vision loss, the presence of a direct response in each eye needs to be assessed and then the swinging-flashlight test performed to assess for a relative afferent pupillary defect (RAPD), i.e., a relative difference in pupillary reaction between the two eyes, which is a very sensitive test for a unilateral or asymmetrical optic neuropathy. Lastly, the retina should be examined. If the pupillary responses do not need to be monitored then this should be performed through dilated pupils to give a better view of the optic discs, the macula, and the peripheral retina.

Imaging modalities

Imaging of the visual pathways, especially with magnetic resonance imaging (MRI), allows for the entire course of the visual pathway from the globe to the primary visual cortex and beyond to be visualized. However, the diagnostic yield of imaging depends on localizing the likely site of the lesion and also deciding on the most likely pathology as these will govern which part of the visual pathway imaging will focus on, the imaging modality, and also the MRI sequences that it is best to employ.

Imaging of the brain in stroke, acute multifocal neurological symptoms, and trauma has been discussed elsewhere in this book in Chapters 12, 13, and 14, respectively. These pathologies can all cause vision loss so the specifics of imaging will not be discussed in this chapter. This chapter will concentrate on imaging of the anterior visual pathways.

(a) MRI of the anterior visual pathways

MRI of the anterior visual pathways presents many challenges [2]. The orbit contains fat, which gives a high signal on both T1 and fast or turbo spin-echo T2-weighted imaging. There are also chemical-shift artifacts at lipid–water boundaries, such as along the cerebrospinal fluid (CSF) of the optic nerve sheath [3]. Fat-suppression techniques can help to reduce these contamination effects [2]. Susceptibility artifacts occur at interfaces between different tissues, due to their different magnetic properties. It is a particular problem in the canalicular portion of the optic nerves due to the bony cavity of the optic canal and air from the adjacent sphenoid and ethmoid sinuses [4]. This is significantly exacerbated when there is pneumatization of the anterior clinoid processes. Metals, particularly iron, can also cause severe image distortion [5]. Artifacts interfering with orbital imaging are commonly seen with metal-containing mascara, tattooed eye-liner [6], and metal

dental work [7]. It is routine practice that patients attending for MRI of the orbits and/or head are asked to remove eye make-up in order to exclude such artifacts. Susceptibility artifacts can be reduced by using spin-echo rather than gradient-echo or echo planar imaging because the spin-echo sequence includes a refocusing pulse [2]. The optic nerves are small and mobile, therefore fast high-resolution imaging is required to image the optic nerves with an acceptable acquisition time [2]. The optic nerves are surrounded by the CSF-containing optic nerve sheaths, which show a high signal on T2-weighted imaging and may obscure the edges of the optic nerve [2].

The orbit can be imaged using a quadrangular routine head coil; however, better image quality can be achieved with some manufacturer-specific configurations of phased array surface coils [8], although the use of surface coils will require the coils to be changed over if the brain needs imaging in the same session. To image the optic nerves in the orbit, fat-saturated imaging sequences are best employed if the patient is compliant. Such sequences that have shown high sensitivity for detecting optic nerve lesions in optic neuritis include short tau inversion recovery (STIR), fat-saturated fast spin echo (FSE), SPIR with fluid-attenuated inversion recovery (SPIR-FLAIR) [9], and extended echo-train acquisition (XETA) FLAIR [10]. The last two sequences have the advantage of suppressing the high signal from the CSF in the optic nerve sheath to increase the conspicuity of optic nerve lesions. Contrast enhancement can be produced by using intravenous gadolinium. It shortens the T1 relaxation time, therefore will show a high signal on T1-weighted imaging [11]. For contrast-enhanced optic nerve imaging fat-saturated T1-weighted or SPIR sequences are best employed [8, 9], as the signal in (abnormal) contrast-enhanced tissues will be suppressed using pulse sequences that are based on T1-relaxation times of water (e.g. STIR). If gadolinium is to be administered it is always prudent to do pre-gadolinium and post-gadolinium fat-saturated T1-weighted or selective partial inversion recovery (SPIR) sequences to ensure that the apparent effects of gadolinium enhancement are not in fact related to failed fat suppression. The combined effects of fat saturation and gadolinium enhancement to increase the ability to detect optic nerve lesions is demonstrated in Figure 6.1. Lesions within the orbit are best appreciated using a combination of fat-saturated heavily T2-weighted imaging,

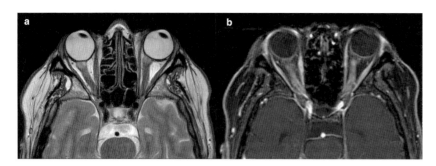

Figure 6.1 Axial (a) T2-weighted, (b) post-gadolinium fat-saturated T1-weighted MRI in a 35-year-old woman who had a 1-week history of progressive bilateral vision loss to perception of light in each eye with bilateral swollen optic disks. A high signal is visible in both optic nerves on the enhanced T1 images, supporting a diagnosis of bilateral optic neuritis. Notice the effect of fat saturation and gadolinium enhancement to make it possible to detect the lesions.

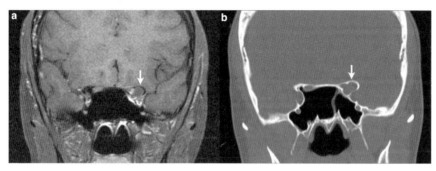

Figure 6.2 (a) Coronal post-gadolinium T1-weighted MRI and (b) coronal bone window CT scan in a 37-year-old woman with a 2-day history of progressive visual loss in her left eye to 20/1200. MRI demonstrates a low signal intensity lesion within the anterior clinoid process extending into the left optic canal, with a rim of peripheral enhancement, compressing the left optic nerve (arrowed). CT shows that there has been expansion of the anterior clinoid process on the left (arrowed) with erosion of the medial wall adjacent to the optic canal. The appearances are of an anterior clinoid mucocele.

T1-weighted imaging and pre- and post-gadolinium fat-saturated T1-weighted imaging [12, 13], although standard T1- and T2-weighted imaging may be useful in imaging the orbit if motion artifact is severe or if there is peri-orbital pathology such as infection or a bone-based mass lesion.

It is essential to image the orbits using the coronal plane. If gadolinium is administered then the pre- and post-gadolinium fat-saturated imaging should be obtained in the same plane, preferably the coronal plane. Sagittal and axial imaging may also be useful, particularly if the pathology is located at the optic nerve head or within the optic canal or cavernous sinus regions.

The optic chiasm is situated at the junction of the floor and anterior wall of the third ventricle, just anterior to the pituitary stalk. It is where the visual pathway fibers undergo partial decussation with crossing of the fibers subserving temporal vision. The optic chiasm lies close to the sphenoid sinus and also the internal carotid arteries. The optic chiasm is best visualized using high-resolution T1, T2, and FLAIR imaging [13].

Additionally, brain MRI should be performed as this adds complementary information, such as showing demyelinating lesions suggestive of multiple sclerosis (MS) in a case of optic neuritis, or meningeal enhancement in neurosarcoidosis.

(b) CT of the anterior visual pathways

Computerized tomography (CT) has a complementary role to MRI in evaluating the anterior visual pathways, as it gives detailed information about the bones surrounding the orbit and optic nerves. When requesting a CT scan it is important to specify whether the study should include the orbit, the head, or both. Head CT scans avoid the orbits to try and minimize the radiation dose to the eyes and, in particular, the lens, which is a highly radiosensitive structure. Orbital CT scans should be acquired using a multi-detector scanner to collect thin-slice (typically 0.7 mm) fast-volume studies. Pre- and post-iodinated contrast images may be acquired unless the history suggests trauma, acute hemorrhage, or there is a contraindication to the use of contrast [14]. Both soft-tissue and bone algorithms should be viewed. Multiplanar reconstruction allows for assessment of the skull base and its foramina, to appreciate fractures, and to detect hemorrhages, foreign bodies, or calcification

[11, 13, 14]. Figure 6.2 shows how MRI and CT compliment each other in the assessment of a clinoid mucocele.

Head and orbital CT scanning is indicated in the acute setting, especially in the unwell patient because images are quicker to acquire and no special MRI-compatible equipment is needed to monitor and/or ventilate the patient. CT is also usually readily available even outside of normal working hours in all acute hospitals.

(c) Ultrasonography

Ultrasonography is quick, well-tolerated, inexpensive, and non-invasive. B-mode ultrasonography can differentiate between solid and cystic orbital lesions and can be of use in demonstrating buried optic disk drusen and papilledema [11]. It can also help to diagnose posterior scleritis, which can present similarly to optic neuritis [15]. Doppler ultrasonography can detect dilatation, arterialization, and reversal of flow in the superior ophthalmic vein in dural carotid cavernous fistulae [16]. It is also of use in assessing for carotid artery stenosis and for measuring intracranial blood flow, as discussed in Chapter 12.

(d) Angiography

The contribution of angiography in the assessment of cerebrovascular disease is discussed in Chapter 12. It is of less use in assessing acute vision loss [13], although aneurysmal compression of the optic nerve or chiasm [17] (Figure 6.3), or cavernous sinus dural arteriovenous fistulae [18] can present with acute vision loss. CT angiography (CTA) or magnetic resonance angiography (MRA) are equivalent first-line investigations, although formal digital subtraction angiography (DSA) will usually also be required [11].

There follows a discussion as to how imaging can help in the management of various patterns of vision loss.

Transient vision loss

An algorithm for how to manage a case of transient visual loss is shown in Figure 6.4. It is important to decide whether the vision loss is truly monocular, is hemianopic, or is binocular [19]. In hemianopia, the loss is often described as being in the eye with the affected temporal visual field (i.e. the larger visual field). However, if half of faces or other objects appear to be missing, or if reading is impaired, this will imply that there is hemianopic rather than monocular visual loss.

(a) Transient monocular vision loss

Transient monocular vision loss (TMVL) may be embolic or non-embolic in origin [20].

Non-embolic TMVL

Non-embolic TMVL is principally caused by decreased retinal or optic nerve head perfusion. This can be due to arterial stenosis secondary to atherosclerosis or vasculitis, which then leads to TMVL at times of relative systemic arterial hypotension. Investigation of these patients will depend on the other presenting features. In all cases of TMVL occurring in the elderly, giant cell arteritis (GCA) needs to be urgently excluded since, if untreated, it can lead to permanent binocular

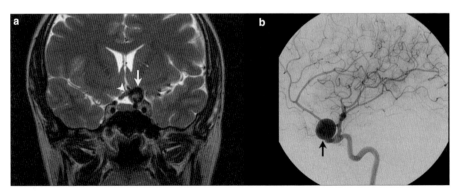

Figure 6.3 (a) Coronal T2-weighted MRI and (b) DSA following left internal carotid contrast injection in a 38-year-old woman with a 6-week history of blurred vision in her left eye. Although she could see 20/20 her color vision was reduced, she had a left relative afferent pupillary defect and a pale left optic disc. MRI demonstrates a lesion with predominantly low signal (flow void) adjacent to the internal carotid artery (arrowed) that distorts and displaces the optic chiasm (shown with an arrowhead). DSA shows this to be a left ophthalmic artery aneurysm (arrowed).

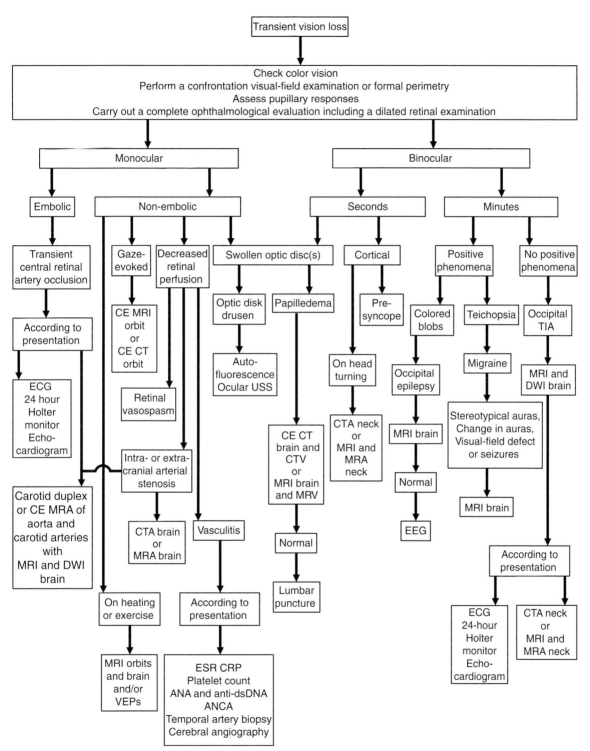

Figure 6.4 Algorithm for the management of transient vision loss. Abbreviations: ANA = antinuclear antibodies; ANCA = antinuclear cytoplasmic antibodies; anti-dsDNA = anti-double-stranded deoxyribonucleic acid antibodies; CE = contrast enhanced; CRP = C reactive protein; CT = computed tomography; CTA = computerized tomographic angiography; CTV = computed tomographic venography; DWI = diffusion-weighted imaging; ECG = electrocardiogram; EEG = electroencephalogram; ESR = erythrocyte sedimentation rate; MRA = magnetic resonance angiography; MRI = magnetic resonance imaging; MRV = magnetic resonance venography; TIA = transient ischemic attack; USS = ultrasound scan; VEPs = visual evoked potentials.

blindness. Atherosclerotic arterial stenosis may be intra- or extracranial. Vascular imaging is therefore required, as discussed in Chapter 12.

Retinal artery vasospasm can also cause TMVL. This may be idiopathic or secondary to vasoconstrictor drugs such as cocaine. If retinal artery vasospasm is observed then further investigation will not be needed, unless vasculitis or another systemic disorder is suspected [20]. Retinal migraine is a diagnosis formerly used in cases of non-embolic TMVL; however, most cases, on close questioning, are probably hemianopic rather than monocular. Truly monocular cases are probably most likely due to vasospasm, since the mechanism behind migraine auras is spreading electrical depression and this has never been demonstrated in the human eye.

Transient arterial occlusion on eye movement can occur due to orbital tumors. The patient may also have proptosis. If an orbital tumor is suspected the patient's orbits need imaging, as discussed above [12]. Transient visual blurring on getting warm or on exercise is called Uhthoff's phenomenon. It occurs due to optic nerve demyelination [15]. It can occur without other symptoms of optic neuritis or MS. Investigations needed for optic neuritis will be discussed below.

Embolic TMVL

Embolic central retinal or branch retinal artery occlusion is the most important cause of TMVL. This was previously termed amaurosis fugax. There is often a typical history of a curtain coming down over one eye with vision going to complete darkness in seconds, before returning to normal, usually within 5 minutes. Embolic central retinal or branch retinal artery occlusion can lead to persisting visual loss if the embolus does not clear. In these circumstances the part of the retina affected will be pale and the macula will have a cherry-red appearance due to the normal choroidal vasculature shining through.

In cases of transient or persisting ischemia in the elderly, GCA needs to be urgently excluded. In cases of transient and persisting visual loss due to embolic arterial occlusion urgent investigation is required to rule out an embolic source from the heart, ascending aorta, or ipsilateral carotid artery. The rapidity of referral for these investigations in TMVL can be calculated from the $ABCD^2$ score [21]. A 12-lead electrocardiogram should be performed and then, according to the presentation, prolonged electrocardiographic

monitoring and echocardiography should be considered to look for a cardiac source of emboli [20]. Carotid imaging needs to be performed in all cases of embolic TMVL to assess for significant ipsilateral carotid artery stenosis, which would trigger consideration for the need for carotid endarterectomy [22]. The imaging required is discussed in Chapter 12.

(b) Transient binocular vision loss

When assessing a patient who complains of transient binocular vision loss (TBVL) it is important to ascertain the duration of symptoms and if any positive phenomena were perceived. Symptoms lasting seconds may be due to transient failure to perfuse the brain, as in pre-syncope, or the optic nerve heads, as in papilledema or optic nerve head drusen. A longer episode lasting minutes without positive phenomena may be due to vertebrobasilar territory transient ischemic attack (TIA). Positive phenomena can occur in migraine and occipital epilepsy.

Pre-syncope

The commonest cause of TBVL lasting seconds is pre-syncope. Neuroimaging is not usually required and investigation should focus on finding a cardiovascular cause. If the TBVL is precipitated by head turning then this will be due to transient vertebral artery compression leading to decreased occipital-lobe perfusion. This is true vertebrobasilar insufficiency. Imaging of the neck vessels is required to find the site of compression [23].

Optic nerve head pathology

Papilledema and optic disk drusen can also cause transient visual loss lasting seconds, termed visual obscurations. Both of these pathologies are usually bilateral, although asymmetrical and monocular cases can occur. The arterial supply to the optic nerve head is via the short posterior ciliary arteries. These will be compromised when there is optic disk swelling. In circumstances where the intracerebral and intraocular pressure rises, such as bending forward or Valsalva maneuvers, or when there is relative arterial hypotension, such as on standing, the arterial supply to the optic nerve head can be temporarily interrupted and visual obscurations result [24, 25]. Buried optic disk drusen can be differentiated from papilledema using B-mode ultrasonography. Optic disk drusen are highly reflective with acoustic shadowing on the medium-gain scan. They can also still be detected on the low-gain scan

[26]. In papilledema there will be a dilated optic nerve sheath with a decrease in optic sheath diameter with abduction (or adduction) of the eye by 30° [11]. Manifest optic disk drusen show characteristic auto-fluorescence on pre-injection photography for fluorescein angiography [26].

Vertebrobasilar territory transient ischemic attack

Transient hemianopia or complete blindness can occur as part of a vertebrobasilar territory TIA. Given the lack of positive phenomena in the majority of cases, the hemianopia may not be recognized by the patient, which may explain in part why TIAs causing hemianopia are relatively rare. Complete bilateral blindness has also been reported to occur, with blindness lasting for 1–15 minutes and vision returning suddenly or within a few seconds [27]. Vertebrobasilar territory TIAs have a higher relative risk of subsequent stroke within 7 days compared with carotid territory TIAs (odds ratio 1.47) so it is important that these cases are urgently managed [28]. If the history suggests the possibility of vertebral dissection then the vertebral arteries need imaging with MRA or CTA, as discussed in Chapter 12. A cardiac source of emboli has to be otherwise ruled out.

Migraine

In migraine, the visual disturbance is usually hemianopic, although complete blindness can result. The visual field defect usually starts as a small scotoma close to fixation and enlarges over minutes surrounded by zigzag lines, termed teichopsia. Hemianesthesia, hemiparesis, and dysphasia can also develop during a migraine aura. The presentation is usually so classical that further investigation is not required. Focal occipital pathology has been reported occasionally with migraine-like visual auras. Neuroimaging with MRI to exclude a focal lesion is recommended if the auras are not completely stereotypical, if there is a change in the migraine pattern, if there is a persisting visual field defect, or if there are coexistent seizures [29].

Occipital seizures

Occipital seizures typically involve auras of multi-colored spots, circles, and balls. They can increase in number, size, or both with progress of the seizure, particularly prior to other, non-visual symptoms. MRI is the first investigation of choice to rule out a tumor, vascular malformation, or cortical malformation. If

imaging is normal then an electroencephalogram (EEG) is required [30].

Acute unilateral vision loss

An algorithm for how to manage a case of acute unilateral visual loss is shown in Figure 6.5.

(a) Ocular causes

Ocular causes will usually be apparent from the history or examination, with OCT and electrophysiology to assess occult cases. Neuroimaging will not usually be required unless the presence of an orbital tumor is suspected if the patient has proptosis or if there is excessive chemosis and raised intraocular pressure to suggest an indirect cavernous sinus dural arteriovenous fistula. Imaging for orbital tumors will be considered below in the investigation of optic neuropathies.

Indirect fistulae tend to occur spontaneously in older patients who have atherosclerotic disease. There is small-volume, slow shunting of blood from the internal carotid artery to the cavernous sinus and then the superior ophthalmic vein. If a fistula is suspected then the simplest investigation is orbital Doppler ultrasonography, which will show dilatation, arterialization, and reversal of the blood flow in the superior ophthalmic vein [16]. A dilated superior ophthalmic vein can also be seen in ophthalmic Graves' disease, Tolosa–Hunt syndrome, orbital pseudotumor, cavernous sinus tumors, and cavernous sinus thrombosis [31]. Although the fistulae can close spontaneously, there is a risk of neovascular glaucoma and also intracranial hemorrhage. Therefore, if a fistula is suspected the investigation of choice is DSA, to assess the extent of the fistula and its drainage to then develop a management plan [32].

(b) Sudden unilateral vision loss

As has been discussed, sudden unilateral visual loss usually implies an ischemic cause.

Central retinal artery occlusion

If there is retinal pallor, attenuated vessels, and a cherry-red macula then the cause will be central retinal artery occlusion. This should be investigated as discussed above in the section on TMVL.

Anterior ischemic optic neuropathy

If there is an altitudinal visual field defect and a swollen optic disk then the most likely cause will be

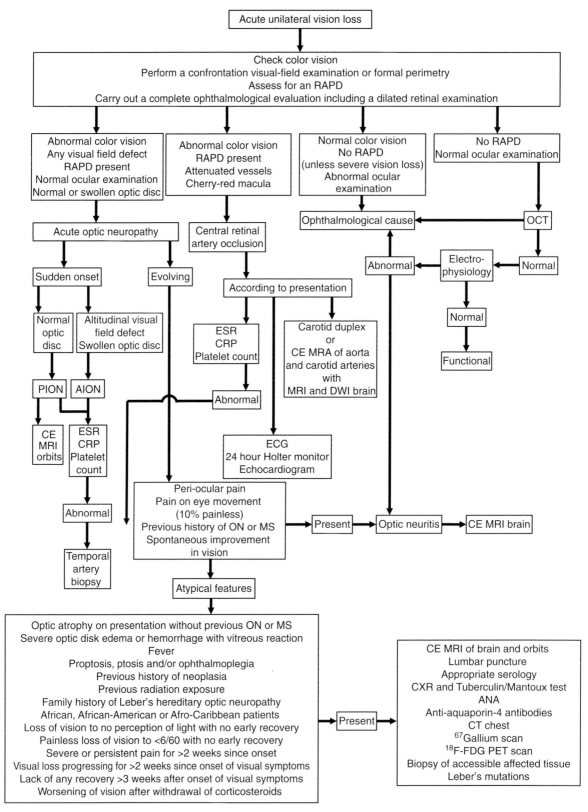

Figure 6.5 Algorithm for the management of acute unilateral vision loss. Abbreviations as per Figure 6.4 and AION = anterior ischemic optic neuropathy; CXR = chest radiograph; 18F-FDG PET = 18F-fluorodeoxyglucose positron emission tomography; MS = multiple sclerosis; OCT = optical coherence tomography; ON = optic neuritis; PION = posterior ischemic optic neuropathy; RAPD = relative afferent pupillary defect.

anterior ischemic optic neuropathy (AION), especially in an older patient in the presence of an optic "disk at risk," which is a small crowded optic disc. Apart from excluding GCA no further investigations are required. If the presentation is not clearly of sudden onset, especially if the patient is at the younger end of the age spectrum for AION, then optic neuritis may need excluding. The predominant MRI feature that distinguishes AION from acute optic neuritis is the gadolinium-enhancement pattern [33]. Gadolinium enhancement is virtually ubiquitous in acute optic neuritis (Figure 6.1), whereas in AION it is much less likely to be seen. In addition, high signal lesions on STIR imaging, or equivalent, are also much more likely to be seen in acute optic neuritis, compared with AION, although an optic nerve high signal tends to develop over time in AION as Wallerian degeneration occurs. Lastly, the lesions in acute optic neuritis tend to be longer than in acute AION, encompassing most of the length of the optic nerve. Recently, it has been shown that diffusion-weighted imaging (DWI) may show restricted diffusion in the affected optic nerve in acute AION [34], although this is not a specific sign as restricted diffusion can also occur in acute optic neuritis [35]. Brain imaging should also be acquired to look for evidence of demyelination to support a diagnosis of optic neuritis, although it is important not to mistake ischemic brain white-matter abnormalities for demyelinating lesions [36].

Posterior ischemic optic neuropathy

Acute unilateral posterior ischemic optic neuropathy (PION) is much rarer than AION. It can occur in GCA, but it is a diagnosis of exclusion, and anterior visual pathway MRI is required to exclude other forms of acute optic neuropathy.

(c) Evolving unilateral vision loss

Optic neuritis

When there is an evolving acute unilateral optic neuropathy then the most likely diagnosis is acute optic neuritis. The presentation and management of optic neuritis has been reviewed elsewhere [15, 37, 38]. In a typical case of demyelinating optic neuritis, as outlined in the algorithm in Figure 6.5, further investigations are not usually required to make the diagnosis. Brain MRI can be requested in order to define the risk for the development of clinically definite MS. Gadolinium-enhanced brain MRI at presentation with acute optic neuritis can also allow for the diagnosis

of MS according to the 2010 McDonald criteria, as outlined in Chapter 13.

Atypical optic neuritis

If atypical features for optic neuritis occur then urgent investigation is mandated as treatment and prognosis may be radically different (Figure 6.5) [15, 37]. Atypical causes of inflammatory optic neuritis include neuromyelitis optica (NMO), neurosarcoidosis, autoimmune optic neuritis, chronic relapsing inflammatory optic neuropathy (CRION), optic perineuritis, and vasculitis. Such cases are more likely to be bilateral, although unilateral presentations do occur. The vision loss tends to be more severe and spontaneous recovery does not occur, or vision can worsen after a short course of corticosteroids. Atypical forms of optic neuritis are more likely in non-white Caucasian populations [37]. The pattern of additional central nervous system lesions tend to be different in NMO compared with MS, as discussed in Chapter 13.

Anterior visual pathway MRI does not always help in differentiating between typical demyelinating and atypical forms of optic neuritis, although some imaging features may be helpful. In NMO, the intracranial optic nerve and optic chiasm are more likely to show T2 high signal and gadolinium enhancement than in demyelinating optic neuritis [39, 40].

In neurosarcoidosis and optic perineuritis, optic-nerve sheath enhancement is prominent [41, 42]. This can occur in demyelinating optic neuritis, although usually in conjunction with more prominent optic-nerve enhancement than in the first two conditions above [43]. In addition, in neurosarcoidosis there may be enhancement of the meninges elsewhere in the brain as well as brain white-matter lesions [41]. The gold standard for diagnosing sarcoidosis is demonstrating non-caseating granulomas histologically. Further imaging with chest CT, ^{67}gallium scanning or ^{18}F-fluorodeoxyglucose positron emission tomography (^{18}F-FDG PET) can help to identify accessible involved tissue for biopsy [41, 44].

Infectious causes

The presence of fever and systemic upset, and/or an inflammatory reaction in the vitreous with a very swollen optic disc, point toward an infectious cause [15]. There may also be a history of exposure to an infectious agent or the patient may live in an endemic area. Most cases are diagnosed with serological testing. Human immunodeficiency virus (HIV) infection needs excluding in all cases of suspected infectious optic neuropathy. Most cases of optic neuropathy in an HIV-positive patient are due to opportunistic infections or tumors, although a direct HIV optic neuropathy can occur. Anterior visual pathway MRI in such cases shows STIR high signal and gadolinium enhancement in the affected optic nerve [45–47].

Tuberculosis (TB) may cause an optic neuropathy by a variety of means including papillitis, retrobulbar optic neuritis, neuroretinitis, tuberculoma either within or compressing the optic nerve, meningeal infection (arachnoiditis), or AION [48, 49]. In addition, acute loss of vision may occur secondary to papilledema if TB meningitis causes raised intracranial pressure [49]. If TB is suspected, then investigations required are a chest radiograph and tuberculin/Mantoux testing. This can be backed up with CSF microscopy and culture, CSF interferon-γ release assay, and biopsy of any accessible involved tissue [48]. Tuberculomas will tend to show restriction on DWI with low central T2 signal, which is more pronounced on gradient-echo T2* or susceptibility-weighted imaging [50]. Tuberculomas and TB arachnoiditis show avid gadolinium enhancement on MRI [51]. In addition, optic nerve tuberculomas can massively expand the optic nerve [52].

In practice, most cases of infectious optic neuropathy are bilateral at onset. An exception to this is neuroretinitis, which is usually unilateral at onset. It causes acute vision loss with a swollen optic disk and a macular star. It can be idiopathic, although it may be caused by an infectious agent, such as Bartonella, Borrelia, TB, syphilis, toxocariasis, toxoplasmosis, or histoplasmosis, which will need excluding with appropriate serology [15]. Neuroretinitis is not associated with MS. Therefore, brain imaging will be normal. The most consistent finding on anterior visual pathway MRI, when an abnormality has been detected, has been enhancement of the optic disk, extending into the anterior optic nerve only. Others have reported optic-sheath enhancement [53].

Acute vision loss can also occur secondary to optic nerve compression from post-septal orbital cellulitis/abscesses. Infection most often spreads to the orbit from the sinuses, though rarely direct extension from the face, via hematogenous spread and from trauma, either with or without foreign-body penetration, can occur [12]. A whole range of infections can cause orbital infections including *Staphylococcus*, *Streptococcus*, TB, and fungi, such as aspergillosis, candidiasis, and mucormycosis [13, 48]. A combination of MRI and CT scanning is usually required to investigate the effects within the orbit and also to assess whether the surrounding bone or sinuses are involved. DWI will usually show restricted diffusion within the abscess [54]. Cavernous sinus thrombosis and, rarely, distant subdural empyema may occur in association with post-septal orbital cellulitis [55].

Compressive causes

If there is optic atrophy on presentation with acute vision loss, in the absence of a previous history of optic neuritis or MS, then this implies that the disease process is more chronic, occurring over at least 4 weeks [56, 57]. It should lead to the suspicion of a tumor causing optic nerve compression [15]. There may be other features of an orbital mass, such as proptosis, ptosis, and/or ophthalmoplegia. The lesions may be inflammatory, such as orbital pseudotumor and thyroid ophthalmopathy, aneurysmal (Figure 6.3), or neoplastic, when there may be a previous history of malignancy [12–14]. Metastases can occur to the optic nerve, optic nerve sheath (Figure 6.6), extraocular muscles, intraorbital fat, lacrimal gland, optic canal, or orbital wall [12, 13]. Mucoceles result from paranasal sinus drainage obstruction by trauma, infection, or tumors. They expand and cause thinning and erosion of the walls of the affected sinus. Compression of the optic nerve may be caused by mucoceles arising in the sphenoid sinus, posterior ethmoid, or clivus, causing bone destruction

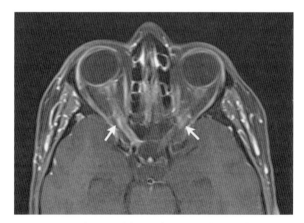

Figure 6.6 Axial post-gadolinium fat-saturated T1-weighted MRI demonstrating bilateral optic nerve sheath infiltration (right > left, arrowed). The abnormal enhancement was from metastatic breast carcinoma in a 49-year-old woman presenting with a two month history of progressive loss of vision initially in her right eye to no perception of light and then in her left eye to 20/600. The vision loss was the first presentation of her breast carcinoma.

of the optic canal (Figure 6.2) [13]. Optic nerve sheath and clival meningiomas usually present with chronic unilateral vision loss, although acute loss of vision can occur, especially in pregnancy, as the tumors are hormonally responsive. The rapidity of onset in pregnancy can mimic demyelinating optic neuritis, but because optic neuritis is unusual in pregnancy an optic nerve sheath meningioma needs to be suspected in a pregnant woman with an optic neuropathy [58]. In a case of optic nerve sheath meningioma the optic nerve head is usually pale, although swelling and optociliary shunt vessels can occur [59]. In all cases of suspected compressive optic neuropathy urgent gadolinium-enhanced MRI of the anterior visual pathways is required [12–14], since surgical resection [60], immunosuppression [61], or radiotherapy [59], depending on the cause, may save sight.

Leber's hereditary optic neuropathy

Leber's hereditary optic neuropathy (LHON) usually presents with acute unilateral painless loss of vision, although bilateral simultaneous onset is possible [62]. The second eye will invariably become affected within the next year. There is often a family history to suggest maternal inheritance. The optic disk will be swollen with peri-papillary telangiectatic vessels and vascular tortuosity. Anterior visual pathway MRI may show swelling and an increased T2 signal centrally in the optic nerves, optic chiasm, and optic tracts [63]. Gadolinium enhancement may be seen in the optic nerves and optic chiasm [64].

Radiation-induced optic neuropathy

Radiation-induced optic neuropathy occurs usually between 10 and 20 months after radiotherapy, but the onset may range from 3 months to 9 years. Cumulative doses of radiation that exceed 50 Gy or single doses to the anterior visual pathway of greater than 10 Gy are usually required for it to develop. The presentation is with acute unilateral or bilateral painless visual loss. It is important to image these patients urgently, to rule out recurrence of the original tumor. In radiation-induced optic neuropathy, MRI typically shows enlargement and gadolinium enhancement of the affected nerve or optic chiasm [65]. Hyperbaric oxygen therapy may help to improve vision in these cases.

Acute bilateral vision loss

The principles for the management of acute bilateral vision loss are similar to those for acute unilateral vision

as described above. An algorithm is presented in Figure 6.7. The principal difference is that bilateral visual loss may be due to a disease process in the optic chiasm or post-chiasmal visual pathways. Once an ocular cause has been ruled out, the two key examination findings are the pupillary responses and the visual field. The afferent pupillary fibers are carried in the optic nerve and decussate in the optic chiasm before continuing in the optic tract. Before the lateral geniculate nucleus the afferent pupillary fibers then pass in the brachium of the superior colliculus to the olivary pretectal nucleus. Therefore, if an abnormality in the pupillary light reflex is detected in the context of acute vision loss then the lesion is anterior to the lateral geniculate nucleus (LGN). If no pupillary abnormality is detected then the lesion is in the posterior visual pathways, or the vision loss is functional in origin. The pattern of the visual field defect will also give a clue as to the possible anatomical location. This has been reviewed elsewhere [66].

(a) Sudden bilateral vision loss

As discussed above, sudden bilateral vision loss will be due to a vascular cause. This can affect both the anterior and posterior visual pathways with differing etiologies according to which parts of the pathway are involved.

Optic nerve heads – bilateral anterior ischemic optic neuropathy

Although AION usually presents with unilateral vision loss, bilateral simultaneous presentations do occur. These are rare when it is spontaneous in onset; however, bilateral AION does occur in GCA and when there is arterial hypotension, such as in acute hemorrhage, renal dialysis, and surgery, particularly prone spinal surgery [67]. The imaging findings in bilateral AION are the same as in unilateral AION described above.

Optic nerves – bilateral posterior ischemic optic neuropathy

The risk factors for bilateral PION are the same as for bilateral AION [67]. There are case reports of bilateral optic nerve FLAIR high signal with restricted diffusion and gadolinium enhancement in acute peri-operative PION [68, 69].

Optic chiasm – apoplexy

Due to its rich blood supply, infarcts of the optic chiasm do not generally happen, although there have

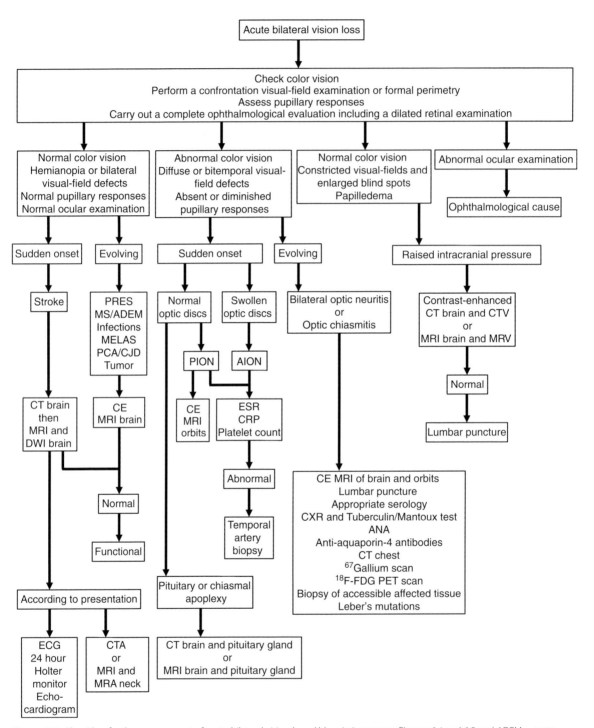

Figure 6.7 Algorithm for the management of acute bilateral vision loss. Abbreviations as per Figures 6.4 and 6.5 and ADEM = acute disseminated encephalomyelitis; CJD = Creutzfeldt–Jakob disease; MELAS = mitochondrial encephalomyelopathy, lactic acidosis, and stroke-like episodes; PCA = posterior cortical atrophy; PRES = posterior reversible encephalopathy syndrome.

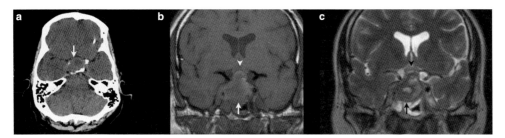

Figure 6.8 (a) Axial CT and subsequent (b) coronal T1-weighted and (c) T2-weighted magnetic MRI in a 46-year-old man with a sudden onset of headache, double vision, and decreased visual acuity down to 20/120 with his right eye and 20/200 with his left eye. The CT scan demonstrates a sellar and suprasellar mass with subtle hemorrhage (arrowed). This is more clearly seen by MRI with signal heterogeneity on both T1- and T2-weighted imaging (arrowed). The MRI also shows optic chiasm displacement and compression (shown with arrowheads).

been occasional case reports of its occurrence, with restricted diffusion in the chiasm on DWI [70, 71]. In addition, chiasmal apoplexy due to hemorrhages secondary to cavernous malformations and tumors have also been reported [72, 73]. Pituitary apoplexy is a clinical syndrome of sudden onset of headache, vomiting, vision loss, and decreased consciousness caused by hemorrhage and/or infarction of the pituitary gland [74]. This is usually into a pre-existing non-functioning pituitary macroadenoma. In the acute setting CT is often performed first as these patients are often systemically unwell. This has been shown to detect a sellar mass in more than 90% of cases, although the diagnosis of apoplexy with high-attenuation acute hemorrhage is found in less than 50% of cases [75]. MRI is more sensitive, with MRI findings correlating with histological or surgical findings in 90% of cases [76]. In the acute phase there is heterogeneous signal intensity on both T1- and T2-weighted MRI (Figure 6.8). In addition, it has recently been reported that T2*-weighted gradient-echo sequences may show early hypointensity within the hemorrhage due to the accumulation of paramagnetic deoxyhemoglobin, or a rim of hypointensity due to a boundary effect based on differences in magnetic susceptibility at the border of tissues and by the deoxygenation of blood occurring at the periphery of the lesion. In time, the low signal intensity of the rim increases as paramagnetic hemosiderin accumulates [77]. Craniopharyngiomas and suprasellar or chiasmatic astrocytomas may present with some of these imaging features on both CT and MRI but the presentation should allow for clinical differentiation. If CT and MRI are inconclusive as to whether the hemorrhage has occurred from a pituitary adenoma or from an aneurysm then CTA or DSA may be required [78].

Post-chiasmal visual pathway strokes

Strokes posterior to the optic chiasm produce visual field defects in both eyes, either a quadrantinopia or hemianopia to the side opposite to the infarct [66]. In one series, 84% occurred due to infarction and 16% due to primary intraparenchymal hemorrhage [79]. The vast majority of these occurred in the occipital cortex or optic radiation, corresponding to the distribution of the posterior cerebral artery. Approximately 6% of the strokes affected the optic tract. The importance of differentiating the two is that the optic tract is supplied by the anterior choroidal artery, which is a branch of the internal carotid artery [80], whereas the posterior cerebral artery receives its supply predominantly from the basilar artery. The source of emboli may therefore be different in infarcts of the two territories. A clue is that in an optic tract infarct there will be an RAPD in the eye which has the temporal (i.e. larger) visual field involved [66], whereas there will not be an RAPD from a more posterior infarct. Occasionally, the posterior cerebral artery will continue to have its fetal origin from the internal carotid artery. If suspected, this should be visible on CTA, MRA, or DSA [81]. Bilateral strokes account for about 6% of strokes causing visual field defects and can result from basilar-artery thromboembolism, transtentorial herniation causing posterior cerebral artery occlusion, and venous sinus thrombosis [66, 79]. Imaging in stroke will be discussed in Chapter 12.

(b) Evolving bilateral vision loss

Papilledema

The vision loss in papilledema occurs due to axonal damage at the optic nerve head. Axoplasmic flow stasis leads to high pressure within the optic nerve head with resultant intraneuronal optic nerve ischemia. The peripherally placed fibers sub-serving peripheral vision are most vulnerable, leading to initial constricted visual fields, although the raised pressure can make the eyes more hypermetropic by flattening the globes. In time, central vision can become irreversibly affected [25]. If raised intracranial pressure is suspected then imaging is urgently required to rule out a space-occupying lesion or cerebral venous sinus thrombosis. The imaging modality chosen will depend on local availability. It has been shown that multidetector-row CTA shows equivalent sensitivity and specificity for detection of venous sinus thrombosis compared with MRI venography [82]. MRI features

of raised intracranial pressure include an empty sella turcica, deformation of the anterior pituitary gland, slit-like ventricles, "tight" subarachnoid spaces, flattening of the posterior globe, protrusion of the optic nerve, enhancement of the optic nerve head, distention of the optic nerve sheath, and vertical tortuosity of the optic nerve, with the most specific sign being posterior globe flattening (Figure 6.9) [83]. The most specific CT finding in chronic raised intracranial pressure is widening of the foramen ovale [84].

Bilateral optic neuritis or optic chiasmitis

The principles of management of bilateral optic neuritis are the same as for unilateral optic neuritis above, although it is much more likely that the optic neuritis is not related to MS and has an atypical cause [37] and should be investigated as laid out in Figure 6.7. Optic chiasmal neuritis is now being increasingly recognized with the more widespread use of MRI [37].

As discussed above, infectious causes of acute optic neuropathy usually affect both optic nerves simultaneously. In addition, meningitis can lead to acute bilateral vision loss due to raised intracranial pressure, or direct effects on the optic chiasm, as seen with optochiasmic arachnoiditis and tuberculomas due to TB (Figure 6.10) [49].

Post-chiasmal visual pathway disease

Many of the diseases discussed in Chapter 13 can affect the posterior visual pathways, either to cause hemianopia or cerebral blindness, if both sides of the brain are affected simultaneously [66]. In addition, mitochondrial encephalomyelopathy, lactic acidosis, and stroke-like episodes (MELAS), posterior cortical

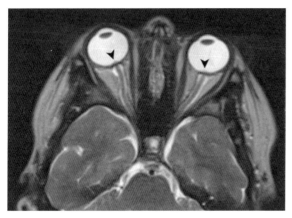

Figure 6.9 Axial T2-weighted MRI in a 19-year-old woman with a one week history of progressive decrease in vision to perception of light in each eye associated with a longer history of headaches. On examination she had bilateral grade 4 papilledema. The imaging shows marked posterior globe flattening (shown with arrowheads) as well as optic nerve sheath dilatation. She was subsequently diagnosed with idiopathic intracranial hypertension.

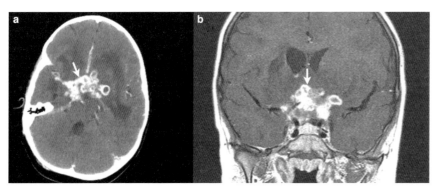

Figure 6.10 (a) Axial post-contrast CT and (b) subsequent coronal post-gadolinium T1-weighted MRI in a 2-year-old girl with a 4-week history of progressive bilateral visual loss down to no perception of light in each eye. The images show multiple suprasellar tuberculomas (arrowed) and areas of cerebral edema.

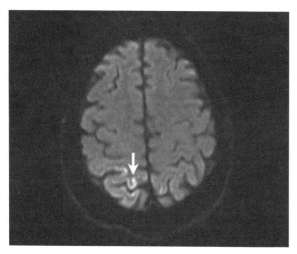

Figure 6.11 Axial diffusion-weighted imaging in a 74-year-old woman with a 3-week history of an evolving left homonymous hemianopia. The images demonstrate high signal in a cortical ribbon pattern, particularly in the right parietal and occipital lobes (arrowed). She died 4 months later and a diagnosis of CJD was confirmed at autopsy.

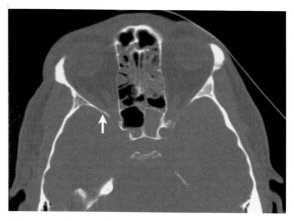

Figure 6.12 Bone window view of an axial CT scan in a 33-year-old man with a traumatic brain injury secondary to a motor-vehicle accident. His right pupil developed decreased reaction to light an hour after admission to the emergency room. On regaining consciousness he could only perceive hand movements with his right eye. The scan shows a right lateral orbital wall fracture (arrowed) as part of more extensive skull base fractures, with an overlying hematoma in the lateral rectus muscle causing optic nerve compression.

atrophy (PCA), and the Heidenhain variant of Creutzfeldt–Jakob disease (CJD) (Figure 6.11) can all present acutely with hemianopia, cerebral blindness, or visuo-perceptual disorders. There are usually characteristic features of each on MRI [85–87], although single photon emission computed tomography (SPECT) and ^{18}F-FDG PET can also be helpful in diagnosing PCA [86]. Tumors, particularly metastases, can also cause acute loss of vision when they affect the posterior visual pathways [88].

Traumatic vision loss

Traumatic loss of vision can occur due to damage at any point along the visual pathway, similar to loss of vision due to medical causes. Trauma to the globe will not be considered further and imaging in cerebral trauma is discussed in Chapter 14. The optic nerve is vulnerable to both direct and indirect traumatic injury. Direct trauma to the optic nerve results from avulsion of the optic nerve, penetrating injury with or without a retained foreign body, or compression from an orbital or optic canal fracture. Indirect traumatic optic neuropathy is thought to be secondary to the transmission of shearing forces to the optic nerve, concentrated at the optic canal, without disruption of the structures neighboring the optic nerve [89]. Orbital CT scanning will demonstrate any fractures (Figure 6.12), orbital hematomas, or metallic orbital foreign bodies as well as any intracranial injuries [13,

90]. MRI is better at detecting radiolucent foreign bodies, such as wood, and is also better than CT in evaluating optic nerve avulsion, axonal injury, or ischemia [13]. The optic chiasm is vulnerable in high-velocity trauma, typically due to motor-vehicle accidents. Injury to the chiasm is usually associated with skull fractures, intracranial hemorrhage, and injuries to other cranial nerves [91]. MRI may show chiasmal contusion [92] or complete chiasmal transection [93]. Traumatic hemianopias have been reported to occur with a range of injuries, although again the majority are due to motor-vehicle accidents. The lesion may affect any part of the post-chiasmal visual pathways with about half the cases having multiple sites of injury [94].

Vision loss can also occur as a secondary consequence of the injury. Major trauma can lead to direct carotid cavernous fistulae with large-volume shunting of blood from the internal carotid artery into the cavernous sinus and superior ophthalmic vein. Presentation is with proptosis, chemosis, orbital bruit, ophthalmoplegia, and decreased visual acuity [95]. DSA is the investigation of choice to plan intervention, which is usually by endovascular or surgical sacrifice of the ipsilateral internal carotid artery. Transtentorial herniation may be a consequence of critically raised intracranial pressure. This can lead to unilateral or bilateral posterior cerebral artery infarction [96].

Pediatric acute vision loss

The principles in investigating acute vision loss in infants and children are the same as in adults [97]. The diseases affecting the pediatric population are similar to adults, although usually at a much reduced prevalence. Clinical assessment is more challenging due to the potential for lack of cooperation and also the difficulties in measuring vision in young children. Observation of behavior and play are therefore extremely important in assessing the level of visual function. Children older than 3 years can often perform simple visual acuity tests to detect shapes or the letters HVOT. Testing children under 3 but over 18-months-old can be performed using small white balls against a black background and observing if the child follows the balls and picks them up (the Stycar rolling-ball test) or with simple object recognition (the BUST-D test) [98]. Testing younger infants can be performed by assessing forced choice preferential looking at grating stimuli with different stripe width [99].

Neuroimaging also presents many challenges. CT is quicker than MRI and does not require high levels of cooperation. It does, however, involve ionizing radiation and it has been estimated that in the 10 years after the first CT scan in patients younger than 10, one excess case of leukemia and one excess case of brain tumor per 10 000 head CT scans will occur [100]. MRI in young and uncooperative children (particularly those younger than 5 years of age) will require sedation or general anesthesia [101]. This requires MRI compatible monitoring, anesthetic supervision, and ventilating equipment and is very time-consuming. Safety of MRI and CT was assessed in a large series of 922 children receiving sedation and 140 given general anesthesia [102]. Hypoxemia occurred in 2.9% of sedated children. Sedation was inadequate in 16% of the children and failed in 7%. One child receiving general anesthesia experienced laryngospasm. Excessive motion artifacts were seen in 12% of images of sedated children and 0.7% of those who had received general anesthesia. It is also likely that imaging protocols will be curtailed in sedated children compared with those receiving an anesthetic, thereby reducing the amount of imaging information obtained.

Optic neuritis in children is frequently bilateral and can occur in isolation or as part of acute disseminated encephalomyelitis (ADEM), MS, or NMO. The differential diagnosis is as broad as it is in adults and therefore neuroimaging with MRI plays a key role in evaluating these cases [103].

Ocular, orbital, and intracranial tumors can also present with acute vision loss in children. Retinoblastoma is the most common intraocular malignant tumor in children. Orbital tumors include rhabdomyosarcoma, metastases from neuroblastoma, plexiform neurofibroma, and Langerhans cell histiocytosis. Gadolinium-enhanced MRI is the imaging modality of choice for the above, with CT providing useful information about bony infiltration, expansion, or destruction [104]. Optic pathway gliomas usually present with slowly progressive visual loss, although rapidly progressive presentations have been reported with sudden deteriorations due to central retinal vein occlusion or chiasmal apoplexy. On MRI, optic pathway gliomas are isointense or hypointense on T1-weighted imaging, hyperintense on T2-weighted imaging, and demonstrate variable enhancement with gadolinium dependent upon disease activity or glioma grade [104, 105].

Vision loss in intracerebral tumors can be secondary to compression of the visual pathways such as in craniopharyngiomas or secondary to raised intracranial pressure in posterior fossa tumors [106]. The other clinical features should provide a guide to localizing the tumor to enable planning of the appropriate MRI sequences required.

Idiopathic intracranial hypertension (IIH) in childhood seems to fall into two groups: pre-pubertal and post-pubertal. In the former group there is not a link with obesity and it is seen in both sexes. Post-pubertal IIH behaves similarly to adult-onset IIH. MRI pre- and post-gadolinium and magnetic resonance venography (MRV) will be the imaging modalities of choice in order to rule out tumors, meningeal infiltration, and venous sinus thromboses [107].

In a series of 852 patients with hemianopia, there were 81 children [108]. The commonest causes in children were traumatic brain injury (34%), tumors (27%), infarction (23%), and cerebral hemorrhage (7%). Some of the etiological factors for infarcts in children include arterial dissection, cardiac disease, particularly related to cardiac repair or catheterization, and inherited disorders such as sickle-cell disease, Marfan syndrome, and homocysteinuria [109, 110].

Encephalitis can also present with acute vision loss in children. The causative infective agents are the same as for adults in most cases. Unusual encephalitides that can cause acute vision loss exclusively in children including acute necrotizing encephalopathy of childhood (ANEC) [111] and subacute sclerosing panencephalitis (SSPE) [112]. In ANEC, brain MRI reveals widespread changes, but typically there are bilateral thalamic lesions with hemorrhage and cavitation [113]. Brain MRI in SSPE can show non-enhancing T1 hypointense and T2 hyperintense changes in the thalami as well as in cortical white and gray matter [112].

Conclusion

Neuroimaging can play a crucial role in elucidating the cause of acute loss of vision as long as the imaging has been targeted to answer the questions raised by the history and examination findings [14]. It is important to have close links with the radiology department in order to discuss which imaging modality to employ and to include on the imaging request all the relevant clinical details and what diseases are being considered, so that the radiologist can protocol the most appropriate imaging. The close links should also include regular meetings to discuss the imaging findings, especially if the imaging is unexpectedly normal or if an abnormality detected on the imaging does not match up with the clinical picture. The area of interest may not have been adequately imaged or may have been obscured by artifact. Initial normal imaging may not exclude pathology, especially in the early stages of a neurodegenerative disorder, such as PCA or CJD, or in optic neuropathies, such as AION. If the clinical picture is evolving then repeating the imaging or using a different imaging modality may bear fruit. Lastly, the loss of vision may be functional (psychological) in origin. Normal imaging in cases where a functional cause is suspected can be very helpful in reassuring the patient that there is not a serious neurological cause for the visual symptoms.

References

1. Kerr NM, Chew SS L, Eady EK, et al (2010). Diagnostic accuracy of confrontation visual field tests. Neurology 74: 1184–1190.

2. Barker GJ (2000). Technical issues for the study of the optic nerve with MRI. J Neurol Sci 172 (suppl 1): S13–16.

3. Soila KP, Viamonte M, Starewicz PM (1984). Chemical shift misregistration effect in magnetic resonance imaging. Radiology 153: 819–820.

4. Farahani K, Sinha U, Sinha S, et al. (1990). Effect of field strength on susceptibility artifacts in magnetic resonance imaging. Comput Med Imaging Graph 14: 409–413.

5. Pusey E, Lufkin RB, Brown RK, et al. (1986). Magnetic resonance imaging artifacts: mechanism and clinical significance. Radiographics 6: 891–911.

6. Weiss RA, Saint-Louis LA, Haik BG, et al. (1989). Mascara and eyelining tattoos: MRI artifacts. Ann Ophthalmol 21: 129–131.

7. Brown BA, Swallow CE, Eiseman AS (2001). MRI artifact masquerading as orbital disease. Int Ophthalmol 24: 343–347.

8. Aviv RI, Casselman J (2005). Orbital imaging: part 1. Normal anatomy. Clin Radiol 60: 279–287.

9. Hickman SJ (2007). Optic nerve imaging in multiple sclerosis. J Neuroimaging 17 (suppl 1): 42S–45S.

10. Aiken AH, Mukherjee P, Green AJ, et al. (2011). MR imaging of optic neuropathy with extended echo-train acquisition fluid-attenuated inversion recovery. AJNR 32: 301–5.

11. Bose S (2007). Neuroimaging in neuroophthalmology. Neurosurg Focus 23: E9.

12. Aviv RI, Miszkiel K (2005). Orbital imaging: part 2. Intraorbital pathology. Clin Radiol 60: 288–307.

13. Becker M, Masterson K, Delavelle J, et al. (2010). Imaging of the optic nerve. Eur J Radiol 74: 299–313.

14. Lee AG, Johnson MC, Policeni BA, et al. (2009). Imaging for neuro-ophthalmic and orbital disease – a review. Clin Experiment Ophthalmol 37: 30–53.

15. Hickman SJ, Dalton CM, Miller DH, et al. (2002). Management of acute optic neuritis. Lancet 360: 1953–1962.

16. Costa VP, Molnar LJ, Cerri GG (1997). Diagnosing and monitoring carotid cavernous fistulas with color Doppler imaging. J Clin Ultrasound 25: 448–452.

17. Optic Neuritis Study Group (1991). The clinical profile of optic neuritis. Experience of the Optic Neuritis Treatment Trial. Arch Ophthalmol 109: 1673–1678.

18. Barry RC, Wilkinson M, Ahmed RM, et al. (2011). Interventional treatment of carotid cavernous fistula. J Clin Neurosci 18: 1072–9.

19. Hickman SJ (2011). Neuro-ophthalmology. Pract Neurol 11: 191–200.

20. Petzold A, Islam N, Hu H-H, et al. (2013). Embolic and nonembolic transient monocular visual field loss: a clinicopathologic review. Surv Ophthalmol 58: 42–62.

21. Johnston SC, Rothwell PM, Nguyen-Huynh MN, et al. (2007). Validation and refinement of scores to predict very early stroke risk after transient ischaemic attack. Lancet 369: 283–292.

22. DH Stroke Policy Team (2008). Implementing the National Stroke Strategy – An Imaging Guide. London: Department of Health.

23. Sell JJ, Rael JR, Orrison WW (1994). Rotational vertebrobasilar insufficiency as a component of thoracic outlet syndrome resulting in transient blindness. Case report. *J Neurosurg* **81**: 617–619.

24. Lee AG, Wall M (2012). Papilledema: are we any nearer to a consensus on pathogenesis and treatment? *Curr Neurol Neurosci Rep* **12**: 334–339.

25. Lam BL, Morais CG, Pasol J (2008). Drusen of the optic disc. *Curr Neurol Neurosci Rep* **8**: 404–408.

26. Auw-Haedrich C, Staubach F, Witschel H (2002). Optic disk drusen. *Surv Ophthalmol* **47**: 515–532.

27. Krasnianski M, Bau V, Neudecker S, et al. (2006). Isolated bilateral blindness as the sole manifestation of transient ischaemic attacks. *Acta Ophthalmol Scand* **84**: 415–418.

28. Floßmann E, Rothwell PM (2003). Prognosis of vertebrobasilar transient ischaemic attack and minor stroke. *Brain* **126**: 1940–1954.

29. Shams, PN, Plant GT (2011). Migraine-like visual aura due to focal cerebral lesions: case series and review. *Surv Ophthalmol* **56**: 135–161.

30. Panayiotopoulos CP (1999). Visual phenomena and headache in occipital epilepsy: a review, a systematic study and differentiation from migraine. *Epileptic Disord* **1**: 205–216.

31. Wei R, Cai J, Ma X, et al. (2002). Imaging diagnosis of enlarged superior ophthalmic vein. *Zhonghua Yan Ke Za Zhi* **38**: 402–404.

32. Miller NR (2007). Diagnosis and management of dural carotid-cavernous sinus fistulas. *Neurosurg Focus* **23**: E13.

33. Rizzo JF, Andreoli CM, Rabinov JD (2002). Use of magnetic resonance imaging to differentiate optic neuritis and nonarteritic anterior ischemic optic neuropathy. *Ophthalmology* **109**: 1679–1684.

34. He M, Cestari D, Cunnane MB, et al. (2010). The use of diffusion MRI in ischemic optic neuropathy and optic neuritis. *Semin Ophthalmol* **25**: 225–232.

35. Spierer, O, Ben Sira L, Leibovitch I, et al. (2010). MRI demonstrates restricted diffusion in distal optic nerve in atypical optic neuritis. *J Neuroophthalmol* **30**: 31–3.

36. Horton JC (2002). Mistaken treatment of anterior ischemic optic neuropathy with interferon beta-1a. *Ann Neurol* **52**: 129.

37. Hickman SJ, Ko M, Chaudhry F, et al. (2008). Optic neuritis: an update of typical and atypical optic neuritis. *Neuroophthalmology* **32**: 237–248.

38. Ko M, Chaudhry F, Hickman SJ, et al. (2009). Optic neuritis: an update II. Optic neuritis and multiple sclerosis. *Neuroophthalmology* **33**: 10–22.

39. Khanna S, Sharma A, Huecker J, et al. (2012). Magnetic resonance imaging of optic neuritis in patients with neuromyelitis optica versus multiple sclerosis. *J Neuroophthalmol* **32**: 216–20.

40. Storoni M, Davagnanam I, Radon M, et al. (2013). Distinguishing optic neuritis in neuromyelitis optica spectrum disease from multiple sclerosis. *J Neuroophthalmol* **33**: 123–127.

41. Zajicek JP, Scolding NJ, Foster O, et al. (1999) Central nervous system sarcoidosis – diagnosis and management. *QJM* **92**: 103–117.

42. Purvin V, Kawasaki A, Jacobson DM (2001). Optic perineuritis: clinical and radiographic features. *Arch Ophthalmol* **119**: 1299–1306.

43. Hickman SJ, Miszkiel KA, Plant GT, et al. (2005). The optic nerve sheath on MRI in acute optic neuritis. *Neuroradiology* **47**: 51–55.

44. Phillips YL, Eggenberger ER (2010). Neuro-ophthalmic sarcoidosis. *Curr Opin Ophthalmol* **21**: 423–429.

45. Sweeney BJ, Manji H, Gilson RJ, et al. (1993). Optic neuritis and HIV-1 infection. *J Neurol Neurosurg Psychiatr* **56**: 705–707.

46. Burton BJ, Leff AP, Plant GT (1998). Steroid-responsive HIV optic neuropathy. *J Neuroophthalmol* **18**: 25–29.

47. Larsen M, Toft PB, Bernhard P, et al. (1998). Bilateral optic neuritis in acute human immunodeficiency virus infection. *Acta Ophthalmol Scand* **76**: 737–738.

48. Davis EJ, Rathinam SR, Okada AA, et al. (2012). Clinical spectrum of tuberculous optic neuropathy. *J Ophthal Inflamm Infect* **2**: 183–189.

49. Sinha MK, Garg RK, Anuradha HK, et al. (2010). Vision impairment in tuberculous meningitis: predictors and prognosis. *J Neurol Sci* **290**: 27–32.

50. Hughes DC, Raghavan A, Mordekar SR, et al. (2010). Role of imaging in the diagnosis of acute bacterial meningitis and its complications. *Postgrad Med J* **86**: 478–485.

51. Aaron S, Mathew V, Anupriya A, et al. (2010). Tuberculous optochiasmatic arachnoiditis. *Neurol India* **58**: 732–735.

52. Sivadasan A, Alexander M, Mathew V, et al. (2013). Radiological evolution and delayed resolution of an optic nerve tuberculoma: challenges in diagnosis and treatment. *Ann Indian Acad Neurol* **16**: 114–117.

53. Purvin V, Sundaram S, Kawasaki A (2011). Neuroretinitis: review of the literature and new observations. *J Neuroophthalmol* **31**: 58–68.

54. Sepahdari AR, Aakalu VK, Kapur R, et al. (2009). MRI of orbital cellulitis and orbital abscess: the role of diffusion-weighted imaging. *AJR* **193**: W244–250.

55. Chaudhry I, Al-Rashed W, Arat Y (2012). The hot orbit: orbital cellulitis. *Middle East Afr J Ophthalmol* **19**: 34–42.

56. Lundström M, Frisén L (1975). Evolution of descending optic atrophy. A case report. *Acta Ophthalmologica* **53**: 738–746.

57. Meier FM, Bernasconi P, Stürmer J, *et al.* (2002). Axonal loss from acute optic neuropathy documented by scanning laser polarimetry. *Br J Ophthalmol* **86**: 285–287.

58. Vukusic S (2004). Pregnancy and multiple sclerosis (the PRIMS study): clinical predictors of post-partum relapse. *Brain* **127**: 1353–1360.

59. Eddleman CS, Liu JK (2007). Optic nerve sheath meningioma: current diagnosis and treatment. *Neurosurg Focus* **23**: E4.

60. Sleep TJ, Hodgkins PR, Honeybul S, *et al.* (2003). Visual function following neurosurgical optic nerve decompression for compressive optic neuropathy. *Eye (Lond)* **17**: 571–578.

61. Swamy BN, McCluskey P, Nemet A, *et al.* (2007). Idiopathic orbital inflammatory syndrome: clinical features and treatment outcomes. *Br J Ophthalmol* **91**: 1667–1670.

62. Yu-Wai-Man P, Chinnery PF (2011). Leber hereditary optic neuropathy – therapeutic challenges and early promise. *ACNR* **11**: 17–19.

63. van Westen D, Hammar B, Bynke G (2011). Magnetic resonance findings in the pregeniculate visual pathways in Leber hereditary optic neuropathy. *J Neuroophthalmol* **31**: 48–51.

64. Vaphiades MS, Phillips PH, Turbin RE (2003). Optic nerve and chiasmal enhancement in Leber hereditary optic neuropathy. *J Neuroophthalmol* **23**: 104–105.

65. Danesh-Meyer HV (2008). Radiation-induced optic neuropathy. *J Clin Neurosci* **15**: 95–100.

66. Hickman SJ (2011). Neurological visual field defects. *Neuroophthalmology* **35**: 242–250.

67. Arnold AC (2005). Ischemic optic neuropathy. In Miller NR, Newman NJ, Biousse V, Kerrison JB, eds. *Walsh and Hoyt's Clinical Neuro-Ophthalmology*, 6th edn. Philadelphia, PA: Lippincott Williams and Wilkins, pp. 349–384.

68. Purvin V, Kuzma B (2005). Intraorbital optic nerve signal hyperintensity on magnetic resonance imaging sequences in perioperative hypotensive ischemic optic neuropathy. *J Neuroophthalmol* **25**: 202–204.

69. Vaphiades MS (2004). Optic nerve enhancement in hypotensive ischemic optic neuropathy. *J Neuroophthalmol* **24**: 235–236.

70. Fabian ID, Greenberg G, Huna-Baron R (2010). Chiasmal stroke following open-heart surgery. *J Neuroophthalmol* **30**: 219–221.

71. Shelton JB, Digre KB, Katz BJ, *et al.* (2012). Chiasmal stroke in patient with atrial fibrillation and complete occlusion of right internal carotid artery. *J Neuroophthalmol* **32**: 189.

72. Liu JK, Lu Y, Raslan AM, *et al.* (2010). Cavernous malformations of the optic pathway and hypothalamus: analysis of 65 cases in the literature. *Neurosurg Focus* **29**: E17.

73. Wright M, Kamal A, Whittle IR, *et al.* (1999). Chiasmal apoplexy, an unusual complication of cerebral glioblastoma. *Eye (Lond)* **13**: 268–269.

74. Rajasekaran S, Vanderpump M, Baldeweg S, *et al.* (2010). UK guidelines for the management of pituitary apoplexy. *Clin Endocrinol* **74**: 9–20.

75. Bills DC, Meyer FB, Laws ER, *et al.* (1993). A retrospective analysis of pituitary apoplexy. *Neurosurgery* **33**: 602–608.

76. Semple PL, Jane JA, Lopes MBS, *et al.* (2008). Pituitary apoplexy: correlation between magnetic resonance imaging and histopathological results. *J Neurosurg* **108**: 909–915.

77. Tosaka M, Sato N, Hirato J, *et al.* (2007). Assessment of hemorrhage in pituitary macroadenoma by T2*-weighted gradient-echo MR imaging. *AJNR* **28**: 2023–2029.

78. Randeva HS, Schoebel J, Byrne J, *et al.* (1999). Classical pituitary apoplexy: clinical features, management and outcome. *Clin Endocrinol* **51**: 181–188.

79. Zhang X, Kedar S, Lynn MJ, *et al.* (2006). Homonymous hemianopia in stroke. *J Neuroophthalmol* **26**: 180–183.

80. Ois A, Cuadrado-Godia E, Solano A, *et al.* (2009). Acute ischemic stroke in anterior choroidal artery territory. *J Neurol Sci* **281**: 80–84.

81. Lochner P, Golaszewski S, Caleri F, *et al.* (2011). Posterior circulation ischemia in patients with fetal-type circle of Willis and hypoplastic vertebrobasilar system. *Neurol Sci* **32**: 1143–1146.

82. Linn J, Ertl-Wagner B, Seelos KC, *et al.* (2007). Diagnostic value of multidetector-row CT angiography in the evaluation of thrombosis of the cerebral venous sinuses. *AJNR* **28**: 946–952.

83. Agid R, Farb RI, Willinsky RA, *et al.* (2006). Idiopathic intracranial hypertension: the validity of cross-sectional neuroimaging signs. *Neuroradiology* **48**: 521–527.

84. Butros SR, Goncalves LF, Thompson D, *et al.* (2012). Imaging features of idiopathic intracranial hypertension, including a new finding: widening of the foramen ovale. *Acta Radiol* **53**: 682–688.

85. Alemdar M, Iseri P, Selekler M, *et al.* (2007). MELAS presented with status epilepticus and Anton–Babinski syndrome; value of ADC mapping in MELAS. *J Neuropsychiatry Clin Neurosci* **19**: 482–483.

86. Crutch SJ, Lehmann L, Schott JM, *et al.* (2012). Posterior cortical atrophy. *Lancet Neurol* **11**: 170–178.

87. Cornelius JR, Boes CJ, Ghearing G, *et al.* (2009). Visual symptoms in the Heidenhain variant of Creutzfeldt–Jakob disease. *J Neuroimaging* **19**: 283–287.

88. Bakar B, Tekkök IH (2008). Primary undifferentiated ovarian carcinoma diagnosed by its metastasis to brain: an unusual case report. *Turk Neurosurg* **18**: 431–435.

89. Hickman SJ, Tomsak RL (2008). The treatment of indirect traumatic optic neuropathy with corticosteroids. *Neuroophthalmology* **35**: 175–180.

90. Kubal WS (2008). Imaging of orbital trauma. *Radiographics* **28**: 1729–1739.

91. Hassan A, Crompton JL, Sandhu A (2002). Traumatic chiasmal syndrome: a series of 19 patients. *Clin Experiment Ophthalmol* **30**: 273–280.

92. Breslau J, Dalley RW, Tsuruda JS, *et al.* (1995). Phased-array surface coil MR of the orbits and optic nerves. *AJNR* **16**: 1247–1251.

93. Segal L, An JA, Gans M (2009). Traumatic disruption of the optic chiasm. *J Neuroophthalmol* **29**: 308–310.

94. Bruce BB, Zhang X, Kedar S, *et al.* (2006). Traumatic homonymous hemianopia. *J Neurol Neurosurg Psychiatr* **77**: 986–988.

95. Malan J, Lefeuvre D, Mngomezulu V, *et al.* (2012). Angioarchitecture and treatment modalities in posttraumatic carotid cavernous fistulae. *Interv Neuroradiol* **18**: 178–186.

96. Hoyt WF (1960). Vascular lesions of the visual cortex with brain herniation through the tentorial incisura. Neuro-ophthalmologic considerations. *Arch Ophthalmol* **64**: 44–57.

97. Hon LQ, Connolly D, Chan J, *et al.* (2012). Pediatric orbit and periorbital pathology: a pictorial review of imaging strategies using CT and MRI. *J Pediatric Neuroradiol* **1**: 7–17.

98. Rydberg A, Ericson B, Lennerstrand G, *et al.* (1999). Assessment of visual acuity in children aged 1 1/2–6 years, with normal and subnormal vision. *Strabismus* **7**: 1–24.

99. Hoyt CS, Nickel BL, Billson FA (1982). Ophthalmological examination of the infant. Developmental aspects. *Surv Ophthalmol* **26**: 177–189.

100. Pearce MS, Salotti JA, Little MP, *et al.* (2012). Radiation exposure from CT scans in childhood and subsequent risk of leukaemia and brain tumours: a retrospective cohort study. *Lancet* **380**: 499–505.

101. Connolly DJA (2006). Imaging developmental abnormalities in children. In Griffiths PD, Paley MNJ, Whitby EH eds. *Imaging the Central Nervous System of the Fetus and Neonate*. New York: Taylor and Francis, pp. 49–62.

102. Malviya S, Voepel-Lewis T, Eldevik OP, *et al.* (2000). Sedation and general anaesthesia in children undergoing MRI and CT: adverse events and outcomes. *Br J Anaesth* **84**: 743–748.

103. Bonhomme GR, Mitchell EB (2011). Treatment of pediatric optic neuritis. *Curr Treat Options Neurol* **14**: 93–102.

104. Rao AA, Naheedy JH, Chen JYY, *et al.* (2013). A clinical update and radiologic review of pediatric orbital and ocular tumors. *J Oncol* Mar 12, doi: 10.1155/2013/795908.

105. Liu GT (2006). Optic gliomas of the anterior visual pathway. *Curr Opin Ophthalmol* **17**: 427–431.

106. Goldenberg-Cohen N, Ehrenberg M, Toledano H, *et al.* (2011). Preoperative visual loss is the main cause of irreversible poor vision in children with a brain tumor. *Front Neur* **2**: 1–6.

107. Ko MW, Liu GT (2010). Pediatric idiopathic intracranial hypertension (pseudotumor cerebri). *Horm Res Paediatr* **74**: 381–389.

108. Kedar S, Zhang X, Lynn MJ, *et al.* (2006). Pediatric homonymous hemianopia. *J AAPOS* **10**: 249–252.

109. Ganesan V, Chong WK, Cox TC, *et al.* (2002). Posterior circulation stroke in childhood: risk factors and recurrence. *Neurology* **59**: 1552–1556.

110. Tsze DS, Valente JH (2011). Pediatric stroke: a review. *Emerg Med Int* **2001**, ID 734506.

111. Bassuk AG, Burrowes DM, McRae W (2003). Acute necrotizing encephalopathy of childhood with radiographic progression over 10 hours. *Neurology* **60**: 1552–1553.

112. Dundar NO, Aralasmak A, Gurer IE, *et al.* Subacute sclerosing panencephalitis case presenting with cortical blindness: early diagnosis with MRI and MR spectroscopy. *Clin Neuroradiol* 2013; Epub ahead of print.

113. Wong AM, Simon EM, Zimmerman RA, *et al.* (2006). Acute necrotizing encephalopathy of childhood: correlation of MR findings and clinical outcome. *AJNR* **27**: 1919–1923.

Dizziness, nystagmus, and disequilibrium

Marianne Dieterich and Thomas Brandt

Introduction

This chapter focuses mainly on current knowledge of imaging in peripheral vestibular disorders as well as in multisensory vestibular structures and their functions in the human brain and how these are influenced by vestibular disorders of different lesion sites [1, 2]. Much of what we know derives from brain activation studies conducted over the last decade with positron emission tomography (PET) and functional magnetic resonance imaging (fMRI). Vestibular stimulation in healthy subjects elicits patterns of signal increases ("activations") and signal decreases ("deactivations") which have been compared with those in patients with acute and chronic peripheral and central vestibular disorders. In this way, much has been learned about the interconnections of vestibular structures, their activations and interactions with other sensory modalities, the correlations of perceptual and motor functions in normal humans, and the abnormalities that result from strategic peripheral and central vestibular lesions such as vestibular neuritis and bilateral vestibular failure, on the one hand, and central vestibular nucleus lesions due to ischemic infarctions of the lateral medulla (Wallenberg's syndrome), on the other.

Vestibular disorders with vertigo and dizziness as key symptoms

Vertigo and dizziness are not unique disease entities. The two terms cover a number of multisensory and sensorimotor syndromes of various etiologies and pathogenesis (for details see: Brandt *et al.* [2]). After headache, vertigo and dizziness are among the most frequent presenting symptoms, not only in neurological conditions. The lifetime prevalence of rotatory and postural vertigo is around 30% [3], and their annual incidence rises with increasing age [4]. Whether caused by physiological irritation (e.g. rotatory vertigo when riding on a merry-go-round, motion sickness, or height intolerance) or a pathological lesion (e.g. unilateral labyrinthine failure or vestibular nuclei lesions), the resulting vertigo syndrome characteristically exhibits similar symptoms and signs – dizziness/vertigo, nystagmus, a tendency to fall, and nausea or vomiting – despite different underlying pathogenetic mechanisms at work. These disorders of perception (vertigo/dizziness), gaze stabilization (nystagmus), postural control (postural imbalance, falling tendency), and the vegetative system (nausea/vomiting) are related to the main functions of the vestibular system, and can be associated with different sites in the brain.

Vertigo/dizziness is also frequently seen in emergency situations. A retrospective study of more than 4000 consecutive emergency neurological consultations in 1 year reported that headache (21%) was the most frequent cardinal symptom, followed by motor deficits (13%), vertigo/dizziness (12%), and epileptic attacks (11%) [5]. In an emergency situation of vertigo/dizziness, one must first and foremost quickly differentiate between central and peripheral causes, since this has immediate diagnostic and therapeutic implications, for example potentially representing an acute stroke within the brainstem or cerebellum. If this is the case, specific diagnostic tests and therapy must be begun without delay. If the main symptom is acute vertigo, the following five-step procedure is recommended for the first examination [2]:

1. perform the head-impulse test,
2. look for a skew deviation (vertical divergence of the eyes) using the cover test,
3. look for peripheral vestibular spontaneous nystagmus (with Frenzel's glasses),

---

4. look for a gaze-evoked nystagmus beating in the opposite direction of a possible spontaneous nystagmus or vertically upward or downward,
5. look for central deficits of smooth pursuit and saccades, especially in the vertical direction.

The presence of a skew deviation, a normal head-impulse test, and a gaze-evoked nystagmus in the opposite direction to that of spontaneous nystagmus in an acute vestibular syndrome indicate a central dysfunction of the brainstem or, less frequently, the cerebellum [6]. This five-step procedure points toward the presence of central ischemia with a sensitivity of more than 90%; this sensitivity is higher than that achievable from performing an early MRI with diffusion-weighted sequences (88%) [7]. It must be stressed that after an acute, isolated episode of vertigo, the risk of stroke is about 6% in the next 4 years. This is three-fold higher than the risk in an age-matched control group; if there are additional vascular risk factors, then the risk is about 5.5-fold greater [8].

Anatomical organization of peripheral and central vestibular structures

The most important functional structure of the vestibular system is the vestibulo-ocular reflex (VOR), which has three major planes of action: (1) horizontal head rotation about the vertical z-axis (yaw); (2) head extension and flexion about the horizontal, binaural y-axis (pitch); and (3) lateral head tilt about the horizontal line of sight, the x-axis (roll). These three planes represent the three-dimensional space in which the vestibular and oculomotor systems responsible for spatial orientation, perception of self-movement, stabilization of gaze, and postural control operate. The neuronal circuitry of the horizontal and vertical semicircular canals as well as of the otolith organs is based on a sensory convergence that takes place within the VOR (Figure 7.1). The VOR connects a set of extraocular eye muscles that are aligned by their primary direction of pull with the same particular spatial plane of the horizontal, anterior, or posterior canal. The canals of both labyrinths form functional pairs in the horizontal and vertical working planes. In other words, the canals are stimulated and inhibited pair-wise: the horizontal right and left pair, as well as the vertical anterior of one side along with the posterior canal of the opposite side, and vice versa.

The most important structures of central vestibular forms of vertigo are the neuronal pathways mediating the VOR. They travel from the peripheral labyrinth over the vestibular nuclei in the medullary brainstem to the ocular motor nuclei (III, IV, VI) and the supra-nuclear integration centers in the pons and midbrain (interstitial nucleus of Cajal (INC) and rostral interstitial nucleus of the medial longitudinal fasciculus (riMLF)) [2]. Compensatory eye movements are generated over this three-neuron reflex arc during rapid head and body movements. Additionally important are the nucleus prepositus hypoglossi together with the vestibular nuclei and the cerebellum as integration centers for horizontal eye movements.

Clinical differentiation of peripheral and central vestibular disorders

Acute peripheral vestibular dysfunction is – as a rule – characterized by an acute strong rotatory vertigo and peripheral vestibular spontaneous nystagmus in one direction, a tendency to fall in the other direction, as well as nausea and vomiting. The most frequent forms of peripheral vestibular vertigo are benign paroxysmal positioning vertigo (BPPV), Ménière's disease, and vestibular neuritis. Bilateral vestibulopathy, vestibular paroxysmia (the neurovascular compression syndrome of the eighth cranial nerve), and perilymph fistulas are more rare.

Central vestibular forms of vertigo arise from lesions in the brainstem or vestibulocerebellum, or of the connections between both, as well as lesions between the vestibular nuclei and the vestibular/ocular motor structures of the brainstem, thalamus, and vestibular cortex. They can manifest as attacks lasting for seconds or minutes (paroxysmal brainstem attacks, vestibular migraine), for hours or up to days (vestibular migraine, episodic ataxia type 2), or as a permanent syndrome (downbeat nystagmus syndrome in cases of degenerative cerebellar diseases). They are most often caused by infarction, hemorrhage, tumor, multiple sclerosis (MS), or degenerative brain diseases. The beginning and duration of the symptoms help in the differential diagnosis of central vestibular forms of vertigo:

– Short rotatory or postural vertigo attacks lasting seconds to minutes or for a few hours are caused by transient ischemic attacks within the vertebrobasilar territory, vestibular migraine, paroxysmal brainstem attacks with ataxia/dysarthria in MS, and, rarely, by vestibular epilepsy.

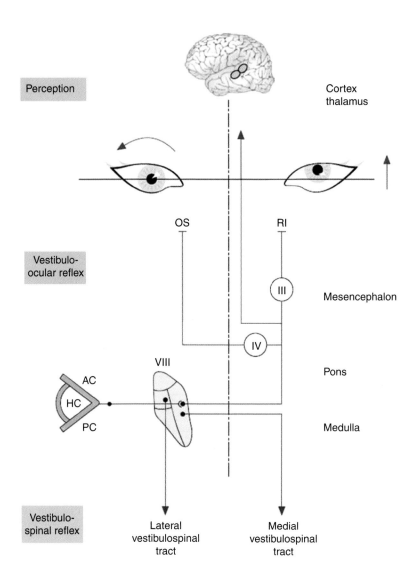

Figure 7.1 Schematic drawing representing the VOR with its three-neuron reflex arc and its mediation of oculomotor, perceptual, and postural functions. A lesion of the vestibular nucleus (VIII) results in an ocular tilt reaction with ocular torsion and vertical divergence of the eyes (i.e. skew deviation) due to a tonus imbalance of the graviceptive pathways. AC, HC, PC = anterior, horizontal, and posterior semicircular canals; OS = superior oblique muscle; RI = inferior rectus muscle; III = oculomotor nucleus; IV = trochlear nucleus.

Perception

Cortex
thalamus

OS   RI

Vestibulo-
ocular reflex

III — Mesencephalon

IV

VIII
AC
HC   Pons
PC   Medulla

Vestibulo-
spinal reflex

Lateral
vestibulospinal
tract

Medial
vestibulospinal
tract

- Attacks of rotatory or postural vertigo lasting hours to several days, generally with additional brainstem deficits, can be caused by infarction, hemorrhage or MS in the brainstem, and, seldom, by a long-lasting attack of vestibular migraine.
- Several days to weeks of persisting postural vertigo (seldom persisting rotatory vertigo), combined with a tendency to fall in a certain direction, is usually caused by permanent damage to the brainstem or the cerebellum bilaterally, e.g. downbeat nystagmus syndrome due to permanently degenerative cerebellar disease or upbeat nystagmus syndrome due to paramedian pontomedullary or ponto-mesencephalic damage (infarction, hemorrhage, tumor, intoxication).

For a simple clinical overview, the central vestibular brainstem syndromes can be classified according to the three major planes of action of the VOR [2].

For differentiating the vertigo syndromes in peripheral or central vestibular disorders the following criteria of the **history** are helpful:

- type of vertigo/dizziness,
- duration of vertigo/dizziness,
- trigger/exacerbation/improvement of vertigo,
- accompanying symptoms (headache, audiological symptoms, central signs)
- illusionary movements of the surroundings (oscillopsia) with head stationary,
- oscillopsia only during head movements,

113

- vertigo with additional brainstem/cerebellar symptoms,
- vertigo with impaired stance and gait.

Besides the detailed patient history, which is the key to diagnosis, systematic **neuro-ophthalmological and neuro-otological examinations** are especially important. In the clinical examination, the physician should at first try to differentiate between peripheral vestibular and central vestibular forms of vertigo as well as between peripheral and central ocular motor disorders since this has immediate diagnostic and therapeutic consequences especially in cases of acute symptoms. The following aspects of the physical examination of patients with vertigo are obligatory and easy to do in the office:

- **Examine the eye position during straight-ahead gaze**, especially with regard to vertical divergence (so-called skew deviation: one eye is higher than the other).
- **Examine the patient for nystagmus**. It is important to use Frenzel's glasses, in particular to differentiate between a peripheral vestibular spontaneous nystagmus that can be suppressed by visual fixation and a central fixation nystagmus; the latter is typically also present during fixation or is even intensified by it.
- **Examine the different types of eye movements** (especially smooth pursuit, saccades, gaze-holding function) for central eye-movement disorders such as saccadic smooth pursuit, gaze palsy, gaze-evoked nystagmus, disorder of saccades, as well as impaired visual-fixation suppression of the VOR. If patients with acute vertigo have central ocular motor disorders, this suggests a central origin, as for example ischemia or inflammation in the brainstem or cerebellum.
- **Perform the head-impulse test according to Halmagyi–Curthoys**, addressing the question of a unilateral or bilateral functional deficit of the VOR [9]. If the patient has acute vertigo with nystagmus but the head-impulse test does not give a pathological result, this indicates a central origin.
- **Perform positioning maneuvers** to determine if there is a positioning nystagmus or positioning vertigo, also to differentiate between a BPPV and a central positional or positioning nystagmus.
- **Examine the patient's stance and gait with the eye open and closed**.

In addition:

- **Determine the subjective visual vertical (SVV)**. A deviation of the SVV occurs in more than 90% of all acute unilateral peripheral and central vestibular disorders. It is thus a very sensitive vestibular sign that can be readily examined in the office using the bucket test [10] but it does not differentiate between a central or peripheral vestibular lesion.
- **Examine the patient's hearing**.

Technical aspects in specific disorders

Imaging of the petrous bone, the cerebellopontine angle, the brainstem, and cerebellum with CT and MRI

In general, with high-resolution magnetic resonance imaging (MRI) and computed tomography (CT) of the petrous bone, it is now possible to reliably identify the following peripheral and central vestibular diseases [2]:

- masses in the cerebellopontine angle and/or internal auditory canal (e.g. vestibular schwannoma) or middle ear (e.g. cholesteatoma);
- post-traumatic forms of vertigo due to petrous bone fractures;
- "vestibular pseudoneuritis" due to fascicular lesions of the vestibular nerve at the entry zone of the brainstem or the vestibulocerebellum (e.g. MS or ischemic lesions).

Imaging is also important for the diagnosis of:

- inflammatory (e.g, labyrinthitis, Cogan's syndrome), hereditary (e.g. Mondini–Alexander dysplasia), or neoplastic (e.g. meningeosis carcinomatosa) inner-ear diseases;
- vestibular paroxysmia (looking for neurovascular cross-compression of the vestibular nerve);
- superior-canal dehiscence syndrome (looking for a defect of the bone over the superior semicircular canal by high-resolution temporal bone CT;
- hemosiderosis affecting the vestibular nerves (Figure 7.2);
- vestibular neuritis due to herpes zoster virus;
- labyrinthine concussion.

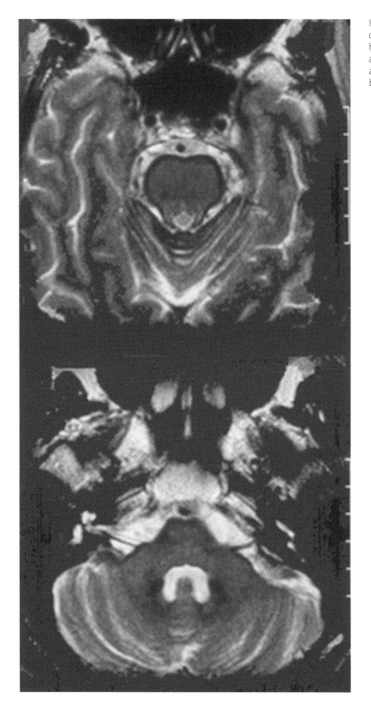

Figure 7.2 MRI scan of the pontomedullary brainstem of a patient with bilateral vestibular failure due to hemosiderosis after subarachnoidal bleeding from an aneurysm (pons, top; medulla, bottom). Hemosiderosis affects the eighth nerves bilaterally and the surface of the brainstem and cerebellar peduncles (black deposition).

Menière's disease

Menière's disease is typically a combination of abruptly occurring attacks that usually last for hours with vestibular and/or cochlear symptoms such as fluctuating, slowly progressive hearing loss, tinnitus, aural fullness, and, in the course of time, vestibular deficits. Monosymptomatic attacks that are purely cochlear or vestibular can occur, particularly at the beginning of Menière's disease. During the course of the disease most patients develop a progressive

115

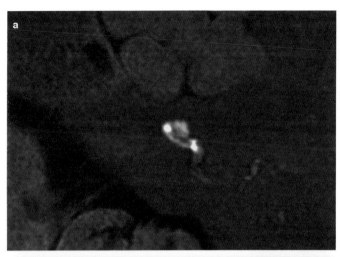

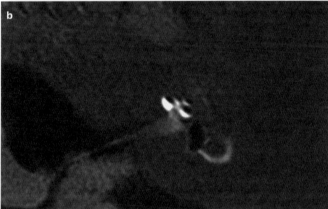

Figure 7.3 Image of endolymphatic hydrops using high-resolution MRI of the petrous bone 24 hours after transtympanic injection of gadolinium contrast, which preferably reaches the perilymph space (Courtesy of Robert Gürkov *et al.* [15]). Labyrinth with cochlea and semicircular canals of a healthy control (a) and of a patient with Menière's disease (b). The hydrops is indicated by the recess of the contrast medium (black areas).

persistent hypoacusis of the affected ear. A relative overproduction or underabsorption of endolymph is thought to be the cause. However, the underlying etiology to date is unknown.

An endolymphatic hydrops can be found in cases of Menière's disease in post-mortem temporal bone studies [11] and also *in vivo* on high-resolution MRI after transtympanic gadolinium (Gd) injection, because Gd diffuses primarily into the perilymphatic space [12]. After the initial descriptions of this approach, this technique has been improved considerably and has been shown to be a supportive diagnostic tool [13, 14, 15] (Figure 7.3). It has also been included in treatment trials to evaluate the effects of different agents on endolymphatic hydrops, although in two small case studies this method has not been found to predict or monitor treatment effects of gentamicin [16] or betahistin [17]. Still, this imaging technique is considered promising for visualizing endolymphatic hydrops [2].

Superior-canal dehiscence syndrome (SCDS)

In the SCDS [18], the bony defect in the superior semicircular canal leads to a third "mobile window" – in addition to the round and oval windows bordering the middle ear (Figure 7.4). With this defect there is pathological transmission of intracranial pressure changes to the perilymphatic space of the labyrinth, thus causing stimulation or inhibition of the superior semicircular canal due to ampullofugal or ampullopetal deviation of the cupula [19]. The symptoms appear as recurrent spells of rotatory or postural vertigo with oscillopsia induced by coughing or increasing the abdominal pressure and sometimes by loud sounds [20]. The clinical diagnosis must be confirmed by thin-slice CT of the petrous bone, which reveals an apical defect of the bony canal. High-resolution CT of the temporal bones may, however, demonstrate a false canal dehiscence [21]. The dehiscence can involve the superior, lateral, or

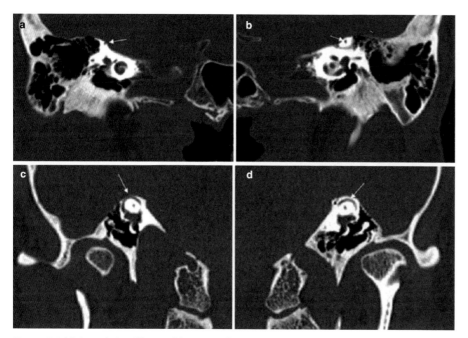

Figure 7.4 High-resolution CT scan of the petrous bone in a patient with an SCDS (left) compared to that of a normal control (right). Coronal slice (a, b) and diagonal slice parallel to the axis of the superior canal (c, d) show the bony defect in the apical part of the right superior canal (a, c) (arrows).

posterior semicircular canals, but the superior is the most relevant clinically [19].

High-resolution CT of the petrous bone

Modern multislice CT instruments allow very high-spatial-resolution imaging of the structures of the petrous bone, in particular the bony labyrinth, the facial nerve canal, and the skull base. For example, an examination in the spiral (helical) mode of operation (with 1-mm slice thickness, 1-mm table feed, 140 kV, 111 mA, and 0.75-s revolution) can yield a local spatial resolution of $0.3 \times 0.3 \times 1$ mm. The data are reconstructed for each side separately. Typically, the study includes multiplanar reconstructions, and three-dimensional (3D) surface reconstructions are also possible. CT of the petrous bone is indicated to evaluate for fractures, malformations (Mondini–Alexander dysplasia), and in particular the SCDS, as well as ossifications of the labyrinth in chronic illnesses (e.g. otosclerosis or Cogan's syndrome) and accompanying bone alterations in benign and malignant growth processes (e.g. cholesteatoma, cholesterol cysts, jugular diverticula, vestibular schwannoma, rhabdomyosarcoma, and metastatic disease).

High-resolution MRI of the petrous bone and the cerebellopontine angle

The MRI examination of the petrous bone and the cerebellopontine angle is most often performed with a circularly polarized head coil. This technique is clearly superior to CT for imaging the non-osseous structures or lesions, e.g. tumors and inflammatory soft-tissue growths, especially in the petrous bone. The numerous anatomical structures confined within a very small space within the petrous bone places high demand on the MRI technology. The examination protocol should include the following (or similar) sequences:

- Transversal (axial) proton-weighted and T2-weighted fast spin-echo sequence with 3-mm-thick slices and an interslice gap of less than 0.8 mm for evaluating the brainstem and cerebellum.
- A transversal T1-weighted sequence (e.g. two-dimensional fast low angle shot, FLASH) with a 2-mm-thick slice and in-plane spatial resolution of about 0.5 mm, before and, if applicable, after intravenous administration of Gd. After the contrast medium is applied, it is advisable to perform additional coronal imaging.

117

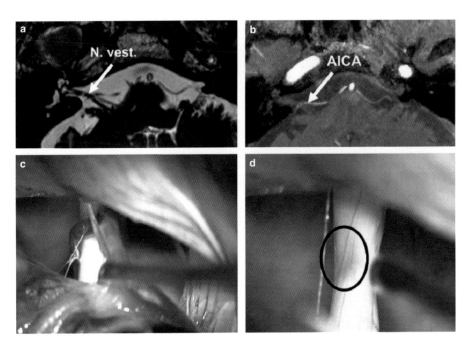

Figure 7.5 Cranial MRI (a: CISS; b: TOF sequence) shows contact between the right vestibular nerve (N. vest) and the anterior inferior cerebellar artery (AICA) (arrows). Intraoperative photographs demonstrate the vascular contact (c) and considerable compression of the nerve (circle) after removal of the arteries (d). (Modified after Strupp et al. [23].)

– A high-resolution, strongly T2-weighted sequence (e.g. 3D constructive interference in steady state (CISS), or 3D fast imaging employing steady-state acquisition (FIESTA)) of about 0.6–0.8 mm slice thickness and 0.5 mm in-plane spatial resolution. This sequence is especially suitable for imaging the cranial nerves and the fluid-filled spaces of the inner-ear structures. It is the method of choice for detecting pathological neurovascular cross-compression. With this high-resolution 3D approach, multiplanar reconstruction is feasible, including parallel to the course of each cranial nerve. By using the maximum intensity projection (MIP) procedure, it is possible to represent the signal-intense structures of the inner ear three-dimensionally and in any orientation.

– If pathological neurovascular cross-compression (i.e. vestibular paroxysmia) is suspected, another complementary examination with magnetic resonance angiography (MRA; e.g. time of flight (TOF)) is performed. If the TOF-MRA is performed before and after intravenous administration of contrast medium, it is possible to identify and differentiate nerve contact with arteries as well as with veins [22–24] (Figures 7.5,

7.6). In the latter study neurovascular contact of the eighth nerve could be detected in all patients at 0.0–10.2 mm distance between brainstem and compressing vessel presenting with vestibular paroxysmia rendering a sensitivity of 100% and a specifity of 82% for the diagnosis of vestibular paroxysmia by MRI.

No imaging recommended

Benign paroxysmal positioning vertigo (BPPV)

BPPV – clinically the most common cause of vertigo, not only in the elderly – usually does not require imaging. It is characterized by brief attacks of rotatory vertigo and simultaneous positioning rotatory-linear nystagmus toward the forehead and toward the under-most ear. BPPV is caused by dislodged particles (probably otoconia) that freely move in the posterior semicircular canal (canalolithiasis) [2]. It may be related to head trauma but more than 95% of all cases are classified as degenerative or idiopathic, especially in older patients. Rotatory vertigo and nystagmus occur after positioning the head or body toward the affected ear with a short latency of seconds in the form of a crescendo/decrescendo course of maximally

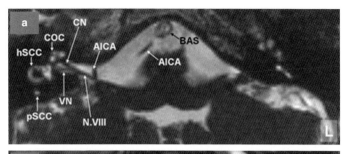
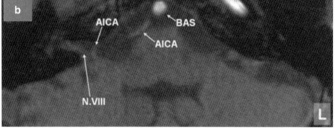
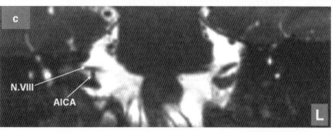
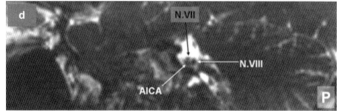

Figure 7.6 Typical illustration of a neurovascular compression of the eighth cranial nerve and the AICA. (a) High-resolution CISS presenting the neurovascular compression between the AICA and the right eighth cranial nerve (N.VIII). On this image the basilar artery (BAS), the cochlear (COC), the posterior semicircular canal (pSCC) as well as the horizontal semicircular canal (hSCC) are also depicted. In addition, the deviation of the eighth cranial nerve into the cochlear nerve (CN) and the vestibular nerve (VN) can be seen. (b) On the TOF sequence without Gd contrast enhancement, the vessel can be identified as artery due to the hyperintensity as well as by retracing it to the parent vessel, the BAS. (c) Coronal reconstruction from the CISS sequences, displaying the contact of nerve and vessel between the AICA and N.VIII. (d) Sagittal reconstruction with illustration of the close relation between N.VIII, N.VII, and the AICA, resulting in a contact of the eighth cranial nerve. (Adopted from Best et al. [24])

30–60 seconds. Complaints and nystagmus are so typical that a diagnosis can often be made solely on the basis of the patient history. The diagnosis requires positioning liberatory maneuvers that result in a canal-specific positional nystagmus of the posterior, horizontal, or anterior semicircular canals (posterior BPPV > horizontal BPPV > anterior BPPV). When correctly performed, the physical liberatory maneuvers according to Semont [25] or Epley [26] are successful in almost all patients. In very rare cases central infratentorial lesions of the cerebellum (nodulus) can mimic BPPV.

Vestibular neuritis

The main symptoms of acute unilateral vestibular neuritis are a sustained violent rotatory vertigo with illusory movements of the surroundings, gait and postural imbalance with a tendency to fall, as well as nausea and vomiting [2]. All of these symptoms have an acute or subacute onset and last for a few days or weeks. Hearing disorders, tinnitus, or other neurological deficits are not part of the clinical picture of the illness. The clinical syndrome is characterized by:

- persistent rotatory vertigo lasting several days;
- horizontal-rotatory spontaneous nystagmus (to the non-affected side), suppressed by visual fixation, increased while looking in the direction of the nystagmus;
- gait deviation and tendency to fall to the affected side;
- nausea and vomiting;

119

- unilateral functional deficit of the horizontal canal, which can be detected by the head-impulse test according to Halmagyi–Curthoys and caloric irrigation [9].

The diagnosis of vestibular neuritis is one of exclusion, ensuring that the patient does not have a central etiology of symptoms such as Wallenberg's syndrome. Structural imaging of the ear is not required for this diagnosis as it gives no positive results. Sometimes it is necessary to exclude or differentiate a central etiology of this acute vestibular syndrome (stroke, MS) by MRI of the brainstem, cerebellum, and brain.

   Treatment is symptomatic for nausea and vomiting (antivertiginous drugs). Some studies indicated that glucocorticoids can improve the course of acute vertigo. However, a recent Cochrane meta-analysis still makes no treatment recommendation for corticosteroids, as the effects on quality of life have not as yet been investigated sufficiently [27].

Structural and functional imaging of the human brain

In this section we describe findings of functional imaging studies during vestibular stimulation in healthy volunteers and the changes caused by vestibular lesions at different sites. Additional detail is available in previously published reviews [1, 28, 29].

The intact vestibular system and its cortical network

Activations during vestibular stimulation in healthy subjects

A complex network of areas has been found mainly in the temporoinsular and temporoparietal cortex in both hemispheres of healthy subjects during caloric irrigation of the horizontal semicircular canals [30–34], during galvanic stimulation of the vestibular nerve [35–38], and even during stimulation of the sacculus otolith (sound induced [39–41]) by means of fMRI or PET techniques. These areas showed signal increases ("activations") in humans located in the posterior insula (first and second long insular gyri) and retroinsular regions; the superior temporal gyrus; parts of the inferior parietal lobule, deep within the intraparietal sulcus; the postcentral and precentral gyrus; the anterior insula and adjacent inferior frontal gyrus; the anterior cingulate gyrus; the precuneus; and

the hippocampus [28]. The area in the posterior insula and the operculum corresponding to the parieto-insular vestibular cortex (PIVC) [42] appears to be a core region of the network. Interestingly, this cortical network was not activated symmetrically in the two hemispheres. Instead, the pattern is determined by three factors as defined in a study of healthy right- and left-handers during caloric irrigation by PET [34]. These are: (1) the subject's handedness, (2) the side of the stimulated ear, and (3) the direction of the induced vestibular nystagmus. Activation was found to be stronger in the non-dominant hemisphere (right hemisphere in right-handers, left hemisphere in left-handers), in the hemisphere ipsilateral to the stimulated ear, and in the hemisphere ipsilateral to the slow phase of vestibular caloric nystagmus [28, 29].

Deactivations during vestibular stimulation in healthy subjects

At the same time as "activations" occurred, there were also signal decreases ("deactivations"), in areas within the visual and somatosensory systems of both hemispheres [34, 36, 43]. The activation–deactivation patterns were opposite to each other. Originally, the patterns were found during visually induced self-motion perception; for example, activations of occipital and parietal visual areas co-occurred with deactivations of the multisensory vestibular cortex, e.g. the PIVC [44] (Figure 7.7). These findings led to the assumption that there is a reciprocal inhibitory cortical interaction between the visual and the vestibular systems. The interaction shifts the dominant sensorial weight from one modality to the other, and so resolves conflicts between incongruent sensory inputs. It was subsequently hypothesized that reciprocal inhibitory interactions between the sensory systems are likely to be a fundamental mechanism of the central nervous system (CNS) [44]. Such interactions also occur between other sensory modalities, e.g., the somatosensory and nociceptive, the nociceptive and the vestibular, the tactile sensory and visual, and the visual and auditory systems [36, 45, 46]. The psychophysical consequences of these interactions were revealed in a study investigating high-resolution visual mental imagery and mental rotation tasks, which were significantly impaired during vestibular caloric stimulation in healthy subjects [47].

   The psychophysical and functional imaging data of an inhibitory interaction within the visual system [48] support the interpretation that the deactivation of

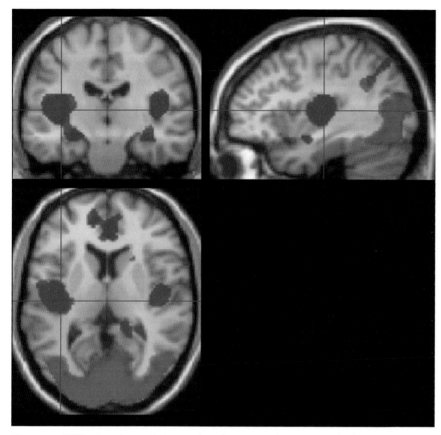

Figure 7.7 fMRI activated areas during visual optokinetic stimulation in seven healthy volunteers. While activations are located in the visual cortex bilaterally, areas with signal decreases are found in the temporal, insular, and parietal cortex areas and the anterior cingulate cortex, i.e., in areas of the multisensory vestibular cortical network. (activations (red): $p \leq 0.001$; deactivations (blue): $p \leq 0.0001$); 1.5 T scanner.

neural activity in the visual system (measured by fMRI and PET) may be associated with a functional decrement in sensitivity needed to perceive motion and orientation. This might reflect transcallosal attentional shifts between the two hemispheres, i.e., so-called "cross-talk," to resolve sensory conflicts. Indeed, negative fMRI responses correlated with decreases in neural activity in the visual area V1 [49]. Taken together, the deactivations found in normal subjects in PET and fMRI studies seem to represent decreases of function at the neural level.

The non-intact vestibular system and the consequences within the cortical network

Acute unilateral lesions of the vestibular nerve

The main symptoms of an acute unilateral vestibular deficit are a sustained violent rotatory vertigo with illusory movements of the surroundings (so-called oscillopsia), gait and postural imbalance with a tendency to fall, as well as nausea and vomiting. All of these symptoms have an acute or subacute onset and last for a few days or weeks [2]. Vestibular neuritis with an incidence of 3.5 per 100 000 persons is the third most frequent cause of peripheral vestibular vertigo after BPPV and Menière's disease and accounts for about 7% of the diagnoses made in a specialized neurological outpatient clinic for vertigo. The disease occurs most frequently in adults between 30 and 60 years of age. The complaints resolve slowly over 1–2 weeks. As a rule the patient is generally symptom-free within 3–5 weeks when at rest, i.e., under static conditions. Recovery is the result of a combination of the following:

- central compensation of the peripheral vestibular tonus imbalance;
- restoration of peripheral vestibular function (generally incomplete)

121

- substitution of the functional loss by the contralateral unaffected vestibular system as well as by somatosensory (neck proprioception) and visual input.

With respect to recovery and compensation several questions are of interest: Which are the neural correlates for this central compensation? Does the acute lesion-induced vestibular tonus imbalance between the two labyrinths lead to a modulation of neural activity within the thalamo-cortical vestibular system? If it does, is this activation pattern asymmetrical, thus reflecting the perceptual correlate of the tonus imbalance at the cortical level?

To answer these questions the cortical activation patterns in patients with unilateral lesions were compared to the functional imaging data of healthy volunteers during unilateral caloric [31–34] or galvanic [36, 37, 45] stimulation. Unilateral vestibular stimulation, on the one hand, and unilateral failure of the vestibular end organ, on the other, should create a vestibular tonus imbalance. However, each occurs at different levels of activity of the vestibular system. A unilateral lesion reduces the resting discharge input, whereas a unilateral stimulation increases the resting discharge input from an end organ.

Activations and deactivations in unilateral peripheral vestibular lesions

During the acute stage of vestibular neuritis (mean: 6.6 days after symptom onset) it was indeed possible to demonstrate that the central vestibular system exhibited a visual–vestibular activation–deactivation pattern similar to that described earlier in healthy volunteers during unilateral vestibular stimulation. Right-handed patients with a right-sided vestibular neuritis were examined with fluorodeoxyglucose (FDG) PET in the acute stage and 3 months later after central vestibular compensation when the patients were symptom-free [50, 51]. The regional cerebral glucose metabolism was significantly increased during the acute stage in multisensory vestibular cortical and subcortical areas such as the PIVC, posterolateral thalamus, anterior cingulate gyrus, ponto-mesencephalic brainstem, and hippocampus (Figure 7.8). Thus, FDG PET could image a cortical activation pattern of the vestibular system, which was induced by unilateral peripheral

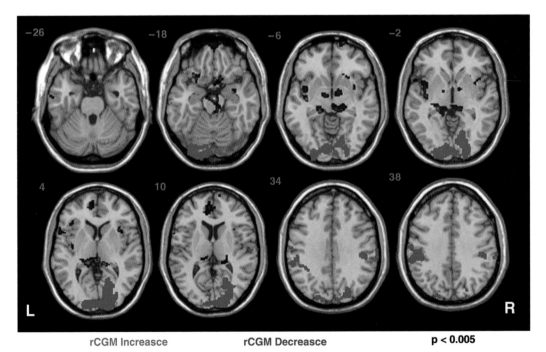

rCGM Increasce   rCGM Decreasce   **p < 0.005**

Figure 7.8 FDG PET imaging. Statistical group analysis based on five patients with vestibular neuritis of the right ear versus the control condition 3 months later (eyes closed, without stimulation). A significant increase (red) of regional cerebral glucose metabolism (rCGM) is seen in the contralateral left vestibular cortex, left superior temporal gyrus, hippocampus, thalamus bilaterally; it is also pronounced in the anterior cingulate gyrus. Simultaneously rCGM decreases (blue) are located in the visual and somatosensory cortex bilaterally. For illustrative purposes, voxels above a threshold of $p \leq 0.005$, uncorrected, are shown.

vestibular loss and may reflect the tonus imbalance. Simultaneously, there was a significant decrease of regional cerebral glucose metabolism in the visual and somatosensory cortex as well as in parts of the auditory cortex (transverse temporal gyrus) [50]. These decreases were very similar to those in the visual and somatosensory systems during vestibular stimulation in healthy subjects. This pattern probably reflects a non-specific inhibition of other sensory areas in response to vestibular activation.

The activation of the PIVC was not bilateral with a dominance of the right side, but unilateral and contralateral (left) to the right labyrinthine failure. This asymmetry of activations within the PIVC can be explained by assuming that the more dominant ipsilateral right-sided ascending projections to the right insular cortex were depressed by the right vestibular neuritis, because the tonic end organ input was absent (resting discharge). Another explanation might be that the vestibular tonus imbalance at the vestibular nuclei level mimics a left-sided vestibular excitation due to a higher resting discharge rate of the unaffected left vestibular nuclei complex.

Chronic bilateral vestibular failure (BVF)

BVF is a rare chronic disorder of the labyrinth or the eighth cranial nerve with various etiologies [2]. Its key symptoms are unsteadiness of gait, particularly in the dark and on unlevel ground, and blurred vision due to oscillopsia, the illusory motion of the visual scene caused by the insufficient VOR. BVF patients do not usually have a vestibular tonus imbalance like patients with vestibular neuritis, and their signs and symptoms can only be elicited by locomotion and head movements, but not at rest.

The etiology of BVF remains unclear in 50% of cases, although these can be assumed to have a degenerative illness. Beyond this group, the three most frequent causes of bilateral vestibulopathy include ototoxic aminoglycosides (13%), Menière's disease (7%), and meningitis (5%). Other causes are bilateral vestibular schwannoma (neurofibromatosis type 2) or autoimmune diseases like Cogan's syndrome. In this syndrome MRI shows typical hemorrhages and an enhanced uptake of contrast medium in the labyrinth and/or cochlea, indicating the activity of the disease [52]. Patients with BVF frequently have a cerebellar syndrome and downbeat nystagmus. Such cases probably involve a neurodegenerative illness that affects the vestibular ganglia cells and the

cerebellum; it often occurs with an additional neuropathy, cerebellar ataxia with neuropathy and vestibular areflexia syndrome (CANVAS) [53].

Since the vestibular input is bilaterally reduced or even absent, the question arises whether compensation of the vestibular deficits is achieved by substitution of another sensory modality.

Activations and deactivations in bilateral vestibular lesions

The differential effects of caloric irrigation in right-handed patients with complete and incomplete BVF are of special interest. These patients exhibit no caloric vestibular nystagmus and do not perceive any illusory self-motion or have vegetative sensations due to caloric irrigation. Their activation–deactivation patterns during vestibular caloric stimulation are generally decreased [54]. In particular, there is only a small area of activation in the PIVC contralateral to the irrigated ear and no significant activation on the side of the irrigated ear. In contrast, healthy right-handers have bilateral activation and the activation on the ipsilateral right side is stronger. BVF patients also largely lack bilateral deactivation of the visual cortex. This general absence suggests that the deactivation depends on a "normal" activation of the vestibular cortex. There is also no evidence of common non-vestibular (e.g. auditory, somatosensory) responses in other cortical areas. Since vestibular input is reduced in these patients, causing them to have reduced or absent vestibular nystagmus and concurrent oscillopsia, there is perhaps no need for a "protective" reduction of visual cortex functions.

An fMRI study on visual optokinetic stimulation in BVF patients provided evidence of visual substitution for vestibular loss [55]. Visual optokinetic stimulation in these patients induced a significantly stronger activation and larger activation clusters of the primary visual cortex bilaterally (inferior and middle occipital gyri, BA 17, 18, and 19); the motion-sensitive area V5 in the middle and inferior temporal gyri (BA 37), and the frontal eye field (BA 8); the right paracentral and superior parietal lobule; and the right fusiform and parahippocampal gyri compared to that of age-matched healthy controls (Figure 7.9). Functionally, the enhanced activations were independent of optokinetic performance, since the mean slow phase velocity of optokinetic nystagmus in the patients did not differ from that in the controls. Furthermore, small areas of signal decreases (deactivations), located primarily in the right posterior insula containing the PIVC, were

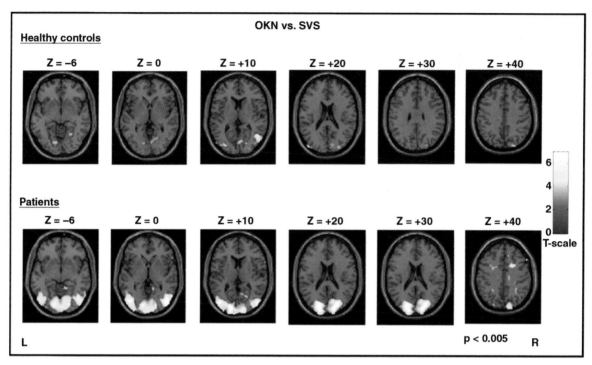

Figure 7.9 Head-to-head display of the activation in the t-contrast optokinetic nystagmus (OKN) vs. stationary visual stimulus (SVS) condition in fMRI for patients with BVF (bottom) and the age-matched healthy control group (top). For illustrative purposes, voxels above a threshold of $p < 0.005$, uncorrected, are shown (modified after Dieterich et al. [55]).

similar to those in healthy controls. These enhanced activations within the visual and ocular motor systems of BVF patients suggest that they might be correlated with an upregulation of visual sensitivity during tracking of visual motion patterns. Also, in structural brain imaging studies (by voxel-based morphometry), a volume increase was seen in the visual motion-sensitive area MT/V5 as well as in the somatosensory area of the nucleus gracilis in the brainstem whereas the vestibular areas of the hippocampus and the superior temporal gyrus showed volume decreases [56] (Figure 7.10). Thus, brain imaging techniques have now complemented the psychophysical and neurophysiological tests showing how sensory loss in one modality leads to a substitutional increase of functional sensitivity in other modalities [57, 58].

Acute unilateral lesions of the vestibular nucleus (infarction of the posterolateral medulla)

Vestibular nucleus lesions due to an acute infarction of the posterolateral medulla (Wallenberg's syndrome) or a plaque in MS affect the medial and/or superior vestibular subnuclei, causing a central vestibular disorder. This central vestibular syndrome is characterized by rotatory vertigo as well as static vestibular signs such as ipsiversive ocular torsion of one or both eyes (82%), skew deviation with the ipsilateral eye lowermost (44%), complete ocular tilt reaction (33%), and tilts of the perceived vertical in most patients (94%). Moreover, dynamic vestibular signs such as ipsilateral lateropulsion of eyes and body [59, 60], torsional nystagmus, and dysmetria of saccades and limbs occur [61]. These vestibular signs due to an infarction are most often combined with other neurological deficits such as Horner's syndrome, impairment of facial pain and temperature sensation, paralysis of the pharynx and larynx with dysphagia and dysphonia, and contralateral impairment of pain and temperature sensation over the trunk and limbs.

How is compensation achieved in central lesions of the vestibular nuclei?

Activations and deactivations in unilateral central lesions of the vestibular nucleus

Caloric irrigation of the ears in patients with Wallenberg's syndrome elicits asymmetrical activations at the cortical level as it does in patients with vestibular neuritis. When examined during warm-

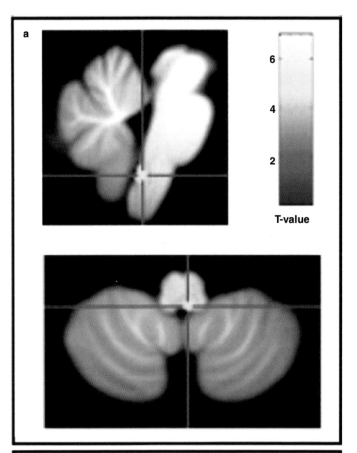

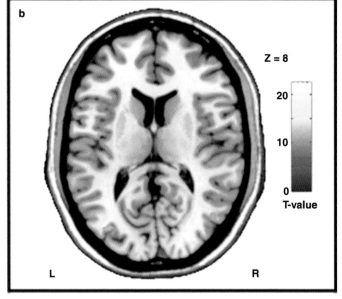

Figure 7.10 Central compensation after vestibular neuritis. (a) Signal increases of the right gracile nucleus in the medullary brainstem in 22 patients with vestibular neuritis; sagittal (top) and transversal (bottom) slices. (b) Vestibular neuritis patients with a residual canal paresis (n = 14) showed a significant increase of the middle temporal visual area V5 bilaterally >2 years after disease onset (modified after zu Eulenburg et al. [56]).

water caloric vestibular stimulation [62], the patients' activation patterns were typically different from those of healthy volunteers. During caloric irrigation of the ear ipsilateral to the side of the lesion, there was either no activation or significantly reduced activation in the contralateral hemisphere, whereas the activation pattern in the ipsilateral hemisphere appeared "normal." These results agree with the existence of bilaterally ascending vestibular pathways from the vestibular nuclei (especially the medial vestibular subnucleus) to vestibular cortex areas in which only the contralateral tract is affected. The novel finding was that the activation patterns support the assumption that mainly the fibers crossing from the medial vestibular subnucleus to the contralateral MLF are lesioned, whereas the ipsilateral vestibular thalamo-cortical projections via the superior vestibular subnucleus may be spared.

Additional findings were reported for right-handed patients with an acute unilateral medullary infarction (six right, six left) when the brain activity was measured during a rest condition with the eyes closed (FDG PET [63]). The patients were examined twice without any stimulation, (1) in the acute phase on day 7 as a mean after symptom onset when they showed vestibular signs and (2) 6 months later after recovery (Figure 7.11). There were widespread *decreases* of regional glucose metabolism not only in the visual cortex (BA 17–19) bilaterally, including the motion-sensitive area MT/V5 and merging into the secondary visual areas in the upper occipital cortex (BA 19/37) but also in the multisensory temporoparietal areas of the medial and superior temporal gyrus (STG) and the inferior parietal lobule (IPL). Interestingly, no relevant activations were seen at the cortical level, in contrast to patients with peripheral vestibular lesions such as vestibular neuritis. However, the findings for deactivations in visual cortex areas parallel the data for vestibular neuritis. This means that the concept of a reciprocally inhibitory interaction between the vestibular and visual systems is modified by the type of central vestibular lesion: areas become deactivated (STG and IPL) which are

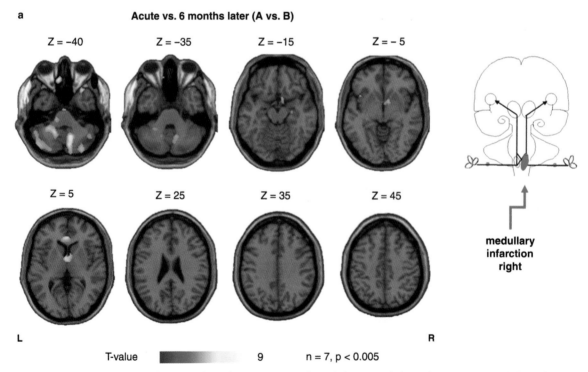

Figure 7.11 (a) FDG PET statistical group analysis of seven patients with vestibular tone imbalance due to an acute medullary infarction affecting the right vestibular nucleus (situated in the right brainstem; i.e., Wallenberg's syndrome) vs. the control scan 6 months later at recovery (contrast A vs. B), and (b) the inverse contrast (B vs. A). The contrast A vs. B (a) mainly showed cerebellar signal differences, whereas the inverse contrast (PET B vs. A (b)) revealed widespread bilateral signal changes in the visual cortex (Brodmann areas [BA] 17–19), including the motion-sensitive area MT/V5 (BA 19/37) and merging into secondary visual areas in the upper occipital cortex (BA 19/39) as well as in temporoparietal areas (GTm/s, LPi, BA 39/40).

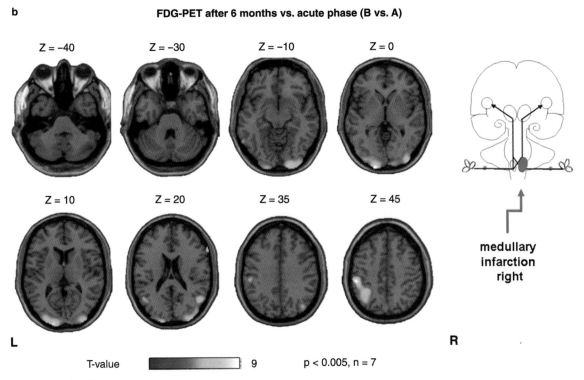

b   **FDG-PET after 6 months vs. acute phase (B vs. A)**

Z = -40   Z = -30   Z = -10   Z = 0

Z = 10   Z = 20   Z = 35   Z = 45

medullary
infarction
right

L   R

T-value ████████ 9   p < 0.005, n = 7

Figure 7.11 (cont.)

normally activated during vestibular stimulation conditions in healthy subjects.

In general, Wallenberg's patients showed signal increases in the acute phase of disease that were located mainly in the medulla and cerebellar peduncle contralateral to the infarction, and also in the vermis, and extensively in both cerebellar hemispheres [51]. The signal increases seem to represent an essential circuit for the central compensation in unilateral central vestibular lesions of the vestibular nuclei, since such relevant cerebellar activations were not observed in the patients with unilateral or bilateral peripheral vestibular lesions.

Acute unilateral lesions along the vestibular pathways in the brainstem

Earlier lesion studies in patients with acute unilateral brainstem infarctions from the medulla to the midbrain provided evidence that the signs of an acute tone imbalance in the roll plane of the VOR – head tilt, skew deviation, and ocular torsion (i.e. ocular tilt reaction) – were associated with perceptual deficits such as tilts of perceived subjective visual vertical (SVV) [60]. These signs were induced by unilateral lesions of the

vestibular nucleus causing ipsilateral deviations or by lesions of the ascending MLF, riMLF, and INC in the ponto-mesencephalic brainstem causing contralateral deviations [60]. Furthermore, ipsilateral tilts of SVV without these other ocular motor signs were elicited by unilateral lesions of the medial lemniscus in the ponto-mesencephalic brainstem [64]. These descriptive data applying paper and pencil mapping were confirmed recently by modern statistical lesion-behavior mapping techniques on a large sample of 79 patients with acute unilateral brainstem strokes [65]. Indeed, a lesion of the medial vestibular nucleus or the medial lemniscus was associated with ipsiversive tilts of SVV; contraversive tilts were associated with lesions of the riMLF, the superior cerebellar peduncle, the oculomotor nucleus, and the INC (Figure 7.12).

Acute unilateral lesions of the vestibular thalamic nuclei

Unilateral lesions of the posterolateral thalamus and – at the cortical level – the superior temporal and the insular cortex (including the PIVC) cause vestibular tonus imbalance without ocular motor signs. These patients, however, have perceptual deficits (e.g.

127

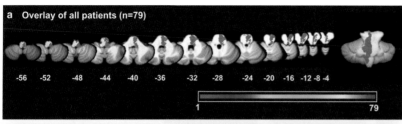

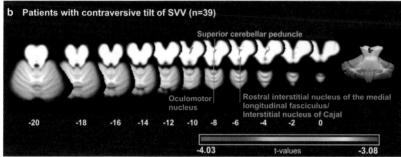

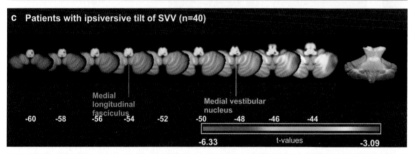

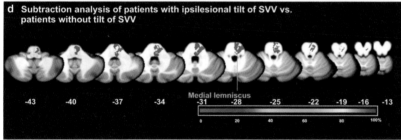

Figure 7.12 (a) Simple overlay of the MRI lesions of all 79 patients with unilateral brainstem infarctions; left-sided lesions are flipped to the right side. The number of overlapping lesions is illustrated by different colors coding increasing frequencies from violet (n = 1) to red (n = max.). Statistical voxelwise lesion-behavior mapping (VLBM) analysis comparing (b) the patients with contraversive tilt of subjective visual vertical (SVV) (n = 39) and (c) the patients with ipsiversive tilt of SVV (n = 40) with respect to absolute SVV tilt (t-test statistic). Presented are all voxels that survived a correction for multiple comparisons using a 5% false-discovery rate (FDR) cut-off threshold. (d) Subtraction analysis of patients with lesions affecting the anteromedial ponto-mesencephalic region with ipsilateral tilt of SVV (tilt >2.5°) vs. patients without tilt of SVV. The percentage of overlapping lesions of the patients with tilt of SVV after subtraction of controls is illustrated by different colors coding increasing frequencies, from violet (0%) to dark red (100%), which reflects the relative frequency of damage, i.e., corresponding percentage more frequently affected in patients with tilt of SVV compared to the control group (modified after Baier et al. [65]).

deviations of the perceived visual vertical) as well as postural deficits, i.e., an imbalance of stance and gait with lateral falls [66, 67]. This type of vestibular imbalance is probably identical to the earlier term "thalamic astasia," a condition of irresistible falls without paresis or sensory or cerebellar signs [68, 69].

In patients with three different types of acute unilateral thalamic infarctions the posterolateral lesions caused transient vestibular signs and symptoms like perceptual deficits with ipsi- or contralateral tilts of the SVV, corresponding deviations of stance and gait, but no ocular motor deficits [66].

Only recently, a lesion study of 37 patients with acute thalamic strokes applying modern statistical lesion-behavior mapping could show two distinct systems for graviceptive vestibular processing by different lesion sites for ipsilateral or contralateral deficits of vertical perception [70]. Whereas contraversive tilts were associated with posterolateral lesions, the regions associated with ipsiversive tilts were located more inferiorly and medially.

These signs of thalamic lesions agree with earlier findings in electrical stimulation studies of the thalamic subnucleus ventro-oralis intermedius in humans.

Patient BS: thalamus infarction left

Calorics right   (H$_2$ ^{15}O-PET)   Calorics left

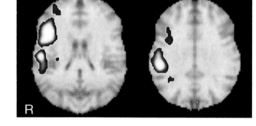
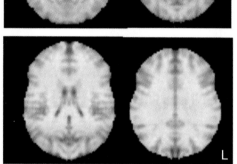

Figure 7.13 Activated areas during caloric stimulation of the right or left ear in a patient with a left-sided posterolateral thalamic infarction (regional cerebral blood flow, RCBF, measured by H$_2$^{15}O-PET; p <0.001). Left: increases of RCBF (activations) for the left-sided lesions during right calorics (non-affected side) occur as large clusters in the posterior and anterior insula, inferior frontal gyrus, superior temporal gyrus, inferior parietal lobule, superior parts of the parietal lobule, hippocampus, paramedian thalamus, midbrain, nucleus ruber, putamen, medial and superior frontal gyrus, and cerebellar vermis of the right hemisphere. Activations of the left hemisphere are found in only the anterior cingulate gyrus, and diagonal frontal gyrus. Right: caloric irrigation of the affected left side shows no significant activations.

Such stimulation elicited a corresponding rotation or spinning of the body, head, or eyes in either a counterclockwise (more often) or clockwise direction [71].

Activations and deactivations in unilateral lesions of the thalamus

In view of the vestibular thalamo-cortical network in both hemispheres, the question arose as to the consequences of a unilateral lesion of the "vestibular relay station" in the posterolateral thalamus. Therefore, the differential effects of unilateral caloric vestibular stimulation (right- or left-ear irrigation with warm water) on the cortical and subcortical activation pattern of both hemispheres were analyzed in right-handed patients who had had an acute unilateral stroke of the posterolateral thalamus [72] (Figure 7.13). It was found that (i) activation of the multisensory vestibular cortex was significantly reduced in the ipsilateral hemisphere, when the ear ipsilateral to the thalamic lesion was stimulated; (ii) activation of multisensory vestibular cortex areas of the hemisphere contralateral to the irrigated ear was also diminished, but to a lesser extent; (iii) the right hemispheric dominance in right-handers was preserved in patients with right and left thalamic lesions. Thus, these data demonstrated the functional importance of the posterolateral thalamus as a gatekeeper of the dominance of ipsilateral ascending pathways, and of the right hemisphere in right-handedness. This asymmetrical pattern of cortical activation during calorics was neither associated with directional asymmetry of caloric nystagmus nor with motion perception for the entire group. The caloric nystagmus tended to be stronger during stimulation of the ear contralateral to the lesion.

Vestibular stimulation in healthy volunteers not only activates vestibular cortex areas but at the same time deactivates visual cortex areas bilaterally [36, 43]. Patients with posterolateral thalamic infarctions generally showed deactivations of the visual cortex areas in only one hemisphere, namely in the hemisphere contralateral to the stimulated ear and contralateral to activated vestibular cortex areas [72]. This suggests a crossed inhibition, i.e., the normal interaction between the vestibular and the visual systems (described earlier as a reciprocal inhibitory interaction in both hemispheres [44]) is disturbed in these patients: their ipsilateral hemisphere was "functionally disconnected."

Conclusion

Although we have learned how certain vestibular disorders from different lesion sites modify visual–vestibular interaction by changing the "normal" cortical activation–deactivation pattern, there remains much to be learned from functional imaging and other studies to determine the neural basis of the underlying disorders. Several vestibular, oculomotor, and cerebellar disorders still await investigation with structural and functional MRI and PET with various ligands. These studies promise to provide further insights into the complex neural networks of the human cortex and the changes occurring during compensatory processes after strategic lesions.

References

1. Dieterich M (2013). Functional imaging of the vestibular system. In Bronstein A, ed. *Oxford Textbook of Vertigo and Imbalance*. Oxford: Oxford University Press, ch.7.

2. Brandt T, Dieterich M, Strupp M (2013). *Vertigo and Dizziness. Common Complaints*, 2nd edn. London: Springer.

3. Neuhauser HK (2007). Epidemiology of vertigo. *Curr Opin Neurol* **20**: 40–46.

4. Davis A, Moorjani P (2003). The epidemiology of hearing and balance disorders. In Luxon LM, Furman JM, Martini A, Stephens D, eds. *Textbook of Audiological Medicine*. London: Dunitz M, pp. 89–99.

5. Royl G, Ploner CJ, Mockel M, Leithner C (2010). Neurological chief complaints in an emergency room. *Nervenarzt* **81**: 1226–1230.

6. Newman-Toker DE, Kattah JC, Alvernia JE, Wang DZ (2008). Normal head impulse test differentiates acute cerebellar strokes from vestibular neuritis. *Neurology* **70**: 2378–2385.

7. Kattah JC, Talkad AV, Wang DZ, Hsieh YH, Newman-Toker DE (2009). HINTS to diagnose stroke in the acute vestibular syndrome: three-step bedside oculomotor examination more sensitive than early MRI diffusion-weighted imaging. *Stroke* **40**: 3504–3510.

8. Lee CC, Suy C, Ho HC, *et al.* (2011). Risk of stroke in patients hospitalized for isolated vertigo. A four year follow-up study. *Stroke* **42**: 48–52.

9. Halmagyi GM, Curthoys IS (1988). A clinical sign of canal paresis. *Arch Neurol* **45**: 737–739.

10. Zwergal A, Rettinger N, Frenzel C, *et al.* (2009). A bucket of static vestibular function. *Neurology* **72**: 1689–1692.

11. Merchant SN, Adams JC, Nadol JB Jr (2005). Pathophysiology of Menière's syndrome: are symptoms caused by endolymphatic hydrops? *Otol Neurot* **26**: 74–81.

12. Nakashima T, Naganawa S, Sugiura M, *et al.* (2007). Visualization of endolymphatic hydrops in patients with Menière's disease. *Laryngoscope* **117**: 415–420.

13. Fiorino F, Pizzini FB, Belramello A, *et al.* (2011). Reliability of magnetic resonance imaging performed after intratympanic administration of gadolinium in the identification of endolymphatic hydrops in patients with Menière's desease. *Otol Neurotol* **32**: 472–477.

14. Pierce NE, Antonelli PJ (2012). Endolymphatic hydrops perspectives 2012. *Curr Opin Otolaryngol Head Neck Surg* **20**: 416–419.

15. Gürkov R, Flatz W, Louza J, *et al.* (2012). In vivo visualized endolymphatic hydrops and inner ear function in patients with electrocochleographically confirmed Menière's disease. *Otol Neurootol* **33**: 1040–1045.

16. Claes G, Van den Hauwe L, Wuyts F, Ven de Heyning P (2012). Does intratympanic gadolinium injection predict efficacy of gentamicin partial chemolabyrinthectomy in Menière's desease patients? *Eur Arch Otorhinolaryngol* **269**: 413–418.

17. Gürkov R, Flatz W, Keeser D, *et al.* (2012). Effect of standard-dose betahistine on endolymphatic hydrops: an MRI pilot study. *Eur Arch Otorhinolaryngol* **270**: 1231–1235.

18. Minor LB, Solomon D, Zinreich JS, Zee DS (1998). Sound- and/or pressure-induced vertigo due to bone dehiscence of the superior semicircular canal. *Arch Otolaryngol Head Neck Surg* **124**: 249–258.

19. Chien WW, Carey JP, Minor LB (2011). Canal dehiscence. *Curr Opin Neurol* **24**: 25–31.

20. Minor LB (2005). Clinical manifestation of superior semicircular canal dehiscence. *Laryngoscope* **115**: 1717–1727.

21. Sequeira SM, Whiting BR, Shimony JS, Vo KD, Hullar TE (2011). Accuracy of computed tomography detection of superior canal dehiscence. *Otol Neurotol* **32**: 1500–1505.

22. Hüfner K, Barresi D, Glaser M, *et al.* (2008). Vestibular paroxysmia: diagnostic features and medical treatment. *Neurology* **71**(13): 1006–1114.

23. Strupp M, Stuckrad-Barre S, Brandt T, Tonn JC (2013). Compression of the eighth cranial nerve causes vestibular paroxysmia. *Neurology* **80**: e77.

24. Best C, Gawehn J, Krämer HH, *et al.* (2013). MRI and neurophysiology in vestibular paroxysmia: contradiction and correlation. *JNNP* **84**: 1349–1356.

25. Semont A, Freyss G, Vitte E (1988). Curing the BPPV with a liberatory maneuver. *Adv Otorhinolaryngol* **42**: 290–293.

26. Epley JM (1992). The canalith repositioning procedure: for treatment of benign paroxysmal positional vertigo. *Otolaryngol Head Neck Surg* **107**: 399–404.

27. Fishman JM, Burgess C, Waddell A (2011). Corticosteroids for the treatment of idiopathic acute vestibular dysfunction (vestibular neuritis). *Cochrane Database Syst Rev* CD008607.

28. Dieterich M, Brandt T (2008). Functional imaging of peripheral and central vestibular disorders. *Brain* **131**; 2538–2552.

29. Dieterich M, Brandt T (2010). Imaging cortical activity after vestibular lesions. *Restor Neurol Neurosci* **28**: 47–56.

30. Bottini G, Karnath HO, Vallar G, *et al.* (2001). Cerebral representations for egocentric space: functional-anatomical evidence from caloric vestibular stimulation and neck vibration. *Brain* **124**: 1182–1196.

31. Suzuki M, Kitano H, Ito R, *et al.* (2001). Cortical and subcortical vestibular response to caloric stimulation detected by functional magnetic resonance imaging. *Cogn Brain Res* **12**: 441–449.

32. Fasold O, von Brevern M, Kuhberg M, *et al.* (2002). Human vestibular cortex as identified with caloric stimulation in functional magnetic resonance imaging. *NeuroImage* **17**: 1384–1393.

33. Naito Y, Tateya I, Hirano S, *et al.* (2003). Cortical correlates of vestibulo-ocular reflex modulation: a PET study. *Brain* **126**: 1562–1578.

34. Dieterich M, Bense S, Lutz S, *et al.* (2003). Dominance for vestibular cortical function in the non-dominant hemisphere. *Cerebral Cortex* **13**: 994–1007.

35. Lobel E, Kleine JF, Le Bihan D, Leroy-Willig A, Berthoz A (1998). Functional MRI of galvanic vestibular stimulation. *J Neurophysiol* **80**: 2699–2709.

36. Bense S, Stephan T, Yousry TA, Brandt T, Dieterich M (2001). Multisensory cortical signal increases and decreases during vestibular galvanic stimulation (fMRI). *J Neurophysiol* **85**: 886–899.

37. Fink GR, Marshall JC, Weiss PH, *et al.* (2003). Performing allocentric visuospatial judgements with induced distortion of the egocentric reference frame: an fMRI study with clinical implications. *NeuroImage* **20**: 1505–1517.

38. Stephan T, Deutschländer A, Nolte A, *et al.* (2005). Functional MRI of galvanic vestibular stimulation with alternating currents at different frequencies. *Neuroimage* **26**: 721–732.

39. Miyamoto T, Fukushima K, Takada T, de Waele C, Vidal PP (2007). Saccular stimulation of the human cortex: a functional magnetic resonance imaging study. *Neurosci Lett* **423**: 68–72.

40. Janzen J, Schlindwein P, Bense S, *et al.* (2008). Neural correlates of hemispheric dominance and ipsilaterality within the vestibular system. *NeuroImage* **42**: 1508–1518.

41. Schlindwein P, Mueller M, Bauermann T, *et al.* (2008). Cortical representation of saccular vestibular stimulation: VEMPs in fMRI. *NeuroImage* **39**: 19–31.

42. Eulenburg zu P, Caspers S, Roski C, Eickhoff SB (2012). Meta-analytical definition and functional connectivity of the human vestibular cortex. *Neuroimage* **60**: 162–169.

43. Wenzel R, Bartenstein P, Dieterich M, *et al.* (1996). Deactivation of human visual cortex during involuntary ocular oscillations. A PET activation study. *Brain* **119**: 101–110.

44. Brandt T, Bartenstein P, Janek A, Dieterich M (1998). Reciprocal inhibitory visual–vestibular interaction: visual motion stimulation deactivates the parieto-insular vestibular cortex. *Brain* **121**: 1749–1758.

45. Laurienti PJ, Burdette JH, Wallace MT, *et al.* (2002). Deactivation of sensory-specific cortex by cross-modal stimuli. *J Cogn Neurosci* **14**: 420–429.

46. Merabet LB, Swisher JD, McMains SA, *et al.* (2007). Combined activation and deactivation of visual cortex during tactile sensory processing. *J Neurophysiol* **97**: 1633–1641.

47. Mast FW, Merfeld DM, Kosslyn SM (2006). Visual mental imagery during caloric vestibular stimulation. *Neuropsychologia* **44**: 101–9.

48. Brandt T, Marx E, Stephan T, Bense S Dieterich M (2003). Inhibitory interhemispheric visuo–visual interaction in motion perception. *Ann NY Acad Sci* **1004**: 283–288.

49. Shmuel A, Augath M, Oeltermann A, Logothetis NK (2006). Negative functional MRI response correlates wuth decreases in neuronal activity in monkey visual area V1. *Nature Neurosci* **9**: 569–577.

50. Bense S, Bartenstein P, Lochmann M, *et al.* (2004). Metabolic changes in vestibular and visual cortices in acute vestibular neuritis. *Ann Neurol* **56**: 624–630.

51. Becker-Bense S, Dieterich M, Buchholz H-G, *et al.* (2013). The differential effects of acute right- vs left-sided vestibular failure on brain metabolism. *Brain Structure and Function*, May 18 [Epub ahead of print]

52. Helmchen C, Jäger L, Büttner U, Reiser M, Brandt T (1998). Cogan's syndrome. High resolution MRI indicators of activity. *J Vestib Res* **8**: 155–167.

53. Szmulewicz DJ, Waterston JA, Halmagyi GM, *et al.* (2011). Sensory neuropathy as part of the cerebellar ataxia neuropathy vestibular areflexia syndrome. *Neurology* **76**: 1903–1910.

54. Bense S, Deutschländer A, Stephan T, *et al.* (2004). Preserved visual–vestibular interaction in patients with bilateral vestibular failure. *Neurology* **63**: 122–128.

55. Dieterich M, Bauermann T, Best C, Stoeter P, Schlindwein P (2007). Evidence for cortical visual substitution of chronic bilateral vestibular failure (an fMRI study). *Brain* **130**: 2108–2116.

56. Eulenburg zu P, Stoeter P, Dieterich M (2010). Voxel-based morphometry depicts central compensation after vestibular neuritis. *Ann Neurol* **68**(2): 241–249.

57. Bles W, de Jong JM, de Wit G (1984). Somatosensory compensation for loss of labyrinthine function. *Acta Otolaryngol (Stockh)* **97**: 213–221.

58. Curthoys IS, Halmagyi GM (1994). Vestibular compensation: a review of the oculomotor, neural, and clinical consequences of unilateral vestibular loss. *J Vest Res* **5**: 67–107.

59. Dieterich M, Brandt T (1992). Wallenberg's syndrome: lateropulsion, cyclorotation, and subjective visual vertical in thirty-six patients. *Ann Neurol* **31**: 399–408.

60. Dieterich M, Brandt T (1993). Ocular torsion and tilt of subjective visual vertical are sensitive brainstem signs. *Ann Neurol* **33**: 292–299.

61. Morrow MJ, Sharpe A (1988). Torsional nystagmus in the lateral medullary syndrome. *Ann Neurol* **24**: 390.

62. Dieterich M, Bense S, Stephan T, *et al.* (2005). Medial vestibular nucleus lesions in Wallenberg's syndrome cause decreased activity of the contralateral vestibular cortex. *Ann NY Acad Sci* **1039**: 1–16.

63. Becker-Bense S, Buchholz H-G, Best C, *et al.* (2013). Vestibular compensation in acute unilateral medullary infarction: FDG PET study. *Neurology* **80**: 1103–1109.

64. Zwergal A, Büttner-Ennever J, Brandt T, Strupp M (2008). An ipsilateral vestibulothalamic tract adjacent to the ML in humans. *Brain* **131**: 2928–2935.

65. Baier B, Thömke F, Wilting J, *et al.* (2012). A pathway in the brainstem for roll-tilt of the subjective visual vertical: evidence from a lesion-behavior mapping study. *J Neurosci* **32**: 14854–14858.

66. Dieterich M, Brandt T (1993). Thalamic infarctions: differential effects on vestibular function in the roll plane (35 patients). *Neurology* **43**: 1732–1740.

67 Brandt T, Dieterich M (1994). Vestibular syndromes in the roll plane: topographic diagnosis from brainstem to cortex. *Ann Neurol* **36**: 337–347.

68. Masdeu JC, Gorelick PB (1988). Thalamic astasia: inability to stand after unilateral thalamic lesions. *Ann Neurol* **23**: 596–602.

69. Elwischger K, Rommer P, Prayer D, *et al.* (2012). Thalamic astasia from isolated centromedian thalamic infarction. *Neurology* **78**: 146–147.

70. Conrad J, Baier B, Dieterich M (2014). The role of the thalamus in the human subcortical vestibular system. *Journal of Vestibular Research* (in press).

71. Tasker RR, Organ LW, Hawrylyshyn PA, eds. (1982). *The Thalamus and Midbrain of Man. A Physiological Atlas using Electrical Stimulation.* Springfield, IL: Charles C Thomas.

72. Dieterich M, Bartenstein P, Spiegel S, *et al.* (2005). Thalamic infarctions cause side-specific suppression of vestibular cortex activations. *Brain* **128**: 2052–2067.

Seizures

Lauren C. Frey and Bronwyn E. Hamilton

Introduction and definitions

What is a seizure?

Seizures are an important cause of visits to an emergency department (ED), accounting for millions of visits annually worldwide. The billions of neurons in the human brain generally communicate with each other via small electrical and chemical signals. However, when networks of neurons function abnormally, they can produce much larger, synchronous, electrical discharges. In general, these highly synchronized discharges are abnormal and when spontaneous and sustained highly synchronous discharges occur, they disrupt otherwise normal brain activity, creating an electrical seizure in the brain. Because this electrical seizure disrupts normal brain activity, a person can experience involuntary experiential or behavioral changes that are the clinical manifestations of a seizure. This chapter will focus on patients presenting with clinical manifestations of seizures. Additional information about seizures occurring alongside symptoms due to other conditions can be found in other chapters of this book.

In general, these involuntary experiential or behavioral changes are highly dependent on the functions of the brain that are located where the abnormal discharge starts and over the area where the abnormal discharge eventually spreads [1]. For example, a complex partial seizure of mesial temporal onset may begin with the patient experiencing a sensation of an unpleasant smell. As the seizure progresses and the abnormal electrical activity spreads within the brain, patients may stare and have abnormal involuntary, often repetitive, movements of their mouth or hands. Seizures with onsets in different areas of the brain will have different manifestations. A list of common clinical manifestations of seizures, along with their suspected regions of onset, can be found in Table 8.1.

How are seizures classified?

Once a seizure is suspected, it can be clinically classified in many different ways. In the emergency setting, the most important classification is whether the seizure is provoked or unprovoked. Provoked seizures are seizures that are secondary to either an identifiable acute insult to the central nervous system (CNS) or to a generalized systemic metabolic disturbance. Provoked seizures are usually a symptom of an acute underlying CNS or systemic illness that requires identification and immediate care within the emergency encounter. A list of common illnesses that can manifest as provoked seizures is included in Table 8.2. In contrast, an unprovoked seizure occurs with no clearly identifiable proximate precipitant. Patients who have had two or more unprovoked seizures can be diagnosed with epilepsy. In one well-regarded study, the age-adjusted incidence rate of epilepsy was as much as one-third lower than the age-adjusted incidence rate for a first unprovoked seizure (1935–1984) in the same population, suggesting that a substantial minority of patients who have one unprovoked seizure will not go on to have a second [2].

A second important classification scheme for seizures is based on the extent of the onset, or beginning, of the seizure. In this scheme, there are two main types of seizures: focal-onset and generalized-onset. In focal-onset seizures, the seizure discharge clearly begins in one specific part of the brain. A focal-onset seizure with preserved consciousness is diagnosed as a **simple partial seizure**. A focal-onset seizure with altered consciousness is referred to as a **complex partial seizure**. A focal-onset seizure that spreads to involve the whole brain and is associated with a generalized convulsion is a **secondarily generalized seizure**. In generalized-onset seizures, the abnormal electrical activity of the seizure is widespread throughout the brain very early

Imaging Acute Neurologic Disease, ed. Massimo Filippi and Jack H. Simon. Published by Cambridge University Press.

Table 8.1 Common clinical manifestations of seizures and potential regions of onset

Onset region	Potential associated clinical manifestations
Frontal-lobe onset seizures	Prominent limb involvement manifests as tonic posturing or clonic Jerking Vocalizations Head and/or eye deviation Urinary incontinence Autonomic signs or symptoms Altered consciousness No or brief post-ictal confusion
Temporal-lobe onset seizures – mesial	Aura of an epigastric sensation, fear or an unpleasant odor or taste Staring Limb or oral automatisms Altered consciousness May be aphasic or confused post-ictally
Temporal-lobe onset seizures – lateral	Aura of auditory hallucination or dizziness Staring Limb or oral automatisms Altered consciousness May be aphasic or confused post-ictally
Parietal	Stereotyped, unexplained sensory experiences Vertigo Choking/sinking sensation Disorientation
Occipital	Elemental visual hallucinations Visual loss Head and/or eye deviation

Table 8.2 Examples of common illnesses that can acutely provoke seizures

CNS infection (meningitis, encephalitis)

Traumatic brain injury

Intoxications

Stroke (hemorrhagic or ischemic)

Metabolic derangements (especially hypoglycemia)

in the seizure. Examples of generalized-onset seizures include **absence seizures** and **primary generalized tonic-clonic seizures** [1].

Assessment algorithm

First priority: Stabilization of patient. When a patient presents with an event that may be a seizure, stabilization of the patient must be the first priority in emergency management. This includes not only ensuring the patient's airway and vital signs, but also implementing measures for bodily safety and administering medications to stop seizures if the patient appears to still be seizing. A patient can be assumed to have stopped seizing if the seizure behavior has stopped and the patient has returned to his or her baseline neurological function. If the seizure behavior has stopped, but the patient has not returned to his or her baseline neurological function, assessment of the patient's brainwave function with an electroencephalogram (EEG) is recommended to ensure that there is no ongoing electrical, but behaviorally asymptomatic, seizure activity in the brain.

Once the patient is stabilized, use patient history and neurological examination to confirm that patient's event was a seizure. The most important element in the diagnosis of a seizure is a detailed history from both the patient and a witness of the event. Typical clinical seizures are brief (1–2 minutes typically), self-limited events of involuntary experiential or behavioral changes. A history of the event should include details about what happened:

(1) . . . before the event occurred.

- Did the patient experience any prodromal symptoms or auras?
- Were there any precipitating factors?

(2) . . . during the event.

- Were there any changes in the patient's responsiveness, orientation, speech, or memory?
- Were there any abnormal motor movements of the face, trunk, or limbs?
- Did the patient complain of any sensory changes?

(3) . . . after the event.

- Did the patient recover immediately or was there a delay?
- Did the patient return to his/her neurological baseline?

These questions can be answered by either the patient or by a witness if the patient cannot recall the details. Neurological examination of the patient may reveal focal neurological deficits suggesting an area of focal structural damage within the brain that can put a person at risk for seizures. A physical examination may also uncover physical manifestations of genetic or other syndromes that can also put a person at higher risk for seizures. Because seizures are episodic events, patients with suspected seizures often do not receive medical attention until after the event is over. For this reason, a diagnosis of seizure often critically depends on the initial history and physical examination, although it can be supported by ancillary studies such as EEG testing or neuroimaging.

It is important to note that while many patients may present to an ED with a seemingly first-time event, their presentation may, instead, reflect the first event that has come to medical attention. Careful history-taking should probe the patient's past to identify any other events or symptoms in the patient's history that might also be seizure-related. Studies of patients who present with a first-time seizure have found that as many as 50% of these patients have had previous events or symptoms that are likely seizure-related [3].

Determine a potential cause for the patient's presumed seizure. Once the patient is stabilized and there is a strong clinical suspicion that the presenting event was, indeed, a seizure, then the next step is to attempt to identify a cause for the seizure. For some patients, information from the comprehensive history and examination will be sufficient in suggesting areas for further etiological evaluation. This step in the assessment algorithm will also help the provider stratify the urgency with which potential etiologies must be screened. Provoked seizures, for example, are often caused by acute physical or metabolic damage to the brain which must be identified with therapy initiated as soon as possible. Underlying seizure etiology may also critically impact decisions about prognosis or long-term anti-seizure treatment regimens. Neuroimaging plays a critical role in this step of the assessment of a patient with seizure in the ED.

Indications for neuroimaging in an ED patient with seizure

The decision about whether or not to perform a neuroimaging study acutely in the ED should be based on the likelihood of discovering a cause of the seizure that requires immediate intervention. A recent practice parameter from the American Academy of Neurology, the American College of Emergency Physicians, the American Association of Neurological Surgeons and the American Society of Neuroradiology was based on review of the relevant literature [4]. Based on this analysis, factors were determined that should prompt acute neuroimaging in the ED in a patient presenting with a seizure. These factors include:

- a higher likelihood of uncovering a specific structural abnormality that must be addressed urgently,
- a higher likelihood of producing change in management with the imaging results.

Most abnormalities on computed tomography (CT) scans in patients with new-onset seizures are due to stroke, neoplasm, or trauma-related lesions. The most urgent conditions associated with seizures are related to hemorrhage, brain swelling, or mass effect from a variety of causes. According to the same practice parameter named above there are a number of historical elements that might predict which patients have a higher likelihood of a specific structural abnormality that must be addressed urgently or that might lead to a change in management [4]. These include:

- patients with a new-onset focal deficit on neurological exam,
- confirmed partial-onset seizure,
- patients with persistent altered mentation,
- presence of fever,
- known recent trauma,
- presence of persistent headache,
- known history of cancer,
- known history of anticoagulation,
- known history of immunosuppression (chronic immunosuppressive medications, AIDS),
- age greater than 40 years.

When in the course of care should neuroimaging be acquired in an ED patient with seizure?

A collaborative group of neurologists, emergency physicians, neurosurgeons, and neuroradiologists performed a comprehensive literature review on the use of CT-based neuroimaging in the emergency setting [4]. Overall, the authors found very little conclusive evidence in the literature on the best timing of neuroimaging in the emergency setting and, instead, used the results of their review as the basis for a consensus-based practice parameter around this topic. This practice parameter was designed to "help define the role and timing of neuroimaging in the spectrum of emergency care of patients with

Table 8.3 Summary of practice-parameter recommendations

Practice-parameter definitions:	Guidelines: "Recommendations for patient management that may identify a particular strategy or range of management strategies and that reflect moderate clinical certainty" Option: "Other strategies for patient management for which the clinical utility is uncertain (i.e., based on inconclusive or conflicting evidence or opinion)" Emergent: Scan immediately. "Essential for a timely decision regarding potential life-threatening or severe disabling entities" Urgent: Make appointment before disposition or scan if follow-up cannot be ensured. "Essential to enable the timely appropriate clinical disposition or discharge of acute condition" Routine: "Indicated for management and diagnosis but not for immediate disposition" Not indicated: "Not indicated for the routine management of the presenting condition"
Recommendations for timing of neuroimaging in patients with a first-time seizure:	Guideline-level recommendations • Emergent neuroimaging (NI) should be performed when a provider suspects a serious structural lesion Option-level recommendations: • Emergent NI should also be considered if any of the following clinical features are present: age > 40 years, partial-onset seizure • Urgent NI should be considered for patients who have completely recovered from their seizure and for whom no clear-cut cause has been identified to help identify a possible structural cause • Consider urgent NI before disposition when timely follow-up cannot be ensured
Recommendations for timing in patients with known epilepsy with a recurrent seizure:	Guideline-level recommendations: • Emergent NI should be performed when a provider suspects a serious structural lesion • Patients with typical febrile seizures or typical recurrent seizure related to previously treated epilepsy are unlikely to have life-threatening structural lesions. These patients do not require emergent or urgent NI Option-level recommendations: • Emergent NI should also be considered if any of the following are present: new seizure pattern or new seizure type or prolonged post-ictal confusion or worsening mental status • Urgent NI should be considered for patients who have completely recovered from their seizure and for whom no clear-cut cause has been identified to help identify a possible structural cause • Consider urgent NI before disposition when timely follow-up cannot be ensured

seizures." The practice parameter specifically did not include patients presenting in status epilepticus (a state of prolonged, continual seizure activity). Because neuroimaging is best used to "determine whether seizures result from a structural abnormality of the brain or its surroundings," the consensus-based recommendations of the practice-parameter group are based on the urgency of clinical presentation, the likelihood of uncovering a specific abnormality, and how important it would be to the patient's overall management that this structural abnormality be found as soon as possible [4]. A summary of the practice-parameters' recommendations for the timing of neuroimaging is given in Table 8.3.

Choosing a modality of neuroimaging for an ED patient presenting with a seizure

The standard neuroimaging work-up for seizures requires non-enhanced head CT (NECT) to rule out a structural abnormality such as an acute intracranial hemorrhage. Negative NECT effectively excludes most of the pathology requiring acute intervention; however, magnetic resonance imaging (MRI) with and without contrast is a more sensitive and specific modality that can be considered as a follow-up investigation as needed [5] and, rarely, more urgently for specific indications as discussed below (e.g. infection). Most visits to the ED for seizures are in the context of epilepsy, where extensive prior clinical and neuroimaging evaluation has previously been performed. Advanced imaging such as high-resolution MRI is not typically necessary in this setting. NECT is adequate to exclude most acute pathology as a cause. First-time seizures, however, deserve special consideration. Enhanced MRI is standard of care in the evaluation of new-onset seizures, although this frequently can be accomplished in the outpatient setting after an initial ED evaluation that includes NECT.

NECT is widely available in all ED settings throughout the USA and Europe. MRI may have limited availability in some geographic areas. Compared to NECT where scans require only a few minutes to complete, MRI often takes half an hour to complete. Longer scan times are not the only impediment to MRI. The scanners are often remote in location to the ED, and require more extensive pre-imaging screening to exclude metallic implants and other safety hazards that are not of concern with NECT. Gadolinium contrast agents also now require pre-imaging renal screening to determine the patient's renal function prior to enhanced MRI, which further increases delays in access. The patient's estimated glomerular filtration rate (eGFR) is determined in many practices prior to contrast administration in order to avoid the risks of a rare but potentially fatal disease related to gadolinium-contrast-agent administration: nephrogenic systemic fibrosis (NSF).

Given these considerations, NECT remains the standard for seizure evaluation in the ED. Knowing when to obtain MRI in the emergent setting is thus important. We review here some of the more common CNS pathology responsible for seizures and compare the relative value of NECT to enhanced MRI.

Spectrum of neuroimaging findings in an ED patient with seizures

Acute traumatic lesions that require immediate aggressive intervention (e.g. neurosurgery) such as extra-axial hematomas, large parenchymal hemorrhages, and cerebral contusions are well visualized with NECT (Figure 8.1). MRI will have far greater sensitivity to non-hemorrhagic and small cerebral contusion, and some small extra-axial blood collections. As discovery of these in adults does not change immediate care, NECT remains the currently accepted standard imaging study to evaluate suspected acute CNS trauma in adults, with its high specificity and good sensitivity to findings that require surgical or more intensive follow-up. In children, consideration of non-accidental trauma may prompt more sensitive MRI, but typically this still follows NECT.

Chronic post-traumatic structural lesions are a common cause of adult epilepsy. These may be apparent by CT as focal areas of encephalomalacia, although MRI tends to be more sensitive to such parenchymal injury. Late sequelae also include post-traumatic cephaloceles, which can be challenging to evaluate with routine NECT, and require dedicated

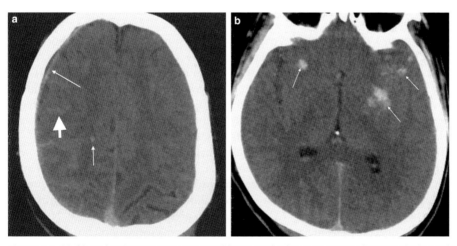

Figure 8.1 (a), (b) Axial NECT images in a 25-year-old man involved in an unrestrained motor-vehicle accident shows extensive hemorrhages (arrows) related to diffuse axonal injury and contusions.

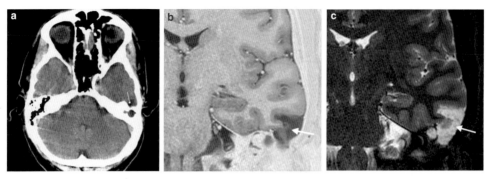

Figure 8.2 NECT obtained in a 36-year-old man with seizures. (a) Subtle and non-specific low density in the temporal lobe (white arrow) and adjacent bone. Coronal high resolution T1-weighted (b) and T2-weighted (c) MRI scans show a left-sided cephalocele herniating into the temporal bone (white arrow, b and c).

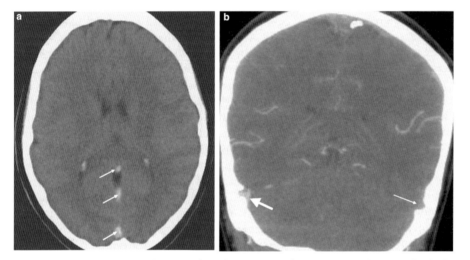

Figure 8.3 Axial NECT. (a) Hyperdense straight and superior sagittal sinuses (arrows), diagnostic for dural sinus thrombosis. The coronal CT venogram reformat (b) confirms the findings with non-enhancement within the left transverse and sagittal sinuses (arrow). Note normally enhancing right transverse sinus for comparison (wide arrow).

MRI usually with high-resolution coronal T2-weighted imaging to confirm (Figure 8.2). Diffusion-weighted (DW) MRI, gradient-echo and susceptibility-weighted MRI provide high sensitivity to traumatic microhemorrhage in the acute and chronic setting.

Cerebrovascular disease is a frequent cause of seizures, particularly in elderly patients. Hypoxic ischemic encephalopathy (HIE) often presents as seizures in neonates and infants. Acute hemorrhagic stroke is well assessed with NECT. NECT is also most commonly used to screen and triage ischemic stroke in the acute setting. MRI with DW MRI is far more sensitive in the first few hours of acute ischemic stroke and HIE, and also better differentiates small-vessel lacunar infarction from large-vessel infarcts.

Venous thrombosis or venous stroke more often present with acute seizures and/or headache in the acute setting than does arterial ischemia (Figure 8.3). NECT may suggest venous thrombosis, but contrast-enhanced CT (CECT) venography or MRI venography is typically required to confirm the finding and characterize its full extent.

Vascular malformations may present with new-onset seizures, with or without acute intracranial hemorrhage. Cavernous malformations frequently present with seizures, although arteriovenous malformations (AVMs) may also present with seizures [6]. NECT can detect larger vascular malformations; however, MRI is a more sensitive modality, and is required for definitive diagnosis.

Subarachnoid hemorrhage (SAH) frequently presents with seizure. The high sensitivity of NECT makes it the imaging test of choice for SAH, although further imaging with CT angiography (CTA), magnetic resonance angiography (MRA), or formal angiography may be required depending on the clinical and NECT findings. AVMs also may present with seizure. These are frequently missed on NECT. CECT and MRI provide far greater sensitivity and improved characterization.

Metabolic disorders may result in seizures. However, the vast majority of the very common metabolic causes of seizure (e.g. hypoglycemia, hyponatremia) and intoxications will have essentially unremarkable CT studies, and the added sensitivity of MRI to rare manifestations of these does not justify its routine use, although MRI will rarely provide benefit after NECT in unusual or otherwise problematic cases.

Posterior reversible encephalopathy syndrome (PRES) is an uncommon but important and treatable cause of acute seizures. Often this syndrome is accompanied by headaches, altered sensorium, and vision changes. PRES should be suspected in the setting of acute hypertensive crisis or with known contributory immunosuppressive medication use, and in the obstetric scenario, but may occur without these classic predisposing factors. NECT can detect PRES when subcortical areas of low density are visible; however, areas of limited involvement can be missed (Figure 8.4). Non-contrast MRI is more sensitive and specific for this diagnosis, and should be the modality of choice if the diagnosis is entertained. This is particularly true for older patients (over 50 years of age), who normally have white-matter hypodensities that are more frequently attributed to "senescent white matter" or "small-vessel" disease on NECT. These findings can mask the findings of PRES, which are more clearly delineated on MRI. Osmotic demyelination, specifically central pontine demyelinosis (CPM) classically presents with areas of increased T2 signal in the central pons by MRI that may progress to encephalomalacia over time. Extra-pontine involvement (thalamus, midbrain, cerebellum) is also common. Most findings will be inapparent on CT, in part as posterior fossa abnormalities are often masked by either small size and/or streak artifacts from beam attenuation on CT.

Infectious causes of acute seizures include meningitis and encephalitis, which should be evaluated on a clinical basis. However, neuroimaging is critical to evaluate for suspected herpes encephalitis. Although NECT may rarely demonstrate findings in encephalitis, enhanced MRI is the modality of choice and should be considered primary in evaluation. Herpes encephalitis has typical MRI findings of hyperintense T2 signal involving the bilateral frontal (often cingulate gyrus) and temporal lobes with mass effect and variable enhancement (Figure 8.5). Such findings in this clinical setting should prompt treatment with intravenous acyclovir, given the low complication rate and significant morbidity and mortality associated with this diagnosis. In the setting of HIV/AIDS, CT may reveal mass lesions or localized swelling from toxoplasmosis, progressive multifocal encephalopathy, or lymphoma.

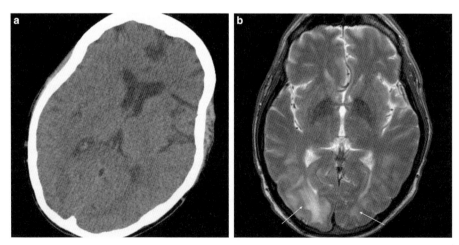

Figure 8.4 (a) Axial NECT in a patient presenting with headaches and seizures is within normal limits. (b) Axial T2-weighted MRI 1 day later shows bioccipital and bitemporal vasogenic edema (arrows) consistent with acute PRES.

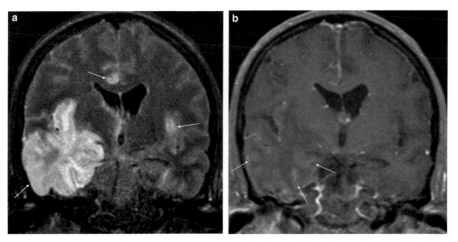

Figure 8.5 (a) Coronal FLAIR MRI shows hyperintense signal and mass effect in the insular cortex bilaterally and right frontal and temporal lobes (arrows). This distribution, although not specific, suggests herpes encephalitis. (b) Coronal T1-weighted post-contrast MRI shows patchy cortical enhancement (arrows).

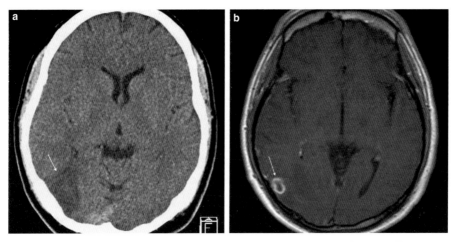

Figure 8.6 (a) Axial NECT in a 27-year-old man with new-onset seizures shows wedge-shaped low attenuation in the right posterior occipital lobe (arrow). This is non-specific and suggests an area of subacute ischemia, edema, or neoplasm. (b) T1-weighted post-contrast MRI scan obtained 1 day later shows a ring-enhancing mass (arrow) concerning for neoplasm or infection. Biopsy disclosed neurocysticercosis.

Unexplained findings may prompt more sensitive follow-up imaging by MRI. Worldwide, the most common infectious cause of seizures is neurocysticercosis. NECT is helpful to identify punctate calcifications that can be a hallmark of healed neurocysticercosis, while enhanced MRI better characterizes active disease (Figure 8.6).

Primary and secondary CNS neoplasms are an important cause of seizures. These include meningioma, primary CNS glial and neuronal neoplasms, and metastatic disease (Figures 8.7, 8.8). Most non-hemorrhagic intraparenchymal tumors will present as a low-density abnormality with mass effect on NECT; however, the imaging is often not specific, and enhanced MRI will be subsequently required in most cases for confirmation. Small meningiomas, when similar to the density of the adjacent brain, can be missed on NECT, and small sub-centimeter-sized intraparenchymal tumors, such as early metastatic disease, can also be missed with screening NECT. Dedicated enhanced MRI is the modality of choice for the evaluation of intracranial neoplastic disease, but often can be accomplished as a follow-up study where indicated after a screening NECT.

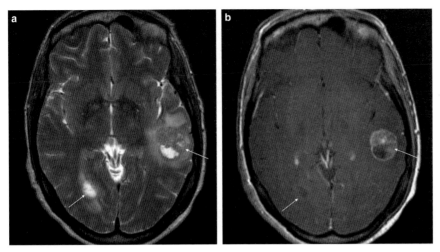

Figure 8.7 Axial T2-weighted (a) and T1-weighted post-contrast MRI (b) shows two heterogeneous and enhancing masses (arrows) in the left temporal and right occipital lobes. Subcortical location and multicentricity favor metastatic disease.

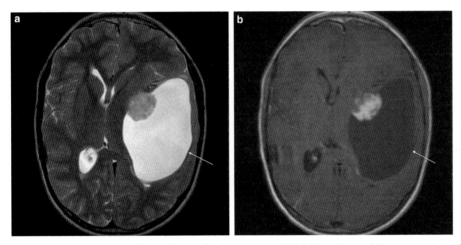

Figure 8.8 Axial T2-weighted (a) and T1-weighted post-contrast MRI (b) in a 13-year-old boy presenting with seziures and 6 months of headache shows a mixed solid and cystic left parietal lobe mass (arrows). Biopsy disclosed ganglioglioma.

Congenital abnormalities that commonly result in seizures include tuberous sclerosis and Sturge Weber syndrome. These are typically diagnosed by clinical features but also have characteristic findings on neuroimaging. Hamartomas are non-neoplastic tumors characterized by normal tissue in abnormal locations that often result in seizure and epilepsy (Figure 8.9).

Patients who present in status epilepticus, particularly over hours to days, may have neuroimaging findings that are an epi-phenomenon thought to be related to hyperperfusion, rather than a primary abnormality. These are sometimes referred to as "ictal changes."

They are only well demonstrated by MRI, but may mimic acute ischemia, CNS neoplasm, or limbic encephalitis in the acute phase (Figure 8.10). Hyperintense T2 signal changes, usually with mild mass effect and variable enhancement, are typically seen involving both hippocampi with variable involvement of the temporal lobes and sylvian cortex. Involvement may be symmetric or asymmetric, and usually resolves within weeks to months after resolution, although long-term atrophy may result. Importantly, these findings must be seen in the expected setting of status epilepticus or non-convulsive status, otherwise more significant pathology must be entertained.

141

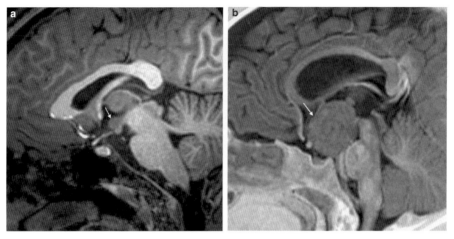

Figure 8.9 (a) Sagittal T1-weighted MRI shows a subtle nodule superior to the mammillary bodies (arrow) characteristic of a tiny hamartoma. A mass this small would routinely be occult on screening NECT. (b) Sagittal T1-weighted MRI in a different patient shows a large hamartoma of the tuber cinereum (arrow). A mass this size would not be missed with screening NECT but requires enhanced MRI for further characterization.

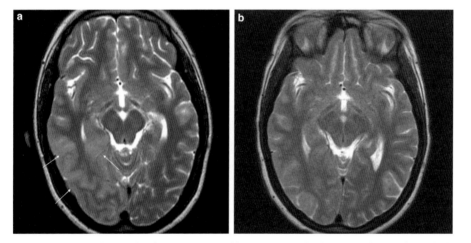

Figure 8.10 (a) Axial T2-weighted MRI in a 17-year-old post-partum girl with status epilepticus shows thickened T2 hyperintense cortex in the right occipital and temporal lobes (arrows), concerning for neoplasm. This finding would likely be occult on NECT. (b) Axial T2-weighted MRI 4 days later shows nearly resolved findings compatible with ictal changes, and excluding neoplastic etiology.

Finally, mesial temporal sclerosis (MTS) is a common finding in epilepsy, with characteristic combined hippocampal volume loss and increased signal on high-resolution T2-weighted imaging [7]. With a seizure presentation, NECT will rarely be sensitive to the volume loss (enlarged temporal horn), and this finding will be non-specific as temporal-horn asymmetry is a frequent normal variant [8]. As most of these patients return for epilepsy evaluation, the missed structural abnormality by NECT will not be immediately consequential. Pediatric febrile seizures have long been associated with subsequent development of MTS. A recent prospective study has shown that febrile status epilepticus places children at risk for hippocampal injury based on acute MRI abnormalities, although the long-term consequences remain to be seen [9].

Summary

Seizures are an important cause of visits to an ED. When a patient presents with an event that may be a seizure, stabilization of the patient must be the first priority in emergency management. The most important element in the diagnosis of a seizure is a detailed history from both the patient and a witness of the event. The decision about whether or not to perform a neuro-imaging study acutely in the ED should be based on the likelihood of discovering a cause of the seizure that requires immediate intervention. The standard neuro-imaging work-up for seizures requires non-enhanced head CT (NECT) to rule out a structural abnormality such as an acute intracranial hemorrhage; however, MRI with and without contrast, is a more sensitive and specific modality that can be considered as a follow-up investigation as needed. Important pathology that can be found on neuroimaging of a patient presenting with seizures includes: acute traumatic lesions, chronic post-traumatic structural lesions, ischemic stroke, intracranial hemorrhage, posterior reversible leukoen-cephalopathy syndrome, CNS infection, neoplasm, MTS, and congenital abnormalities.

References

1. Ebersole JS, Pedley TA, eds. (2003). *Current Practice of Clinical Electroencephalography*. New York: Lippincott Williams and Wilkins.

2. Hauser WA (1997). Incidence and prevalence. In Engel J, Pedley T, eds. *Epilepsy: A Comprehensive Textbook*. Philadelphia: Lippincott-Raven, pp. 47–57.

3. Jallon P, Loiseau P, *et al.* (2011). Newly diagnosed unprovoked epileptic seizure: presentation at diagnosis in CORALE study. *Epilepsia* **42**: 464–475.

4. AAN (1996). Report of the Quality Standards Subcommittee of the American Academy of Neurology: Practice parameter: a guideline for discontinuing antiepileptic drugs in seizure-free patients. *Neurology* **47**: 600–602.

5. Hess C, Barkovich A (2010). Seizures: emergency neuroimaging. *Neuroimagin Clin N Am* **20**: 619–637.

6. Garcin B, Houdart E, Porcher R, *et al.* (2012). Epileptic seizures at initial presentation in patients with brain arteriovenous malformation. *Neurology* **78**: 626–631.

7. Gilliam F, Faught E, Martin R, *et al.* (2002). Predictive value of MRI-identified mesial temporal sclerosis for surgical outcome in temporal lobe epilepsy: an intent-to-treat analysis. *Epilepsia* **41**: 963–966.

8. Kasasbeh A, Hwang EC, Steger-May K, *et al.* (2012). Association of magnetic resonance imaging identification of mesial temporal sclerosis with pathological diagnosis and surgical outcomes in children following epilepsy surgery. *J Neurosurg Pediatr* **9**: 552–561.

9. Shinnar S, Bello JA, Chan S, *et al.* (2012). MRI abnormalities following febrile status epilepticus in children: the FEBSTAT study. *Neurology* **79**: 871–877.

Acute and subacute ataxia

Chapter

9

Bart P. van de Warrenburg, Judith van Gaalen, Andrea Ginestroni,
and Mario Mascalchi

Introduction

Cerebellar ataxia is a syndrome of disturbed coordination, affecting various domains of voluntary motor control. Several oculomotor disturbances can occur, such as dysmetria of fast saccades, gaze-evoked nystagmus, and fixation instability. These problems are caused by degenerative processes or lesions that affect the flocculonodular lobe (vestibulocerebellum). Ataxic or cerebellar dysarthria is a slurred, scanning speech, due to involvement of the superior paravermal region and intermediate cerebellar cortex (spinocerebellum). When the cerebellar vermis is affected, this results in truncal and gait ataxia, noticeable as a broad-based gait with irregularity of steps and speed. The lateral cerebellar cortex and deep cerebellar nuclei regulate limb movements, and deficits in these regions cause loss of dexterity, dysmetria, and tremor [1].

Cerebellar ataxia has numerous causes, but the onset of disease is an important clue towards the underlying etiology (Figure 9.1). Ataxias are commonly divided into genetic and non-genetic ataxias, and the latter is split into acquired versus degen-

erative. In this chapter, we will cover the major causes – which are all acquired – of acute and subacute cerebellar ataxia, with an emphasis on imaging characteristics.

Stroke

Ataxia is a common feature in cerebral ischemia or hemorrhage. Of all strokes, 2 to 3% involve the cerebellum [2]. Symptoms of ataxia are frequently accompanied by nausea, vomiting, and headache. Rapid deterioration due to severe complications can occur from hydrocephalus or brainstem compression because of the mass effect. Pure cerebellar hemorrhage or ischemic stroke can occur due to occlusion of one of the three pairs of cerebellar arteries (posterior inferior cerebellar artery, anterior inferior cerebellar artery, and superior cerebellar artery) (Figure 9.2). Additionally, specific stroke syndromes can be distinguished.

Unenhanced computed tomography (CT) is the initial imaging examination in a patient with suspected brainstem or cerebellar stroke since it promptly reveals hemorrhagic lesions as hyperdense areas. Once

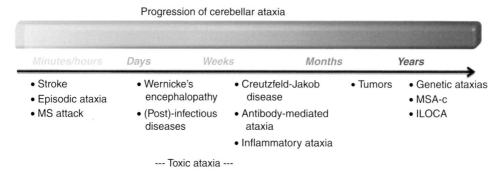

Progression of cerebellar ataxia

Minutes/hours	Days	Weeks	Months	Years
• Stroke • Episodic ataxia • MS attack	• Wernicke's encephalopathy • (Post)-infectious diseases	• Creutzfeld-Jakob disease • Antibody-mediated ataxia • Inflammatory ataxia	• Tumors	• Genetic ataxias • MSA-c • ILOCA

--- Toxic ataxia ---

Figure 9.1 **Timeline**. Rate of onset for the different causes of cerebellar ataxia. MS = multiple sclerosis; MSA-c = multiple system atrophy – cerebellar type; ILOCA = idiopathic late-onset cerebellar ataxia.

Imaging Acute Neurologic Disease, ed. Massimo Filippi and Jack H. Simon. Published by Cambridge University Press.
© Cambridge University Press 2014.

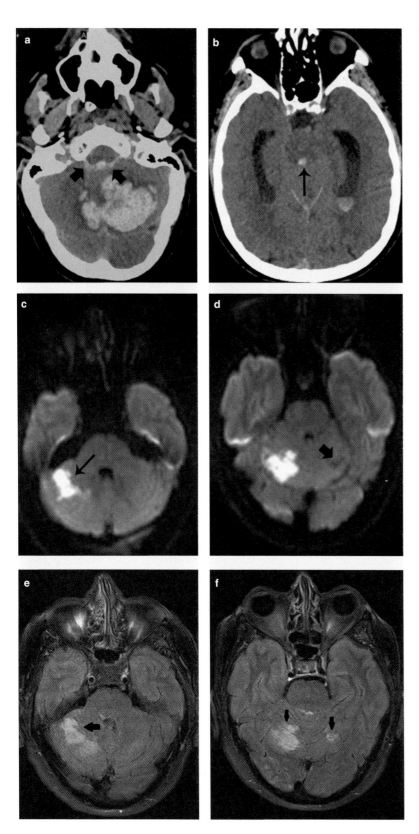

Figure 9.2 Cerebellar strokes.
Unenhanced CT (a, b) shows massive hemorrhage in the left cerebellar hemisphere appearing as a hyperdense collection with perilesional hypodense edema. Note the extension of the hyperdense blood to the subarachnoid space around the medulla (black arrowheads in a) and the cerebral aqueduct (black arrow in b) and the obstructive pattern dilatation of the temporal horns of the lateral ventricles. There is a clot in the left lateral ventricle (b). MRI (c–f) shows two infarcts in the territories of the superior cerebellar arteries. The high signal on the diffusion-weighted image indicates that the larger lesion in the right cerebellar hemisphere (black arrow in c) is recent, whereas the cerebrospinal fluid-like low signal on the diffusion weighted image demonstrates that the smaller lesion in the left cerebellar hemisphere (black arrowhead in d) is old corresponding to a focal area of tissue loss. The two lesions exhibit similar high signal intensity on axial FLAIR images (black arrows in e and f).

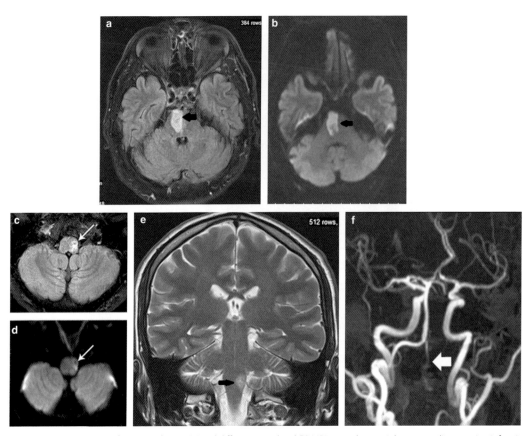

Figure 9.3 **Brainstem infarcts**. Axial FLAIR (a) and diffusion-weighted (b) MRI scans show a right paramedian pontine infarction appearing as a well-defined area of high signal typically extending to the surface of the pons (black arrow in a) and attributed to atheromatous changes of the wall of the basilar artery (b). Axial FLAIR (c), diffusion-weighted (d), and coronal T2-weighted MRI scans show a recent infarct in the posterior lateral portion of the left medulla appearing as an area of high signal intensity (black arrow in e). Note that both axial FLAIR and diffusion-weighted images reveal a small hypointense dot (white arrows in c, d) just anteriorly to the recent lesion consistent with an old infarct. Coronal oblique view of MRA demonstrates lack of flow in the intracranial portion of the left vertebral artery (white arrowhead in f).

hemorrhagic stroke has been excluded, magnetic resonance imaging (MRI) enables demonstration of an ischemic lesion in the first few hours after the onset of symptoms as a well demarcated area of high signal in diffusion-weighted images reflecting restricted diffusion of water protons. The same area will subsequently become hyperintense on T2-weighted images [3]. Importantly, in the same examination, magnetic resonance angiography (MRA) may reveal abnormal flow or narrowed lumen of the vertebrobasilar arteries often underlying the brainstem or cerebellar ischemic stroke, or a mural hematoma from arterial dissection, appearing as a hyperintense crescent on T1-weighted images.

Clinical features

Ataxic hemiparesis

One of the well-known lacunar stroke syndromes is ataxic hemiparesis, which is most often due to a lacunar

infarction in the pons, internal capsule, or thalamus (Figure 9.3). Patients develop acute ipsilateral ataxia and hemiparesis. Dysmetria is present in almost all patients, but it is not always accompanied by dysdiadochokinesis or hypotonia. Lacunar infarcts are small subcortical infarcts caused by occlusion of a small penetrating artery and are strongly associated with small-vessel disease.

Isolated hemiataxia caused by a supratentorial stroke is rare, but has been observed in patients with ischemia in the posterior limb of the internal capsule or in the thalamus [4].

Isolated acute vertigo (pseudoneuritis)

Vestibular migraine, vestibular neuritis, cerebellar stroke, and benign paroxysmal positional vertigo are only some of the many disorders that can cause acute vertigo. When additional symptoms, like tinnitus or dysarthria, are also present it is easier to make a distinction between a peripheral or central disorder. Sometimes it is difficult to differentiate between a peripheral versus central origin, particularly vestibular neuritis versus cerebellar stroke. Both disorders have a rather acute onset and can have vertigo as the only presenting symptom. There are some clinical symptoms and signs that can help in the differential, such as a negative head-thrust test that should raise suspicion of a central cause of vertigo [5]. Similarly, a hyperacute onset, old age, and a history of cerebrovascular disease also favor a vascular origin. However, these clinical features have no complete discriminative value, and therefore an MRI brain scan should be requested in such patients.

A stroke from posterior inferior cerebellar artery (PICA) stenosis or occlusion, which supplies the nodulus and uvula, is most frequently associated with isolated vertigo. The uvula is part of the vestibulocerebellum and receives input from the vestibular system. The nodulus lies in the midline cerebellum between the inferior medullary velum and uvula. Together with the flocculus, paraflocculus, and ventral uvula, it is called the vestibulocerebellum. The nodulus receives input from the vestibular system and is involved in controlling eye movements and in postural adjustments to gravity. In patients with this stroke subtype, vertigo, imbalance, and nystagmus resolve within a few days from onset and patients usually fully recover over the following weeks [6].

Bilateral ataxia with unilateral brainstem infarction

A strategic unilateral infarction that affects both efferent cerebellar pathways, before and after the decussation of the superior cerebellar peduncle, can cause bilateral ataxia. While ataxia is often accompanied by hemiparesis or hypesthesia, it can also be the sole symptom [7].

Prognosis and treatment

Patients should be treated in accordance with international stroke guidelines. In the acute phase, intravenous thrombolysis and intra-arterial thrombolysis/thrombectomy need to be considered [8]. Also, neurosurgical intervention might be necessary in patients with a decreased level of consciousness, loss of brainstem reflexes, hydrocephalus, or obliterated fourth ventricle or basal cisterns. When a cerebellar hemorrhage is more than 3 cm in diameter, surgical evacuation should be considered, although outcome in these patients even after intervention remains poor.

Patients who have suffered from a cerebellar hemorrhage have a worse long-term functional outcome compared to those who have a cerebellar infarction. Indicators for a poor prognosis are: systolic blood pressure greater than 200 mmHg, decreased level of consciousness, and a gaze palsy [9].

CT features that correlate with a poor prognosis include: midline location, obliterated fourth ventricle or basal cisterns, intraventricular hemorrhage, and hydrocephalus (Figure 9.2).

After the acute phase, patients should be treated with life-long dual antiplatelet therapy.

Other risk factors for stroke, such as hypertension and hyperlipidemia, should be assessed and targeted.

Key points: Stroke

Clinical features

- Acute onset within minutes
- History of cardiovascular risk factors
- Often lateralized symptoms

Neuroimaging

- CT: hyperdensity in hemorrhagic lesions
- MRI: restricted diffusion and over time high signal on T2-weighted images in ischemic lesions
- MRA or CT angiography (CTA): occlusion or narrowing of cervical or intracranial arteries supplying vascular territories

Treatment

- < 4.5–6 hours after onset: intravenous or intra-arterial thrombolysis
- Secondary prevention: antiplatelet therapy; reduction of cardiovascular risk

Toxic and metabolic causes

Drugs

Acute ataxia due to intoxication can occur with lithium, phenytoin, amiodarone, and the cystostatics 5-fluorouracil and cytosine arabinoside (Table 9.1).

Toxic agents

Poisoning with heavy metals such as mercury, thallium, and lead also causes ataxia. Methylmercury, more than the other forms of mercury, has an effect on the central nervous system (CNS). Methylmercury poisoning is

Table 9.1 Ataxia due to (drug) intoxications

Drugs – anticonvulsants	Heavy metals
– Phenytoin	– Mercury
– Carbamazapine	– Lead
– Barbiturates	– Manganese
– Vigabatrin	– Thallium
– Gabapentin	– Germanium
– Topiramate	
– Lamotrigine	
Drugs – antineoplastics	**Insecticides and herbicides**
– 5-fluorouracil	– Chlordecone
– Cytosine arabinoside	– Phosphin
– Methotrexate	– Carbon disulfide
Drugs – other	**Various toxic agents**
– Lithium	– Eucalyptus oil – Saxitoxin (shellfish poisoning)
– Amiodarone	– Nicotine
– Cyclosporin	– Cyanide
– Bismuth	
– Bromides/ bromverylurea	
– Mefloquine	
– Isoniazid	
– Lindane	
– Perhexiline maleate	
– Cimetidine	
Drug abuse	**Other**
– Cocaine	– Toluene/benzene derivatives
– Heroin	– Carbon monoxide (CO)
– Phencyclidine	

also known as Minamata disease, named after the region in Japan where poisoning occurred at a large scale through the ingestion of fish contaminated by methylmercury. Intoxication leads to severe generalized ataxia and visual disturbances. If possible, quick elimination of the toxic compounds, for example with hemodialysis, is the best treatment [10, 11]. Additional causes of acute ataxia following intoxication include methanol, methadone, and methyl bromide.

Generally, MRI after acute drug intoxication or poisoning can demonstrate a non-specific pattern of cortical cerebellar atrophy variably combined with symmetric high signal intensity of the subcortical white matter of the cerebellar hemispheres and dentate nuclei, as well as signal changes in other parts of the brain. Some intoxications show more specific MRI patterns, such as atrophy of the visual cortex, postcentral cortex, and cerebellum with mercury intoxication,

or hyperintensities on T2-weighted MRI in the basal ganglia, insula, and pons with lead intoxication [12–15].

Electrolyte disturbances

Various electrolyte disturbances can result in subacute ataxia. It has been described in patients with hyponatremia, hypocalcemia, and hypomagnesemia [16–19]. Hypomagnesemia can be caused by malnutrition or diarrhea. It can lead to a variety of neurological symptoms, including seizures, altered mental status, and hemiplegia. Hypomagnesemia has also been described as the cause of subacute cerebellar ataxia with T2-weighted abnormalities in the cerebellum on MRI. The clinical and radiological features appeared to be reversible, after correction of the low magnesium levels.

Note that ataxia is not usually part of pontine and extra-pontine myelinolysis, which occurs after overly rapid correction of hyponatremia.

Key points: Toxic and metabolic ataxia

Clinical features

- Acute or subacute onset
- Patient history: prescribed drugs, exposure to toxins, underlying diseases that may cause metabolic problems

Treatment

- Elimination of responsible drugs or toxic compounds
- Treatment of underlying disease/electrolyte disturbance

Wernicke–Korsakoff's encephalopathy

Epidemiology and clinical features

In the general population, brain lesions typical for Wernicke–Korsakoff's encephalopathy are present in 1–3% of cases on autopsy, but are mainly seen in alcoholics. This percentage is higher than reported in clinical studies, indicating that this entity can remain undetected with clinical examination. A study on alcohol-related deaths revealed typical brain lesions in 30–60% of these cases. Besides chronic alcohol abuse in combination with poor nutrition, bariatric surgery, and cancer are risk factors for the development of Wernicke–Korsakoff's encephalopathy.

Wernicke–Korsakoff's encephalopathy is a clinical syndrome consisting of the triad of encephalopathy, oculomotor disturbances, and gait ataxia. However, absence of one of the symptoms does not exclude the diagnosis, as only one-third of the patients display the full triad. Severe thiamine (vitamin B1) deficiency leads to this subacute disorder, which arises within days. Because the vermis of the cerebellum is mainly affected, gait ataxia without dysarthria or limb ataxia is characteristic. Within the spectrum of oculomotor disturbances, nystagmus is most frequent and is evoked by horizontal gaze more than with vertical gaze. Ophthalmoplegia is mainly caused by a lesion of the abducens nerve resulting in a lateral rectus palsy. The encephalopathic features are apathy, indifference, and disorientation.

Further investigations

MRI is relevant for the diagnosis of Wernicke–Korsakoff's encephalopathy, given the non-specific and often subtle clinical signs. Symmetric abnormal hyperintensities on T2-weighted and fluid-attenuated inversion recovery (FLAIR) images are typically observed in the mammillary bodies, periaqueductal gray matter, tectum of the midbrain (quadrigeminal plate), dorsal medulla, medial thalami, and frontal cortex. Variable contrast enhancement on gadolinium T1-weighted images in the areas of signal change is observed, more frequently in cases associated with alcohol abuse (Figure 9.4) [20–22].

Thiamine deficiency is the cause of Wernicke–Korsakoff's encephalopathy. Thiamine is a crucial cofactor for several enzymes involved in energy metabolism. Approximately 3 weeks after thiamine depletion, enzymatic activity is disturbed and blood levels of thiamine are decreased. Thiamine also has a role in biochemical processes in the CNS relevant to energy production by adenosine triphosphate (ATP), lipid metabolism, and the production of neurotransmitters.

Treatment and prognosis

Treatment with high-dose thiamine results in rapid improvement of symptoms. Patients should be treated with 500 mg of thiamine intravenously three times a day for 3 days, followed by 250 mg of thiamine three times a day for 3–5 days. Long-term supplementation of vitamin C and vitamin B-complex is advised [23]. After the start of high-dose thiamine, improvement of oculomotor disturbances usually occurs within hours to days. Although the symptoms and MRI signal abnormalities improve after treatment, residual deficits are seen in virtually every patient. Gaze palsies recover completely in more than half of the patients, but only about 40% recover completely from ataxia, leaving many patients with gait disturbances. After the symptoms of acute encephalopathy have declined, patients begin to notice deficits in learning and memory. Most of the patients eventually suffer from a permanent anterograde amnesia, referred to as Korsakoff's syndrome.

Key points: Wernicke–Korsakoff's encephalopathy

Clinical features

- Onset within days
- Patients with alcohol abuse and poor nutrition, bariatric surgery, and cancer
- Triad of encephalopathy, oculomotor disturbances, and gait ataxia

Neuroimaging

- MRI: symmetric hyperintensities on T2-weighted and FLAIR images in the mammillary bodies, periaqueductal region, tectum of the midbrain, dorsal medulla and medial thalamic nuclei with variable contrast enhancement

Treatment

- Acute phase: thiamine 500 mg intravenous three times a day, for 3 days
- Chronic treatment: supplementation of vitamin C and vitamin B-complex

Inflammatory diseases

Steroid-responsive encephalopathy associated with autoimmune thyroiditis (SREAT)

Epidemiology and clinical features

SREAT, also known as Hashimoto's encephalopathy, is an autoimmune syndrome characterized by cognitive impairment, seizures, ataxia, and myoclonus with positive thyroperoxidase (anti-TPO) antibodies. Ataxia is seen in up to 65% of the patients. In some cases, progressive cerebellar ataxia can be the sole manifestation of this syndrome [24, 25].

The exact prevalence of SREAT is not known and the number of reported cases and case series is limited.

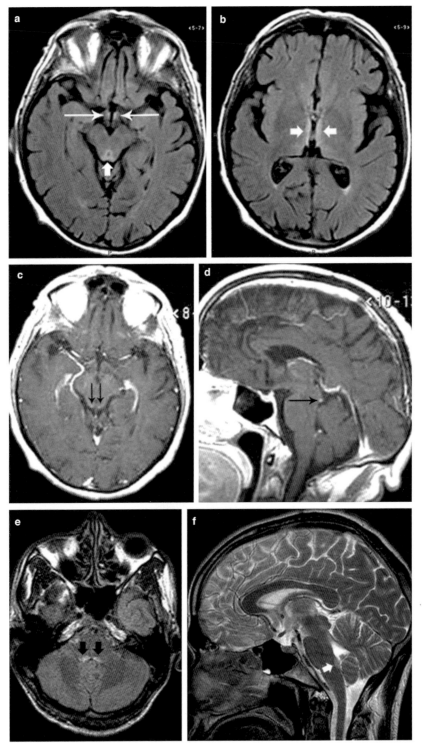

Figure 9.4 **Wernicke–Korsakoff's encephalopathy**. Axial FLAIR images show increased signal in the mammillary bodies (white arrows in a), periaqueductal gray matter and tectum of the midbrain and medial thalami (white arrowheads in b). Axial (c) and sagittal (d) T1-weighted images after intravenous contrast administration show enhancement in the inferior tectum (black arrows in c, d). Case provided courtesy of Professor Massimo Gallucci, University of l'Aquila, Italy. Axial FLAIR MRI shows symmetric hyperintensity in the posterior portion of the medulla oblongata (black arrowheads in e) in another case. The signal change in the posterior medulla (white arrowhead in f) is confirmed on the sagittal T2-weighted image.

However, this diagnosis is often unrecognized. In a hospital-based study, involving extensive screening for SREAT in patients with an unexplained neurologic syndrome with possibly compatible clinical features, 6% of the 143 screened patients fulfilled the criteria for the diagnosis [26].

Further investigations

MRI is generally normal, but can display non-specific focal, or diffuse increased signal in the cerebral subcortical white matter on T2 or FLAIR scans in about 25% of cases [27]. The presence of hypo- or hyperthyroidism is not a prerequisite for the diagnosis. In fact, a high percentage of patients have a normal thyroid status at the time of diagnosis.

Besides anti-TPO, antithyroglobulin (anti-TG) antibodies are also frequently found. The role of these thyroid autoantibodies in the pathogenesis of SREAT is not clear, since (1) a raised titer of anti-TPO antibodies is found in about 10% of healthy adults, (2) these antibodies may also be present in patients with other autoimmune disorders, and (3) these antibodies do not have any biological activity. Anti-TPO antibodies are present in serum and in the thyroid gland, but there is no evidence that they have any effect on neuronal tissue. Therefore, these antibodies may rather be non-specific markers or epiphenomena of an autoimmune disorder that affects the CNS.

Treatment and prognosis

When SREAT is suspected, patients should be treated with high doses of steroids, most commonly 0.5 to 1 g of intravenous methylprednisone per day for 5 days. Most patients show marked improvement of cognitive and neurological symptoms after treatment. Several patients require more than one course of steroids; some patients need another short course of methylprednisone when they have a relapse, other patients need continuous treatment with lower doses of oral steroids to stay in remission. When patients do not respond to treatment, a re-evaluation of the diagnosis should be considered, as on autopsy some "non-responders" with SREAT turned out to have Creutzfeldt–Jakob disease (CJD) or diffuse Lewy body disease [27].

After immunomodulatory treatment, the prognosis is good, with absence of recurrence in more than half of the patients. In about 30% of cases, withdrawal of corticosteroids will lead to a relapse. The remaining group of patients had a relapse despite continuous treatment. A delay of diagnosis and treatment is associated with a worse outcome and leaves about one-quarter of patients with residual cognitive deficits.

Key points: SREAT

Clinical features
- Onset within weeks to months
- Cognitive impairment, seizures, ataxia, and myoclonus

Immunology
- Raised titer of anti-TPO and/or anti-TG antibodies

Neuroimaging
- MRI: mostly normal, but may show non-specific focal or diffuse increased signal of the cerebral subcortical white matter on T2 or FLAIR

Treatment
- High doses of steroids

Prognosis
- In general, rapid improvement after treatment, sometimes relapses when treatment is discontinued

Chronic lymphocytic inflammation with pontine perivascular enhancement responsive to steroids (CLIPPERS)

Clinical features

CLIPPERS is a rare, chronic inflammatory syndrome affecting the CNS and runs a relapsing–remitting course. To date, only a few cases have been described [28, 29]. Patients suffer from gait ataxia, intermittent diplopia, nystagmus, and perioral and facial paresthesia.

Further investigations

On MRI, a characteristic punctuate pattern of patchy contrast enhancement is seen, referred to as "peppering."

Originally, these lesions were found predominantly in the pons and cerebellum, but a phenotype with lesions in the spinal cord, basal ganglia, or cerebral cortex has recently been described (Figure 9.5) [30].

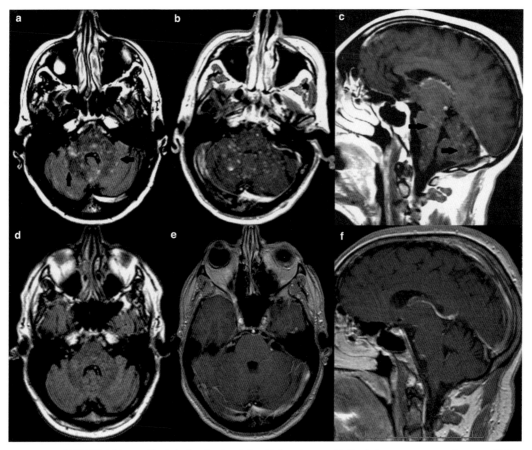

Figure 9.5 **CLIPPERS**. MRI scan of brain before (a–c) and after (d–f) corticosteroids. Typical punctuate or patchy areas of T2 hyperintensities (a) and contrast enhancement (b,c) are observed in the pons, cerebellum, and medulla oblongata (black arrows in a and c). Hyperintensities are less evident (d) and contrast enhancement is lacking (e,f) after corticosteroids. (a,d) Axial T2-weighted images; axial (b,e) and sagittal (c,f) T1-weighted images after gadolinium intravenous administration. Reproduced from Biotti *et al.* [28] with permission from BMJ Publishing Group Ltd.

Analysis of cerebral spinal fluid in most cases will reveal an increased number of lymphocytes and increased protein levels.

The imaging features of CLIPPERS are fairly unique. The main differential diagnosis on MRI of CLIPPERS includes capillary telangiectasia, which, however, is usually restricted to the basis pontis and shows characteristic low signal on T2*-weighted gradient-echo images, and patchy contrast enhancement, sometimes associated with an enlarged draining vein [31].

Treatment and prognosis

Rapid clinical improvement with treatment by high-dose corticosteroids is typical. Treatment should be initiated as soon as the diagnosis is estab-lished. A course of 1 g of methylprednisone per day during 5 days is generally the first step, followed by oral prednisone. However, after tapering, most patients experience a relapse. Therefore, several other immuno-suppressive drugs have been used in these patients, such as cyclophosphamide, methotrexate, and dexametha-sone, followed by maintenance treatment with oral immunosuppressive agents.

In addition to the beneficial clinical response to treatment, prompt resolution of contrast-enhancing lesions on MRI is also seen after the first course of methylprednisone. In many patients, however, cere-bellar atrophy can be seen despite improvement of clinical symptoms. After long-term follow-up all patients suffer from residual symptoms, hence the label "chronic" in the CLIPPERS acronym [29, 30].

Clinical features

- Onset within weeks to months
- Gait ataxia, intermittent diplopia, nystagmus, and perioral and facial paresthesia

Neuroimaging

- MRI: punctuate or patchy areas of T2 hyperintensity and contrast enhancement in pons/cerebellum, spinal cord, basal ganglia, and cerebral cortex

Treatment

- Methylprednisone 1000 mg per day for 5 days

Prognosis

- Rapid clinical and radiological response after treatment
- Residual symptoms in all patients

Bickerstaff encephalitis

Clinical features

Bickerstaff encephalitis shares some features with Miller Fisher syndrome (a variant of acute inflammatory demyelinating polyradiculoneuropathy, i.e., Guillain–Barré syndrome – GBS) but, in addition to progressive ophthalmoplegia and ataxia, there are symptoms reminiscent of CNS involvement, like disturbed consciousness and hyperreflexia. Some patients with Bickerstaff encephalitis complain of sensory disturbance at the distal extremities. Antecedent infectious symptoms are often seen, mainly fever, diarrhea, and upper-respiratory-tract complaints.

Further investigations

In about one-third of the patients, MRI shows high intensity on T2-weighted images in the brainstem, thalamus, cerebral white matter, and cerebellum (Figure 9.6) [32].

In up to two-thirds of patients, serum anti-GQ1b antibodies can be positive.

Cerebrospinal fluid analysis shows increased cell count and protein in approximately 40% of patients.

Nerve conduction studies show motor nerve dysfunction, predominantly axonal, possibly reflecting the overlap within the spectrum of the motor axonal neuropathy variant of GBS.

Treatment and prognosis

Like GBS and Miller Fisher syndrome, Bickerstaff encephalitis is treated with intravenous immunoglobulins (IVIG) or plasmapheresis. Combination therapy with steroids has also been applied in some cases.

After treatment, two-thirds of the patients recover without residual symptoms. The patients with remaining symptoms most frequently report dysesthesia, limb weakness, and diplopia.

The abovementioned features shared between GBS, Miller Fisher syndrome, and Bickerstaff encephalitis suggest that they are part of a spectrum of autoimmune disorders that have overlapping symptoms, which is sometimes referred to as the *anti-GQ1b antibody syndrome* [33].

Clinical features

- Shares clinical features with Miller Fisher syndrome and Guillain-Barré syndrome
- Besides ophthalmoplegia and ataxia, also CNS symptoms (disturbed consciousness, hyperreflexia)

Laboratory features

- Two-thirds of patients positive serum anti-GQ1b antibodies

Neuroimaging

- MRI: up to one-third of patients show increased signal on T2-weighted images in the brainstem, cerebellum, and thalamus

Treatment

- Treatment with intravenous immunoglobulins (IVIG) and/or plasmapheresis

Prognosis

- Two-thirds recover without residual symptoms

Rhombencephalitis

Clinical features

The term rhombencephalitis was originally used to describe an inflammatory syndrome of the brainstem and cerebellum. *Listeria monocytogenes* is the most common cause of rhombencephalitis, but all kinds of viral and bacterial infections, like Epstein–Barr virus

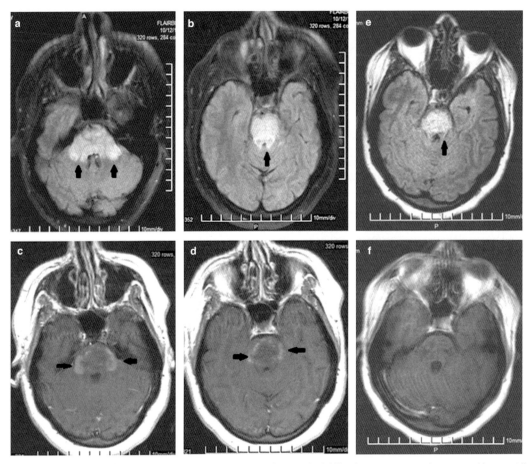

Figure 9.6 **Bickerstaff encephalitis**. (a)–(f) Axial FLAIR images show marked diffuse hyperintensity in the pons and lower midbrain extending to the middle and superior cerebellar peduncles (black arrows in a, b). Axial T1-weighted images after intravenous administration of gadolinium demonstrate a slightly irregular band of contrast enhancement at the periphery of the lesion (black arrows in c, d). Three weeks after corticosteroid treatment the extension of the area of hyperintensity in the lower midbrain and superior cerebellar peduncles is decreased on a FLAIR image (black arrow in e) and no contrast enhancement is seen (f).

(EBV), herpes simplex, and tuberculosis can give rise to this syndrome. There are also non-infectious causes of this syndrome, such as Behçet disease and other systemic disorders, and also paraneoplastic diseases.

The initial symptoms are non-specific, like headache, nausea, vomiting, and fever. The disease has a biphasic course with cranial nerve palsies, ataxia, tremor, and decreased consciousness developing over the following days [34].

Further investigations

MRI typically demonstrates high-signal lesions on proton density, T2-weighted, and FLAIR images (Figure 9.7) with variable nodular or ring contrast enhancement [35].

Blood and cerebrospinal fluid cultures are positive for the abovementioned microbiologic agents in about 60% of cases.

Treatment and prognosis

In patients who have fever, empirical treatment with ampicillin is recommended. In patients with a systemic disease who receive immunosuppressive drugs, ampicillin should also be added as these patients may not be able to produce fever. If tuberculosis or herpes simplex is suspected based on the clinical symptoms, tuberculostatic drugs or acycloguanosine (acyclovir), respectively, should be started. If toxoplasmosis is suspected in a human immunodeficiency virus (HIV)-positive patient, cotrimoxazole should be started.

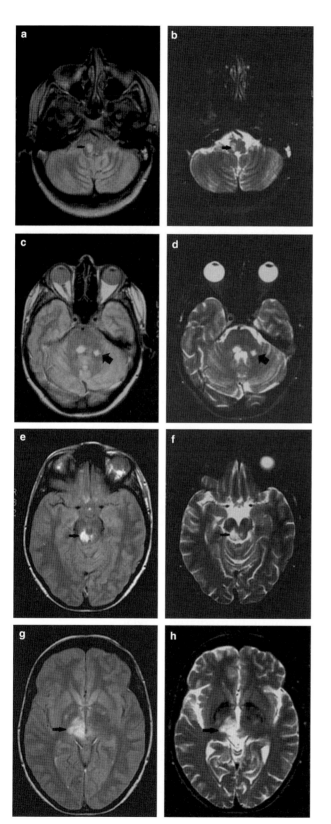

Figure 9.7 **Rhombencephalitis due to Toxoplasma gondii in AIDS**. Axial proton-density (a, c, e, g) and T2-weighted (b, d, f, h) images show a wide area of high signal intensity in the right brainstem, extending from the medulla (black arrow in a and b) to the dorsal midbrain (black arrow in e and f) and thalamus (black arrow in g, h) and a single focus of high signal intensity in the left middle cerebellar peduncle (black arrowhead in c and d).

Prognosis is poor with a high mortality of up to 50% of cases, but differs among the various etiologies. Patients with a paraneoplastic rhombencephalitis have a poorer outcome than patients with an infectious origin. Although 70% of patients who were treated with antibiotics survived [36], morbidity was high with neurologic sequelae in two-thirds of patients.

Key points: Rhombencephalitis

Clinical features

- Cranial nerve palsies, ataxia, tremor, and decreased consciousness
- Most frequently associated with infection by *Listeria monocytogenes*

Neuroimaging

- MRI: homogeneous, hyperintense areas in the brainstem with variable annular or nodular contrast enhancement

Treatment

- Treatment of underlying disease

Prognosis

- High mortality and morbidity

Parainfectious cerebellitis

Clinical features

Cerebellar ataxia can be a complication of several viral infections. Typically, there is a prodromal infectious phase, often caused (in adults) by the EBV, followed by subacute cerebellar symptoms. In adults, it is most frequently seen in males under the age of 30 years. In addition to an isolated cerebellar syndrome, cranial nerve palsies or a diffuse encephalitis can occur. Other associated infections are influenza, para-influenza, polio, and West–Nile virus.

Further investigations

Although there have been recent claims of early findings of restricted diffusion in the cerebellum, in general, MRI shows no abnormalities in the first days after onset. Subsequently, symmetric increased signal on T2-weighted images variably combined with swelling of the cerebellar folia and contrast enhancement can be observed (Figure 9.8) [37].

In patients with neurologic sequelae, cerebellar atrophy has been found with degeneration of Purkinje cells on autopsy.

Cerebrospinal fluid shows mild lymphocytic pleocytosis and moderate elevation of protein.

There might be serological evidence of a viral infection, such as EBV or varicella-zoster virus.

Treatment and prognosis

If clinical features suggest an active infection, the underlying disease should be treated accordingly. There are no reports that favor the use of immuno-modulatory drugs.

Overall, parainfectious cerebellitis has a favorable prognosis and clinical symptoms resolve within a few weeks. However, in patients older than 60 years prognosis is worse and they may suffer from persistent ataxia [38].

Key points: Parainfectious cerebellitis

Clinical

- Onset within days to weeks
- Mainly in young males with evidence of a concurrent/preceding EBV infection

Neuroimaging

- MRI: normal in the first few days after onset (besides symmetrically restricted diffusion); subsequently, symmetric T2 hyperintensity of the cerebellar folia variably combined with swelling and contrast enhancement

Treatment

- Treatment of underlying disease

Antibody-mediated ataxias

In the recent literature, there is accumulating evidence for several forms of ataxia associated with the presence of specific antibodies. The best known example is paraneoplastic cerebellar degeneration (PCD), but there are other CNS syndromes that are associated with specific antibodies. In addition to the onconeural antibodies that are directed to intracellular proteins, another group of antibodies bind to cell-surface determinants of membrane-associated proteins. These are also referred to as "neuronal surface antibodies" (NSAbs) [39]. The syndromes caused by antibodies to intracellular antigens can be distinguished from

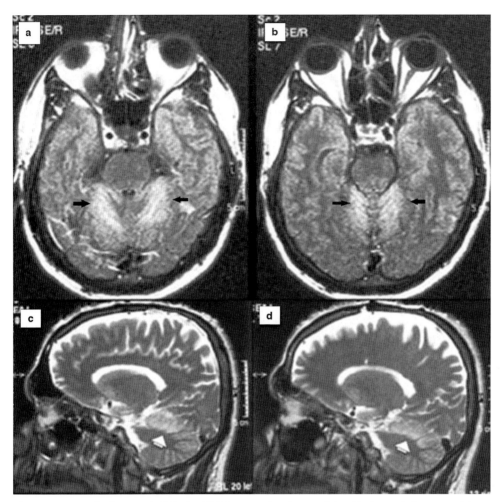

Figure 9.8 **Parainfectious cerebellitis**. Axial FLAIR images show increased signal in the cerebellar cortex of the superior vermis and paravermian cerebellar lobules (black arrows in a, b). The areas of signal change are confirmed in (left and right) parasagittal T2-weighted spin-echo images (white arrowheads in c, d). Reprinted with permission from Mascalchi M, Vella A (2012). *Handbook of Clinical Neurology* 103: 85–110.

those related to NSAbs; the latter group can occur at any age, are usually not associated with tumors, and can have a very good response to immunotherapy.

A possible immune-mediated cause of ataxia should be considered in patients with an acute or subacute onset of symptoms and an inflammatory response in the cerebrospinal fluid, such as pleocytosis, cerebrospinal fluid specific oligoclonal bands, or an elevated IgG index. MRI is usually negative.

Patients with a history of other autoimmune diseases have a higher risk of developing additional immune-mediated diseases. Frequently, the onset of symptoms is preceded by an infectious prodrome.

In patients in whom there is suspicion of an immune-mediated cause of ataxia, several antibodies can be tested, which will be discussed below.

Key points: Antibody-mediated ataxias

- Paraneoplastic ataxia with onconeural antibodies to intracellular antigens: anti-Hu, anti-Yo, anti-Tr
- Ataxia with non-onconeural antibodies to intracellular antigens: anti-Glutamate decarboxylase (anti-GAD), Homer-3
- Ataxia with identified neuronal surface antibodies against: metabotropic glutamate receptor 1 (mGluR1), voltage-gated potassium channel (VGCC), contactin associated protein 2 (CASPR2)

Clinical

- Acute or subacute onset
- Evidence of CNS inflammation

157

Neuroimaging

- MRI: usually negative

Treatment

- Treatment with immunotherapy

Prognosis

- Onconeural antibodies: poor, mainly determined by tumor treatment
- Other antibodies: variable, generally good, can show a good response to treatment; spontaneous remission possible

Paraneoplastic ataxia with onconeural intracellular antigens

Epidemiology and clinical features

Neurological paraneoplastic syndromes are caused by onconeural antigens that are released by apoptotic tumor cells. Antibodies to onconeural antigens in the nervous system lead to neurological symptoms. This autoimmune reaction is seen in less than 1% of all cancer patients. Cerebellar degeneration is one of the most frequent paraneoplastic syndromes of the CNS.

In patients with a known malignancy who develop rapidly progressive ataxia, the suspicion of PCD should be raised. But it is also possible for the cerebellar symptoms to precede the clinical manifestation of cancer by months to years and tumor screening can be negative initially. Consequently, tumor screening should be repeated several times when onconeural antigens or a classic paraneoplastic syndrome are present.

Patients usually present with subacute vertigo, nausea, and vomiting. In the following days, they develop oculomotor disturbances, such as downbeat nystagmus and jerky pursuit, dysarthria, dysphagia, and cerebellar ataxia; the latter is frequently asymmetric. These symptoms initially run a progressive course before reaching a static phase after several months.

PCD is mainly associated with small-cell lung cancer, gynecological and breast tumors, and Hodgkin's lymphoma.

Further investigations

In most patients, the initial MRI scan is normal, but can show cerebellar cortical atrophy and diffuse symmetric T2 hyperintensity in the cerebellar white matter

and cortex [40, 41]. The main differential diagnosis is with intra-axial masses and leptomeningeal metastases, the latter appearing as nodular or diffuse areas of contrast enhancement (see below). Since negative tests for serum antibodies do not exclude this diagnosis, whole-body fluorodeoxyglucose positron emission tomography (FDG PET) is recommended to detect a possibly underlying occult primary malignancy (typically ovarian, breast, or lung) in patients with suspected PCD and unknown cancer. In paraneoplastic degeneration, FDG PET of the brain usually demonstrates diffuse hypometabolism of the cerebellar cortex [42].

In small-cell lung cancer, anti-Hu is frequently found and additional paraneoplastic syndromes like sensory neuropathy or diffuse encephalomyelitis can be seen. A relatively pure cerebellar syndrome is found in patients with breast cancer or gynecological malignancies and is associated with anti-Yo antibodies. In patients with a Hodgkin lymphoma, PCD often develops only after the diagnosis has been made or may occur in patients who are in remission. Anti-Tr can be detected in serum, but antibodies can also be absent or present only in cerebrospinal fluid.

Treatment and prognosis

Treating the underlying tumor and/or immunosuppressive therapy are indicated, but generally they do not improve the cerebellar symptoms. Some patients, however, do benefit from immunosuppressants when given in the very early stages of the disease.

Neurologic outcome and median survival for the different onconeural antigens are as follows: 75–80% of patients with anti-Hu and anti-Yo antigens become wheelchair-bound and they have a median survival, from time of diagnosis, of 7 months for anti-Hu and of 13 months for anti-Yo. The outcome in anti-Tr is somewhat better with approximately 40% of patients remaining ambulatory and a median survival of 117 months [43, 44].

Key points: Paraneoplastic cerebellar degeneration (PCD)

Clinical features

- Onset and severe disability within weeks
- Mainly associated with small-cell lung cancer, gynecological and breast tumors, and Hodgkin's lymphoma
- Cerebellar symptoms can precede the clinical manifestation or detection of cancer

Neuroimaging

- MRI: often negative; rarely cerebellar atrophy or symmetric high signal on T2-weighted and FLAIR images of the cerebellar cortex and underlying white matter
- Whole-body FDG PET: detection of the underlying primary cancer (breast, ovarian, and lung)

Onconeural antibodies

- Mainly anti-Yo, anti-Hu, anti-Tr

Treatment

- Immunosuppressive drugs very early in the course of the disease might be beneficial

Prognosis

- Median survival: anti- Hu: 7 months; anti-Yu: 13 months: anti-Tr: 117 months

Ataxia with non-onconeural intracellular antigens

Epidemiology and clinical features

Recently, anti-GAD antibodies have been found in patients with cerebellar ataxia. The onset can be subacute, but also more insidious. It is characterized by a pancerebellar syndrome, but gait is often the most severely affected. GAD is an enzyme that catalyzes the conversion of glutamic acid in the neurotransmitter GABA. Anti-GAD antibodies are present in 60–90% of patients with type 1 diabetes and are also present in most patients with stiff person syndrome [45].

Another non-onconeural intracellular antigen is Homer-3, which is predominantly expressed in the dendritic spines of the Purkinje cells.

Further investigations

MRI usually reveals cerebellar atrophy in patients with high titers of anti-GAD antibodies, but also imaging abnormalities compatible with limbic encephalitis have occasionally been reported. Cerebellar cortical atrophy was also observed in patients with ataxia and low-titer anti-GAD antibodies [46].

A lumbar puncture is recommended in patients with high GAD antibody titers in serum to calculate the index for the presence or absence of actual intrathecal synthesis of anti-GAD antibodies. This index can be calculated with the following formula (CSF is cerebral spinal fluid):

$$\frac{CSF\ GAD - antibody\ titer / serum\ GAD - antibody\ titer}{CSF\ albumin\ (mg/1) / serum albumin (mg/1)}$$

Index values higher than the IgG index suggest an autoimmune reaction to GAD, caused by intrathecal synthesis of specific anti-GAD IgG. In patients with other autoimmune (endocrine) syndromes associated with anti-GAD antibodies, such as diabetes, this index is particularly important, because high anti-GAD antibody levels in serum could be related to the autoimmune disorder from diabetes or other autoimmune disorders and not specifically to the ataxia.

Treatment and prognosis

Immunotherapy, such as with steroids or intravenous immunoglobulins, leads to improvement of neurological symptoms in some patients with anti-GAD ataxia regardless of the level of anti-GAD antibodies.

Ataxia with identified NSAbs

VGCC antibodies: In patients with cerebellar ataxia, various NSAbs have been identified. Brain MRI is usually negative or demonstrates a non-specific cerebellar cortical atrophy pattern [47]. In a study of 39 patients with PCD and lung cancer, 41% had increased levels of P/Q-type voltage-gated potassium channel (VGCC) antibodies. These are also the culprits in Lambert–Eaton myasthenic syndrome (LEMS). Of this 41%, only half of the patients suffered from concurrent LEMS. Usually patients with syndromes caused by NSAbs show a good response when treated with immunotherapy, but they do not show improvement of their ataxia. A possible explanation might be that the Purkinje cells are already irreversibly damaged in an early phase of the disease or that the immunotherapy is unable to eliminate the pathogenic antibodies.

mGlur1 antibodies: mGlur1 antibodies have been identified in three patients with subacute cerebellar ataxia. mGluR1 is a cell-surface receptor in the cerebellar Purkinje cells.

CASPR2 antibodies: In 10% of 88 patients with either subacute or chronic, idiopathic late-onset ataxia, CASPR2 antibodies were identified. This was significantly higher than the percentages found in the control groups of patients with multiple sclerosis (MS) and dementia. CASPR2, a VGKC-associated protein, is highly expressed in the axons of the granule cells of the cerebellum [48].

Treatment and prognosis

In patients who suffer from a possible antibody-mediated ataxia, treatment should be started promptly, even before the results of the antibody screening have been returned.

Various forms of immunotherapy, like intravenous corticosteroids, intravenous immunoglobulins, or plasma exchange have led to an improvement of symptoms. If patients do not respond to these forms of immunotherapy, rituximab or cyclophosphamide are second-line options.

The outcome is generally good and patients may even experience a spontaneous remission [39].

Multiple sclerosis (MS)

MS is the most common autoimmune inflammatory demyelinating disease of the CNS. Strategically located plaques in MS are a frequent cause of unilateral ataxia of subacute onset in young adults. They are usually accompanied by further white-matter lesions elsewhere in the brain (Figure 9.9) and spinal cord. Because ataxia is only one of the many symptoms caused by MS, and MS is covered in detail in other chapters, this will not be further discussed here.

Creutzfeldt–Jakob disease (CJD)

Epidemiology and clinical features

CJD is the most frequent of human prion diseases, but is very rare, with an incidence of about one case per 1 000 000 people per year. Eighty-five percent of the cases are sporadic, 5–15% are familial, and less than 1% are iatrogenic. In regions with clustering of familial CJD, the incidence is increased 30 to 100-fold.

CJD is a neurodegenerative prion disease with rapid progression of dementia and myoclonus as the most prominent features. Additional symptoms include visual disturbances, cerebellar ataxia, and pyramidal or other extrapyramidal features. Akinetic mutism frequently develops in the course of the disease. This clinical constellation in combination with typical electroencephalogram (EEG) changes (periodic synchronous bi- or triphasic sharp-wave complexes), the presence of the 14–3–3 protein and increased levels of tau in cerebrospinal fluid, and typical MRI abnormalities, are in general sufficient to diagnose CJD, but brain biopsy remains the gold standard.

The mean age of onset is 60 years (range 40–80 years). A small subgroup of patients initially suffer from a pure cerebellar variant and develop other symptoms in later stages of the disease. This subtype is associated with a molecular variant within the *PRNP* gene (valine homozygosity at position 129; VV2) [49].

Familial CJD patients have a *PRNP* mutation, which is inherited as an autosomal dominant trait.

More than 50 different mutations in *PRNP* have been described in CJD families. Variant CJD is very rare and associated with consumption of infected beef. A few cases have been reported in Europe, mainly the United Kingdom and France. The mean age of onset is 29 years and patients suffer from early psychiatric and

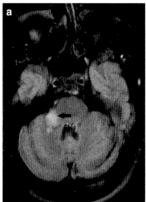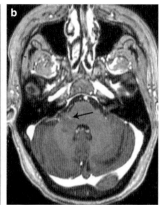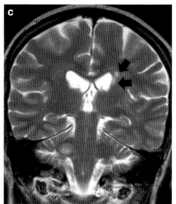

Figure 9.9 **Acute multiple sclerosis plaque**. The axial FLAIR image shows two juxtaposed hyperintense lesions in the right middle cerebellar peduncle (black arrow in a). The anterior portion of the largest lesion exhibits some mild enhancement (black arrow in b) in an axial T1-weighted image after gadolinium intravenous administration. The coronal T2-weighted image confirms the lesion in the right middle cerebellar peduncle and discloses two additional lesions near the frontal horn of the left lateral ventricle (black arrowheads in c).

painful sensory symptoms [50]. Lastly, iatrogenic CJD has been reported in patients who received a human cadaveric dura mater graft. Some of these patients also present with an ataxic phenotype, mainly affecting gait. Lumping these different subtypes of CJD, younger patients more often display a cerebellar phenotype and this subtype is associated with a longer mean survival.

Further investigations

MRI significantly contributes to the diagnosis by showing high signal changes on T2-weighted images, best seen with FLAIR imaging within the cerebral cortex, pulvinar, head of caudate, and putamen [51]. These cortical and deep gray-matter abnormalities are even better outlined as high-intensity areas on diffusion-weighted images reflecting restricted diffusion (Figure 9.10). The cortical

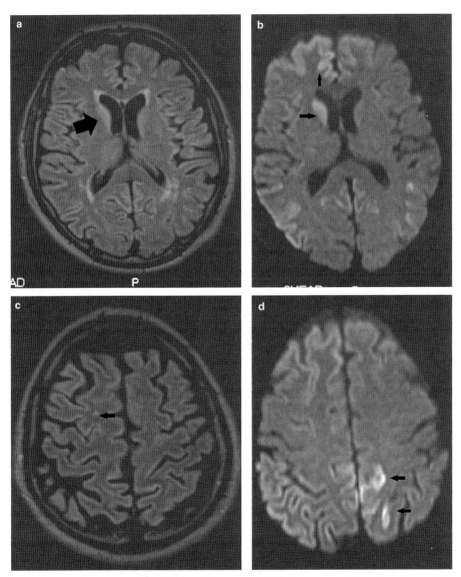

Figure 9.10 Creutzfeld–Jakob disease. Axial FLAIR images (a,c) show non-specific symmetric areas of increased signal in the peritrigonal white matter of the cerebral hemispheres and in the subcortical white matter of the right frontal lobe (black small arrow in c) as well as subtle hyperintensity of the right head of caudate (black large arrowhead in a). Axial diffusion-weighted images (b,d) confirm the abnormality in the right head of caudate (black small arow in b) and reveals additional areas of diffusion restriction in the right frontal cortex (black small arrow in b) and the mesial left parietal cortex (black small arrows in d).

and basal ganglia involvement may be asymmetric initially and becomes symmetric later in the course of the disease. Contrast enhancement is lacking.

Specific cerebrospinal fluid markers can be found in patients with suspected CJD. The presence of the 14–3–3 protein has a sensitivity of about 92%, but a specificity of 40%. False-positive results have been reported in patients with herpes simplex encephalitis, metabolic and hypoxic encephalopathies, and paraneoplastic syndromes.

Elevated levels of tau is another marker; while slightly less sensitive (87%) than 14–3–3, it has a specificity of 67%. Both tests are only of additional value on top of a clinical suspicion of CJD. Their positive predictive value drops considerably if they are used in patients with a low a-priori chance of CJD [52].

In CJD patients, the EEG shows periodic synchronous bi- or triphasic sharp-wave complexes. However, these complexes are not seen in all patients, the sensitivity is only approximately 40–67%. Furthermore, these EEG findings are seen only relatively late in the course of the disease.

Treatment and prognosis

There is currently no treatment for CJD. Therapeutic interventions are being explored, such as vaccines, RNA-interference, and anti-inflammatory agents.

After onset of the first symptoms, the mean survival in sporadic CJD is 4 months. Those with the VV2-variant have a longer mean survival of 9 months. The mean survival in variant CJD is 14 months.

Familial CJD is associated with the longest mean survival, ranging from 5 to 11 years.

Key points: Creutzfeldt–Jakob disease

Clinical features

- Rapid progression of dementia and myoclonus
- Cerebellar ataxia can be a dominant disease feature in early stages

Neuroimaging

- MRI: high signal changes on T2-weighted (especially FLAIR) images and restricted diffusion in the cortical gray matter, basal ganglia, and pulvinar; changes may be asymmetric in the early phase.

Prognosis

- Mean survival 4 to 14 months, longer in familial cases

Leptomeningeal carcinomatosis

Epidemiology and clinical features

Tumors outside the CNS can metastasize to the leptomeninges through hematogenous spread, in continuum from vertebral, subdural, or epidural metastases, direct spread along peripheral nerves to the subarachnoid space, or perivenous dissemination from the bone marrow within the skull. Leptomeningeal carcinomatosis is found in 5% of patients with a metastatic malignancy, but this percentage is higher in autopsy studies, as it can remain asymptomatic. It is most frequently found in patients with breast cancer, lung cancer, melanoma, and gastrointestinal malignancies. Patients can present with symptoms such as nuchal rigidity, headache, nausea, and vomiting. Focal symptoms can occur if intra-axial metastases are also present. Isolated cerebellar ataxia has also been described [53].

Further investigations

On MRI, diffuse or multinodular contrast-enhancing lesions can be detected in the subarachnoid space, cerebellar folia, or cortical surface (Figure 9.11), which typically can be missed on non-contrast-enhanced MRI examination.

Because leptomeningeal carcinomatosis frequently results in elevated intracranial pressure, a lumbar puncture generally shows a high opening pressure. Analysis of cerebrospinal fluid can reveal lymphocytic pleocytosis, low glucose, and high protein concentration. Malignant cells in the cerebrospinal fluid can be found with cytology and confirm the diagnosis.

Treatment and prognosis

Before treatment is started, patients should be clinically evaluated to assess their functional status. The Karnofsky performance status [54], a scoring system used to classify patient functional impairment, is an important indicator to decide whether the patient should undergo further treatment. Patients can be treated aggressively with radiotherapy, and intrathecal or systemic chemotherapy, but in those with a poor functional status and high risk of serious adverse events, treatment is more targeted at pain reduction and relief of symptoms. Despite treatment, prognosis is poor with a median survival of 2 to 10 months.

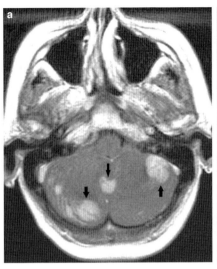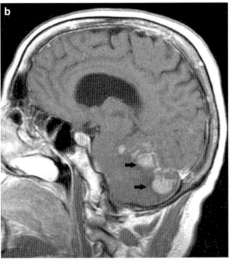

Figure 9.11 **Leptomeningeal carcinomatosis from gastric cancer**. Axial (a) and sagittal (b) T1-weighted images after intravenous administration of gadolinium reveal multiple nodules of homogeneous contrast enhancement in the subarachnoid spaces of the posterior cranial fossa (black arrows in a, b).

Key points: Leptomeningeal carcinomatosis

Clinical features

- Onset within weeks
- Patients with a known malignancy
- Nuchal rigidity, headache, vomiting, focal neurological symptoms

Neuroimaging

- MRI with gadolinium: multi-nodular or diffuse contrast enhancement in the subarachnoid spaces of the posterior cranial fossa, cerebellar folia, or cortical surface

Treatment

- Palliative treatment; radiotherapy and chemotherapy can be considered in patients with a good Karnofsky score

References

1. Grimaldi G, Manto M. (2012). Topography of cerebellar deficits in humans. *Cerebellum* **11**: 336–351.

2. Amarenco P. (1991). The spectrum of cerebellar infarctions. *Neurology* **41**: 973–979.

3. Mascalchi M, Filippi M, Floris R, *et al.* (2005). Diffusion-weighted MR of the brain: methodology and clinical application. *Radiol Med* **109**: 155–197.

4. Moulin T, Bogousslavsky J, Chopard JL, *et al.* (1995). Vascular ataxic hemiparesis: a re-evaluation. *J Neurol Neurosurg Psychiatry* **58**: 422–427.

5. Newman-Toker DE, Kattah JC, Alvernia JE, Wang DZ. (2008). Normal head impulse test differentiates acute cerebellar strokes from vestibular neuritis. *Neurology* **70**: 2378–2385.

6. Lee H, Sohn SI, Cho YW, *et al.* (2006). Cerebellar infarction presenting isolated vertigo: frequency and vascular topographical patterns. *Neurology* **67**: 1178–1183.

7. Moon IS, Kim JS, Choi KD, *et al.* (2009). Isolated nodular infarction. *Stroke* **40**: 487–491.

8. Kirmani JF, Alkawi A, Panezai S, Gizzi M. (2012). Advances in thrombolytics for treatment of acute ischemic stroke. *Neurology* **79**: S119–S125.

9. St Louis EK, Wijdicks EF, Li H, Atkinson JD. (2000). Predictors of poor outcome in patients with a spontaneous cerebellar hematoma. *Can J Neurol Sci* **27**: 32–36.

10. Satoh H. (2000). Occupational and environmental toxicology of mercury and its compounds. *Ind Health* **38**: 153–164.

11. Korogi Y, Takahashi M, Okajima T, Eto K. (1998). MR findings of Minamata disease – organic mercury poisoning. *J Magn Reson Imaging* **8**: 308–316.

12. Kuruvilla T, Bharucha NE. (1997). Cerebellar atrophy after acute phenytoin intoxication. *Epilepsia* **38**: 500–502.

13. Roy M, Stip E, Black D, Lew V, Langlois R. (1998). Cerebellar degeneration following acute lithium intoxication. *Rev Neurol (Paris)* **154**: 546–548.

14. Suwanlaong K, Phanthumchinda K (2008). Neurological manifestation of methyl bromide intoxication. *J Med Assoc Thai* **91**: 421–426.

15. Xiao L, Lin X, Cao J, Wang X, Wu L (2011). MRI findings in 6 cases of children by inadvertent ingestion of diphenoxylate-atropine. *Eur J Radiol* **79**: 432–436.

16. Boulos MI, Shoamanesh A, Aviv RI, Gladstone DJ, Swartz RH (2012). Severe hypomagnesemia associated with reversible subacute ataxia and cerebellar hyperintensities on MRI. *Neurologist* **18**: 223–225.

17. Sedehizadeh S, Keogh M, Wills AJ (2011). Reversible hypomagnesaemia-induced subacute cerebellar syndrome. *Biol Trace Elem Res* **142**: 127–129.

18. Nguyen HV, Gan SK (2005). Neurological sequelae of chronic profound hypocalcaemia. *Med J Aust* **182**: 123.

19. Asokumar P, Gogate YV, Gangadhar P, Bhansali A (2011). Reversible cerebellar ataxia: a rare presentation of depletional hyponatremia. *Neurol India* **59**: 631–632.

20. Mascalchi M, Simonelli P, Tessa C, *et al.* (1999). Do acute lesions of Wernicke's encephalopathy show contrast enhancement? Report of three cases and review of the literature. *Neuroradiology* **41**: 249–254.

21. Zuccoli G, Pipitone N (2009). Neuroimaging findings in acute Wernicke's encephalopathy: review of the literature. *AJR Am J Roentgenol* **192**: 501–508.

22. Zuccoli G, Santa CD, Bertolini M, *et al.* (2009). MR imaging findings in 56 patients with Wernicke encephalopathy: nonalcoholics may differ from alcoholics. *AJNR Am J Neuroradiol* **30**: 171–176.

23. Sechi G, Serra A (2007). Wernicke's encephalopathy: new clinical settings and recent advances in diagnosis and management. *Lancet Neurol* **6**: 442–455.

24. Nakagawa H, Yoneda M, Fujii A, Kinomoto K, Kuriyama M (2007). Hashimoto's encephalopathy presenting with progressive cerebellar ataxia. *J Neurol Neurosurg Psychiatry* **78**: 196–197.

25. Tang Y, Chu C, Lin MT, *et al.* (2011). Hashimoto's encephalopathy mimicking spinocerebellar ataxia. *J. Neurol* **258**: 1705–1707.

26. Ferracci F, Bertiato G, Moretto G (2004). Hashimoto's encephalopathy: epidemiologic data and pathogenetic considerations. *J Neurol Sci* **217**: 165–168.

27. Castillo P, Woodruff B, Caselli R, *et al.* (2006). Steroid-responsive encephalopathy associated with autoimmune thyroiditis. *Arch Neurol* **63**: 197–202.

28. Biotti D, Deschamps R, Shotar E, *et al.* (2011). CLIPPERS: chronic lymphocytic inflammation with pontine perivascular enhancement responsive to steroids. *Pract Neurol* **11**: 349–351.

29. Pittock SJ, Debruyne J, Krecke KN, *et al.* (2010). Chronic lymphocytic inflammation with pontine perivascular enhancement responsive to steroids (CLIPPERS). *Brain* **133**: 2626–2634.

30. Simon NG, Parratt JD, Barnett MH, *et al.* (2012). Expanding the clinical, radiological and neuropathological phenotype of chronic lymphocytic inflammation with pontine perivascular enhancement responsive to steroids (CLIPPERS). *J Neurol Neurosurg Psychiatry* **83**: 15–22.

31. Scaglione C, Salvi F, Riguzzi P, *et al.* (2001). Symptomatic unruptured capillary telangiectasia of the brain stem: report of three cases and review of the literature. *J Neurol Neurosurg Psychiatry* **71**: 390–393.

32. Odaka M, Yuki N, Yamada M, *et al.* (2003). Bickerstaff's brainstem encephalitis: clinical features of 62 cases and a subgroup associated with Guillain–Barré syndrome. *Brain* **126**: 2279–2290.

33. Shahrizaila N, Yuki N (2012). Bickerstaff brainstem encephalitis and Fisher syndrome: anti-GQ1b antibody syndrome. *J Neurol Neurosurg Psychiatry* **84**: 576–583

34. Moragas M, Martinez-Yelamos S, Majos C, *et al.* (2011). Rhombencephalitis: a series of 97 patients. *Medicine (Baltimore)* **90**: 256–261.

35. Mrowka M, Graf LP, Odin P (2002). MRI findings in mesenrhombencephalitis due to *Listeria monocytogenes*. *J Neurol Neurosurg Psychiatry* **73**: 775.

36. Armstrong RW, Fung PC (1993). Brainstem encephalitis (rhombencephalitis) due to *Listeria monocytogenes*: case report and review. *Clin Infect Dis* **16**: 689–702.

37. Guerrini L, Belli G, Cellerini M, Nencini P, Mascalchi M (2002). Proton MR spectroscopy of cerebellitis. *Magn Reson Imaging* **20**: 619–622.

38. Klockgether T, Doller G, Wullner U, Petersen D, Dichgans J (1993). Cerebellar encephalitis in adults. *J Neurol* **240**: 17–20.

39. Zuliani L, Graus F, Giometto B, Bien C, Vincent A (2012). Central nervous system neuronal surface antibody associated syndromes: review and guidelines for recognition. *J Neurol Neurosurg Psychiatry* **83**: 638–645.

40. Schlake HP, Husstedt IW, Grotemeyer KH, Potter R (1989). Paraneoplastic subacute cerebellar degeneration in Hodgkin's disease. Report of three cases and review of the literature. *Clin Neurol Neurosurg* **91**: 329–335.

41. Gilmore CP, Elliott I, Auer D, Maddison P (2010). Diffuse cerebellar MR imaging changes in anti-Yo positive paraneoplastic cerebellar degeneration. *J Neurol* **257**: 490–491.

42. Basu S, Alavi A (2008). Role of FDG PET in the clinical management of paraneoplastic neurological syndrome: detection of the underlying malignancy and the brain PET–MRI correlates. *Mol Imaging Biol* **10**:131–137.

43. Gozzard P, Maddison P (2010). Which antibody and which cancer in which paraneoplastic syndromes? *Pract Neurol* **10**: 260–270.

44. Shams'ili S, Grefkens J, de LB, *et al.* (2003). Paraneoplastic cerebellar degeneration associated with antineuronal antibodies: analysis of 50 patients. *Brain* **126**: 1409–1418.

45. Saiz A, Blanco Y, Sabater L, *et al.* (2008). Spectrum of neurological syndromes associated with glutamic acid decarboxylase antibodies: diagnostic clues for this association. *Brain* **131**: 2553–2563.

46. Honnorat J, Saiz A, Giometto B, *et al.* (2001). Cerebellar ataxia with anti-glutamic acid decarboxylase antibodies: study of 14 patients. *Arch Neurol* **58**: 225–230.

47. Hoftberger R, Sabater L, Ortega A, Dalmau J, Graus F (2013). Patient with Homer-3 antibodies and cerebellitis. *JAMA Neurol* **70**: 506–509.

48. Becker EB, Zuliani L, Pettingill R, *et al.* (2012). Contactin-associated protein-2 antibodies in non-paraneoplastic cerebellar ataxia. *J Neurol Neurosurg Psychiatry* **83**: 437–440.

49. Cooper SA, Murray KL, Heath CA, Will RG, Knight RS (2006). Sporadic Creutzfeldt–Jakob disease with cerebellar ataxia at onset in the UK. *J Neurol Neurosurg Psychiatry* **77**: 1273–1275.

50. Johnson RT (2005). Prion diseases. *Lancet Neurol* **4**: 635–642.

51. Newey CR, Sarwal A, Wisco D, Alam S, Lederman RJ (2013). Variability in diagnosing Creutzfeldt–Jakob disease using standard and proposed diagnostic criteria. *J Neuroimaging* **23**: 58–63.

52. Hamlin C, Puoti G, Berri S, *et al.* (2012). A comparison of tau and 14–3–3 protein in the diagnosis of Creutzfeldt–Jakob disease. *Neurology* **79**: 547–552.

53. Lahiri RP, Burnand KM, Bandi A, Farooq N, Sathesh-Kumar T (2011). Colorectal cancer presenting with dysarthria and ataxia: a case of isolated leptomeningeal metastasis. *Ann R Coll Surg Engl* **93**: e133–e135.

54. Yates JW, Chalmer B, McKegney FP (1980). Evaluation of patients with advanced cancer using the Karnofsky performance status. *Cancer* **45**: 2220–2224.

Chapter 10

Syncope

C. T. Paul Krediet and Horacio Kaufmann

Introduction

Syncope is a transient loss of consciousness (TLOC) and postural tone due to global cerebral hypoperfusion with spontaneous recovery and no neurological sequelae. Although syncope is arguably the most frequent cause of TLOC, not all episodes of TLOC are due to syncope [1]. Indeed, seizures, head trauma, metabolic abnormalities, and psychogenic disorders may also present as TLOC. Thus, until a diagnosis of syncope can be established it is useful to refer to these events as TLOC. TLOC is a common medical problem. It accounts for 0.6–3% of visits to the emergency department and up to 6% of hospital admissions [2].

The diagnostic approach to a patient with TLOC should be aimed at stratifying risks: i.e., identifying patients with a potentially serious, or lethal, underlying pathology causing TLOC while, at the same time, applying diagnostic tests in a rational manner that prevents unnecessary costs and needless medical involvement. The initial diagnostic considerations should distinguish syncope from seizures and from other causes, such as metabolic and psychogenic disorders.

Global cerebral hypoperfusion causing syncope can result from (1) a temporary fall in systemic blood pressure (e.g. orthostatic hypotension in patients with chronic autonomic failure – either isolated or in the setting of a neurodegenerative disease or polyneuropathies, or neurally mediated syncope), (2) a fall in cardiac output (e.g. severe brady- or tachy-arrhythmia), or (3) episodic increases in intracranial pressure compromising global cerebral blood flow [3]. Contrary to the *global* cerebral hypoperfusion that causes syncope, *local* cerebral hypoperfusion causes specific neurological deficits depending on the area of the brain that is affected, and is referred to as "transient ischemic attacks" (TIA)

and rarely, if ever, presents as isolated TLOC. Table 10.1 presents an overview of causes of TLOC.

Epidemiological considerations

TLOC in the general population is very common. TLOC events often do not reach medical attention, particularly in the young in whom most episodes are considered to be benign vasovagal faints (i.e. neurally mediated or reflex syncope) [4]. Studies in teenagers and young adults show a strikingly high incidence of TLOC; e.g. in medical students, 20–25% of males and 40–50% of females report that they have experienced at least one such episode [5]. The majority of the TLOC triggers identified in these students involved stresses or conditions that affect orthostatic blood-pressure control. Neurally mediated syncope was therefore a likely cause of the symptoms in these young subjects.

In senior subjects, cardiac causes of syncope, as well as orthostatic and postprandial hypotension and presumed carotid sinus hypersensitivity are more frequent [6]. Older age, structural heart disease, or a history of coronary artery disease should be considered as risk factors for adverse outcome, with a 1-year mortality ranging up to 27% [7].

Emergency room diagnostic work-up on TLOC

Initial evaluation of TLOC should include a thorough clinical history, physical examination with blood pressure and heart rate measurements while supine and standing, and a 12-lead ECG [7, 8] (Figure 10.1).

The first diagnostic step is to ascertain whether the episode of TLOC is actually syncope or something else. Neurally mediated syncope, also referred to as reflex syncope, frequently has a characteristic history that includes premonitory symptoms such as yawning,

 Imaging Acute Neurologic Disease, ed. Massimo Filippi and Jack H. Simon. Published by Cambridge University Press.
© Cambridge University Press 2014.

Table 10.1 Causes of TLOC

SYNCOPE	Cardiac arrhythmia	Bradyarrhythmias	*Sinus node dysfunction*
			Atrioventricular (AV) blocks
		Tachyarrhythmias	*Supraventricular*
			Ventricular
	Neurally mediated	Vasovagal	
		Carotid sinus syncope	
		Situational syncope	*Cough syncope*
			Micturition syncope
			Defecation syncope
			Deglutition syncope
	Orthostatic hypotension	Volume depletion	*Diuretics/Polyuria*
			Adrenal insufficiency
			Gastrointestinal volume loss
		Loss of vasoconstrictor capacity	*Antihypertensives*
			Autonomic failure
	Block in minor circulation	Pericardial effusion	
		Pulmonary embolism	
		Atrial myxoma	
	Paroxysmal increased intracerebral pressure	Meningocele	
SEIZURES			
METABOLIC			
PSYCHOGENIC			

light-headedness, visual disturbances, nausea, or epigastric discomfort. Often there is also a typical appearance (pallor, sweating) and syncope occurs during characteristic settings such as with strong emotions, unexpected pain, or during prolonged standing. Conversely, in patients with autonomic failure and chronic orthostatic hypotension, premonitory symptoms are absent and syncope occurs usually after meals or during maneuvers that impede venous return to the heart (e.g. Valsalva maneuver). In these patients, orthostatic hypotension is a reproducible phenomenon and heart-rate increase is blunted. Neurological examination may show parkinsonism, cerebellar ataxia, or signs of a peripheral neuropathy. Occasionally, orthostatic hypotension is the sole presenting feature of these disorders [9].

Syncope preceded by chest pain suggests a myocardial infarction and blood levels of cardiac enzymes should be obtained. Ventral chest pain also accompanies type A aortic dissections that may present with syncope due to cardiac tamponade [10]. Syncope during exercise or the finding of a systolic ejection bruit suggests ventricular outflow obstruction. An echocardiogram will characterize the anatomy and confirm the diagnosis. Syncope preceded by palpitations without other prodromes suggests a cardiac arrhythmia. When the episodes are frequent, Holter monitoring may reveal the arrhythmia. In some cases, these patients may be candidates for prolonged ECG monitoring with an implantable device. Exercise stress testing can unravel myocardial ischemia or exercise-induced arrhythmias. In patients with organic heart disease and diminished ejection fraction that are at high risk for ventricular arrhythmias, electrophysiologic studies of the heart should be considered [8].

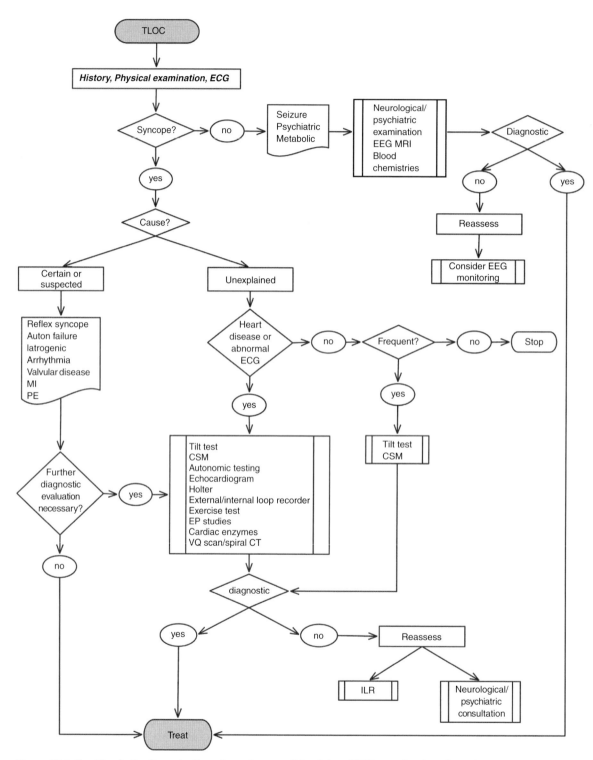

Figure 10.1 Algorithm for the diagnosis of loss of consciousness. Abbreviations: TLOC = transient loss of consciousness; ECG = electrocardiogram; EEG = electroencephalogram; MRI = magnetic resonance imagining; MI = myocardial infarction; PE = pulmonary embolism; CSM = carotid sinus massage; EP studies = electrophysiological studies; VQ scan = ventilation perfusion scan; CT = computed tomography; ILR = insertable loop recorder (based on Kaufmann and Wieling [1]).

In summary, when ECG, history or physical examination suggest or indicate that the patient has structural heart disease, cardiac enzymes, echocardiogram, Holter monitoring and exercise testing or intracardiac electrophysiological studies may be indicated [8]. Patients with the long QT syndrome, a rare but potentially deadly cause of syncope, have a characteristic ECG and often a typical family history as well. Ventricular tachy- and bradyarrhythmias that potentially explain syncope may appear in the initial ECG.

Iatrogenic causes, most commonly polypharmacy in the elderly, are easily uncovered by a careful history-taking. In these cases, no further diagnostic tests are necessary and treatment can be instituted. In summary, a characteristic history and ECG finding can establish the diagnosis of neurally mediated/reflex syncope, chronic autonomic failure, long QT syndrome, and iatrogenic syncope, among others.

If neurological deficits such as diplopia, limb weakness, sensory deficits, or speech difficulties occurred in conjunction with TLOC, the episode is not syncope. A neurological deficit indicates an abnormality in a particular brain area, probably caused by a TIA, a seizure, or, rarely, a migraine attack. Upward turning of the eyes, asynchronous myoclonic jerks, and brief automatisms can occur frequently during syncope, but aura, prolonged tonic clonic convulsions, synchronous myoclonic jerks, and prolonged automatisms are restricted to seizures [1]. In the medical history the presence of post-ictal confusion differentiates syncope best from seizures. In a patient with syncope, the duration of such confusion, if at all present, does not exceed the duration of the TLOC [3]. In patients who have had a seizure, the confusion can be prolonged and does exceed the TLOC duration. Urinary incontinence is uncommon in syncope but frequent in epileptic as well as psychogenic seizures (more than 40% of patients). When seizures are suspected, the patient should undergo an EEG and brain imaging.

Imaging in patients with TLOC

In general, imaging should be used very conservatively in patients with TLOC and only be applied to selected patients [7].

Cardiopulmonary imaging

In the patient with suspected syncope from cardiac arrhythmias, cardiac imaging is indicated, as well as rhythm observation during radiological examinations [8]. Echocardiography can be helpful to assess possible gross structural and/or valve abnormalities (e.g., aortic valve stenosis predisposes to ventricular arrhythmias) and/or the presence of cardiomyopathies. Echocardiography may also be helpful to assess causes of a block in the minor circulation, such as pericardial effusion or increased right-ventricle pressure in the setting of pulmonary embolism. If ruling out pulmonary embolism CT angiography (CTA) is indicated. Ventilation perfusion lung scan (VQ scan) may be used when contrast agents are not appropriate, such as in patients with renal failure.

Cerebral and vascular imaging

When a diagnosis of neurally mediated or reflex syncope can be ascertained, the patient does not require brain imaging. There are exceptions, however, such as when the person suffered head trauma during unconsciousness, particularly in the elderly in whom a subdural hematoma may be suspected [7].

In patients with suspected intermittent intra-cranial hypertension leading to syncope, MRI or CT scanning of the brain and spine may be of diagnostic help to find abnormalities that may lead to paroxysmal (e.g. positional) increases of intracranial pressure. In patients with a seizure, brain imaging studies can exclude a structural brain abnormality, particularly when the patient's first seizure was clearly not a provoked seizure. In patients with orthostatic hypotension due to autonomic failure, brain MRI can show signs suggestive of a neurodegenerative disorder.

Clinical vignette 1: syncope from pericardial effusion

A 50-year-old man presented with brief TLOC and sinus tachycardia. Recently, he had been diagnosed with lung carcinoma with pleural and pericardial metastases and was to receive palliative therapy. Loss of consciousness and collapse had occurred while standing and lasted less than a minute. There was no post-ictal confusion or other residual neurological deficits. On physical examination he was in moderate distress. Blood pressure was 90/60 mmHg, pulse was 120 beats/minute and there was distension of the jugular vein and pulsus paradoxus. Cardiac examination revealed muffled heart sounds and an ECG showed sinus tachycardia with low voltages.

169

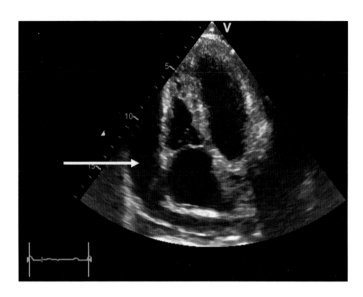

Figure 10.2 Echocardiography showing cardiac tamponade from pericardial effusion (arrow) in metastatic pericarditis. (Courtesy of Dr. Frederik J. de Lange MD PhD, Academic Medical Center at the University of Amsterdam.)

Imaging: Echocardiography showed a prominent pericardial effusion, blocking right atrial inflow. After emergency pericardial drainage, producing sero-sanguinolent liquid, tachycardia disappeared. Cytological examination confirmed the clinical diagnosis of metastatic pericarditis.

Comments: Malignant pericardial effusions leading to sub-tamponade can present with syncope, due to the impediment of right atrial influx (Figure 10.2) [11] for which ultrasonography is the preferred imaging technique. Tamponade is a medical emergency that requires prompt evacuation of the pericardial fluid. The etiology of pericardial effusion includes pericarditis (e.g. metastatic, bacterial, viral, uremic, autoimmune in patients with systemic lupus erythematosus), hypothyroidism, trauma, and myocardial rupture (e.g. from infarction or after pacemaker lead implantation). Type A aortic dissections may also present with syncope due to tamponade [10].

Clinical vignette 2: syncope due to pulmonary embolism

A 32-year-old woman presented with TLOC that had occurred while standing, taking a hot shower. Medical history included hypermenorrhea, presumably caused by uterine myomatosis, with subsequent iron-deficiency anemia. Apart from iron supplements and an oral contraceptive she took no other medications. Loss of consciousness lasted for about 30 seconds and was preceded by brief light-headedness. She suffered no head trauma and on coming to she was not confused. A review of systems revealed progressive shortness of breath during mild exercise.

On examination, blood pressure while supine was 100/70 mmHg with a regular heart rate of 110 beats/minute. Respiration rate was 20 respiratory cycles per minute and hemoglobin–oxygen saturation was 95% while breathing room air. The central venous pressure was elevated. A cardiac examination revealed an S3. In the lower abdomen a mass could be palpated consistent with a uterine myoma. There was no edema or signs of deep venous thrombosis on either extremity. An ECG showed sinus tachycardia with signs of right-ventricle overload. Hemoglobin level was 4.0 mmol/l.

Imaging: CTA of the thorax showed bilateral pulmonary emboli in the right pulmonary artery (Figure 10.3). The patient was admitted to hospital and treated with low-molecular-weight heparin. She made an uneventful recovery. Subsequent work-up did not reveal any pro-coagulatory abnormalities.

Comments: Pulmonary embolism can present with syncope, which should be considered as a prognostic risk factor for mortality [12, 13]. The blockade in the lung circulation compromises left ventricular filling and thereby systemic arterial pressure that cannot be fully overcome by arterial baroreflex function (i.e. tachycardia and vasoconstriction). During triggers such as taking a hot shower, which decrease peripheral vascular resistance, and which should normally result in an increased cardiac output, this leads to episodic

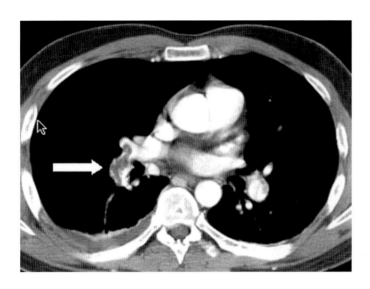

Figure 10.3 CTA shows a large thrombus (white arrow) in the right main pulmonary artery. (Courtesy of Professor Dr. Saskia Middeldorp MD PhD, Academic Medical Center at the University of Amsterdam.)

hypotension and possibly syncope. It has also been suggested that pulmonary embolisms contribute to the occurrence of a vasovagal reflex by unloading left-ventricular volume receptors [12]. The risk of syncope may be augmented by concomitant anemia such as in this case.

Clinical vignette 3: syncope due to increased intracranial pressure

An 81-year-old man presented with recurrent episodes of brief TLOC following an L3–4 discectomy with multiple post-operative complications including meningitis. The TLOC episodes occurred while in the supine position when laying on his back. Loss of consciousness lasted less than 30 seconds and was frequently preceded by headaches. On coming to, he was usually fully alert but occasionally remained obtunded with slurred speech lasting up to 30 minutes.

An ECG and Holter monitor were normal. Blood pressure while supine was 150/85 mmHg with a heart rate of 76 beats/minute, and while standing 140/80 mmHg with a heart rate of 85 beats/minute. Neurological examination showed distal sensory loss but was otherwise normal. Examination of his back revealed a palpable mass, 2 inches in diameter.

Imaging. MRI of the brain showed diffuse atrophy. MRI of the lumbar spine revealed a spinal pseudomeningocele containing approximately 200 cc of cerebrospinal fluid (CSF), the result of inadvertent dural tear during his discectomy (Figure 10.4). Transcranial Doppler (TCD) of his right middle cerebral artery (MCA) during manual compression of the pseudomeningocele (in the sitting position) showed that systolic pressure was maintained, but there was absent diastolic blood flow and systemic blood pressure was unchanged.

Comments: The absence of blood pressure changes and the observed TCD pattern in the MCA, which is consistent with collapse of the artery during diastole, indicate that the episodes of loss of consciousness were due to increased intracranial pressure (ICP) [14].

The cranium and the vertebral canal with the inelastic dura form a rigid box that contains the brain, blood, and CSF. Therefore as the Monro–Kellie hypothesis states: "If the sum of volumes of the brain, CSF, and intracranial blood is constant, an increase in one should cause a decrease in one or both of the remaining two" [15, 16]. As the brain tissue is relatively non-compressible, changes in CSF volume are compensated by changes in blood volume. When the accommodative mechanisms fail, ICP rises.

When the pseudomeningocele is compressed its CSF content is mechanically pushed into the head [14]. The syncopal episodes in this patient are explained as the result of displacement of CSF from the pseudomeningocele towards the cranium causing a sudden rise in ICP. In patients with syncopal episodes following discectomies the possibility of a pseudomeningocele should be considered.

171

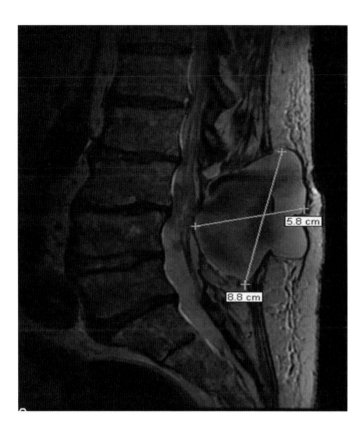

Figure 10.4 MRI of the post-operative spine showing a lumbar mass, at L3–4 level, measuring 8.8 × 5.8 × 4.0 cm. A total volume of 204 cc of CSF was collected in this pseudomeningocele.

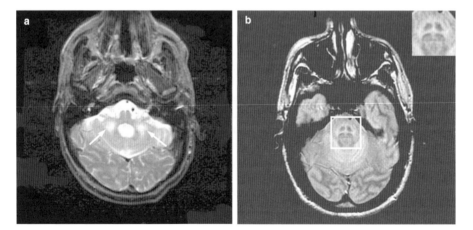

Figure 10.5 T2-weighted brain magnetic resonance imaging shows increased signal in the middle cerebellar peduncles (arrows, a). The proton-density-weighted image (b) shows the classic "hot-cross-bun sign" (square) of MSA in the pons (magnified in the insert) (from Bhattacharya et al. [17]).

Clinical vignette 4: syncope due to chronic autonomic failure

A 56-year-old high school teacher consulted for a brief episode of TLOC. He had finished having breakfast when he stood up from his chair and collapsed to the floor. He came to in around 40 seconds, surprised but not confused, and was able to stand up unassisted. Three years prior he had noted erectile dysfunction, urinary frequency, and nocturia. In the last 6 months he felt tired particularly in the mornings and noted clumsiness.

On examination, blood pressure while supine was 160/90 mmHg with a heart rate of 78 beats/minute. After standing for 3 minutes blood pressure fell to 105/70 mmHg with a heart rate of 85 beats/minute.

Neurological examination showed him alert with no cognitive difficulties. He had very mild limb ataxia on all limbs and mild increase in muscle tone with cogwheel phenomena on both arms. Rapid alternating movements were impaired bilaterally. Myotatic reflexes were brisk and plantar responses were flexor.

Imaging: Brain MRI showed increased signal in the middle cerebellar peduncles and a "hot-cross-bun sign" in the pons (Figure 10.5). These imaging changes are characteristic of multiple system atrophy (MSA) (see Chapter 17).

Comments: Syncope was the event that made the patient seek medical attention. Neurological examination showed orthostatic hypotension and additional neurological features, namely mild cerebellar and parkinsonian features. This combination of findings suggested the diagnosis of MSA. The brain MRI findings of increased signal in the middle cerebellar peduncles and a hot-cross-bun sign in the pons helped confirm the diagnosis.

MSA is a sporadic, progressive neurodegenerative disease with sometimes-insidious onset of autonomic failure and different combinations of parkinsonism, and cerebellar ataxia [18]. It has a poor prognosis with a mean life expectancy of around 8 years from the time of diagnosis [19].

MRI of the brain is used as a supportive feature for the diagnosis of MSA [17]. Several MRI features are very characteristic of the disease, namely putaminal, pontine, and middle cerebellar peduncle (MCP) atrophy, posterior putaminal hypointensity, hyperintense lateral putaminal rim, signal abnormality on T2-weighted imaging within the central brainstem, and MCP in a characteristic pattern with sparing of the motor tracts (hot-cross-bun sign) [18].

A recent study shows gradient-echo three-dimensional T1-weighted magnetic resonance volumetry is useful in following MSA disease progression over time and thus may serve as a surrogate marker in clinical trials to measure disease progression [20].

References

1. Kaufmann H, Wieling W (2004). Syncope: a clinically guided diagnostic algorithm. *Clin Auton Res* **14** (suppl 1): 87–90.

2. Sun BC, Emond JA, Camargo CA, Jr (2004). Characteristics and admission patterns of patients presenting with syncope to U.S. emergency departments, 1992–2000. *Acad Emerg Med* **11**: 1029–1034.

3. Wieling W, Thijs RD, van DN, *et al.* (2009). Symptoms and signs of syncope: a review of the link between physiology and clinical clues. *Brain* **132**; 2630–2642.

4. Colman N, Nahm K, Ganzeboom KS, *et al.* (2004). Epidemiology of reflex syncope. *Clin Auton Res* **14** (suppl 1): 9–17.

5. Ganzeboom KS, Colman N, Reitsma JB, Shen WK, Wieling W (2003). Prevalence and triggers of syncope in medical students. *Am J Cardiol* **91**: 1006–1008.

6. Kapoor WN (1994). Syncope in older persons. *J Am Geriatr Soc* **42**: 426–436.

7. Huff JS, Decker WW, Quinn JV, *et al.* (2007). Clinical policy: critical issues in the evaluation and management of adult patients presenting to the emergency department with syncope. *Ann Emerg Med* **49**: 431–444.

8. Moya A, Sutton R, Ammirati F, *et al.* (2009). Guidelines for the diagnosis and management of syncope (version 2009): the Task Force for the Diagnosis and Management of Syncope of the European Society of Cardiology (ESC). *Eur Heart J* **30**(21): 2631–2671.

9. Jecmenica-Lukic M, Poewe W, Tolosa E, Wenning GK (2012). Premotor signs and symptoms of multiple system atrophy. *Lancet Neurol* **11**: 361–368.

10. Imamura H, Sekiguchi Y, Iwashita T, *et al.* (2011). Painless acute aortic dissection – diagnostic, prognostic and clinical implications. *Circ J* **75**: 59–66.

11. Cheng MF, Tsai CS, Chiang PC, Lee HS (2005). Cardiac tamponade as manifestation of advanced thymic carcinoma. *Heart Lung* **34**: 136–141.

12. Wolfe TR, Allen TL (1998). Syncope as an emergency department presentation of pulmonary embolism. *J Emerg Med* **16**: 27–31.

13. Koutkia P, Wachtel TJ (1999). Pulmonary embolism presenting as syncope: case report and review of the literature. *Heart Lung* **28**: 342–347.

14. Bekavac I, Halloran JI (2003). Meningocele-induced positional syncope and retinal hemorrhage. *AJNR* **24**: 838–839.

15. Miller JD, Stanek A, Langfitt TW (1972). Concepts of cerebral perfusion pressure and vascular compression during intracranial hypertension. *Prog Brain Res* **35**: 411–432.

16. Davson H, Hollingsworth G, Segal MB (1970). The mechanism of drainage of the cerebrospinal fluid. *Brain* **93**: 665–678.

17. Bhattacharya K, Saadia D, Eisenkraft B, *et al.* (2002). Brain magnetic resonance imaging in multiple-

system atrophy and Parkinson disease: a diagnostic algorithm. *Arch Neurol* **59**: 835–842.

18. Gilman S, Wenning GK, Low PA, *et al.* (2008). Second consensus statement on the diagnosis of multiple system atrophy. *Neurology* **71**: 670–676.

19. Schrag A, Wenning GK, Quinn N, Ben-Shlomo Y (2008). Survival in multiple system atrophy. *Mov Disord* **23**: 294–296.

20. Hauser TK, Luft A, Skalej M, *et al.* (2006). Visualization and quantification of disease progression in multiple system atrophy. *Mov Disord* **21**: 1674–1681.

Chapter 11

Fever

Felix Benninger and Israel Steiner

Introduction

Akkadian cuneiform inscriptions from the sixth century BC were the first to refer to fever in writing [1]. Only a couple of centuries later the ancient Greeks, including Hippocrates, developed the first theoretical concepts about the pathophysiology of fever. Fever then was believed to be a beneficial sign during infection [2]. This concept was maintained even into the seventeenth century. The English physician Thomas Sydenham (1624–1689) claimed that "Fever is Nature's engine which she brings into the field to remove her enemy" [3]. Nevertheless, starting from the late nineteenth century the beneficial effect of fever was questioned. Writings by the German physician Carl von Liebermeister were the first to claim that fevers were dangerous if they were too high or persisted for too long [4]. If in fact fever in itself is beneficial or destructive (and thus an adaptive or maladaptive response) is not yet decided. From an evolutionary point of view, Mackowiak stated that "the febrile response and its mediators may have evolved both as a mechanism for accelerating the recovery of infected individuals with localized or mild to moderately severe systemic infections and for hastening the demise of hopelessly infected individuals, who pose a threat of epidemic disease to the species" [5].

Since the central mechanism for the regulation of body temperature is hosted by the brain, almost all illnesses that cause fever must interact with the central nervous system (CNS). In the CNS, circumventricular organs (CVOs) located around the third and fourth ventricles are vascularized structures characterized by the lack of a blood–brain barrier (BBB). Blood, the brain parenchyma, and the cerebrospinal fluid (CSF) are able to communicate here. Sodium and water balance, cardiovascular regulation, energy metabo-

lism, immunomodulation, and, last but not least, the fever response are regulated via interconnections with the hypothalamus and brainstem.

Circulating "endogenous pyrogens" like interleukin-6 (IL-6) activates the inducible cyclooxygenase-2 pathway within astrocytes leading to the production of prostaglandin E2, which acts at the level of the medial preoptic area to increase body temperature [6]. Other pathways involve Toll-like receptors on macrophage-like cells which lead to microglial cell activation and secretion of prostaglandin E2 and thus to a rise in body temperature [7].

For the clinician, a febrile patient with neurologic impairment might represent a medical emergency (Figure 11.1). Fever in association with neurologic disease can be divided into: (i) neurologic impairment resulting from fever itself as is commonly seen in the very young and elderly population, (ii) CNS infections which present with fever, (iii) systemic febrile disorders which also manifest with CNS signs, and (iv) primary neurologic diseases with fever as a presenting sign. Here we will focus especially on the last category and try to give an overview of imaging tools helpful in the diagnosis. We present selected cases from our daily practice and add differential diagnoses and discussion. We do not claim that these cases are a representative selection but rather are useful in conveying the diagnostic approach using imaging tools.

Neurological dysfunction caused by fever

As emphasized above, the elevation of body temperature seems to be of advantage in conditions like infection or inflammation, possibly by inhibiting pathogen growth and by augmenting the immune response.

Imaging Acute Neurologic Disease, ed. Massimo Filippi and Jack H. Simon. Published by Cambridge University Press.
© Cambridge University Press 2014.

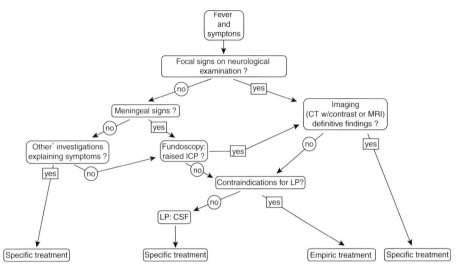

Figure 11.1 Flow chart for decision-making in case of patients with fever and neurological symptoms. ICP, intracranial pressure; LP, lumbar puncture; CSF, cerebrospinal fluid; *, whole blood count, CRP, urine examination, chest X-ray.

On the other hand, excessive temperature can cause endothelial damage, rhabdomyolysis, and neurological alterations as seen in the syndromes of malignant hyperthermia, neuroleptic malignant syndrome, or heatstroke. Interestingly, mortality of patients with extreme temperatures of diverse causes was related to the underlying illness rather than elevation of the temperature [8]. The accompanying metabolic stress may be cardiotoxic and lead to congestive heart failure, angina, or arrhythmias especially in patients with cardiac, pulmonary, or peripheral vascular diseases. However, most patients can tolerate excessive temperatures with little damage from the fever itself.

Fever in the elderly

Confusion, delirium, and change in the level of consciousness can occur in every age group but are frequently present in the elderly and very old. Patients with underlying chronic neurologic abnormalities like Alzheimer's disease, Parkinson's disease, and multi-infarct states are especially susceptible to develop mental changes as a reaction to increased body temperature. Of note is the fact that 20–30% of elderly patients with serious bacterial or viral infections will present with a blunted or entirely absent fever response [9]. The elderly in general may present with lower temperatures in the context of serious infections like meningitis [10], meriting caution in the decision about a diagnostic lumbar puncture (LP) in the elderly.

Seizures and fever

Fever has long been associated with lowering of seizure threshold especially in the young. In infants, elevation in body temperature can result in febrile seizures. They occur in infancy and early childhood, usually between the ages of 3 months and 5 years, with a peak incidence at 9–20 months. Febrile seizures remain the most common childhood neurological emergency [11]. Febrile seizures are associated with fever but without evidence of intracranial infection or a defined cause for the seizure [12]. The fever is at least 38 °C and seizures are more likely to occur during the rise of temperature or at the maximal rate of temperature increase. Febrile seizures may be defined as simple or complex [13]. Although they are frightening to parents, febrile seizures are rarely associated with long-term morbidity or mortality [14]. However, complex febrile seizures, defined as of longer duration, with focal semiology and/or recurrence within 24 h, carry a higher risk for later development of epilepsy not necessarily as a consequence of the febrile seizure, but possibly as the first presentation of epilepsy [15]. In Dravet syndrome, febrile seizures are not a cause but part of the phenotype. Typically prolonged seizures, usually focal, which may require intensive care unit admission and usually present at 4–8 months of age, are seen in Dravet syndrome [16]. From the second year of life, additional focal and generalized seizures develop and the prognosis for seizure control and development is poor.

There is a high association with SCN1A gene mutations [17]. A further entity also linking febrile seizures to SCN1A gene mutations is "genetic epilepsy with febrile seizures plus" (GEFS+) where febrile seizures are associated with the development of other epilepsy syndromes in later life [18]. Other mutations associated with GEFS+ include those of the sodium channel beta 1 subunit SCN1B and the GABA(A) receptor gamma 2 subunit GABRG2.

Lastly, fever has to be mentioned as one of many known triggers of seizures in patients with epilepsy. In questionnaires, most young and adult patients (53–65%) report seizures at times or exclusively provoked by internal or external precipitants like stress, fatigue, sleep deprivation, and fever [19, 20]. Fever alone is rarely a cause of neurologic dysfunction. Rather, the presence of an abnormally elevated body temperature should cause the clinician to initiate a search for the underlying disorder. Even in the presence of a documented infection not associated with a CNS source, one should be hesitant to ascribe alterations in mental status to the fever alone, and consideration should be given to ruling out the presence of a CNS infection by LP if findings might result in a change in therapy.

CNS infections and fever

Infections of the nervous system are commonly accompanied by fever. The combination of elevated body temperature and non-specific neurological signs like headache, lethargy, or altered level of consciousness, irritability, nausea, vomiting, and photophobia warrant thorough neurological examination and high suspicion. Neurologic deficits in combination with fever should lead to imaging of the CNS. Bacterial meningitis in children is accompanied by fever in 97% of cases [21] and any of the described non-specific signs and evidence of meningeal irritation, such as nuchal rigidity, should prompt the clinician to initiate a search for meningitis. Although nuchal rigidity is present in approximately 80% of patients with bacterial meningitis, this sign is not universal and may occur only late in the disease especially in children. The absence of nuchal rigidity should not exclude the diagnosis of meningitis. Meningitis should also be considered when fever is accompanied by changes in behavior or mental status, even without signs of meningeal irritation or complaints of headache or stiff neck. Many elderly patients have cervical spondylosis or suffer from rigidity accompanying extra pyramidal diseases, which may be confused with nuchal rigidity. With meningeal irritation, the neck resists passive flexion in the anterior–posterior direction. In the patient with cervical disease, the neck resists passive motion in all directions. Imaging in the patient suspected to suffer from bacterial meningitis is usually warranted before LP to exclude contraindications especially if there are focal neurological deficits or in patients with a history of traumatic head injury. Imaging should not delay the start of empirical antibiotic treatment in suspected bacterial meningitis. Most commonly, computed tomography (CT) scanning is performed as the initial imaging but it has to be remembered that CT scanning may not be sufficient to exclude elevated intracranial pressure in bacterial meningitis (especially in children).

CT scans in uncomplicated bacterial meningitis usually demonstrate normal findings or small ventricles and effacement of sulci. To exclude complications that require prompt neurosurgical intervention, such as symptomatic hydrocephalus, subdural empyema, and cerebral abscess contrast-enhanced CT imaging might be warranted. Fever is found less commonly in patients who have a brain abscess and only approximately 40% of adults with brain abscess have temperatures of 38.0°C or higher. Afebrile patients with brain abscess might present in a subacute fashion and the most common findings in patients with brain abscess are (i) hemicranial or generalized headache reported in approximately 70% of patients, (ii) generalized seizures in approximately one-third of patients, and (iii) focal neurologic findings in approximately 50% of those with intracerebral abscess (see Box 11.1).

Symptoms of meningitis and positive CSF findings can be present in patients with parameningeal infectious foci such as epidural abscesses. These are commonly located in the spinal epidural space and only in 10% above the foramen magnum [23]. They may produce minimal symptoms and are often slow growing. Therefore, diagnosis is often delayed for several weeks. Infection may occur following sinusitis, facial cellulitis, skull fracture, or neurosurgical procedures and attention is often focused onto these primary disorders, missing the secondary infection. Focal neurological signs can develop with continued expansion of the infected mass and the extension of infection can result in venous thrombosis of intracranial veins, subdural empyema, or brain abscess. MRI of the entire neuro axis is warranted in patients with non-improving meningeal signs under antibiotic treatment (see Box 11.2).

Box 11.1 – Stroke?

A 57-year-old female patient, right handed, married, and mother of three children with a 2-week history of fatigue and apathy was admitted due to sudden left-sided weakness beginning 8 hours before presenting to the emergency department. The patient was known to suffer from recurrent oral apthous disease, fatty liver, dyslipidemia, hypothyroidism, allergy to penicillin, and was currently treated with prednisone 75 mg once per day for pemphigus vulgaris. On initial examination, the patient's temperature was 36.9 °C with a blood pressure of 152/99. She was fully oriented and had no meningeal signs but on examination a left central facial palsy, pronation and drift of the left arm, and no movement of the leg was noticed. Reflexes were enhanced asymmetrically on the left body side. The plantar response was flexor on the right and indifferent on the left side. The initial laboratory work showed leukocytosis of 23 000 which was chronically elevated, a C-reactive protein (CRP) of 3.58 (maximum 0.9), erythrocyte sedimentation rate of 45, and raised glutamate pyruvate transaminase (GPT), gamma-glutamyl transpeptidase (GGT), and lactate dehydrogenase (LDH). Clinically she was suspected to have a cerebral vascular event (National Institutes of Health Stroke Scale (NIHSS): 7). Initial imaging was ordered.

CT without contrast, as seen in Figure 11.2, showed a hypodense lesion in the area of the right internal capsule highly suspicious for a vascular event. The patient was started on antiplatelet therapy and admitted to the neurology department. A day later her level of consciousness deteriorated with increased tiredness with episodes of stupor. No worsening of the left hemiparesis was noted but an evolution of the stroke was suspected and a CT angiogram (CTA) was performed, which did not reveal any narrowing of the extra- or intracranial arteries. There was no change in the hypodense lesion initially seen. At this point LP was performed, which indicated a cell count of 110/ml (85% mononuclear), protein, glucose, and chloride within normal range, and initial microscopy and bacterial culture was negative. An electroencephalogram (EEG) showed diffuse slowing in the theta range without focus. The patient was started on acyclovir and rocephine and, owing to a known allergy to penicillin, additionally meropenem and septrim, with a rapid improvement of her mental status and the left-sided weakness. This was accompanied by a decrease of the pleocytosis in the CSF (23 cells/ml).

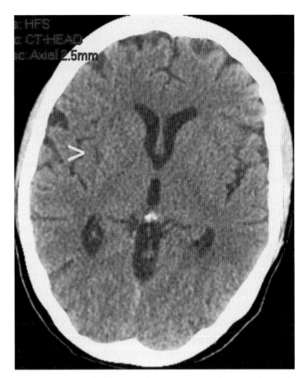

Figure 11.2 Initial CT brain without contrast. Right external capsule shows a hypodense lesion.

HSV polymerase chain reactions (PCRs) turned out to be negative and acyclovir was discontinued. At this time magnetic resonance imaging (MRI) of the brain was performed (Figure 11.3). The MRI scan was atypical for a localized vascular event, and suggested a differential diagnosis including septic emboli, *in situ* infection (coccidiomycosis, toxoplasma), or ADEM.

Serology testing for *Listeria monocytogenes* returned positive from serum and CSF and the patient was treated with an appropriate antibiotic (see also reference [22]).

Similar to bacterial abscesses, fever is not necessarily a presenting sign of encephalitis. The most common symptom is headache in 62% of patients suffering from encephalitis, with only 41% having fever [26–28]. Encephalitis may present as an acute confusional state, often after several days of a hemicranial headache. This is followed by a change in behavior, new-onset seizure activity, or focal neurologic deficits. Treatment with acyclovir should be initiated even before confirmation of PCR results

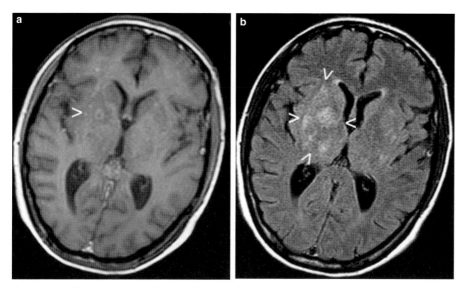

Figure 11.3 (a). Enhancement of the right basal ganglia. (b). Fluid-attenuated inversion recovery (FLAIR) series shows hyperintensity of the internal and external capsule, basal ganglia, and thalamus

Box 11.2 – Meningitis without clinical improvement

A 59-year-old female patient was admitted after a previous admission to another hospital for continuous and worsening neck pain and fever. The patient had a history of multiple myeloma and underwent an autologous bone-marrow transplant 4 years earlier, was currently in remission, and was not undergoing any immunosuppressive treatment. For 10 days she suffered from fever up to 38.5 °C and neck pain without headaches. On previous laboratory examinations no leukocytosis was present but CRP was elevated to 37 mg/dl (range 0.0–0.5 mg/dl). At the previous admission no neck stiffness was noticed and X-ray of the cervical spine was unremarkable (Figure 11.4). She was treated with opioid analgesics and released to ambulatory care. She presented to our emergency department 10 days later due to worsening neck pains with an intact neurological status and no neck stiffness. A head and neck CT without contrast did not show any abnormality and LP was performed with an opening pressure of 14 cm water level, 100 cells (50% segmentary and 50% mononuclear), an elevated protein of 423 mg/dl, and glucose of 49 mg/dl (blood glucose 132 mg/dl). On microscopic examination of the CSF, no bacteria were noted, India ink staining and Cryptococcal antigen were negative, and she was admitted to our department with a suspicion of viral meningitis without any

further antibiotic treatment. In the next 2 days the neurologic examination was without change but due to the non-improving neck pains, which could only be controlled with opiates, MRI of the neck was performed. As seen in Figure 11.5, at the cervical vertebra C4–C5, a space-occupying, gadolinium-enhancing epidural mass was noted involving the vertebra bodies and the intervertebral disc. The finding was compatible with an infectious process and was diagnosed by the MRI as discitis–osteomyelitis. Broad-spectrum antibiotic treatment was initiated and since there was no neurological deficit, no surgical intervention or biopsy for definite diagnosis was performed. The patient improved rapidly.

This is a case, not commonly seen, of a parameningeal infectious focus causing CSF pleocytosis. Here, imaging was essential for diagnosis and treatment. Previous cases have been reported [24, 25].

for herpes simplex virus (HSV). Imaging is warranted in all patients suspected of encephalitis initially, with CT scanning as described above to exclude contraindications for LP, but the diagnosis can usually be made by a combination of LP, EEG, and MRI. Mimics of encephalitis should be kept in mind and MRI imaging is necessary to reach a definite diagnosis (see Box 11.3).

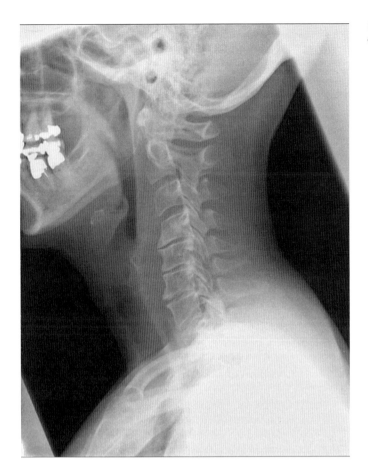

Figure 11.4 Initial X-ray of the cervical spine. No bony changes were noticed to explain the neck pain.

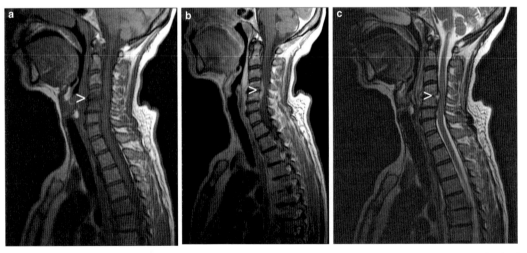

Figure 11.5 MRI of the cervical spine. T1 weighted images without (a) and with (b) gadolinium contrast show an epidural enhancing lesion at C4–C5 highly suspicious for osteomyelitis and discitis. (c). T2-weighted image.

Box 11.3 – HSV encephalitis?

A 63-year-old woman with a history of mild sensineural hearing loss, diabetes mellitus (diagnosed over three decades previously), and polyneuropathy with atrophy of the leg muscles and foot drop presented to the emergency room with acute confusion, cognitive impairment, and two generalized tonic clonic seizures. Initially a CT was performed and showed a hypodense lesion in the right temporal lobe (Figure 11.6). She was transferred to the neurosurgery department due to a suspected space-occupying lesion. Acyclovir was initiated because of the possibility of HSV encephalitis and LP revealed elevated protein (69mg/dl) but no pleocytosis and PCRs for HSV turned out to be negative. Acyclovir was discontinued. The brain MRI showed bilateral asymmetric temporal lesions (see Figure 11.7) mimicking HSV encephalitis but LP showed no signs of inflammation or infection. Her family medical history revealed that her son was diagnosed with mitochondrial encephalomyopathy, lactic acidosis, and stroke-like episodes (MELAS) at the age of 4 and subsequently died at the age of 14 years following an episode of seizures, coma, and gastrointestinal hemorrhage. The lactate blood levels in our patient were increased and electromyography (EMG) showed myopathic changes. Open-muscle biopsy revealed ragged red fibers and confirmed the suspicion of a mitochondrial disease. Genetic testing of muscle cells revealed a heteroplasmy of 95% for MELAS A3243G mutation. It is known that neurologic symptom onset can be delayed in some patients with MELAS until late adulthood. The reasons for the delay are still unclear but might be explained by the mosaic distribution of affected mitochondria with a lower mutation load in the brain. Particularly interesting in this case is the extreme age difference of presentation between the two family members suffering from the same disease. Three other children have not shown any clinical symptoms. Furthermore, the presence of hearing loss, diabetes, and neurologic deficit can be indicative of a mitochondrial disorder even in an elderly patient.

Neuroimaging features can be diagnostic, may help direct further work-up, and aid in characterizing the underlying brain abnormalities. Neurologic symptom onset might be delayed until late adulthood in MELAS and neurologists should be alerted to this possible etiology in unusual presentations [29, 30].

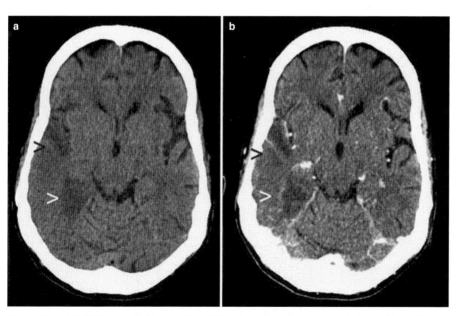

Figure 11.6 Initial CT scan with (a) and without (b) contrast showing hypodense lesions of the right temporal lobe.

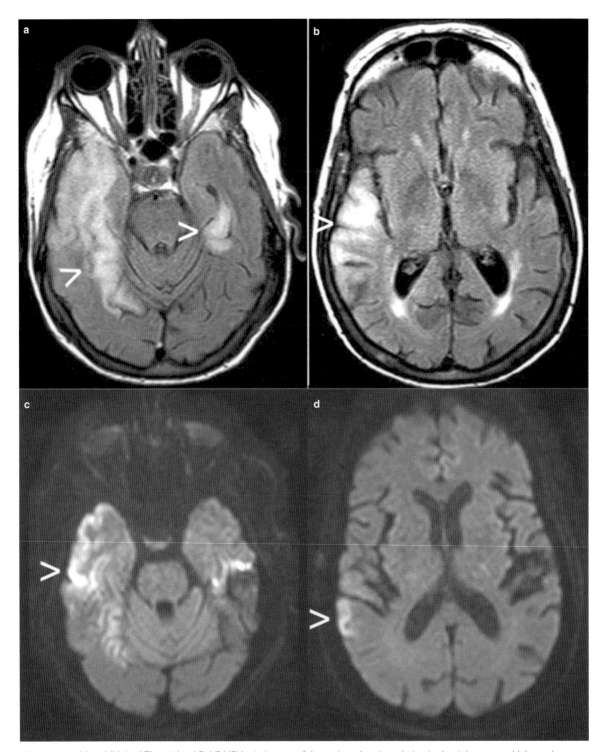

Figure 11.7 (a) and (b) Axial T2-weighted FLAIR MRI brain images of the patient showing a lesion in the right temporal lobe and a smaller lesion in the mesial left temporal lobe. (c) and (d). Diffusion-weighted images with asymmetric high signal within the cortex in the temporal lobes as well as the right parietal cortex.

Systemic disorders with fever and neurological alterations

Sepsis and septic shock lead to organ hypoperfusion and, as a consequence, to lactic acidosis and oliguria, often resulting in acute changes of mental status. Fever is a cardinal symptom of sepsis. The mental status changes are part of a septic encephalopathy with unknown pathophysiology, but micro-abscesses, central pontine myelinolysis, and purpuric lesions in the brain have been found on biopsies. Cytokines such as tumor necrosis factor (TNF) and interleukins can alter the permeability of the BBB and thus be responsible for encephalopathic changes as well. Finally, the metabolic consequences in sepsis may contribute to the observed changes in mental status. The evaluation of patients with mental status changes and sepsis should therefore include a CT scan of the head to exclude structural abnormalities, LP to rule out meningitis, and an EEG [31].

Vasculitis that affects the CNS is a diagnostic and therapeutic challenge. Two categories have to be separated: primary CNS vasculitis (also referred to as primary angiitis of the CNS (PACNS)) when it is confined to the CNS and secondary when associated with various other disorders. Secondary CNS vasculitis has been described in association with multiple conditions including systemic vasculitides, connective tissue disease, sarcoidosis, infections, and lymphoproliferative diseases. Pathologically, the angiitis consists of granulomatous inflammation of small meningeal and parenchymal arteries, veins, arterioles, venules, and capillaries confined to the CNS. Patients usually present with subacute encephalopathy, with fever, chills, and weight loss occurring in 10–25% and might hint more towards a secondary rather than primary CNS vasculitis. Seizures, hemiparesis, and visual loss can occur. CSF findings are abnormal in 80–90% of cases and reflect aseptic meningitis, with pleocytosis, normal glucose, elevated protein levels, and occasionally the presence of oligoclonal bands [32]. The gold standard for diagnosis of CNS vasculitis is biopsy but imaging plays a major part in the diagnostic process. CT is less sensitive than MRI in assessment of lesions of cerebral vasculitis, apart from cerebral hemorrhage. Several studies have reported the sensitivity of MRI to be close to 100%, but patients with primary CNS vasculitis and normal MRI have been reported. Common findings on MRI include cortical/subcortical infarctions, leptomeningeal enhancement, tumor-like mass lesions, or hemorrhages but usually findings on MRI are nonspecific. Cerebral angiography can be highly supportive for the diagnosis. Findings of primary CNS vasculitis include alternating segments of stenosis with normal or dilated intervening segments, and arterial occlusions. These findings are however not specific as they can be seen in vasospasm, CNS infection, cerebral arterial emboli, and atherosclerosis. Even with these limitations, cerebral angiography is the gold standard imaging modality to identify primary CNS vasculitisis [33, 34].

Fever, arthritis, arthralgia, skin lesions, and serositis are the most common systemic clinical abnormalities in systemic lupus erythematosus (SLE). In general, a chronic inflammatory condition of unclear cause that most commonly affects young women, it is associated with neurological abnormalities in approximately 75% of patients [35]. CNS abnormalities tend to occur early in the course of the illness, appearing in the first year in approximately 63% of patients. Dementia, psychosis, and seizures are the most common CNS findings [36, 37]. Neuroradiologic evaluation favors MRI over CT, because subtle ischemia or cerebritis may be seen with greater sensitivity. The most common findings with either modality are ischemic zones that may correspond to cortical or subcortical infarcts and can be large or small according to the size of vessel involved and the mechanism of stroke. One to three percent of patients with CNS involvement might present with myelitic syndromes (see Box 11.4 [38–40]).

Box 11.4 – Longitudinally extensive transverse myelitis and SLE

A 20-year-old female patient was seen in the emergency department three times during 1 week initially for fever and neck pains without headaches. Body temperature was 38.6 °C and the patient was released home with analgesic treatment. Due to worsening pains and vomiting she was admitted to the hospital. CT of the cervical spine was unremarkable. On repeated examination, there was no neck stiffness, but CSF analysis showed 170 cells and elevated protein of 107 mg/dl. Upon admission, progressive weakness of the legs was noted without any signs of incontinence and without sensory levels. MRI (Figure 11.8) showed a massive diffuse white- and gray-matter lesion with gadolinium enhancement involving the spinal cord from the cervical to the lumbar region and a diagnosis of longitudinally extensive transverse myelitis was made. On further blood testing ANA antibodies were increased (1:160) and Lupus anticoagulant was elevated five times above upper normal limits. She was treated with intravenous steroids and motor strength returned to normal levels.

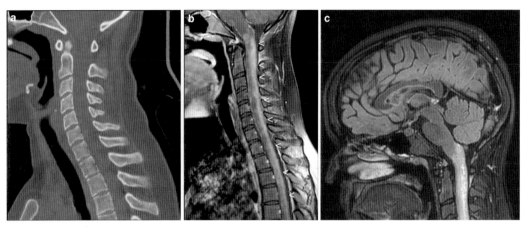

Figure 11.8 (a) Unremarkable CT of the cervical spine. Contrast-enhanced (b) and FLAIR MRI images (c) of the spine show longitudinally extensive spinal cord pathology.

Fever as a presentation of primary neurologic diseases

Fever can occur in ischemic as well as hemorrhagic stroke, reported in about 22% of ischemic strokes, and more common with large infarcts [41]. Pyrexia after stroke onset is associated with a marked increase in morbidity and mortality but the effect of treatment and temperature reduction on mortality is not settled [42, 43]. In hemorrhagic stroke, and especially with subarachnoid bleeds, the inflammatory reaction of the meninges causes a rise in body temperature. Intraventricular bleeds are associated with immediate temperature increases from the blood itself or by prostaglandin release [44, 45]. Imaging is guided by the management of the cerebrovascular accident. Endocarditis as a source of emboli should be ruled out in all patients with sudden onset of neurologic deficits and fever. Transesophageal echocardiography is the test of choice and should be urgently applied.

Damage to the hypothalamus can result in loss of control over body temperature regulation. The most common response to abnormalities in the hypothalamus is hypothermia, but hyperthermia has been described. Imaging is mandatory to identify the underlying cause including penetrating head injuries, tumor (e.g. craniopharyngiomas, astrocytomas), vascular lesions (A–V malformations), congenital hamartomas, vasculitis, traumatic hemorrhages, malformations of the third ventricle, hypothalamic hypopituitarism resulting from encephalitis, and various forms of encephalopathy (acute intermittent porphyria, Wernicke's).

A long list of neurological diseases can cause fever but there are several disorders in which imaging is necessary or can help establish the diagnosis. Fabry disease, central anticholinergic syndrome, neuroleptic malignant syndrome, and others cause fever and neurological symptoms but imaging is less helpful.

Seizures can be a cause of elevated body temperature but, as mentioned above, it might be difficult to establish the exact timing of the fever occurrence and the combination of seizures and fever should always raise special concern. Imaging in first seizure episodes include MRI or CT with contrast irrespective of raised temperature. In a post-ictal patient with a reduced level of consciousness or focal neurological deficits and elevated temperature, even if the diagnosis of epilepsy is established, LP might be indicated and exclusion of raised intracranial pressure by CT is recommended. Acute spinal cord syndromes are an emergency and require immediate imaging and diagnosis to avoid long-term disability due to delayed treatment.

Patients with spinal cord injuries at the T8 level and above may be unable to regulate body temperature. The loss of afferent pathways from peripheral temperature sensors, as well as a loss of hypothalamic thermoregulatory control over parts of the body below the level of the lesion can result in hypo- or hyperthermia. The absence of CNS input results in decreased sweating and muscular activity below the level of the lesion and fevers in these patients might be difficult to control [46–48]. MRI of the spinal cord is far superior to CT imaging and recommended for suspected spinal cord syndromes.

Conclusions

The various syndromes that present with fever and neurologic impairment are best approached with a careful history and physical examination to differentiate between them. Family members are essential and of great help in many cases as these patients may be obtunded and unable to offer information. Preceding symptoms, the pace of the illness, physical symptoms, and ingestion of medications can be of prime importance.

Many of the disease entities are diagnoses of exclusion and the clinician should always be careful before excluding infectious causes in a patient who presents with fever and neurologic findings. In this context, LP is often indispensable in excluding the diagnosis of meningitis, which can be quickly lethal if left untreated. LP is relatively contraindicated in patients with focal neurologic findings, and CT or MRI should be performed prior to CSF examination in such circumstances. Antibiotic treatment for the possible causes of meningitis, however, should not be withheld while awaiting the results of a scan.

Overall, the take-home messages may be summarized as follows:

- The elderly with serious bacterial or viral infections will present with a blunted or entirely absent fever response.
- Complex febrile seizures, defined as of longer duration, with focal semiology and/or recurrence within 24 h, carry a higher risk for later development of epilepsy.
- The absence of nuchal rigidity should not exclude the diagnosis of meningitis.
- Imaging should not delay the start of empirical antibiotic treatment in suspected bacterial meningitis.
- MRI imaging of the entire neuro axis is warranted in patients with non-improving meningeal signs under antibiotic treatment.
- Mimics of encephalitis should be kept in mind and MRI is necessary to reach a definite diagnosis.

References

1. Majno G (1991). *The Healing Hand: Man and Wound in the Ancient World*. Cambridge, MA: Harvard University Press.

2. Coxe Jr (1846). *The Writings of Hippocrates and Galen*. Philadelphia, PA: Lindsay and Blakiston.

3. Payne H (1900). *Thomas Sydenham*. London: T Fisher Unwin.

4. Fichtner G (1985). Carl von Liebermeister. *Neue Deutsche Biographie*: **486**.

5. Mackowiak P (1994). Fever: blessing or curse? A unifying hypothesis. *Ann Intern Med* **120**: 1037–1040.

6. Rummel C, Sachot C, Poole S (2006). Circulating interleukin-6 induces fever through a STAT3-linked activation of COX-2 in the brain. *Am J Physiol* **291**: R1316–R1326.

7. Chakravarty S, Herkenham M (2005). Toll-like receptor 4 on nonhematopoietic cells sustains CNS inflammation during endotoxemia, independent of systemic cytokines. *J Neurosci* **25**: 1788–1796.

8. McCarthy P, Dolan T, Schachtel B (1976). Hyperpyrexia in children: eight-year emergency room experience. *Am J Dis Child* **130**: 845–851.

9. Norman D, Yoshikawa T (1996). Fever in the elderly. *Infect Disease Clin N Am* **10**: 93–99.

10. Gorse G, Thrupp L, Nudleman K (1984). Bacterial meningitis in the elderly. *Arch Intern Med* **144**: 1603–1607.

11. Anon (2000). Pediatric emergency preparedness in the office. *Am Family Physician* **61**: 3333–3342 Available at: http://eutils.ncbi.nlm.nih.gov/entrez/eutils/elink.fcgi?dbfrom=pubmed&id=10865928&retmode=ref&cmd=prlinks.

12. APP (2008). Febrile seizures: clinical practice guideline for the long-term management of the child with simple febrile seizures. *Pediatrics* **121**: 1281–1286.

13. Nelson K, Ellenberg J (1976). Predictors of epilepsy in children who have experienced febrile seizures. *N Engl J Med* **295**: 1029–1033.

14. Nelson K, Ellenberg J (1978). Prognosis in children with febrile seizures. *Pediatrics* **61**: 720–727.

15. Verity C, Golding J (1991). Risk of epilepsy after febrile convulsions: a national cohort study. *BMJ* **304**: 147.

16. Dravet C, Bureau M, Oguni H (2005). Severe myoclonic epilepsy in infancy (Dravet syndrome). In Roger J, Bureau M, Dravet C, Genton P, eds. *Epileptic Syndromes in Infancy, Childhood, and Adolescence*. Montrouge: John Libbey Eurotext, ch. 7.

17. Scheffer I, Zhang Y, Jansen F (2009). Dravet syndrome or genetic (generalized) epilepsy with febrile seizures plus? *Brain Dev* **31**: 394–400.

18. Scheffer I, Berkovic S (1997). Generalized epilepsy with febrile seizures plus. A genetic disorder with heterogeneous clinical phenotypes. *Brain* **120**: 479–490.

19. Nakken K, Solaas M, Kjeldsen M, Friis M (2005). Which seizure-precipitating factors do patients with epilepsy most frequently report? *Epilepsy Behavior* **6**: 85–89.

20. Fang P, Chen Y, Lee I (2008). Seizure precipitants in children with intractable epilepsy. *Brain Development* **30**: 527–532.

21. Valmari P, Peltola H, Ruuskanen O, Korvenranta H (1987). Childhood bacterial meningitis: initial symptoms and signs related to age, and reasons for consulting a physician. *Eur J Pediatr* **146**: 515–518.

22. Clauss HE, Lorber B (2008). Central nervous system infection with *Listeria monocytogenes*. *Curr Infect Dis Rep* **10**: 300–306.

23. Harris LF, Haws FP, Triplett JN Jr (1987). Subdural empyema and epidural abscess: recent experience in a community hospital. *S Med J* **80**: 1254–1258.

24. Pasqualini L, Mencacci A, Scarponi AM, *et al.* (2008). Cervical spondylodiscitis with spinal epidural abscess caused by *Aggregatibacter aphrophilus*. *J Med Microbiol* **57**: 652–655.

25. McCormick A (2012). Severe neck pain with fever: is it meningitis? *West J Emerg Med* **13**: 505–506.

26. Kennard C, Swash M (1981). Acute viral encephalitis: its diagnosis and outcome. *Brain* **104**: 129–148.

27. Whitley RJ (1990). Viral encephalitis. *N Engl J Med* **323**: 242.

28. Granerod J, Tam CC, Crowcroft NS, *et al.* (2010). Challenge of the unknown. A systematic review of acute encephalitis in non-outbreak situations. *Neurology* **75**: 924–932.

29. Hirano M, Pavlakis SG (1994). Mitochondrial myopathy, encephalopathy, lactic acidosis, and strokelike episodes (MELAS): current concepts. *J Child Neurol* **9**: 4–13.

30. Friedman SD, Shaw DWW, Ishak G, Gropman AL, Saneto RP (2010). The use of neuroimaging in the diagnosis of mitochondrial disease. *Dev Disabil Res Rev* **16**: 129–135.

31 Wijdicks EFM (2009). *Neurologic Complications of Critical Illness*, 3rd edn. New York: Oxford University Press.

32. Reik L, Grunnet ML, Spencer RP, Donaldson JO (1983). Granulomatous angiitis presenting as chronic meningitis and ventriculitis. *Neurology* **33**: 1609–1612.

33. Küker W (2007). Cerebral vasculitis: imaging signs revisited. *Neuroradiology* **49**: 471–479.

34. Salvarani C, Brown RD, Hunder GG (2012). Adult primary central nervous system vasculitis. *Lancet* **380**: 767–777.

35. Voss EV, Stangel M (2012). Nervous system involvement of connective tissue disease: mechanisms and diagnostic approach. *Curr OpinNeurol* **25**: 306–315.

36. Tay CH, Khoo OT (1971). Neurological involvement in systemic lupus erythematosus. *Singapore Med J* **12**: 18–23.

37. Gotkine M, Vaknin-Dembinsky A (2012). Neurologic manifestations of systemic immunopathological diseases. *Curr Treat Options Neurol* **14**: 276–292.

38. Krishnan AV, Halmagyi GM (2004). Acute transverse myelitis in SLE. *Neurology* **62**: 2087.

39. Birnbaum J, Petri M, Thompson R (2009). Distinct subtypes of myelitis in systemic lupus erythematosus. *Arthr Rheum* **60**: 3378–3387.

40. Pawate S, Sriram S (2009). Isolated longitudinal myelitis: a report of six cases. *Spinal Cord* **47**: 257–261.

41. Hindfelt B (1976). The prognostic significance of subfebrility and fever in ischaemic cerebral infarction. *Acta Neurol Scand* **53**: 72–79.

42. Hajat C, Hajat S, Sharma P (2000). Effects of poststroke pyrexia on stroke outcome: a meta-analysis of studies in patients. *Stroke* **31**: 410–414.

43. Georgilis K, Plomaritoglou A, Dafni U (1999). Aetiology of fever in patients with acute stroke. *J Internal Med* **246**: 203–209

44. Azzimondi G, Bassein L, Nonino F, Fiorani L (1995). Fever in acute stroke worsens prognosis: a prospective study. *Stroke* **26**: 2040–2043.

45. Filho JO, Ezzeddine MA, Segal AZ (2001). Fever in subarachnoid hemorrhage. *Neurology* **56**: 1299–1304.

46. Essiet A, Onuba O (1992). Hyperpyrexia in spinal injury patients. *Spinal Cord* **30**: 339–342.

47. Tow AP-E, Kong KH (1995). Prolonged fever and heterotopic ossification in a C4 tetraplegic patient. Case report. *Spinal Cord* **33**: 170–174.

48. Ulger F, Dilek A, Karakaya D, Senel A (2009). Fatal fever of unknown origin in acute cervical spinal cord injury: five cases. *J Spinal Cord Med* **32**: 343–348.

Chapter 12

Acute, focal neurological symptoms

Megan C. Leary and Louis R. Caplan

Introduction – The modus operandi of the clinician seeking a diagnosis

When seeing a patient with acute, focal neurological symptoms, it is critically important to remember that both the history and the neurological examination are typically the keys to ordering further testing and in making a correct diagnosis. There is a wide range of potential causes of focal neurological symptoms in the central and peripheral nervous systems, including, but not limited to, stroke, migraine, seizure, infection, demyelination, tumor, trauma, psychiatric, and toxic-metabolic etiologies. An appropriate ordering of neuroimaging cannot even begin without taking a detailed history.

The effective clinician must find answers to two different queries to arrive at a diagnosis. *What* is the disease mechanism and *where* is it located? These two queries should be pursued concurrently and from the very beginning of the patient encounter [1].

This chase is hypothesis-driven. The clinician generates and tests hypotheses, gradually refining them at each phase of the clinical encounter. Hypothesis generation begins early and should proceed throughout the encounter. The *what* and *where* hypotheses derived after the history is taken are pursued and clarified during the general and neurological examinations. The examination should be planned to answer the queries and should not be a rote mechanical procedure. After the examination, the imaging and laboratory procedures are also planned sequentially depending on the hypotheses that have been generated by the history and examinations. During and after the history, during and after the general and neurological examinations, and after each planned series of investigations, the skilled clinician models and refines the anatomical and disease diagnoses much like a sculptor gradually chips away at the marble, slowly allowing a face to emerge [1–4].

History

The chief complaint is the start of the history-taking process. The clinician starts the wheels turning by making hypotheses from the opening complaint. For example, a 58-year-old man is brought to the emergency department after he has developed left-sided weakness. The clinician must next decide what further questions are useful to determine *where* the lesion causing this man's weakness is located and *what* its cause could be [1–4].

Different information is used to answer these two quite different questions. In determining stroke mechanism – the *what* question – the following clinical bedside data are most helpful:

1. Ecology – the past and present personal and family illnesses.
2. Presence and nature of past medical illnesses especially strokes or transient ischemic attacks (TIAs).
3. Activity at the onset of the symptoms.
4. Temporal course and progression of the findings. Was the onset sudden with the deficit maximal at onset? Or did it develop gradually over hours, days, weeks, months, or years? Did the deficit improve, worsen, or remain the same after onset? If it worsened, did this occur in a stepwise, remitting or a gradually progressive fashion? Were there fluctuations or intervals between normal and abnormal?
5. Accompanying symptoms such as headache, vomiting, weight loss, fatigue, fever, pain, and change in level of consciousness.

Imaging Acute Neurologic Disease, ed. Massimo Filippi and Jack H. Simon. Published by Cambridge University Press. © Cambridge University Press 2014.

The most important information used to answer the *where* question are:

1. Any localized head, neck, body, or limb pain or tenderness.
2. The presence and localization of any symptoms referable to the nervous system.
3. The findings on carefully planned and thorough general and neurological examinations.

A detailed historical account of the onset and progression of the symptoms provides clues about the location of the pathology as well as its etiology [1–4]. Returning to our patient vignette, if you determined that his symptoms developed while he was at work and were sudden and maximal at or very near onset and that he also had a history of hypertension, hypercholesterolemia, and diabetes, then stroke would be considered the most likely cause. If, however, the patient had a history of fever and chills for weeks, increasing headaches, and human immunodeficiency virus (HIV) positivity, then infection would be a stronger consideration. If the patient had a history of known seizure disorder, and awoke with his acute left-sided weakness, as well as a bitten tongue and incontinence, then seizure would rank higher on your list of possible causes. If he smoked and had a bad cough and his weakness had developed gradually with headache as an additional symptom, then a brain metastasis from lung cancer would likely head the list of probabilities.

Anatomic hypotheses are also generated. A left hemiparesis raises the possibility of a right cerebral or brainstem lesion, so the clinician asks about accompanying visual, sensory, or brainstem symptoms that would help make a more specific anatomic localization. The process of anatomic diagnosis is much like locating a missing person. First, the clinician must determine whether the person is in the United States before limiting the whereabouts to Massachusetts, then the Boston vicinity, then to a specific street in a neighborhood. Suppose that this patient reported that the major problem was using his arm or hand. The clinician first thinks of a local process in the hand or arm, such as a median or ulnar neuropathy. He or she asks about the distribution of the numbness. Was it primarily the thumb and adjacent two fingers (median) or the little finger and adjacent half of the fourth finger (ulnar) or both? Was there pain in the wrist or arm? Knowing that carpal tunnel syndrome is the commonest cause of neuropathy in the hand, the physician asks about precipitation or relief of numbness by various positions or activities and about past wrist trauma. The patient responds that the distribution is the entire hand and the numbness is constant and not altered by position or activity and that his upper arm is also weak. The physician should now explore an alternate hypothesis, having not confirmed the original idea. Could the lesion be at the neck, affecting the left cervical roots or the spinal cord? Questions now relate to the presence of neck or shoulder pain, past cervical arthritis, past neck injury, or wearing of a collar. Is there weakness or numbness of the legs or feet, difficulty walking or a change in gait, urinary dysfunction, decreased potency? Any of these symptoms suggests a myelopathy. If the patient responds negatively, the neurologist pursues another anatomical hypothesis: the brainstem. The clinician asks about dizziness, double vision, staggering, and other brainstem symptoms. Then pursuing a cerebral localization, the clinician asks about headache and numbness or weakness of the left face or lower extremity. Now, when asked specifically, the patient recalls minor tingling of his left cheek and left tongue.

Knowing now that the lesion is most likely right cerebral, the medical sleuth focuses in on anatomical subdivisions of the cerebral hemisphere. Numbness suggests a post-Rolandic localization. The presence of symptoms of a hemianopia would localize the process far posteriorly in the occipital lobe or occipitoparietal junction, or in the deeper temporal lobe structures adjacent to the geniculocalcarine tract. Did the patient have difficulty seeing to the left? Did he bump into things? Was there difficulty reading? The neurologist recalls that right parietal lesions often cause visual spatial problems. Did the patient have difficulty finding his way, did he get lost? The clinician does not simply wait and listen but switches to an active hypothesis-generated inquiry mode. In this patient who describes a left hemiparesis, the clinician can localize the process to involve the right cerebral hemisphere, but the right brainstem is also a possible site. The clinician makes a mental note to pursue the functions of these areas during the neurological examination and subsequently during investigations [1–4].

The technique of localization can be likened to finding a son or daughter's car that has somehow conked out. A telephone call informs the parent that the car is non-operative. "Come and get me," the driver says. The parent responds "Where is it?" "Somewhere on Route 9," comes the reply. The parent, knowing various landmarks and intersections on Route 9 then proceeds to interrogate the driver – "Where on Route 9?" "Before the Route 128 turnoff?" "Near Route 16?" And so on. Similarly, knowing one finding, the clinician asks about other findings known to be in the near vicinity or pathway of a symptom, e.g. weakness of the left limbs.

At the end of the history-taking process, the clinician should have a potential location (and list of causes) in mind. The examinations should be planned to both test these hypotheses and to revise them; even to generate other new hypotheses if there are unexpected findings not noted during the history, e.g. clubbed fingers, a loud heart murmur, fever, irregular heart rhythm [1–4].

The general and neurological examinations

The nervous system can be involved in many systemic medical diseases. Thus, after airway, breathing, circulation, and the vital signs are assessed, a brief but thorough neurological examination should go hand in hand with a basic general physical examination (Figure 12.1). The general physical examination is critical in identifying other potential causes of the presenting symptoms, coexisting comorbidities, or other issues that may impact the neurological patient's management [4]. For example, facial examination may

---

Mental-status examination: Assess general cognitive function during history-taking. Consider further formal testing or performing MiniMental Status Exam based on history

Cranial nerves: Generally not tested unless facial trauma
Visual acuity, visual field examination, fundoscopy

    III, IV, V. Pupil reaction to light, extraocular movement
    VI. Pinprick and light touch to face
    VII. Raise eyebrows, close eyes tight, smile, puff cheeks
    VIII. Finger rub, repeat a whispered number each ear
    IX, X. Palate elevates symmetrically, gag present
    X, XI. Shoulder shrug, head turn bilaterally
    XII. Tongue protrusion

Motor: Test muscle tone in each limb separately. Observe for fasciculations, atrophy, tremor. Test strength in all four limbs and grade accordingly.
Sensory: Test pinprick, light touch, proprioception, and vibration in all four limbs. Test for neglect with double simultaneous stimulation.
DTR: Deep tendon reflexes in all four limbs. Check plantar responses.
Coordination: Finger to nose, heel to shin. Tandem gait. Romberg.
Gait: Baseline gait. Observe for wide base, shuffle, flexing or circumduction of limbs, foot drop.

Figure 12.1 Basic screening neurologic examination.

---

reveal signs of trauma or tongue bite caused during a seizure. Neck examination may disclose a carotid bruit or jugular venous distention consistent with congestive heart failure. Chest auscultation can provide information about comorbid cardiac or pulmonary disease, such as a heart murmur or an irregular heart rate consistent with atrial fibrillation. Examination of the lower extremity pulses and skin may suggest co-existing vascular disease. Dermatologic examination can reveal a host of comorbidities that can relate to a neurological diagnosis, including signs of emboli or coagulopathy, signs of rheumatologic disease or infection, as well as evidence of trauma. However, while both the general and neurological examinations can suggest the suspected pathology of the patient's symptoms, only the neurological examination can provide clues into the location of the suspected lesion [1–4].

Both the suspected location of the symptoms, and its cause, should be considered during the neurological examination, just as they were during the history-taking process. Like the history, the examination should be hypothesis-driven and planned to clarify and reinforce or challenge the hypotheses raised from the history. When the examinations are completed, the clinician should have a strong suspicion for where the lesion is located within the nervous system [1–4]. This is important because some acute focal neurological symptoms do not warrant neuroimaging. For example, if a patient has weakness of his face, but the weakness pattern is consistent with a peripheral seventh-nerve impairment, or Bell's palsy, no diagnostic neuroimaging is needed. Additionally, if a patient was found to have severe pain in the upper arm or shoulder after a fall while horseback riding, which acutely had transitioned to weakness and/or numbness in the muscles of the affected arm or shoulder, then brachial plexopathy would be a suspected cause. Neuroimaging of the brain or spine would not be indicated for that condition either, although chest imaging potentially could be, as well as EMG or nerve conduction studies to determine the specific nature and extent of the nerve damage. Imaging could focus on the shoulder and brachial plexus region. For the purposes of this chapter, we will focus on lesions (and their causes) that are expected to specifically involve the central nervous system (CNS).

Differential diagnosis

After the history-taking and the examinations are completed and a particular location and cause are suspected, the clinician must develop a differential diagnosis: a list of potential illnesses that could be causing the patient's symptoms. The most likely culprit is at the top of the list, with lesser likely suspects found lower down. This list-making is important, because the diagnostic testing protocol performed first is the scan that would confirm or refute the possibility of the most likely disease causing the patient's symptoms [1–3]. Stroke is the most common cause of acute focal neurological deficits [2–5]. However, stroke mimics such as seizure, migraine, toxic-metabolic issues (such as hypo- or hyperglycemia), and conversion disorder, as well as other pathologies, need to be considered in the acute setting as well [3–8]. A different neuroimaging protocol may be ordered in a patient with focal weakness thought to be due to suspected stroke, versus weakness thought to be secondary to other causes. For example, in a patient with multiple stroke risk factors and headache who awakens with left-sided numbness and weakness, a head computed tomography (CT) scan would be appropriate. However, in a patient with a known history of multiple sclerosis who awakens with new hemi-body symptoms, magnetic resonance imaging (MRI) with and without contrast would likely be a more appropriate first choice of imaging.

Brain parenchyma imaging techniques

General considerations

It is important to determine the location of the pathology as well as its suspected cause because, in turn, these two factors will direct the choice of neuroimaging tests ordered. There are some important generalities to be aware of in choosing brain imaging. Typically, MRI is considered to be superior to CT for assessing the brain's parenchyma and is also more sensitive to the presence of ischemia. However, CT is thought to be superior to MRI for the evaluation of acute subarachnoid hemorrhage [9, 10]. Timely neuroimaging is critical during the rapid evaluation and diagnosis of patients with acute focal neurological symptoms, particularly in those thought to be due to acute ischemic stroke [4, 5, 9]. Brain imaging findings, such as the size, location, and vascular distribution of an infarct, presence of hemorrhage, and presence of large-vessel occlusion will absolutely affect both short- and long-term treatment decisions. Additionally,

information regarding the degree of possible reversible ischemic injury and cerebral blood flow can be obtained from imaging and will also affect urgent patient management. Either CT or MRI may be used as the initial imaging study in patients with acute focal neurological deficits [6, 10]. The Massachusetts General Hospital stroke imaging algorithm suggests the utilization of CT as a first line test in acute stroke patients unless one of the following exceptions are present: poor renal function preventing use of contrast for CT angiography (CTA), young patients with stroke, or patients more likely to have a non-ischemic etiology such as mass, seizure, multiple sclerosis, or migraine [9].

Non-contrast-enhanced and contrast-enhanced head CT

Non-contrast CT

Non-contrast CT scanning of the brain can identify the majority of intracranial hemorrhage cases and can also screen for non-vascular causes of neurological symptoms, such as brain tumor or abscess. Non-contrast CT may show subtle parenchymal damage suggestive of acute ischemic stroke, including loss of gray–white differentiation or sulcal effacement within 3 hours [10–14]. Another useful CT sign to look for is an increased density within an occluded artery (e.g. the hyperdense middle cerebral artery (MCA) sign), which is indicative of large-vessel occlusion (Figure 12.2) [4, 15]. Large-vessel occlusion typically causes severe stroke, independently predicts poor neurological outcome, and is a stronger predictor of "neurological deterioration" (91% positive predictive value) than even early CT evidence of > 50% MCA involvement (75% positive predictive value) [15–18]. The hyperdense MCA sign, however, is seen in only one-third to one-half of ischemic stroke cases with angiographically proven thromboses; hence, it is an appropriate indicator of clot when present [4, 18, 19]. A similar CT sign to search for in patients with focal acute neurological deficits is the hyperdense MCA "dot" sign [4, 20]. The MCA dot sign is an indication of a clot within a branch, rather than the trunk of the MCA. Barber et al. found that patients with the MCA dot sign alone had better outcomes than patients with an accompanying hyperdense MCA sign [4, 20]. Validation for the MCA dot sign has been performed with digital subtraction angiography (DSA), with the conclusion that

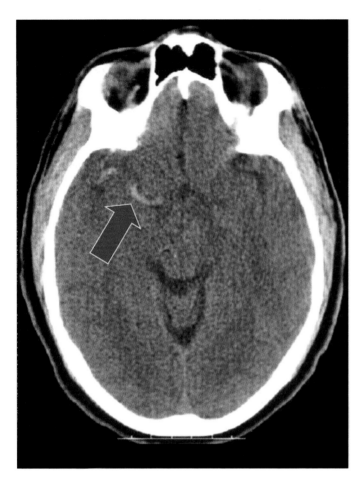

Figure 12.2 An example of a hyperdense MCA sign is seen on a non-contrast head CT scan, as indicated with the red arrow.

the sensitivity is low (38%) but the specificity is 100% [4, 21]. The hyperdense basilar artery sign has also been described with similar implications as the hyperdense MCA sign [4, 22, 23].

Non-contrast CT is also used in other urgent clinical situations. It can also exclude midline or downward shift prior to a lumbar puncture, or to screen for hydrocephalus. One limitation of non-contrast CT is its lack of sensitivity in detecting early small acute cortical or subcortical infarcts, especially those within the posterior fossa [4, 24–27]. Despite that, its widespread immediate availability, ease to interpret, and acquisition speed make non-contrast CT the most common initial study used to image patients with acute focal neurological deficits. Non-contrast CT is certainly sufficient to quickly identify contradictions to intravenous t-PA (tissue plasminogen activator) in patients with potential ischemic stroke, including parenchymal hemorrhage or widespread hypoattenuation [4, 28–30].

Contrast CT

Contrast CT of the head is not usually ordered as part of a routine stroke work-up, unless it is being used for the purpose of obtaining a CTA scan of the blood vessels. A head CT scan with contrast is classically not included in the acute stroke protocol imaging. Rather, a CT scan of the head with contrast is performed in addition to a non-contrast CT scan in situations where acute focal neurological deficits are thought to be secondary to inflammatory, infectious, neoplastic, or demyelinating causes [8, 31]. For example, if a patient had a known history of breast cancer and awoke with new-onset face and hand weakness, a CT scan with and without contrast would assess for the presence of possible brain metastases. Additionally, contrast CT is also important in identifying skull base pathology contributing to acute CNS infection, such as mastoiditis [31].

MRI of the brain

There are several different MRI sequences to consider, and ultimately the sequences chosen are based upon clinical suspicion. The standard MRI sequences include T1-weighted, T2-weighted, and fluid-attenuated inversion recovery (FLAIR) sequences. The selection of additional MRI sequences to add to a standard MRI scan varies, depending on the suspected cause of the patient's acute focal neurological deficits. To put it simplistically, specific MRI sequences are typically only helpful for certain clinical situations. For example, the magnetic resonance (MR) diffusion-weighted imaging (DWI) sequence is generally used to assess patients with possible acute stroke as the cause of their symptoms. Fat-suppressed T1 axial images are ordered when there is a suspected cervicocerebral arterial dissection. Adding proton MR spectroscopy to a standard MRI can be considered for brain neoplasms [8].

Diffusion-weighted MRI

As mentioned, DWI is the MRI sequence that is sensitive to acute ischemia (Figure 12.3) [4, 8, 32]. DWI has emerged over the past decade as the most sensitive and specific imaging technique for acute infarct, far superior to non-contrast CT or any other MRI sequence. It has a high sensitivity at 88% to 100%, with a 95% to 100% specificity for detecting acute ischemic stroke, even within minutes of symptom onset [4, 8, 33–42]. DWI allows identification of the lesion size, location, and, when combined with appropriate image acquisition/processing (to generate a diffusion coefficient map), provides information regarding lesion age. DWI can detect relatively small cortical lesions and subcortical lesions, including those in the brainstem or cerebellum (areas often poorly visualized with non-contrast CT) [4, 43–46]. DWI can identify additional subclinical ischemic lesions, which in turn provides information on stroke mechanism [4, 34, 37, 40, 47–58]. For example, if acute strokes are seen bilaterally in the brain cortex as well as in the cerebellum, the stroke obviously could not come from an isolated carotid artery stenosis. Rather, a cardiac source such as atrial fibrillation or aortic arch atheromatous embolism might be the culprit, given that acute infarcts were noted bilaterally, as well as in the anterior and

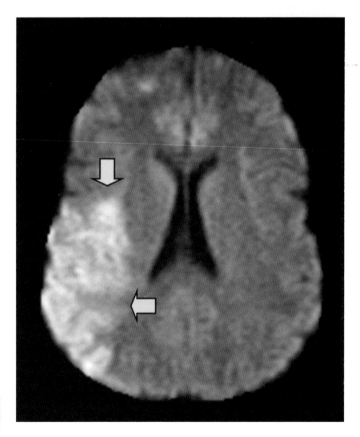

Figure 12.3 DWI of a patient with an acute ischemic stroke. Yellow arrows indicate an area of hyperintensity or "brightness" on the DWI scan consistent with an acute ischemic injury.

posterior circulation territories. It should be noted that the DWI positive lesions in early acute stroke patients may include both areas of irreversible infarction (i.e. permanently damaged brain) and regions of salvageable penumbra (i.e. areas of brain and potential function that may be salvageable if blood flow is restored).

Gradient refocused echo MRI

There is an MRI equivalent of the hyperdense MCA seen on non-contrast CT known as the "artery susceptibility sign". A study comparing both CT and MRI in patients with an occluded proximal middle cerebral artery found that 54% of patients demonstrated this sign on non-contrast CT, while 82% of the same patients had clot on MRI seen with the gradient refocused echo (GRE) sequence [4, 19]. GRE MRI or MR susceptibility-weighted imaging (SWI) sequences are the MRI sequences that screen for symptomatic intracranial bleeding as well as asymptomatic microhemorrhages (Figure 12.4). The appearance of hemorrhage on MRI depends on both the age of the blood and the pulse sequences used [4, 59–66]. Two prospective studies have shown GRE sequences to be as accurate as non-contrast CT in detecting hyperacute intraparenchymal hemorrhage in symptomatic patients presenting within 6 hours of onset [4, 63, 67]. As a result, some centers now use standard MRI scans with DWI, GRE, and magnetic resonance angiography (MRA) sequences added into it as the sole initial brain-imaging modality to evaluate acute stroke patients, including candidates for thrombolysis.

MRI with contrast

MRI with contrast is generally not performed during the work-up of a patient with acute focal neurological deficits thought to be due to stroke. Contrast is typically used with MRI in situations where acute focal neurological deficits are thought to be due to inflammatory, infectious, neoplastic, or demyelinating causes [8]. While contrast MRI is generally not performed for patients with uncomplicated bacterial meningitis, in more complex patients with suspected CNS infections (e.g. those with fever, seizures, and evolving acute neurological deficits), MRI is superior to CT in demonstrating parenchymal lesions due to meningoencephalitis or vasculitis [31]. Additionally, MRI is superior to CT in depicting certain other infectious or inflammatory conditions such as subdural/epidural empyema, and pyogenic abscess [31].

Compared with CT, advantages of MRI for brain imaging include the ability to distinguish acute, small cortical, small deep, and posterior fossa infarcts; the ability to distinguish acute from chronic ischemia; identification of subclinical satellite ischemic lesions that provide information on stroke mechanism; the avoidance of exposure to ionizing radiation; and greater spatial resolution. As mentioned, GRE MRI sequences also have the ability to detect clinically silent prior microbleeds, although it is uncertain whether microbleeds represent markers for increased risk of cerebral hemorrhage after thrombolytic therapy [4, 8, 68–71]. The limits of MRI in the acute hospital setting include cost, limited availability of the test, long duration of the test, increased vulnerability to motion

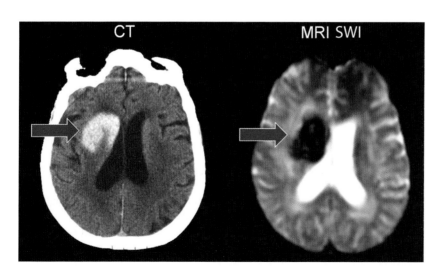

Figure 12.4 Hemorrhage is indicated by red arrows on both a non-contrast head CT scan as well as with SWI MRI.

artifact, and patient contraindications such as claustrophobia, cardiac pacemakers, or metal implants. Additionally, in approximately 10% of MRI patients, an inability to remain still may obliterate the ability to obtain quality imaging [4, 8].

Blood-vessel imaging techniques

Because stroke is the most common cause of acute focal neurological deficits, it is also important to discuss vascular imaging techniques. An integral part of the work-up of patients with stroke, TIA, or other suspected cerebrovascular disease involves imaging the intra- and extracranial blood vessels. Most devastating ischemic strokes are caused by occlusion of one or more large intracranial vessels [4, 16, 17, 72–84]. Detecting large-vessel occlusion with non-invasive intracranial vascular imaging is easily done, and it can greatly improve one's clinical decision-making [4, 72, 74, 76, 85, 86]. It is also important to rapidly identify the cause of a stroke or TIA to prevent additional strokes in the future [4, 87, 88]. Imaging the blood vessels of the head and neck is an integral part of the work-up for any patient with acute focal neurological deficits thought to be due to stroke or TIA.

In addition, certain treatments to prevent stroke recurrence, such as carotid endarterectomy (CEA) or carotid angioplasty and stenting are sometimes performed in the acute setting, and these procedures also require appropriate vessel imaging beforehand. The major intra- and extracranial cervicocephalic vessels can be imaged via several non-invasive techniques, including ultrasound, CTA, time-of-flight and contrast-enhanced MRA, as well as with the more invasive DSA [4, 89–91]. Although each technique has certain advantages in specific clinical situations, the non-invasive techniques such as MRA and CTA show general agreement to DSA in 85% to 90% of cases.

Ultrasound

Extracranial Doppler

B-Mode ultrasound coupled with Doppler (duplex ultrasound) is a safe and inexpensive screening technique for imaging the carotid and vertebral arteries in the neck and measuring blood velocities, respectively, within the common carotid, internal carotid, and external carotid arteries [4, 89, 92]. Doppler test results are influenced by various factors, such as the equipment, the specific laboratory, and the technologist performing the test [4, 93, 94]. For these reasons, it is

recommended that each laboratory validate its own Doppler criteria for clinically relevant stenosis [4, 95, 96]. Sensitivity and specificity of carotid ultrasound for detecting stenotic lesions greater than 70% are less than for other modalities, with an 83–86% sensitivity and an 87–99% specificity [4, 97–99]. Another limitation to carotid ultrasound is its limited ability to image the extracranial vasculature proximal or distal to the carotid bifurcation. Additionally, information about the posterior circulation's extracranial vasculature (the cervicocephalic vertebral arteries) cannot be reliably obtained with this test. Thus, in a patient with a stroke or TIA symptoms localized to a territory perfused by the posterior circulation, CTA or MRA of the neck vasculature would be preferable to carotid Doppler.

The vertebral arteries in the neck can also be well studied using ultrasound. The origin of the vertebral arteries is an important locus of atherosclerotic narrowing and occlusion especially in Caucasian men. The frequency of severe disease at this location parallels that of carotid artery disease. The vertebral artery serves as an important source of intra-arterial embolism to the intracranial posterior circulation arteries. The origin of the vertebral arteries from the subclavian can be imaged using B-mode ultrasound and the arteries can be followed in the neck using a Doppler probe.

Transcranial Doppler of the intracranial vasculature

Transcranial Doppler (TCD) ultrasonography has been used to detect intracranial occlusions, cerebral vasospasm, and stenosis [4, 100–102]. Like carotid Doppler in the neck, the accuracy of TCD in doing so is less than that of CTA and MRA. The sensitivity and specificity of TCD ranges from 55–90% and from 90–95%, respectively [4, 103–110]. In an attempt to better define the accuracy of TCD for intracranial stenoses (a common cause of stroke), the Stroke Outcomes and Neuroimaging of Intracranial Atherosclerosis (SONIA) trial was designed, with 407 patients enrolled at 46 sites [4, 110]. For 50–99% of the stenoses that were angiographically confirmed with conventional cerebral angiography (the "gold standard"), TCD was only able to positively predict 55% of these lesions. This multi-institutional study suggested less than optimal TCD accuracy [4, 100].

TCD has been shown to predict, as well as enhance, outcomes in acute ischemic stroke patients treated with t-PA [4, 111]. TCD provides continuous, real-time imaging and can thus determine the timing of recanalization and the occurrence of reocclusion of vessels [4, 112–114]. Additionally, TCD can also detect microembolic signals, which are a sign of embolism from a more proximal location [4, 115–118]. TCD performed with a "bubble study" can identify the presence of a right to left shunt as a potential cause of ischemic stroke [118]. TCD performed with a vasomotor reactivity study can record changes in cerebral blood flow velocity in response to hypercapnia and hypocapnia, with vasoreactivity of the vessels being assessed to screen for the possibility of migraine [102]. It has been suggested that migraineurs have a different degree of vasomotor reactivity than patients without headache; however, conflict in the literature does remain regarding this issue [102]. The negative points of TCD include its accuracy compared to CTA and MRA, its poor visualization in patients with suboptimal bone windows, and its overall accuracy being dependent on the experience of the technician, the interpreter, and the patient's vascular anatomy [4].

CTA

CTA of the head (intracranial vasculature)

Helical CTA is one way to rapidly and non-invasively assess the intra- and extracranial vasculature in acute, subacute, and chronic stroke settings. CTA is a highly accurate test for evaluating large-vessel intracranial stenoses and occlusions [4, 77, 119–123], and in some cases its overall accuracy approaches or exceeds that of the more invasive conventional cerebral DSA [4, 120, 124]. The sensitivity and specificity of CTA for the detection of intracranial occlusions ranges between 92% and 100% and between 82% and 100%, respectively [4, 77, 125–127]. Because CTA provides only a static image of vascular anatomy, it is inferior to DSA for demonstrating flow rates and direction.

CTA of the neck (extracranial vasculature)

CTA is also a sensitive, specific, and accurate technique for imaging the extracranial vasculature. It is clearly superior to carotid ultrasound in differentiating a carotid occlusion from a very high-grade stenosis [4, 128]. CTA also has an excellent (100%) negative predictive value for excluding greater than 70% carotid stenosis compared with conventional catheter angiography, thereby functioning well as a screening test [4, 129]. A large meta-analysis found it to have a sensitivity greater than 90% and a specificity greater than 95% for detecting significant lesions compared with DSA [4, 98, 122, 130–133].

MRA

MRA of the head

As mentioned above, intracranial MRA can play an important role in a stroke or TIA patient's work-up. Additionally, MRA can be performed in combination with brain MRI in the setting of acute stroke to guide therapeutic decision-making [4, 134]. There are several different MRA techniques that are used for imaging intracranial vessels. They include two-and three-dimensional time of flight, refinements such as multiple overlapping thin-slab acquisition, and contrast-enhanced MRA [4, 135]. Intracranial MRA with non-enhanced time-of-flight techniques has a sensitivity ranging from 60–85% for stenoses and from 80–90% for occlusions compared with CTA or DSA [4, 120, 125]. Typically, time-of-flight MRA is useful in identifying acute proximal large-vessel occlusions but cannot reliably identify distal or branch occlusions [4, 136].

MRA of the neck

Two-dimensional and three-dimensional time-of-flight MRA used for the detection of extracranial carotid disease (with a threshold stenosis typically of 70%) showed a mean sensitivity of 93% and a mean specificity of 88% [135]. Contrast-enhanced MRA is more accurate than non-enhanced time-of-flight techniques, with specificities and sensitivities of 86–97% and 62–91%, respectively, compared with DSA [4, 99, 137–143]. Craniocervical arterial dissections of the carotid and vertebral arteries can often be detected with MRA [4, 144–146]. Contrast-enhanced MRA may improve the detection of arterial dissections [4, 147], although there are few large, prospective studies to prove its accuracy versus catheter angiography. Non-enhanced T1-weighted MRI with fat-saturation techniques can frequently depict a subacute hematoma within the wall of an artery, which is highly suggestive of a recent dissection [4, 148, 149]. However, an acute intramural hematoma may not be well visualized on fat-saturated T1-weighted MRI until the blood is metabolized to methemoglobin, which may require a few days to develop. MRA is also helpful for detecting other less-common causes of ischemic stroke or TIAs such as fibromuscular dysplasia, venous thrombosis, and some cases of vasculitis [4, 147].

Conventional catheter angiography or DSA

Conventional catheter angiography, also known as DSA, is the "gold standard" for the detection of many types of cerebrovascular lesions that affect both the intra- and extracranial vessels [4, 150–152]. For most types of cerebrovascular disease, the resolution, sensitivity, and specificity of DSA equal or exceed those of the non-invasive techniques [4, 150, 152–156]. However, if non-invasive imaging provides a clear diagnostic finding, cerebral angiography is not usually required. This is because DSA is an invasive test and inherent risks of the procedure include serious complications such as vascular injury, stroke, and death, although advances over the past two decades have made cervicocerebral angiography safer. Most large series have reported rates of stroke or death in <1% of DSA procedures, although the largest series of cases to date reported a rate of stroke or death of <0.2% [4, 157–159]. DSA should not be the initial imaging modality for emergency intracerebral evaluation of large-vessel occlusion in stroke because of the time necessary to perform the test; a CTA or MRA can be performed with only an additional 2 to 4 minutes during initial stroke evaluation (in a multimodal evaluation in process) and can eliminate the need for catheter angiography [4, 150, 152].

That being said, when making decisions regarding invasive treatments such as surgical or endovascular revascularization, DSA still remains the most informative technique for imaging the cervical carotid and vertebral arteries. In addition to providing specific information about a vascular lesion, DSA can provide valuable information about collateral flow, perfusion status, and other occult vascular lesions (e.g. dural fistula) that may affect decisions about patient care [4, 150–156]. In particular, DSA can be useful in cases of vascular dissection, both to image the dissection and to delineate the collateral supply to the brain (Figure 12.5).

In summary, for any patient with acute focal neurological deficit thought to be due to stroke or TIA, there are a variety of imaging modalities available to assess the intracranial and extracranial vasculature. In our view, CTA of the head and neck or MRA of the head and neck are generally appropriate. For evaluating the degree of stenosis and for determining patient eligibility for either CEA or carotid angioplasty and stenting, DSA is still the "gold standard" imaging modality. However, the use of two concordant non-invasive techniques (among ultrasound, CTA, and MRA) to assess treatment candidacy can also be done, and has the advantage of avoiding catheterization risks [4, 160, 161]. CTA (in the absence of heavy calcifications) and multimodal MRI (including MRA and fat-saturation axial T1 imaging) are both highly accurate for detecting dissection; for subtle dissections, DSA and multimodal MRI appear to be complementary, and there have been reports of dissections detected by one modality but not the other [4, 162, 163]. A very high-grade stenosis ("string sign") is most accurately detected by DSA, followed closely by CTA and contrast-enhanced MRA [4, 164].

Perfusion imaging techniques

Perfusion CT and perfusion MRI

Given that stroke is the most common cause of acute focal neurological deficits, it is also important to review brain perfusion imaging techniques. Perfusion imaging is a means of imaging cerebral blood flow. Theoretically, perfusion imaging such as CT perfusion or MR perfusion (in conjunction with other sequences in the non-contrast CT or stroke protocol MRI scans) can help physicians distinguish which areas of the brain have diminished blood flow, but are salvageable (the "ischemic penumbra"), and which areas of the brain are permanently damaged by stroke. In the past, physicians only had a "time clock" (a patient's "last known well" time) to determine if patients were eligible for treatments such as intravenous t-PA, to attempt to reverse their focal neurological deficit and/or improve outcome from stroke [4, 9]. Perfusion imaging was an incredibly important development in acute stroke care, because it brought with it the potential to change how physicians view which patients are eligible for acute stroke treatments. The advent of perfusion imaging brought with it the possibility of using a "tissue physiology clock," rather than a "time clock" for therapeutic guidance [164, 165]. Current literature notes that the ischemic, but potentially salvageable, penumbra tissue is an ideal target for reperfusion and neuroprotective therapies, but that these treatments require proper patient selection [4, 17, 82, 112, 166–171]. Perfusion imaging provides a way to select which patients may be appropriate for certain interventions.

Brain perfusion imaging provides information about regional cerebral hemodynamics in the form of such parameters as cerebral blood flow, cerebral blood volume, and mean transit time [9]. Perfusion

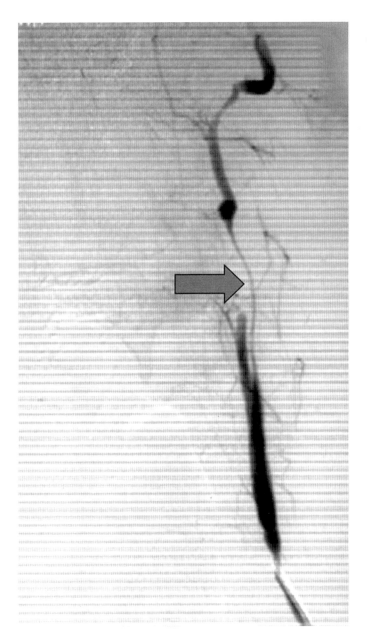

Figure 12.5 Conventional angiogram: left vertebral artery dissection is indicated with a gray arrow.

CT and perfusion-weighted MRI have been widely incorporated into acute multimodal stroke imaging protocols at many institutions. Combined with brain parenchymal imaging, both perfusion-weighted MRI and perfusion CT imaging allow delineation of the ischemic penumbra [4, 9, 172–180]. Perfusion imaging can also indicate areas that are severely and probably irretrievably infarcted. On MRI, the ischemic penumbra (or salvageable brain) is roughly outlined as the area of "mismatch" between the area of abnormal perfusion seen with perfusion-weighted imaging and the area of infarct seen with DWI (Figure 12.6) [4, 37, 181–183]. On perfusion CT imaging, the penumbra is indexed as the area of mean transit time–cerebral blood volume mismatch [4, 184–187]. "Core" ischemia (or permanently damaged brain) can be defined accurately by perfusion CT depending on equipment and programming.

Of note, in the acute stroke setting there is also a trade-off between the increased information provided

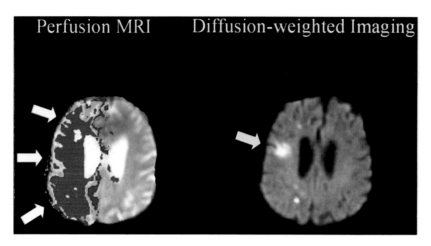

Figure 12.6 MR perfusion and MR DWI images in acute ischemic stroke. The white arrows in the perfusion image point to areas where perfusion is affected. The yellow arrow in the DWI image points to a hyperintense area, which is considered to be acutely ischemic. The difference between the two areas is the "ischemic penumbra", or potentially salvageable brain.

by perfusion imaging and the increased time needed to acquire additional imaging sequences. The Massachusetts Hospital acute stroke imaging algorithm suggests that perfusion CT and perfusion MRI are unnecessary for the safe and effective triage of patients with severe anterior circulation arterial occlusions [9]. Current 2013 American Heart Association (AHA) guidelines suggest that performance of these additional imaging sequences should not unduly delay treatment with intravenous t-PA within the ≤4- and 0.5-hour window in appropriate patients [4, 9, 150, 155–159]. However, the 2013 AHA guidelines also state that in patients beyond the 4- and 0.5-hour time window, CT perfusion and MRI perfusion, and diffusion imaging, including measures of infarct core and penumbra, may be considered for the selection of patients for acute reperfusion therapies [4]. Perfusion imaging provides additional information that may improve diagnosis, mechanism, and severity of ischemic stroke, allowing more informed clinical decision-making.

Advantages and disadvantages of perfusion CT
Advantages of the multimodal CT approach over MRI include wider availability of emergency CT imaging, more rapid imaging, and fewer contraindications to CT versus MRI [4, 188–190]. Additionally, perfusion CT parameters of cerebral blood volume, cerebral blood flow, and mean transit time can be more easily quantified than their perfusion-weighted MRI counterparts. Because of its availability and greater degree of quantification, perfusion CT has the potential to increase patient access to new treatments and imaging-based clinical trials.

Disadvantages of the CT approach over MRI include the use of ionizing radiation and iodinated contrast, which carries a small risk of nephrotoxicity. Use of low-osmolar or iso-osmolar contrast minimizes the risk of contrast-induced nephropathy [4, 191, 192]. A recent study of CTA in patients with acute ischemic and hemorrhagic stroke demonstrated a rate of contrast-induced nephropathy at 3%, with no patients requiring dialysis [3, 193]. Another disadvantage of perfusion CT is limited brain coverage, typically a 4-cm-thick slab per contrast bolus [4, 77, 126, 194, 195]. Developments such as the toggling-table technique allow doubling of the perfusion CT coverage (typically up to 8 cm) [4, 196]. Finally, the latest generations of the 256- and 320-slice CT scanners afford whole-brain coverage but are limited in availability.

Advantages and disadvantages of perfusion MRI
The major advantages of perfusion MRI over perfusion CT include its ability to be incorporated into a stroke protocol MRI, which can effectively evaluate many aspects of the parenchyma, including the presence of infarction with DWI, and the avoidance of ionizing radiation. Of note, the whole-brain coverage offered by perfusion MRI comes at the cost of a limited resolution. Disadvantages of perfusion MRI include limited availability in emergency settings, duration of the study, and patient contraindications such as claustrophobia, motion, cardiac pacemakers, or metal implants. Gadolinium-based MR contrast reactions are less common than CT contrast dye reactions but can be dangerous [4, 190, 197, 198]. Nephrogenic systemic fibrosis/nephrogenic fibrosing dermopathy can be caused by gadolinium-based contrast agents used for

MRI [4, 196]. Gadolinium-based MR contrast media generally should be avoided in the presence of advanced renal failure with estimated glomerular filtration rate <30 ml·min·m [4, 196, 197]. Arterial spin labeling is a different MRI method that assesses brain perfusion without the need to inject gadolinium contrast material, but it is not currently widely available [4].

Several recent trials have studied MRI perfusion/diffusion mismatch. EPITHET (Echoplanar Imaging Thrombolytic Evaluation Trial) was designed to answer the question of whether intravenous t-PA given 3 to 6 hours after stroke onset promotes reperfusion and attenuates infarct growth in patients who have a "mismatch" between perfusion-weighted and diffusion-weighted MRI. Intravenous t-PA was non-significantly associated with lower infarct growth but significantly associated with increased reperfusion in patients who had mismatch [4, 122, 199]. In the Diffusion-Weighted Imaging Evaluation for Understanding Stroke Evolution (DEFUSE) study, a target mismatch pattern of small core and large penumbra was associated with greater clinical response to reperfusion [4, 176, 177, 200, 201]. DEDAS (Dose Escalation of Desmoteplase for Acute Ischemic Stroke) [4, 178] appeared to show intravenous desmoteplase to be safe and led to two pivotal studies: Desmoteplase in Acute Ischemic Stroke (DIAS) 1 and DIAS 2 trials, which tested the concept of using advanced MR or CT for intravenous fibrinolysis triage in the 3- to 9-hour time window [4, 180, 202]. Unfortunately, there was no clinical benefit demonstrated, although favorable trends were seen in the MR-selected patients [4, 202]. Newer studies are currently under way, incorporating lessons from these published trials, and hopefully may help identify those subsets of patients who would benefit from an intervention after the typical time window for treatment has passed.

Imaging protocol selection

As discussed above, brain, vascular, and perfusion imaging can all be components of the emergency assessment of patients with acute focal neurological deficits. Information about multimodal CT and MRI of the brain suggests that these diagnostic studies provide important information about the etiology and prognosis, and may even help to determine appropriate treatment of patients with acute focal neurological deficits.

Either CT or MRI may be used as the initial imaging test. MRI is more sensitive to the presence of ischemia, but at most institutions CT remains the most practical initial brain imaging test. A physician skilled in assessing CT or MRI studies should be available to promptly examine the initial scan. In particular, the scan should be evaluated for evidence of early signs of infarction, vessel thrombosis, or bleed in any patient with an acute focal neurological deficit thought to be due to stroke. For ischemic stroke patients, both CT and MRI platforms offer powerful multimodal imaging capabilities. For patients with rapidly transient acute focal neurological symptoms, diffusion MRI provides a unique insight into whether a stroke has occurred and is the preferred modality if available.

Important points when selecting imaging protocols

Current 2013 AHA guidelines recommend the following in patients with persistent acute focal neurological deficits due to suspected cerebral ischemia [4]:

- Emergency imaging of the brain is recommended before initiating any specific therapy to treat acute ischemic stroke. In most instances, a non-contrast head CT will provide the necessary information to make decisions about emergency management.
- Either non-contrast head CT or MRI with GRE is recommended before intravenous t-PA administration to exclude intracerebral hemorrhage (an absolute contraindication to treatment) and to determine whether CT hypodensity or MRI hyperintensity of ischemia is present.
- A non-invasive intracranial vascular study such as CTA or MRA is strongly recommended during the initial imaging evaluation of the acute stroke patient if either intra-arterial chemical or mechanical thrombolysis is considered for management. These studies should not delay intravenous t-PA if indicated.
- In intravenous t-PA candidates, the brain imaging study should be interpreted within 45 minutes of patient arrival in the emergency department by a physician with expertise in reading CT and MRI studies of the brain.
- Frank hypodensity on non-contrast head CT may increase the risk of hemorrhage with t-PA and should be considered in treatment decisions. If frank hypodensity involves more than one-third of the middle cerebral artery territory, intravenous t-PA treatment should be withheld.

199

The AHA recommendations for patients with cerebral ischemic symptoms that have resolved include [4]:

- Non-invasive imaging of the cervical vessels should be performed routinely as part of the evaluation of patients with suspected TIAs.
- Non-invasive imaging by means of CTA or MRA of the intracranial vasculature is recommended to exclude the presence of proximal intracranial stenosis and/or occlusion and should be obtained when knowledge of intracranial steno-occlusive disease will alter management. Reliable diagnosis of the presence and degree of intracranial stenosis requires the performance of catheter angiography to confirm abnormalities detected with non-invasive testing.
- Patients with transient ischemic neurological symptoms should undergo neuroimaging evaluation within 24 hours of symptom onset or as soon as possible in patients with delayed presentations. MRI with DWI is the preferred brain diagnostic imaging modality. If MRI is not available, head CT should be performed.

In general, an institution can adopt one neuroimaging protocol as its primary strategy and optimize systems operations to attain rapid and reliable scan perform-ance. For example, the Massachusetts General Hospital Neuroradiology Division employed an expe-rience- and evidence-based approach to develop an imaging algorithm to best select patients with possible severe ischemic strokes caused by anterior circulation occlusions for treatment with either intravenous t-PA or endovascular therapy (Figure 12.7) [9]. Methods

Step 1: All patients undergo non-contrast head CT. CT is performed and read.*
Step 2: CTA is done (t-PA is prepared while CTA is being performed).
Step 3: CTA is assessed for an accessible proximal occlusion and patient assessed for MRI eligibility.
Step 4: If occlusion present, and MRI eligible, DWI is done. If the DWI lesion is small, the patient is immediately triaged to endovascular therapy (if eligible) or a CT or MRI perfusion is ordered (if the DWI lesion is large or if the patient was ineligible for endovascular therapy).

If occlusion is not present, or if patient is not MRI eligible, CT perfusion is done.
*Only the first step in this algorithm and the time from stroke onset are needed for the decision to treat with intravenous t-PA. The remaining steps are used to determine eligibility for endovascular therapies such as chemical or mechanical thrombolysis [9].

Figure 12.7 Massachusetts General Hospital acute stroke imaging algorithm

found to be of value in this article included performing a National Institutes of Health Stroke Scale known as the NIHSS (to assess the severity of a suspected stroke), a non-contrast CT (to identify hemorrhage and large hypodensity), a CTA of the neck and head (to identify the anterior circulation occlusion), and the DWI component of an MRI (to estimate the ischemic core of the infarct in conjunction with the NIHSS).

Conclusions

In summary, two factors of primary importance to keep in mind when assessing patients with acute focal neurological deficits are the location of the potential pathology as well as its suspected cause. The history and the examination are key factors in guiding a physician toward appropriate choices of imaging. Both history and the examination will direct the choice of whether neuroimaging tests are ordered, as well as which types of neuroimaging and the rapidity with which they are needed. There are some important generalities to be aware of in the choice of brain imaging. Either CT or MRI may be used as the initial imaging study in patients with acute focal neurological deficits [4]. Contrast is typically used in a brain paren-chymal study when acute focal neurological deficits are thought to be secondary to inflammatory, infectious, neoplastic, or demyelinating causes. Imaging of the brain's parenchyma as well as its vasculature and, potentially, perfusion imaging are performed when the acute neurological deficits are thought to be sec-ondary to cerebral ischemia. Rapid neuroimaging is critical during the emergent evaluation of patients with acute focal neurological symptoms thought to be due to acute ischemic stroke [4, 8, 9]. Brain imaging findings, including the size, location, and vascular dis-tribution of an infarct, presence of hemorrhage, pres-ence of large-vessel occlusion, possible degree of reversible ischemic injury, and cerebral hemodynamic status can be obtained from imaging and will affect both short-term and long-term patient management.

References

1. Bradley WG, Daroff RB, Fenichel GM, Marsden CD (2000). Diagnosis of neurological disease. In Bradley WG, Daroff RB, Fenichel GM, Marsden CD, eds. *Neurology in Clinical Practice*, 3rd edn. New York: Marcel Dekker, pp. 3–8.

2. Caplan LR (2000). Diagnosis and the clinical encounter. In Caplan LR, ed. *Caplan's Stroke*, 3rd edn. Boston: Butterworth-Heinemann, pp. 51–71.

3. Caplan LR, Hollander J (2011). The general systemic and neurological examinations. In Shelton CT, ed. *The Effective Clinical Neurologist*, 3rd edn. Shelton, CT: People's Medical Publishing House-USA, pp. 63–103.

4. Jauch EC, Saver JL, Adams HP, *et al.*, on behalf of the American Heart Association Stroke Council, Council on Cardiovascular Nursing, Council on Peripheral Vascular Disease, and Council on Clinical Cardiology (2013). Guidelines for the early management of patients with acute ischemic stroke: a guideline for healthcare professionals from the American Heart Association/American Stroke Association. *Stroke* 44: 870–947.

5. Winkler DT, Fluri F, Fuhr P, *et al.* (2009). Thrombolysis in stroke mimics: frequency, clinical characteristics, and outcome. *Stroke* 40: 1522–1525.

6. Scott PA, Silbergleit R (2003). Misdiagnosis of stroke in tissue plasminogen activator-treated patients: characteristics and outcomes. *Ann Emerg Med* 42: 611–618.

7. Chernyshev OY, Martin-Schild S, Albright KC, Barreto A, *et al.* (2010). Safety of tPA in stroke mimics and neuroimaging – negative cerebral ischemia. *Neurology* 74: 1340–1345.

8. Cochrane Miller J (2006). Neuroimaging for headaches. In Lee SI, ed. *Radiology Rounds: A Newsletter for Referring Physicians*. Massachusetts, MA: Massachusetts General Hospital, Department of Radiology, vol 4, issue 10.

9. González RG, Copen WA, Schaefer PW, *et al.* (2013). The Massachusetts General Hospital acute stroke imaging algorithm: an experience and evidence based approach *J NeuroInterventional Surg* 5: i7–i12.

10. Noguchi K, Ogawa T, Inugami A, *et al.* (1995). Acute subarachnoid hemorrhage: MR imaging with fluid-attenuated inversion recovery pulse sequences. *Radiology* 196: 773–777.

11. Sames TA, Storrow AB, Finkelstein JA, Magoon MR (1996). Sensitivity of new-generation computed tomography in subarachnoid hemorrhage. *Acad Emerg Med* 3: 16–20.

12. Tomura N, Uemura K, Inugami A, *et al.* (1988). Early CT finding in cerebral infarction: obscuration of the lentiform nucleus. *Radiology* 168: 463–467.

13. Truwit CL, Barkovich AJ, Gean-Marton A, Hibri N, Norman D (1990). Loss of the insular ribbon: another early CT sign of acute middle cerebral artery infarction. *Radiology* 176: 801–806.

14. von Kummer R, Meyding-Lamade U, Forsting M, *et al.* (1994). Sensitivity and prognostic value of early CT in occlusion of the middle cerebral artery trunk. *AJNR* 15: 9–15.

15. Moulin T, Cattin F, Crépin-Leblond T, *et al.* (1996). Early CT signs in acute middle cerebral artery infarction: predictive value for subsequent infarct locations and outcome. *Neurology* 47: 366–375.

16. Manno EM, Nichols DA, Fulgham JR, Wijdicks EF (2003). Computed tomographic determinants of neurologic deterioration in patients with large middle cerebral artery infarctions. *Mayo Clin Proc* 78: 156–160.

17. Smith WS, Tsao JW, Billings ME, *et al.* (2006). Prognostic significance of angiographically confirmed large vessel intracranial occlusion in patients presenting with acute brain ischemia. *Neurocrit Care* 4: 14–17.

18. Tomsick T, Brott T, Barsan W, *et al.* (1996). Prognostic value of the hyperdense middle cerebral artery sign and stroke scale score before ultraearly thrombolytic therapy. *AJNR* 17: 79–85.

19. Flacke S, Urbach H, Keller E, *et al.* (2000). Middle cerebral artery (MCA) susceptibility sign at susceptibility-based perfusion MR imaging: clinical importance and comparison with hyperdense MCA sign at CT. *Radiology* 215: 476–482.

20. Barber PA, Demchuk AM, Hudon ME, *et al.* (2001). Hyperdense sylvian fissure MCA "dot" sign: a CT marker of acute ischemia. *Stroke* 32: 84–88.

21. Leary MC, Kidwell CS, Villablanca JP, *et al.* (2003). Validation of computed tomographic middle cerebral artery "dot" sign: an angiographic correlation study. *Stroke* 34: 2636–2640.

22. Arnold M, Nedeltchev K, Schroth G, *et al.* (2004). Clinical and radiological predictors of recanalisation and outcome of 40 patients with acute basilar artery occlusion treated with intra-arterial thrombolysis. *J Neurol Neurosurg Psychiatr* 75: 857–862.

23. Goldmakher GV, Camargo EC, Furie KL, *et al.* (2009). Hyperdense basilar artery sign on unenhanced CT predicts thrombus and outcome in acute posterior circulation stroke. *Stroke* 40: 134–139.

24. Demchuk AM, Hill MD, Barber PA, *et al*; National Institute of Neurological Disorders and Stroke rtPA Stroke Study Group, NIH (2005). Importance of early ischemic computed tomography changes using ASPECTS in NINDS rtPA Stroke Study. *Stroke* 36: 2110–2115.

25. Dzialowski I, Hill MD, Coutts SB, *et al.* (2006). Extent of early ischemic changes on computed tomography (CT) before thrombolysis: prognostic value of the Alberta Stroke Program Early CT Score in ECASS II. *Stroke* 37: 973–978.

26. Patel SC, Levine SR, Tilley BC, *et al*; National Institute of Neurological Disorders and Stroke rt-PA Stroke Study Group, NIH (2001). Lack of clinical significance of early ischemic changes on computed tomography in acute stroke. *JAMA* 286: 2830–2838.

27. Kidwell CS, Alger JR, Di Salle F, *et al.* (1999). Diffusion MRI in patients with transient ischemic attacks. *Stroke* 30: 1174–1180.

28. von Kummer R, Bourquain H, Bastianello S, *et al.* (2001). Early prediction of irreversible brain damage after ischemic stroke at CT. *Radiology* **219**: 95–100.

29. The European Stroke Organisation (ESO) Executive Committee and the ESO Writing Committee (2008). Guidelines for management of ischaemic stroke and transient ischaemic attack 2008. *Cerebrovasc Dis* **25**: 457–507.

30. Larrue V, von Kummer R, del Zoppo G, Bluhmki E (1997). Hemorrhagic transformation in acute ischemic stroke: potential contributing factors in the European Cooperative Acute Stroke Study. *Stroke* **28**: 957–960.

31. Kastrup O, Wanke I, Maschke M (2005). Neuroimaging of infections. *NeuroRx*: **2**: 324–332.

32. Mohr JP, Biller J, Hilal SK, *et al.* (1995). Magnetic resonance versus computed tomographic imaging in acute stroke. *Stroke* **26**: 807–812.

33. Barber PA, Darby DG, Desmond PM, *et al.* (1999). Identification of major ischemic change: diffusion-weighted imaging versus computed tomography. *Stroke* **30**: 2059–2065.

34. Fiebach JB, Schellinger PD, Jansen O, *et al.* (2002). CT and diffusion-weighted MR imaging in randomized order: diffusion-weighted imaging results in higher accuracy and lower interrater variability in the diagnosis of hyperacute ischemic stroke. *Stroke* **33**: 2206–2210.

35. González RG, Schaefer PW, Buonanno FS, *et al.* (1999). Diffusion-weighted MR imaging: diagnostic accuracy in patients imaged within 6 hours of stroke symptom onset. *Radiology* **210**: 155–162.

36. Ay H, Buonanno FS, Rordorf G, *et al.* (1999). Normal diffusion-weighted MRI during stroke-like deficits. *Neurology* **52**: 1784–1792.

37. Barber PA, Darby DG, Desmond PM, *et al.* (1998). Prediction of stroke outcome with echoplanar perfusion- and diffusion-weighted MRI. *Neurology* **51**: 418–426.

38. Lee LJ, Kidwell CS, Alger J, Starkman S, Saver JL (2000). Impact on stroke subtype diagnosis of early diffusion-weighted magnetic resonance imaging and magnetic resonance angiography. *Stroke* **31**: 1081–1089.

39. Lövblad KO, Laubach HJ, Baird AE, *et al.* (1998). Clinical experience with diffusion-weighted MR in patients with acute stroke. *AJNR* **19**: 1061–1066.

40. Lutsep HL, Albers GW, DeCrespigny A, *et al.* (1997). Clinical utility of diffusion-weighted magnetic resonance imaging in the assessment of ischemic stroke. *Ann Neurol* **41**: 574–580.

41. van Everdingen KJ, van der Grond J, Kappelle LJ, Ramos LM, Mali WP (1998). Diffusion-weighted magnetic resonance imaging in acute stroke. *Stroke* **29**: 1783–1790.

42. Warach S, Chien D, Li W, Ronthal M, Edelman RR (1992). Fast magnetic resonance diffusion-weighted imaging of acute human stroke. *Neurology* **42**: 1717–1723.

43. Albers GW, Lansberg MG, Norbash AM, *et al.* (2000). Yield of diffusion-weighted MRI for detection of potentially relevant findings in stroke patients. *Neurology* **54**: 1562–1567.

44. Bryan RN, Levy LM, Whitlow WD, *et al.* (1991). Diagnosis of acute cerebral infarction: comparison of CT and MR imaging. *AJNRl* **12**: 611–620.

45. Perkins CJ, Kahya E, Roque CT, Roche PE, Newman GC (2001). Fluid-attenuated inversion recovery and diffusion- and perfusion-weighted MRI abnormalities in 117 consecutive patients with stroke symptoms. *Stroke* **32**: 2774–2781.

46. Wiener JI, King JT Jr., Moore JR, Lewin JS (2001). The value of diffusion-weighted imaging for prediction of lasting deficit in acute stroke: an analysis of 134 patients with acute neurologic deficits. *Neuroradiology* **43**: 435–441.

47. Arauz A, Murillo L, Cantú C, Barinagarrementeria F, Higuera J (2003). Prospective study of single and multiple lacunar infarcts using magnetic resonance imaging: risk factors, recurrence, and outcome in 175 consecutive cases. *Stroke* **34**: 2453–2458.

48. Ay H, Oliveira-Filho J, Buonanno FS, *et al.* (1999). Diffusion-weighted imaging identifies a subset of lacunar infarction associated with embolic source. *Stroke* **30**: 2644–2650.

49. Baird AE, Lövblad KO, Schlaug G, Edelman RR, Warach S (2000). Multiple acute stroke syndrome: marker of embolic disease? *Neurology* **54**: 674–678.

50. Caso V, Budak K, Georgiadis D, Schuknecht B, Baumgartner RW (2005). Clinical significance of detection of multiple acute brain infarcts on diffusion weighted magnetic resonance imaging. *J Neurol Neurosurg Psychiatr* **76**: 514–518.

51. Etgen T, Gräfin von Einsiedel H, Röttinger M, *et al.* (2004). Detection of acute brainstem infarction by using DWI/MRI. *Eur Neurol* **52**: 145–150.

52. Gerraty RP, Parsons MW, Barber PA, *et al.* (2002). Examining the lacunar hypothesis with diffusion and perfusion magnetic resonance imaging. *Stroke* **33**: 2019–2024.

53. Keir SL, Wardlaw JM, Bastin ME, Dennis MS (2004). In which patients is diffusion-weighted magnetic resonance imaging most useful in routine stroke care? *J Neuroimaging* **14**: 118–122.

54. Mullins ME, Schaefer PW, Sorensen AG, *et al.* (2002). CT and conventional and diffusion-weighted MR imaging in acute stroke: study in 691 patients at presentation to the emergency department. *Radiology* **224**: 353–360.

55. Seifert T, Enzinger C, Storch MK, *et al.* (2005). Acute small subcortical infarctions on diffusion weighted MRI: clinical presentation and aetiology. *J Neurol Neurosurg Psychiatr* **76**: 1520–1524.

56. Takahashi K, Kobayashi S, Matui R, Yamaguchi S, Yamashita K (2002). The differences of clinical parameters between small multiple ischemic lesions and single lesion detected by diffusion-weighted MRI. *Acta Neurol Scand* **106**: 24–29.

57. Wessels T, Röttger C, Jauss M, *et al.* (2005). Identification of embolic stroke patterns by diffusion-weighted MRI in clinically defined lacunar stroke syndromes. *Stroke* **36**: 757–761.

58. Wityk RJ, Goldsborough MA, Hillis A, *et al.* (2001). Diffusion- and perfusion-weighted brain magnetic resonance imaging in patients with neurologic complications after cardiac surgery. *Arch Neurol* **58**: 571–576.

59. Bradley WG Jr., Schmidt PG (1985). Effect of methemoglobin formation on the MR appearance of subarachnoid hemorrhage. *Radiology* **156**: 99–103.

60. Edelman RR, Johnson K, Buxton R, *et al.* (1986). MR of hemorrhage: a new approach. *AJNR* **7**: 751–756.

61. Gomori JM, Grossman RI, Goldberg HI, Zimmerman RA, Bilaniuk LT (1985). Intracranial hematomas: imaging by high-field MR. *Radiology* **157**: 87–93.

62. Hayman LA, Taber KH, Ford JJ, Bryan RN (1991). Mechanisms of MR signal alteration by acute intracerebral blood: old concepts and new theories. *AJNR* **12**: 899–907.

63. Kidwell CS, Chalela JA, Saver JL, *et al.* (2004). Comparison of MRI and CT for detection of acute intracerebral hemorrhage. *JAMA* **292**: 1823–1830.

64. Linfante I, Llinas RH, Caplan LR, Warach S (1999). MRI features of intracerebral hemorrhage within 2 hours from symptom onset. *Stroke* **30**: 2263–2267.

65. Patel MR, Edelman RR, Warach S (1996). Detection of hyperacute primary intraparenchymal hemorrhage by magnetic resonance imaging. *Stroke* **27**: 2321–2324.

66. Schellinger PD, Jansen O, Fiebach JB, Hacke W, Sartor K (1999). A standardized MRI stroke protocol: comparison with CT in hyperacute intracerebral hemorrhage. *Stroke* **30**: 765–768.

67. Fiebach JB, Schellinger PD, Gass A, *et al* (2004). Stroke magnetic resonance imaging is accurate in hyperacute intracerebral hemorrhage: a multicenter study on the validity of stroke imaging. *Stroke* **35**: 502–506.

68. Chalela JA, Kang DW, Warach S (2004). Multiple cerebral microbleeds: MRI marker of a diffuse hemorrhage-prone state. *J Neuroimaging* **14**: 54–57.

69. Kidwell CS, Saver JL, Villablanca JP, *et al.* (2002). Magnetic resonance imaging detection of microbleeds before thrombolysis: an emerging application. *Stroke* **33**: 95–98.

70. Wong KS, Chan YL, Liu JY, Gao S, Lam WW (2003). Asymptomatic microbleeds as a risk factor for aspirin-associated intracerebral hemorrhages. *Neurology* **60**: 511–513.

71. Kakuda W, Thijs VN, Lansberg MG, *et al*; DEFUSE Investigators (2005). Clinical importance of microbleeds in patients receiving IV thrombolysis. *Neurology* **65**: 1175–1178.

72. Kharitonova T, Thorén M, Ahmed N, *et al*; SITS investigators (2009). Disappearing hyperdense middle cerebral artery sign in ischaemic stroke patients treated with intravenous thrombolysis: clinical course and prognostic significance. *J Neurol Neurosurg Psychiatr* **80**: 273–278.

73. Linfante I, Llinas RH, Selim M, *et al.* (2002). Clinical and vascular outcome in internal carotid artery versus middle cerebral artery occlusions after intravenous tissue plasminogen activator. *Stroke* **33**: 2066–2071.

74. Manelfe C, Larrue V, von Kummer R, *et al.* (1999). Association of hyperdense middle cerebral artery sign with clinical outcome in patients treated with tissue plasminogen activator. *Stroke* **30**: 769–772.

75. Tan IY, Demchuk AM, Hopyan J, *et al.* (2009). CT angiography clot burden score and collateral score: correlation with clinical and radiologic outcomes in acute middle cerebral artery infarct. *AJNR* **30**: 525–531.

76. Nichols C, Khoury J, Brott T, Broderick J (2008). Intravenous recombinant tissue plasminogen activator improves arterial recanalization rates and reduces infarct volumes in patients with hyperdense artery sign on baseline computed tomography. *J Stroke Cerebrovasc Dis* **17**: 64–68.

77. Lev MH, Farkas J, Rodriguez VR, *et al.* (2001). CT angiography in the rapid triage of patients with hyperacute stroke to intraarterial thrombolysis: accuracy in the detection of large vessel thrombus. *J Comput Assist Tomogr* **25**: 520–528.

78. Lin K, Rapalino O, Law M, *et al.* (2008). Accuracy of the Alberta Stroke Program Early CT Score during the first 3 hours of middle cerebral artery stroke: comparison of noncontrast CT, CT angiography source images, and CT perfusion. *AJNR* **29**: 931–936.

79. Ryoo JW, Na DG, Kim SS, *et al.* (2004). Malignant middle cerebral artery infarction in hyperacute ischemic stroke: evaluation with multiphasic perfusion computed tomography maps. *J Comput Assist Tomogr* **28**: 55–62.

80. Mattle HP, Arnold M, Georgiadis D, *et al.* (2008). Comparison of intraarterial and intravenous thrombolysis for ischemic stroke with hyperdense middle cerebral artery sign. *Stroke* **39**: 379–383.

81. Zaidat OO, Suarez JI, Santillan C, *et al.* (2002). Response to intra-arterial and combined intravenous and intra-arterial thrombolytic therapy in patients with distal internal carotid artery occlusion. *Stroke* **33**: 1821–1826.

82. Sims JR, Rordorf G, Smith EE, *et al.* (2005). Arterial occlusion revealed by CT angiography predicts NIH stroke score and acute outcomes after IV tPA treatment. *AJNR* **26**: 246–251.

83. Coutts SB, Lev MH, Eliasziw M, *et al.* (2004). ASPECTS on CTA source images versus unenhanced CT: added value in predicting final infarct extent and clinical outcome. *Stroke* **35**: 2472–2476.

84. Torres-Mozqueda F, He J, Yeh IB, *et al.* (2008). An acute ischemic stroke classification instrument that includes CT or MR angiography: the Boston Acute Stroke Imaging Scale. *AJNR* **29**: 1111–1117.

85. Furlan A, Higashida R, Wechsler L, *et al.* (1999). Intra-arterial prourokinase for acute ischemic stroke: the PROACT II study: a randomized controlled trial: Prolyse in Acute Cerebral Thromboembolism. *JAMA* **282**: 2003–2011.

86. Hacke W, Kaste M, Bluhmki E, *et al.* (2008). Thrombolysis with alteplase 3 to 4.5 hours after acute ischemic stroke. *N Engl J Med* **359**: 1317–1329.

87. Easton JD, Saver JL, Albers GW, *et al.* (2009). Definition and evaluation of transient ischemic attack: a scientific statement for healthcare professionals from the American Heart Association/American Stroke Association Stroke Council; Council on Cardiovascular Surgery and Anesthesia; Council on Cardiovascular Radiology and Intervention; Council on Cardiovascular Nursing; and the Interdisciplinary Council on Peripheral Vascular Disease. *Stroke* **40**: 2276–2293.

88. Adams RJ, Albers G, Alberts MJ, *et al.* (2008). Update to the AHA/ASA recommendations for the prevention of stroke in patients with stroke and transient ischemic attack [published correction appears in *Stroke* 2010;41: e455]. *Stroke* **39**: 1647–1652.

89. Buskens E, Nederkoorn PJ, Buijs-Van Der Woude T, *et al.* (2004). Imaging of carotid arteries in symptomatic patients: cost-effectiveness of diagnostic strategies. *Radiology* **233**: 101–112.

90. Lovett JK, Dennis MS, Sandercock PA, *et al.* (2003). Very early risk of stroke after a first transient ischemic attack. *Stroke* **34**: e138–e140.

91. Rothwell PM, Giles MF, Flossmann E, *et al.* (2005). A simple score (ABCD) to identify individuals at high early risk of stroke after transient ischaemic attack. *Lancet* **366**: 29–36.

92. Carroll BA (1989). Duplex sonography in patients with hemispheric symptoms. *J Ultrasound Med* **8**: 535–540.

93. Alexandrov AV, Brodie DS, McLean A, *et al.* (1997). Correlation of peak systolic velocity and angiographic measurement of carotid stenosis revisited. *Stroke* **28**: 339–342.

94. Ranke C, Trappe HJ (1997). Blood flow velocity measurements for carotid stenosis estimation: interobserver variation and interequipment variability. *VASA* **26**: 210–214.

95. Curley PJ, Norrie L, Nicholson A, Galloway JM, Wilkinson AR (1998). Accuracy of carotid duplex is laboratory specific and must be determined by internal audit. *Eur J Vasc Endovasc Surg* **15**: 511–514.

96. Kuntz KM, Polak JF, Whittemore AD, Skillman JJ, Kent KC (1997). Duplex ultrasound criteria for the identification of carotid stenosis should be laboratory specific. *Stroke* **28**: 597–602.

97. Blakeley DD, Oddone EZ, Hasselblad V, Simel DL, Matchar DB (1995). Noninvasive carotid artery testing: a meta-analytic review. *Ann Intern Med* **122**: 360–367.

98. Long A, Lepoutre A, Corbillon E, Branchereau A (2002). Critical review of non- or minimally invasive methods (duplex ultrasonography, MR- and CT-angiography) for evaluating stenosis of the proximal internal carotid artery. *Eur J Vasc Endovasc Surg* **24**: 43–52.

99. Nederkoorn PJ, Elgersma OE, van der Graaf Y, *et al.* (2003). Carotid artery stenosis: accuracy of contrast-enhanced MR angiography for diagnosis. *Radiology* **228**: 677–682.

100. Babikian VL, Pochay V, Burdette DE, Brass ML (1991). Transcranial Doppler sonographic monitoring in the intensive care unit. *J Intensive Care Med* **6**: 36–44.

101. Newell DW, Aaslid R (1992). Transcranial Doppler: clinical and experimental uses. *Cerebrovasc Brain Metab Rev* **4**: 122–143.

102. Nowak A, Kacinski M (2009). Transcranial Doppler evaluation in migraineurs. *Neurol Neurochir Pol* **43**: 162–172.

103. Baumgartner RW, Mattle HP, Aaslid R (1995). Transcranial color-coded duplex sonography, magnetic resonance angiography, and computed tomography angiography: methods, applications, advantages, and limitations. *J Clin Ultrasound* **23**: 89–111.

104. de Bray JM, Joseph PA, Jeanvoine H, *et al.* (1988). Transcranial Doppler evaluation of middle cerebral artery stenosis. *J Ultrasound Med* **7**: 611–616.

105. Demchuk AM, Christou I, Wein TH, *et al.* (2000). Accuracy and criteria for localizing arterial occlusion with transcranial Doppler. *J Neuroimaging* **10**: 1–12.

106. Rorick MB, Nichols FT, Adams RJ (1994). Transcranial Doppler correlation with angiography in detection of intracranial stenosis. *Stroke* **25**: 1931–1934.

107. Sloan MA, Alexandrov AV, Tegeler CH, *et al.* (2004). Assessment: transcranial Doppler ultrasonography: report of the Therapeutics and Technology Assessment Subcommittee of the American Academy of Neurology. *Neurology* **62**: 1468–1481.

108. Wong KS, Li H, Lam WW, Chan YL, Kay R (2002). Progression of middle cerebral artery occlusive disease and its relationship with further vascular events after stroke. *Stroke* **33**: 532–536.

109. Zanette EM, Fieschi C, Bozzao L, *et al.* (1989). Comparison of cerebral angiography and transcranial Doppler sonography in acute stroke. *Stroke* **20**: 899–903.

110. Feldmann E, Wilterdink JL, Kosinski A, *et al.* (2007). The Stroke Outcomes and Neuroimaging of Intracranial Atherosclerosis (SONIA) trial. *Neurology* **68**: 2099–2106.

111. Alexandrov AV, Molina CA, Grotta JC, *et al.* (2004). Ultrasound-enhanced systemic thrombolysis for acute ischemic stroke. *N Engl J Med* **351**: 2170–2178.

112. Saqqur M, Uchino K, Demchuk AM, *et al.* (2007). Site of arterial occlusion identified by transcranial Doppler predicts the response to intravenous thrombolysis for stroke. *Stroke* **38**: 948–954.

113. Christou I, Alexandrov AV, Burgin WS, *et al.* (2000). Timing of recanalization after tissue plasminogen activator therapy determined by transcranial Doppler correlates with clinical recovery from ischemic stroke. *Stroke* **31**: 1812–1816.

114. Demchuk AM, Burgin WS, Christou I, *et al.* (2001). Thrombolysis In Brain Ischemia (TIBI) transcranial Doppler flow grades predict clinical severity, early recovery, and mortality in patients treated with intravenous tissue plasminogen activator. *Stroke* **32**: 89–93.

115. Imray CH, Tiivas CA (2005). Are some strokes preventable? The potential role of transcranial Doppler in transient ischaemic attacks of carotid origin. *Lancet Neurol* **4**: 580–586.

116. Markus HS, Droste DW, Kaps M, *et al.* (2005). Dual antiplatelet therapy with clopidogrel and aspirin in symptomatic carotid stenosis evaluated using Doppler embolic signal detection: the Clopidogrel and Aspirin for Reduction of Emboli in Symptomatic Carotid Stenosis (CARESS) trial. *Circulation* **111**: 2233–2240.

117. Poppert H, Sadikovic S, Sander K, Wolf O, Sander D (2006). Embolic signals in unselected stroke patients: prevalence and diagnostic benefit. *Stroke* **37**: 2039–2043.

118. Goutman SA, Katzan IL, Gupta R (2012). Transcranial Doppler with bubble study as a method to detect extracardiac right-to-left shunts in patients with ischemic stroke. *J Neuroimaging* Aug 28. doi:10.1111/j.1552-6569.2012.00738.x. [Epub ahead of print]

119. Esteban JM, Cervera V (2004). Perfusion CT and angio CT in the assessment of acute stroke. *Neuroradiology* **46**: 705–715.

120. Bash S, Villablanca JP, Jahan R, *et al.* (2005). Intracranial vascular stenosis and occlusive disease: evaluation with CT angiography, MR angiography, and digital subtraction angiography. *AJNR* **26**: 1012–1021.

121. Graf J, Skutta B, Kuhn FP, Ferbert A (2000). Computed tomographic angiography findings in 103 patients following vascular events in the posterior circulation: potential and clinical relevance. *J Neurol* **247**: 760–766.

122. Moll R, Dinkel HP (2001). Value of the CT angiography in the diagnosis of common carotid artery bifurcation disease: CT angiography versus digital subtraction angiography and color flow Doppler. *Eur J Radiol* **39**: 155–162.

123. Suwanwela NC, Phanthumchinda K, Suwanwela N (2002). Transcranial Doppler sonography and CT angiography in patients with atherothrombotic middle cerebral artery stroke. *AJNR* **23**: 1352–1355.

124. Nguyen-Huynh MN, Wintermark M, English J, *et al.* (2008). How accurate is CT angiography in evaluating intracranial atherosclerotic disease? *Stroke* **39**: 1184–1188.

125. Hirai T, Korogi Y, Ono K, *et al.* (2002). Prospective evaluation of suspected stenoocclusive disease of the intracranial artery: combined MR angiography and CT angiography compared with digital subtraction angiography. *AJNR* **23**: 93–101.

126. Lev MH, Segal AZ, Farkas J, *et al.* (2001). Utility of perfusion-weighted CT imaging in acute middle cerebral artery stroke treated with intra-arterial thrombolysis: prediction of final infarct volume and clinical outcome. *Stroke* **32**: 2021–2028.

127. Skutta B, Fürst G, Eilers J, Ferbert A, Kuhn FP (1999). Intracranial stenoocclusive disease: double-detector helical CT angiography versus digital subtraction angiography. *AJNR* **20**: 791–799.

128. Lubezky N, Fajer S, Barmeir E, Karmeli R (1998). Duplex scanning and CT angiography in the diagnosis of carotid artery occlusion: a prospective study. *Eur J Vasc Endovasc Surg* **16**: 133–136.

129. Gladstone DJ, Kapral MK, Fang J, Laupacis A, Tu JV (2004). Management and outcomes of transient ischemic attacks in Ontario. *CMAJ* **170**: 1099–1104.

130. Anderson GB, Ashforth R, Steinke DE, Ferdinandy R, Findlay JM (2000). CT angiography for the detection and characterization of carotid artery bifurcation disease. *Stroke* **31**: 2168–2174.

131. Berg MH, Manninen HI, Räsänen HT, Vanninen RL, Jaakkola PA (2002). CT angiography in the assessment of carotid artery atherosclerosis. *Acta Radiol* **43**: 116–124.

132. Leclerc X, Godefroy O, Lucas C, *et al.* (1999). Internal carotid arterial stenosis: CT angiography with volume rendering. *Radiology* **210**: 673–682.

133. Randoux B, Marro B, Koskas F, *et al.* (2001). Carotid artery stenosis: prospective comparison of CT, three-dimensional gadolinium-enhanced MR, and conventional angiography. *Radiology* **220**: 179–185.

134. Schellinger PD, Jansen O, Fiebach JB, *et al.* (2000). Feasibility and practicality of MR imaging of stroke in the management of hyperacute cerebral ischemia. *AJNR* **21**: 1184–1189.

135. Yucel EK, Anderson CM, Edelman RR, *et al.* (1999). AHA scientific statement: magnetic resonance angiography: update on applications for extracranial arteries. *Circulation* **100**: 2284–2301.

136. Qureshi AI, Isa A, Cinnamon J, *et al.* (1998). Magnetic resonance angiography in patients with brain infarction. *J Neuroimaging* **8**: 65–70.

137. Cosottini M, Pingitore A, Puglioli M, *et al.* (2003) Contrast-enhanced three-dimensional magnetic resonance angiography of atherosclerotic internal carotid stenosis as the noninvasive imaging modality in revascularization decision making. *Stroke* **34**: 660–664.

138. Goyal M, Nicol J, Gandhi D (2004). Evaluation of carotid artery stenosis: contrast-enhanced magnetic resonance angiography compared with conventional digital subtraction angiography. *Can Assoc Radiol J* **55**: 111–119.

139. Huston J 3rd., Fain SB, Wald JT, *et al.* (2001). Carotid artery: elliptic centric contrast-enhanced MR angiography compared with conventional angiography. *Radiology* **218**: 138–143.

140. Remonda L, Heid O, Schroth G (1998). Carotid artery stenosis, occlusion, and pseudo-occlusion: first-pass, gadolinium-enhanced, three-dimensional MR angiography: preliminary study. *Radiology* **209**: 95–102.

141. Serfaty JM, Chirossel P, Chevallier JM, *et al.* (2000). Accuracy of three-dimensional gadolinium-enhanced MR angiography in the assessment of extracranial carotid artery disease. *AJR* **175**: 455–463.

142. Westwood ME, Kelly S, Berry E, *et al.* (2002). Use of magnetic resonance angiography to select candidates with recently symptomatic carotid stenosis for surgery: systematic review. *BMJ* **324**: 198.

143. Berletti R, Cavagna E, Cimini N, Moretto G, Schiavon F (2002). Dissection of epiaortic vessels: clinical appearance and potentiality of imaging techniques [in English, Italian]. *Radiol Med* **107**: 35–46.

144. Clifton AG (2000). MR angiography. *Br Med Bull* **56**: 367–377.

145. Patel MR, Edelman RR (1996). MR angiography of the head and neck. *Top Magn Reson Imaging* **8**: 345–365.

146. Phan T, Huston J 3rd., Bernstein MA, Riederer SJ, Brown RD Jr (2001). Contrast-enhanced magnetic resonance angiography of the cervical vessels: experience with 422 patients. *Stroke* **32**: 2282–2286.

147. Okumura A, Araki Y, Nishimura Y, *et al.* (2001). The clinical utility of contrast-enhanced 3D MR angiography for cerebrovascular disease. *Neurol Res* **23**: 767–771.

148. Gelal FM, Kitis O, Calli C, *et al.* (2004). Craniocervical artery dissection: diagnosis and follow-up with MR imaging and MR angiography. *Med Sci Monit* **10**: MT109–MT116.b

149. Keller E, Flacke S, Gieseke J, *et al.* (1997). Craniocervical dissections: study strategies in MR imaging and MR angiography [in German]. *Rofo* **167**: 565–571.

150. Barr JD (2004). Cerebral angiography in the assessment of acute cerebral ischemia: guidelines and recommendations. *J Vasc Interv Radiol* **15**: S57–S66.

151. Citron SJ, Wallace RC, Lewis CA, *et al.* (2003). Quality improvement guidelines for adult diagnostic neuroangiography: cooperative study between ASITN, ASNR, and SIR [republished from *AJNR* 2000; 21: 146–150 and *J Vasc Interv Radiol* 2000 **11**: 129–134]. *J Vasc Interv Radiol* **14**: S257–S262.

152. Culebras A, Kase CS, Masdeu JC, *et al.* (1997). Practice guidelines for the use of imaging in transient ischemic attacks and acute stroke: a report of the Stroke Council, American Heart Association. *Stroke* **28**: 1480–1497.

153. Räsänen HT, Manninen HI, Vanninen RL, *et al.* (1999). Mild carotid artery atherosclerosis: assessment by 3-dimensional time-of-flight magnetic resonance angiography, with reference to intravascular ultrasound imaging and contrast angiography. *Stroke* **30**: 827–833.

154. Schenk EA, Bond MG, Aretz TH, *et al.* (1988). Multicenter validation study of real-time ultrasonography, arteriography, and pathology: pathologic evaluation of carotid endarterectomy specimens. *Stroke* **19**: 289–296.

155. Trystram D, Dormont D, Gobin Metteil MP, Iancu Gontard D, Meder JF (2002). Imaging of cervical arterial dissections: multi-center study and review of the literature [in French]. *J Neuroradiol* **29**: 257–263.

156. Warren DJ, Hoggard N, Walton L, *et al.* (2001). Cerebral arteriovenous malformations: comparison of novel magnetic resonance angiographic techniques and conventional catheter angiography. *Neurosurgery* **48**: 973–982.

157. Hankey GJ, Warlow CP, Sellar RJ (1990). Cerebral angiographic risk in mild cerebrovascular disease. *Stroke* **21**: 209–222.

158. Kaufmann TJ, Huston J 3rd., Mandrekar JN, *et al.* (2007). Complications of diagnostic cerebral

angiography: evaluation of 19,826 consecutive patients. *Radiology* **243**: 812–819.

159. Willinsky RA, Taylor SM, TerBrugge K, *et al.* (2003). Neurologic complications of cerebral angiography: prospective analysis of 2, 899 procedures and review of the literature. *Radiology* **227**: 522–528.

160. Johnston DC, Goldstein LB (2001). Clinical carotid endarterectomy decision making: noninvasive vascular imaging versus angiography. *Neurology* **56**: 1009–1015.

161. Nederkoorn PJ, Mali WP, Eikelboom BC, *et al.* (2002). Preoperative diagnosis of carotid artery stenosis: accuracy of noninvasive testing. *Stroke* **33**: 2003–2008.

162. Flis CM, Jäger HR, Sidhu PS (2007). Carotid and vertebral artery dissections: clinical aspects, imaging features and endovascular treatment. *Eur Radiol* **17**: 820–834.

163. Goyal MS, Derdeyn CP (2009). The diagnosis and management of supraaortic arterial dissections. *Curr Opin Neurol* **22**: 80–89.

164. Lev MH, Romero JM, Goodman DN, *et al.* (2003). Total occlusion versus hairline residual lumen of the internal carotid arteries: accuracy of single section helical CT angiography. *AJNR* **24**: 1123–1129.

165. Koroshetz WJ, Gonzalez G. (1997). Diffusion-weighted MRI: An ECG for "Brain Attack" (editorial, comment). *Annals Neurol* **41**:565–6.

166. Schramm P, Schellinger PD, Klotz E, *et al.* (2004). Comparison of perfusion computed tomography and computed tomography angiography source images with perfusion-weighted imaging and diffusion-weighted imaging in patients with acute stroke of less than 6 hours' duration. *Stroke* **35**: 1652–1658.

167. Agarwal P, Kumar S, Hariharan S, *et al.* (2004) Hyperdense middle cerebral artery sign: can it be used to select intra-arterial versus intravenous thrombolysis in acute ischemic stroke? *Cerebrovasc Dis* **17**: 182–190.

168. Bendszus M, Urbach H, Ries F, Solymosi L (1998). Outcome after local intra-arterial fibrinolysis compared with the natural course of patients with a dense middle cerebral artery on early CT. *Neuroradiology* **40**: 54–58.

169. Dittrich R, Kloska SP, Fischer T, *et al.* (2008). Accuracy of perfusion-CT in predicting malignant middle cerebral artery brain infarction. *J Neurol* **255**: 896–902.

170. Kakuda W, Hamilton S, Thijs VN, *et al.* (2008). Optimal outcome measures for detecting clinical benefits of early reperfusion: insights from the DEFUSE Study. *J Stroke Cerebrovasc Dis* **17**: 235–240.

171. Olivot JM, Mlynash M, Thijs VN, *et al.* (2008). Relationships between infarct growth, clinical outcome, and early recanalization in diffusion and perfusion imaging for understanding stroke evolution (DEFUSE). *Stroke* **39**: 2257–2263.

172. Thomalla G, Schwark C, Sobesky J, *et al.* (2006). Outcome and symptomatic bleeding complications of intravenous thrombolysis within 6 hours in MRI-selected stroke patients: comparison of a German multicenter study with the pooled data of ATLANTIS, ECASS, and NINDS tPA trials. *Stroke* **37**: 852–858.

173. Warach S (2001). New imaging strategies for patient selection for thrombolytic and neuroprotective therapies. *Neurology* **57**: S48–S52.

174. Warach S (2003). Measurement of the ischemic penumbra with MRI: it's about time. *Stroke* **34**: 2533–2534.

175. Wintermark M, Albers GW, Alexandrov AV, *et al.* (2008). Acute stroke imaging research roadmap. *Stroke* **39**: 1621–1628.

176. Albers GW, Thijs VN, Wechsler L, *et al.* (2006). Magnetic resonance imaging profiles predict clinical response to early reperfusion: the Diffusion and Perfusion Imaging Evaluation for Understanding Stroke evolution (DEFUSE) study. *Ann Neurol* **60**: 508–517.

177. Davis SM, Donnan GA, Parsons MW, *et al.* (2008). Effects of alteplase beyond 3 h after stroke in the Echoplanar Imaging Thrombolytic Evaluation Trial (EPITHET): a placebo-controlled randomised trial. *Lancet Neurol* **7**: 299–309.

178. Furlan AJ, Eyding D, Albers GW, *et al.* (2006). Dose Escalation of Desmoteplase for Acute Ischemic Stroke (DEDAS): evidence of safety and efficacy 3 to 9 hours after stroke onset. *Stroke* **37**: 1227–1231.

179. Grotta J (2002). Neuroprotection is unlikely to be effective in humans using current trial designs. *Stroke* **33**: 306–307.

180. Hacke W, Albers G, Al-Rawi Y, *et al.* (2005). The Desmoteplase in Acute Ischemic Stroke Trial (DIAS): a phase II MRI-based 9-hour window acute stroke thrombolysis trial with intravenous desmoteplase. *Stroke* **36**: 66–73.

181. Baird AE, Benfield A, Schlaug G, *et al.* (1997). Enlargement of human cerebral ischemic lesion volumes measured by diffusion-weighted magnetic resonance imaging. *Ann Neurol* **41**: 581–589.

182. Beaulieu C, de Crespigny A, Tong DC, *et al.* (1999). Longitudinal magnetic resonance imaging study of perfusion and diffusion in stroke: evolution of lesion volume and correlation with clinical outcome. *Ann Neurol* **46**: 568–578.

183. Tong DC, Yenari MA, Albers GW, *et al.* (1998). Correlation of perfusion- and diffusion-weighted MRI with NIHSS score in acute (< 6.5 hour) ischemic stroke. *Neurology* **50**: 864–870.

184. Arakawa S, Wright PM, Koga M, *et al.* (2006). Ischemic thresholds for gray and white matter: a diffusion and perfusion magnetic resonance study. *Stroke* **37**: 1211–1216.

185. Schaefer PW, Roccatagliata L, Ledezma C, *et al.* (2006). First-pass quantitative CT perfusion identifies thresholds for salvageable penumbra in acute stroke patients treated with intra-arterial therapy. *AJNR* **27**: 20–25.

186. Sobesky J, Zaro Weber O, Lehnhardt FG, *et al.* (2005). Does the mismatch match the penumbra? Magnetic resonance imaging and positron emission tomography in early ischemic stroke. *Stroke* **36**: 980–985.

187. Wintermark M, Flanders AE, Velthuis B, *et al.* (2006). Perfusion-CT assessment of infarct core and penumbra: receiver operating characteristic curve analysis in 130 patients suspected of acute hemispheric stroke. *Stroke* **37**: 979–985.

188. Gleason S, Furie KL, Lev MH, *et al.* (2001). Potential influence of acute CT on inpatient costs in patients with ischemic stroke. *Acad Radiol* **8**: 955–964.

189. Smith WS, Roberts HC, Chuang NA, *et al.* (2003). Safety and feasibility of a CT protocol for acute stroke: combined CT, CT angiography, and CT perfusion imaging in 53 consecutive patients. *AJNR* **24**: 688–690.

190. Josephson SA, Dillon WP, Smith WS (2005). Incidence of contrast nephropathy from cerebral CT angiography and CT perfusion imaging. *Neurology* **64**: 1805–1806.

191. Aspelin P, Aubry P, Fransson SG, *et al.*; Nephrotoxicity in High-Risk Patients Study of Iso-Osmolar and Low-Osmolar Non-Ionic Contrast Media Study Investigators (2003). Nephrotoxic effects in high-risk patients undergoing angiography. *N Engl J Med* **348**: 491–499.

192. Rudnick MR, Goldfarb S (2003). Pathogenesis of contrast-induced nephropathy: experimental and clinical observations with an emphasis on the role of osmolality. *Rev Cardiovasc Med* **4**: S28–S33.

193. Krol AL, Dzialowski I, Roy J, *et al.* (2007). Incidence of radiocontrast nephropathy in patients undergoing acute stroke computed tomography angiography [correction appears in *Stroke* 2007; 38: e97]. *Stroke* **38**: 2364–2366.

194. Wintermark M, Reichhart M, Cuisenaire O, *et al.* (2002). Comparison of admission perfusion computed tomography and qualitative diffusion- and perfusion-weighted magnetic resonance imaging in acute stroke patients. *Stroke* **33**: 2025–2031.

195. Wintermark M, Reichhart M, Thiran JP, *et al.* (2002). Prognostic accuracy of cerebral blood flow measurement by perfusion computed tomography, at the time of emergency room admission, in acute stroke patients. *Ann Neurol* **51**: 417–432.

196. Roberts HC, Roberts TP, Smith WS, *et al.* (2001). Multisection dynamic CT perfusion for acute cerebral ischemia: the "toggling-table" technique. *AJNR* **22**: 1077–1080.

197. Kribben A, Witzke O, Hillen U, *et al.* (2009). Nephrogenic systemic fibrosis: pathogenesis, diagnosis, and therapy. *J Am Coll Cardiol* **53**: 1621–1628.

198. Perez-Rodriguez J, Lai S, Ehst BD, Fine DM, Bluemke DA (2009). Nephrogenic systemic fibrosis: incidence, associations, and effect of risk factor assessment: report of 33 cases. *Radiology* **250**: 371–377.

199. Karnik R, Stelzer P, Slany J (1992). Transcranial Doppler sonography monitoring of local intra-arterial thrombolysis in acute occlusion of the middle cerebral artery. *Stroke* **23**: 284–287.

200. Butcher K, Parsons M, Allport L, *et al.* (2008). Rapid assessment of perfusion–diffusion mismatch. *Stroke* **39**: 75–81.

201. Butcher KS, Lee SB, Parsons MW, *et al.* (2007). Differential prognosis of isolated cortical swelling and hypoattenuation on CT in acute stroke. *Stroke* **38**: 941–947.

202. Hacke W, Furlan AJ, Al-Rawi Y, *et al.* (2009). Intravenous desmoteplase in patients with acute ischaemic stroke selected by MRI perfusion-diffusion weighted imaging or perfusion CT (DIAS-2): a prospective, randomised, double-blind, placebo-controlled study. *Lancet Neurol* **8**: 141–150.

Chapter 13

Acute, multifocal neurological symptoms

Joanna Kitley, Jacqueline A. Palace, Maria A. Rocca, and Massimo Filippi

Introduction

When a patient presents with multiple neurological symptoms not referable to a single anatomical location, they are said to have multifocal neurological symptoms. Although common in chronic disorders, where disease burden increases and spreads over time leading to progressive accumulation of symptoms and signs, multifocal neurological symptoms occurring acutely are relatively rare. When they do occur, they are usually caused by disorders of the central nervous system (CNS). Occasionally, peripheral nervous system disorders can also give rise to acute multifocal symptoms, for example in the context of mononeuritis multiplex. However, imaging plays little role in the evaluation of such patients and thus this chapter will focus primarily on acute CNS disorders.

CNS disorders causing multifocal neurological symptoms are usually inflammatory in nature. Although "dissemination in space," a term synonymous with multifocal CNS involvement, is usually reserved for multiple sclerosis (MS), many other inflammatory disorders can cause dissemination in space. The most frequent of these are acute disseminated encephalomyelitis (ADEM) and neuromyelitis optica (NMO), and these three disorders will form the bulk of this chapter. However, we will also briefly touch upon other inflammatory and non-inflammatory disorders that may also present with multifocal neurological symptoms.

Imaging is an essential tool in the work-up of patients presenting with acute inflammatory disorders of the CNS. Magnetic resonance imaging (MRI) is by far the most useful imaging modality for such patients, although occasionally computed tomography (CT) and other techniques such as non-invasive magnetic resonance angiography (MRA) can add valuable information. MRI is not only sensitive in detecting

inflammation, it also enables lesion localization and differentiation of inflammatory lesions from mimics such as neoplastic and vascular disease; some patterns of MRI abnormalities are characteristic of a disease almost to the point of being diagnostic, e.g. snowball lesions in Susac's syndrome. Thus, MRI is recommended as the mainstay of imaging for acute multifocal neurological symptoms.

Multiple sclerosis and clinically isolated syndromes

MS is the most common demyelinating disorder of the CNS. It presents most frequently in the third or fourth decades but onset can occur in childhood and later life. There is a female preponderance, which seems to be increasing, and the disease is more common in Caucasian populations. Although the disease can present insidiously as progressive neurological deterioration, the majority of adults – around 85% – and almost all pediatric patients present with acute or subacute neurological symptoms as a clinically isolated syndrome (CIS) and subsequently follow a relapsing remitting course.

Although a hallmark of MS is dissemination in space, i.e. multifocal inflammation of the CNS, the majority of clinically isolated syndromes are unifocal. However, a multifocal CIS can occur and some studies have suggested that this may increase the risk of developing clinically definite MS and be associated with greater disability over time.

A CIS most frequently involves the optic nerve, brainstem/cerebellum, or spinal cord. Typical presenting clinical features therefore are blurred vision with reduced color vision due to optic neuritis, and brainstem/cerebellar presentations with diplopia due to an internuclear ophthalmoplegia or VI cranial nerve

Imaging Acute Neurologic Disease, ed. Massimo Filippi and Jack H. Simon. Published by Cambridge University Press.
© Cambridge University Press 2014.

palsy, nystagmus, vertigo, or ataxia. Incomplete (partial) transverse myelitis frequently presents with lower limb paresthesia with or without limb weakness. Occasionally, symptomatic cerebral lesions can cause hemisensory disturbance or hemiparesis. Around 20% of adult patients will have a multifocal presentation with symptoms attributable to multiple anatomical locations, usually with a combination of features described above. Evidence of multifocal involvement on examination is more common than symptomatic multifocal presentations. For example, a patient presenting with optic neuritis may be found to have brisk reflexes on examination.

A multifocal presentation of MS is more common in children than in adults, occurring in up to 50% of patients. As is seen in adults, the typically affected regions are the optic nerves, spinal cord, brainstem, and/or cerebellum. Additionally, an ADEM-like presentation with encephalopathy occurs in around 25% of patients; this is particularly common in very young children. Moreover, many children presenting with multifocal symptoms and no encephalopathy never experience a recurrence of their neurological inflammation (i.e. never develop MS). Thus, it is extremely difficult at first presentation of a demyelinating CNS disorder to tell whether a child has ADEM or has a CIS and is likely to go on to develop MS.

Optic neuritis in CIS/MS is nearly always unilateral, is usually retrobulbar and thus not associated with disk swelling, and, even when severe, tends to recover well. Spinal cord lesions generally cause an incomplete transverse myelitis, which is usually sensory predominant and causes mild gait and/or sphincter disturbance. Severe paralysis or severe sphincter impairment are unusual at presentation. Brainstem presentations can be more troublesome and lead to disabling vertigo and ataxia. However, respiratory impairment, significant bulbar dysfunction, and impaired consciousness (except in young children) are rare.

Imaging in a CIS

MRI is the imaging modality of choice in patients presenting with a CIS. MRI can visualize the symptomatic lesion, exclude MS mimics such as vascular events and neoplasms, and also provides diagnostic and prognostic information – information on the likelihood of conversion to clinically definite MS and possibly also information on subsequent accumulation of disability.

Around 50–70% of patients presenting with a CIS have brain lesions at presentation that are not responsible for their clinical symptoms, i.e. they have asymptomatic brain lesions. These patients undoubtedly have a higher risk of subsequently developing MS than those whose brain scans lack asymptomatic lesions. Patients with a CIS and a normal scan have a roughly 20% chance of converting to clinically definite MS over time whilst those with MS-like lesions have around an 80% chance of developing MS, which will usually occur within 10 years.

MRI is highly important in the diagnosis of MS and various diagnostic criteria have been proposed. The most commonly used are the McDonald criteria, first established by an International Panel on the Diagnosis of MS in 2001. These criteria have recently been revised and simplified and now enable a diagnosis of MS to be made at presentation in CIS patients who have radiological evidence of dissemination in space and time (Table 13.1).

MRI brain lesions in MS are characteristically small and multiple T2 hyperintensities, though large and even tumefactive lesions can occur. These T2 hyperintensities have a predilection for the periventricular and juxtacortical white matter, corpus callosum, and posterior fossa. Lesions are often ovoid and orientated perpendicular to the lateral ventricles and corpus callosum, so called Dawson's fingers. Hypointensities or "black holes" may be seen on T1-weighted images, and acute lesions typically show post-contrast enhancement; this can be nodular, diffuse, or partially or completely ring-enhancing.

In patients presenting with a suspected CIS, spinal MRI can also be helpful. Spinal cord lesions are usually of short length (< 2 vertebral bodies), located

Table 13.1 2010 McDonald criteria

Dissemination in space	Clinically silent lesions in at least two of the following locations: • juxtacortical • periventricular • infratentorial • spinal cord
Dissemination in time	Presence of at least one clinically asymptomatic gadolinium-enhancing lesion and at least one clinically asymptomatic non-enhancing lesion on a scan, which can be the initial scan, OR A new lesion on a follow-up scan (timing of scan unimportant)

peripherally, and are most commonly seen in the cervical cord. Additionally, cord lesions are useful diagnostic features for MS when the brain MRI has white-matter lesions, which may be vascular or inflammatory in nature. Asymptomatic spinal cord lesions are common in patients with a CIS but rare in aging as well as in other inflammatory disorders, infections, and malignancies. Thus, asymptomatic spinal cord lesions are highly suggestive of a diagnosis of MS and may also predict conversion to clinically definite MS in patients presenting with a monofocal non-spinal CIS.

Other investigations in CIS/MS

Cerebrospinal fluid (CSF) examination can provide supportive evidence for a diagnosis of MS, since intrathecal synthesis of oligoclonal bands is seen in the majority; this holds true in both children and adults. A CSF pleocytosis may also be seen during an acute attack, but is usually mild (< 10 white-cell count), and a markedly elevated CSF white-cell count (>50) should prompt a search for an alternative diagnosis. The optic nerves may be affected subclinically and delayed visual-evoked potentials are also suggestive of the diagnosis in the appropriate clinical context.

Acute disseminated encephalomyelitis

ADEM is an acute inflammatory demyelinating disorder of the CNS that by definition is multifocal. Although more common than MS in childhood, it is rare in adults. The neurological features are preceded by infection in 50 to 75% of patients; this is usually a non-specific upper respiratory tract infection or flu-like illness. Less commonly, the neurological syndrome may be preceded by vaccination.

Clinical features of ADEM

ADEM can occur at any age and is most common in children and young adults, with a mean age at presentation of around 5 to 8 years. There may be a slight male preponderance though most studies report fairly equal gender distribution.

ADEM presents with a variety of neurological symptoms referable to the brain, brainstem, optic nerves, and spinal cord. Onset of symptoms occurs acutely or subacutely over hours to days. Where there is a history of preceding infection or vaccination, the neurological manifestations occur after a delay

of 2 to 28 days. Encephalopathy is considered a prerequisite for a diagnosis of ADEM and is included in the pediatric diagnostic criteria, defined as altered consciousness, behavior, or cognition [1]. However, encephalopathy may be lacking in adults, thus making ADEM difficult to distinguish from the first attack of MS. Even in children, studies that do not require encephalopathy for a diagnosis of ADEM have found this feature to be lacking in a substantial proportion of patients [2]. Encephalopathy in ADEM can be mild, manifesting only as irritability or lethargy, or can be severe and cause reduced conscious level and even coma. The common focal neurological symptoms of ADEM are motor and sensory deficits in the limbs, together with brainstem symptoms and signs such as diplopia, dysarthria, and ataxia. Optic-nerve involvement can cause unilateral or, more commonly, bilateral optic neuritis with visual loss and deficits in color vision with or without pain on eye movement. Spinal cord involvement is also relatively common and can result in sphincter disturbance and para- or quadraparesis. Seizures may also occur, particularly in children; these are usually partial motor seizures and can cause status epilepticus. Meningismus is seen in up to 30% of patients and fever is also common. Less frequently, extrapyramidal signs occur due to basal ganglia or thalamic involvement. Peripheral nervous system involvement causing polyradiculoneuropathy may also be seen in ADEM, though it is not a typical feature and is considered to be rare, particularly in childhood ADEM.

Imaging in ADEM

Although CT may demonstrate abnormalities, MRI is the radiological investigation of choice in patients with suspected ADEM. MRI lesions are best seen as hyperintensities on T2-weighted or fluid-attenuated inversion recovery (FLAIR) sequences. Lesions are usually numerous, widespread, poorly demarcated, involve both white and gray matter, occur supra- and infratentorially and are usually bilateral but asymmetric. Involvement of deep-gray-matter nuclei, particularly the basal ganglia and thalamus, is typical. Mild mass effect is common, but mass effect may be severe enough to cause raised intracranial pressure and rarely tentorial herniation. Although one would expect all lesions in ADEM to be of the same age, and this is considered a typical appearance, lesions can evolve over weeks and thus it is not uncommon to see some that enhance post contrast and others that do not.

Contrast enhancement of ADEM lesions may be completely or partially ring enhancing or more focal and patchy.

Proposed diagnostic criteria for ADEM [3] suggest that MRI shows only acute lesions, which are typically multiple, include at least one large lesion, are supra- and infra-tentorial and may or may not involve the basal ganglia or enhance after administration of gadolinium.

Involvement of the spinal cord is also common radiologically. Lesions are typically longitudinally extensive and may involve the entire cord. Edema and post-contrast enhancement within the cord are common. Idiopathic acute transverse myelitis is probably an anatomically limited ADEM phenotype.

Differentiating ADEM from MS

A few studies have directly compared the radiological features of ADEM and MS [4, 5]. However, it is important to note that the age of presentation may influence MRI appearances; a study comparing the imaging features in childhood to adult ADEM noted more cerebellar and spinal cord, and less medullary and periventricular abnormalities in children. Thus, some observed differences between MS and ADEM may not be pathological distinguishers unless the groups are age-matched. It is generally accepted that ADEM lesions are ill-defined and diffuse whilst MS lesions are more sharply demarcated. However, in clinical practice, particularly in the acute setting, we often observe fluffy, ill-defined lesions in MS. Although ADEM lesions are typically numerous, one study comparing MRI features of ADEM and MS in children [5] found that the number of T2 lesions did not differ between the groups, although MS scans had a significantly higher number of periventricular lesions. This same study found that the frequency of involvement of cortical gray matter and deep gray nuclei, a feature typically associated with ADEM, was not different between ADEM and MS pediatric patients. Additionally, the presence and number of large lesions was also not a differentiating factor. Factors that did differentiate ADEM from MS scans were a diffuse bilateral distribution and the absence of chronic or non-enhancing black holes in ADEM. This group proposed the Callen criteria for differentiating ADEM from MS, which require the presence of two out of three of: $\geq$ two periventricular lesions, presence of black holes, and absence of diffuse bilateral lesion distribution for a diagnosis of

MS over ADEM. This model has been found to have a specificity and sensitivity for MS of 95% and 81%, respectively, and has been validated by an independent group who found a sensitivity of 75% and specificity of 95% [2]. Other criteria that have been assessed in differentiating MS from ADEM include: the KIDMUS criteria, which require the presence of either lesions perpendicular to the long axis of the corpus callosum or the sole presence of well-defined lesions and have a high specificity for MS but only moderate sensitivity; and the Barkhof criteria with a sensitivity of 61% and specificity of 91%. In clinical practice, we would also consider the presence of hemorrhage specific to ADEM over MS, although clearly other diagnoses including vasculitis and malignancy would need to be excluded. Additionally, lesions of different ages are in favor of a diagnosis of MS rather than an acute monophasic disorder, as are development of new lesions at a different site once the acute phase is settling; substantial or complete resolution of lesions without development of new lesions on follow-up imaging is more suggestive of ADEM.

Using magnetization transfer (MT) MRI and diffusion tensor (DT) MRI, in pooled groups of patients, no abnormalities of the normal-appearing brain tissue and spinal cord have been detected in ADEM patients after the acute phase of the disease [6], whereas mild DT MRI abnormalities of the basal ganglia have been described [7]. Proton magnetic resonance spectroscopy (^{1}H-MRS) studies provided conflicting results in ADEM: some authors found no metabolic abnormalities in the acute stage of the disease, and others described a transient decrease of N-acetylaspartate (NAA) in regions corresponding to T2 lesions on the ^{1}H-MRS results obtained during the acute phase, which normalized after clinical recovery [8, 9]. Note that these advanced quantitative measures are not currently routinely used in the individual patient.

Other investigations in ADEM

The CSF in ADEM is usually inflammatory, with a mild to moderate lymphocytic pleocytosis (typically < 200) and moderately elevated protein count. An elevated IgG index may occur and oligoclonal bands may also be seen in the acute setting and thus cannot be used to differentiate ADEM from a CIS; nor can they be used to predict recurrent disease. Peripheral blood markers of inflammation, such as C-reactive protein and erythrocyte sedimentation rate, may be elevated and there may be a pleocytosis. Some patients may have serological evidence of an infectious trigger, such as positive mycoplasma pneumoniae or influenza serology. Antibodies to myelin oligodendrocyte glycoprotein, a CNS-specific myelin antigen, have recently been described in childhood ADEM. However, they have also been reported in pediatric MS and patients with NMO spectrum disorders, and thus, although high serum titers of this autoantibody are suggestive of ADEM, further studies defining their role are necessary before they can be used reliably as a biomarker.

Neuromyelitis optica

NMO is an autoimmune disorder of the CNS caused by autoantibodies against aquaporin-4, the most abundant water channel in the CNS. Although NMO was originally described as a brain-sparing monophasic inflammatory disorder in which optic neuritis and transverse myelitis occurred simultaneously or sequentially (Devic's syndrome), it is now recognized that the majority of NMO patients follow a relapsing course, usually have optic neuritis and myelitis attacks that are separated by months or years, and not infrequently have involvement of the brain. The original "Devic's phenotype" of simultaneous or rapidly sequential optic neuritis and myelitis is now known to be relatively rare; such patients are usually negative for aquaporin-4 antibodies, and monophasic NMO may represent an "opticospinal" form of ADEM.

Demographic and clinical features of NMO

NMO can occur at any age, with a mean age at onset of around 40 years, though patients without aquaporin-4 antibodies may be younger. NMO with aquaporin-4 antibodies has a strong female preponderance (up to 10:1), whilst the sex ratio is almost equal in antibody-negative patients with monophasic NMO. Although occurring worldwide in all ethnic groups, NMO with aquaporin-4 antibodies is over-represented in Afro-Caribbean and Asian populations.

As mentioned, a classic "Devic's NMO" phenotype of simultaneous optic neuritis and myelitis is rare in NMO patients with aquaporin-4 antibodies, occurring in less than 10% of such patients. Nevertheless, NMO patients with aquaporin-4 antibodies can still present with acute multifocal polysymptomatic presentations, for example with acute brain lesions or with brain

or brainstem lesions plus myelitis or optic neuritis. In fact, symptomatic brain lesions as the first presentation of NMO have been shown to occur in 16% of children and brain involvement as the first clinical manifestation is also common in Asians, occurring in 18% of patients. The clinical manifestations of brain lesions in NMO include: vomiting, hiccups, ataxia, and tetraparesis caused by periaqueductal lesions and lesions around the third and fourth ventricles; diplopia, bulbar dysfunction, and facial sensory disturbance from lesions involving the midbrain, anterior pons, middle cerebellar peduncles, and medulla; and ataxia, diplopia, internuclear ophthalmoplegia, hemisensory loss, and hemiparesis from lesions of the dorsolateral pons and superior cerebellar peduncle. Hypothalamic disturbance manifesting as hypersomnolence, hyperphagia, or hyponatremia may also be seen, and encephalopathy can occur, particularly in children and non-Caucasian patients.

Optic neuritis in aquaporin-4 antibody-positive NMO is typically unilateral and severe but may be bilateral in up to one-third of cases. Recovery is often poor, with up to 40% of patients being left blind in one eye after a single attack. Myelitis in NMO is also usually severe, with limb weakness and marked sphincter involvement, and, in contrast to the myelitis attacks in MS, patients are often unable to walk at nadir. Another striking feature of myelitis in NMO is association with severe back, neck, or trunk pain, which may be the presenting feature. Painful dystonic spasms may also occur. Table 13.2 summarizes the clinical feature of CIS/MS, ADEM and MS.

Imaging in NMO

Since the discovery of aquaporin-4 antibodies, there has been a wealth of studies describing brain MRI findings in NMO. It is now clear that, in contrast to original beliefs that NMO was a brain-sparing disease, a substantial proportion of patients have brain involvement, at least radiologically. By far the most common abnormalities in NMO are multiple T2 white-matter lesions that are "non-specific" or "MS-like"; many patients even fulfill radiological MS diagnostic criteria. These non-specific lesions seem to occur in around two-thirds of NMO patients, on average in most series, and sometimes greater. Studies looking more closely at these lesions have revealed important differences when compared to lesions seen in MS. NMO lesions are predominantly

Table 13.2 Clinical features differentiating CIS/MS, ADEM, and NMO

Clinical feature	CIS/MS	ADEM	NMO
Onset age	Mean 30, rare in < 10 or > 50 years	Children or young adults, mean 5–7 years	Any age, mean 40 years
Male:female	Female preponderance	Equal	Strong female preponderance
Ethnicity	Rare in non-Caucasian populations	All ethnicities	All ethnicities but over-represented in non-Caucasian populations
Coexisting autoimmune disorders	Uncommon	Rare	Common (thyroid disease, myasthenia, SLE, Sjogren's syndrome)
Preceding illness	Uncommon	Common	Uncommon
Fever	Rare	Common	Rare
Encephalopathy	Rare except in children	Common	Uncommon except in children
Seizures	Rare	Can occur	Rare
Optic neuritis	Common, nearly always unilateral and associated with good recovery	Common, usually bilateral	Common, usually unilateral and severe, although bilateral not uncommon
Myelitis	Usually sensory predominant with mild sphincter disturbance	May be severe with limb paresis and sphincter involvement	Often severe with limb paresis, severe sphincter involvement, loss of multiple sensory modalities
Brain and brainstem involvement	Vertigo, diplopia, internuclear ophthalmoplegia, hemisensory disturbance	Headache, hemisensory disturbance, hemiparesis, altered level of consciousness	Brainstem involvement common with hiccups and vomiting, diplopia, bulbar and respiratory dysfunction

Abbreviations: ADEM, acute disseminated encephalomyelitis; CIS, clinically isolated syndrome; MS, multiple sclerosis; NMO, neuromyelitis optica; SLE, systemic lupus erythematosus.

located in the subcortical and deep white matter, in contrast to MS lesions, which are largely periventricular. Absence of cortical lesions can also help differentiate NMO from MS. Large lesions are more common in NMO than MS in the splenium of the corpus callosum. Recently, it was shown that the presence of at least one lesion both adjacent to the body of the lateral ventricle and in the inferior temporal lobe, or either a Dawson's finger-like lesion perpendicular to the lateral ventricle or a subcortical U-fiber lesion distinguished MS from NMO with a greater than 90% specificity and sensitivity, whereas 27% of abnormal NMO brain scans fulfilled the Barkhof criteria for MS [10]. Figure 13.1 compares the characteristic white-matter lesions of MS, ADEM, and NMO.

Whilst small T2 white-matter lesions are the common brain MRI finding in NMO, they are not specific for the disease. However, other brain abnormalities have been identified that are highly characteristic for NMO (Figure 13.2). These include lesions around the third and fourth ventricles in the hypothalamus and area postrema and surrounding the aqueduct of Sylvius; these areas are rich in aquaporin-4.

Lesions in the area postrema at the floor of the fourth ventricle are thought to be responsible for the characteristic prodrome of vomiting and hiccups that occurs in around 10% of NMO patients at first presentation. This region lacks an intact blood–brain barrier and has also been implicated as the entry site for serum aquaporin-4 antibodies into the CNS. However, whilst highly characteristic for NMO, these lesions in aquaporin-4-rich regions only occur in between 5 and 10% of patients.

Other brain abnormalities seen in NMO include brainstem lesions, particularly of the centro-dorsal medulla and the pons, and large, even tumefactive, hemispheric lesions, which are seen relatively commonly in children and may also be more frequent in non-Caucasian populations.

Longitudinally extensive transverse myelitis, defined as T2 hyperintensity on spinal MRI extending beyond three vertebral segments, has long been recognized as a hallmark of NMO, and is incorporated into the clinical diagnostic criteria [11]. The fact that the majority of NMO patients have such lesions has been confirmed in many studies, though it is recognized

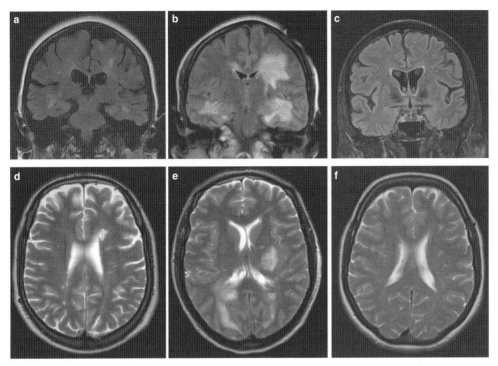

Figure 13.1 Comparison of brain lesions in a CIS/MS, ADEM, and NMO; (a)–(c): coronal FLAIR images, (d)–(f) axial T2-weighted images. MS lesions (a, d) tend to be small, numerous, and well defined and occur adjacent to the lateral ventricles, often with a perpendicular orientation. ADEM lesions (b, e) are often large, numerous, bilateral but asymmetrical, fluffy, and involve both gray and white matter. Lesions in NMO (c, f) are usually small, round, and well defined and occur in subcortical or deep white matter locations.

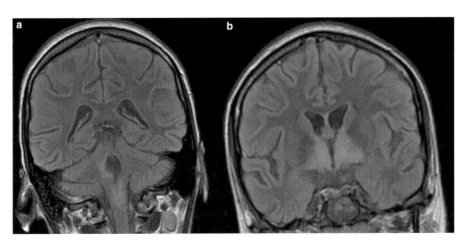

Figure 13.2 Classic brain lesions of aquaporin-4 antibody-positive NMO showing high signal on coronal FLAIR images around the fourth ventricle (a) and in the hypothalamus and surrounding the third ventricle (b). Such lesions occur in less than 10% of NMO patients but are very characteristic.

that short cord lesions of less than three vertebral segments can also occur. The spinal lesions in NMO have a propensity to involve the central gray matter, with relative sparing of peripheral white matter, are often associated with cord edema, tend to occur in the cervical and upper- to mid-thoracic cord, and may be associated with hypointensity on T1-weighted imaging in the acute setting (Figure 13.3). In contrast, MS lesions tend to be posterior or lateral, are of short length, and are rarely associated with T1

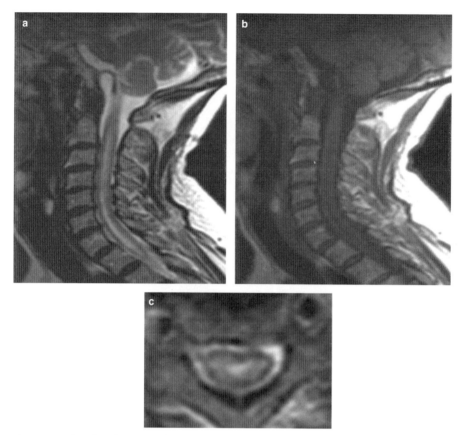

Figure 13.3 Spinal-cord MRI scan of a patient with aquaporin-4 antibody-positive NMO showing classic findings of: (a) longitudinally extensive signal change in the the cervical cord with (b) hypointensity on T1-weighted images and (c) involvement of the central gray matter with relative peripheral sparing on axial imaging.

hypointensity. Table 13.3 summarizes the MRI features of CIS/MS, ADEM and NMO.

MT MRI studies in patient groups have suggested that this technique can contribute to distinguish patients with NMO from those with MS, since focal T2 lesions of the brain (whenever present) have higher MTR values in NMO than in MS patients [12], and, in contrast to MS, NMO patients have no abnormalities in the normal-appearing brain tissue [12]. Conversely, cervical cord damage, quantified using MT MRI, is similar in NMO and MS patients [12]. However, a DT MRI study disclosed more severe cervical cord damage in NMO than in MS patients [13]. The assessment of brain normal-appearing white matter and gray-matter damage in NMO patients gave conflicting results: some authors found an isolated involvement of the gray matter [14], and others described an involvement of several white-matter tracts [15], which was more severe in the optic radiation and the corticospinal tracts [16].

Other investigations in NMO

CSF in NMO is often inflammatory with a pleocytosis that is usually lymphocytic but which may also contain neutrophils and eosinophils. The pleocytosis is usually moderate. A CSF cell count of > 200 would be unusual. CSF protein may also be moderately elevated but rarely is above 1g/dl. CSF oligoclonal bands can occur in the acute setting but usually disappear if repeated when the disease is quiescent. Both organ-specific and non-organ-specific autoimmune disorders may coexist in NMO patients, including myasthenia gravis, Sjögren's syndrome, systemic lupus erythematosus (SLE), and thyroid disease. Thus, the presence of other auto-antibodies, particularly antinuclear antibody (ANA), is common and can be an important diagnostic clue.

Other inflammatory disorders

The majority of patients presenting with acute multi-focal inflammation of the CNS will have one of the

Table 13.3 MRI features of CIS/MS, ADEM, and NMO

MRI brain features	CIS/MS	ADEM	NMO
Lesion location and characteristics	Periventricular white matter, juxtacortical, cerebellum, brainstem, corpus callosum, ovoid, small and well demarcated	White and gray matter, particularly basal ganglia and thalamus; diffuse, poorly demarcated lesions	Deep white matter, brainstem, hypothalamus; lesions usually small and well demarcated
Periventricular lesions	Common, usually adjacent to lateral ventricles	Uncommon	Uncommon, but when occurring are characteristic and seen adjacent to third and fourth ventricles and aqueduct
Symmetry of lesions	Asymmetrical in brain and cord	Can be symmetrical	Asymmetrical in brain but cord lesions usually central and symmetrical
Chronic or non-enhancing hypointensity on T1-weighted images	Common	Rare	Rare
Lesion size	Usually small	Often large and confluent	Usually small, but unusual appearances and large not uncommon
Post-gadolinium enhancement	Common, often nodular	Common, often extensive and in multiple lesions	Relatively uncommon except in acutely symptomatic brain lesions, and with unusual patterns
MRI cord features			
Axial location	Usually lateral	Any	Usually central > lateral
Sagittal location	Cervical > thoracic	Any	Cervical and thoracic
Lesion length	Short ≤ two segments	Long to very long	Long to very long
Cord edema	Rare	Common	Common
Post-contrast enhancement	Less common	Common	Common
Hypointensity on T1-weighted images	Very rare	Can occur	Common
Asymptomatic lesions	Common	Uncommon	Rare

Abbreviations: ADEM, acute disseminated encephalomyelitis; CIS, clinically isolated syndrome; MS, multiple sclerosis; NMO, neuromyelitis optica.

three disorders described above. However, there are many other inflammatory disorders that can mimic MS and which should be included in the differential diagnosis of acute CNS inflammation. Most of these present more insidiously but occasionally acute presentations may be seen.

Neurosarcoidosis

Sarcoidosis is a multisystem granulomatous disorder that often affects the lungs, lymph nodes, skin, and eyes, but which can affect virtually any organ. It frequently presents between the ages of 20 and 40 years and is more common in patients of African ethnicity. CNS involvement occurs in between 5 and 10% of patients and can occasionally be the presenting feature. However, evidence of involvement of other systems is usually seen and isolated neurosarcoidosis accounts for less than 1% of cases of sarcoidosis.

Although neurosarcoidosis can affect any part of the nervous system, it has a predilection for the base of the brain; cranial neuropathies are therefore the

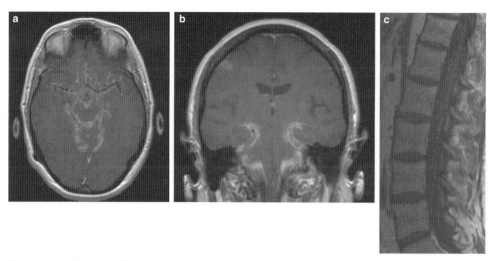

Figure 13.4 (a) Axial and (b) coronal post-gadolinium T1-weighted images demonstrating florid basal leptomeningeal enhancement surrounding the brainstem and cerebellum. (c) Post-contrast sagittal spinal cord imaging in neurosarcoidosis demonstrating nodular enhancement of the surface of the conus medullaris and nerve roots of the cauda equina.

most frequent manifestation. The most commonly affected nerves are the facial and optic nerves, followed by the cranial nerves III, VI, and VIII. Aseptic meningitis causing headaches, nausea, and vomiting is also relatively common. Symptomatic CNS parenchymal lesions are a less common presentation although these do occasionally occur.

Spinal sarcoidosis is not infrequent but, in contrast to most other inflammatory disorders, intramedullary lesions are rare; arachnoiditis and extramedullary granulomas are more common and can give rise to radiculopathies and cauda equina syndrome.

The characteristic MRI abnormality in neurosarcoidosis is basal leptomeningeal enhancement (Figure 13.4), although this is seen in less than half of cases. More commonly, periventricular white-matter lesions occur, which are similar to those seen in MS. Intraparenchymal lesions can also occur and hydrocephalus may be seen as a complication of basal meningitis.

CSF is usually abnormal; the most common abnormality is a raised CSF protein, which may be massively elevated. A lymphocytic pleocytosis occurs in around half of patients and occasionally a low glucose level is seen. Oligoclonal bands are rare. Sarcoidosis should be suspected in patients with concurrent respiratory or systemic symptoms. All patients should undergo a chest radiograph to look for pulmonary involvement and, if clinical suspicion remains high, a high-resolution chest CT and pulmonary function tests should be performed.

Sjögren's syndrome

Sjögren's syndrome is an autoimmune disease that characteristically causes xerophthalmia and xerostomia due to lymphocytic infiltration of exocrine glands. It is more common in women and usually manifests in middle age. The peripheral nervous system is commonly involved; this usually causes a slowly progressive sensory-predominant axonal neuropathy, small-fiber neuropathy, or sensory ataxic neuropathy but can occasionally present acutely with mononeuritis multiplex. The CNS features of Sjögren's syndrome are less well characterized. Probably the most common CNS manifestation is acute myelitis, which is often associated with longitudinally extensive signal change on MRI. Optic neuritis is also fairly common. Optic neuritis and myelitis in Sjögren's syndrome are usually associated with aquaporin-4 antibodies and probably represent coexisting NMO, since Sjögren's patients lacking these features have been shown to be aquaporin-4 antibody-negative. Occasionally Sjögren's syndrome can present with acute focal or multifocal brain lesions, which may be "stroke-like" or resemble MS. MRI often shows "MS-like" white-matter lesions, but the corpus callosum is rarely involved and there may be prominent involvement of deep-gray-matter structures, particularly the basal ganglia. In contrast to MS, CSF oligoclonal bands are only found in a minority. Up to half of patients with Sjögren's syndrome and CNS involvement will be positive for anti-Ro or anti-La antibodies and a positive ANA or rheumatoid factor may also occur. Schirmer's tear test or the Rose-Bengal test looking for keratoconjunctivitis are often positive and biopsy of the minor salivary glands usually shows infiltration by mononuclear cells.

Neurolupus

SLE is a multisystem autoimmune disease that can cause a variety of clinical symptoms as a result of involvement of organs including the skin, joints, lungs, and kidneys. It is over-represented in Afro-Caribbean populations and has a female preponderance. The neurological manifestations are usually neuropsychiatric; behavioral and psychiatric disturbance with or without cognitive impairment occur, and seizures are also common. Focal neurological symptoms due to vascular occlusion occur less commonly but may result in acute presentations. Histological analysis of neurolupus in general is more in keeping with vascular than inflammatory pathology. Opticospinal syndromes can also occur in SLE but, as is seen in Sjögren's syndrome, this is normally in association with aquaporin-4 antibodies and probably represents co-occurrence of NMO. Most patients with SLE have a positive ANA, and anti-double-stranded DNA (anti-dsDNA) antibodies are positive in around 70% of patients. Antiphospholipid antibodies may also be positive.

MRI abnormalities are commonly indistinguishable from those of MS. However, the predominance of lesions located at the cortical or subcortical junction (Figure 13.5), as well as the concomitant finding of brain infarcts, calcification, or hemorrhages, should always raise the suspicion of neuropsychiatric systemic immune-mediated diseases, small-vessel vasculitides, or antiphospholipid antibody syndrome (either primary or secondary to systemic immune-mediated diseases). In these latter disorders, enhancing lesions and T1 black holes are much less common than in MS and this could also be a suggestive feature. By contrast to MS, spinal cord lesions are rare in systemic immune-mediated diseases, and can completely disappear after steroid or immunosuppressive treatment.

Neuro-Behçet's disease

Behçet's disease is a multisystem inflammatory disorder of unknown cause, which occurs most commonly in the Middle and Far East and in the Mediterranean basin. It is rare in Europe and North America. It is more common in males than females and usually presents in the third or fourth decade. Recurrent oral ulceration is a pre-requisite for diagnosis and patients often have other systemic manifestations such as arthralgia, anterior or posterior uveitis, skin lesions such as folliculitis or erythema nodosum, or genital ulcers. Neurological involvement in Behçet's disease is rare, and usually occurs in patients with a history of systemic Behçet's symptoms; neurological involvement as the first manifestation is infrequent.

There are two types of neurological involvement in Behçet's – parenchymal disease and non-parenchymal disease. Whilst non-parencyhmal disease generally presents chronically with a syndrome of raised intracranial pressure due to venous sinus thrombosis, parenchymal disease usually presents acutely or subacutely with a meningoencephalitis that can cause multifocal

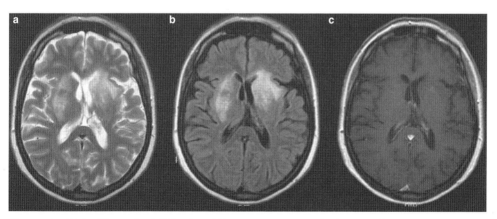

Figure 13.5 (a) Axial T2-weighted, (b) FLAIR, and (c) post-contrast T1-weighted images of the brain from a patient with neurolupus. Diffuse bilateral abnormalities of the basal ganglia are visible, with partial mass effect on the left lateral ventricle. No enhancement is detected after gadolinium administration.

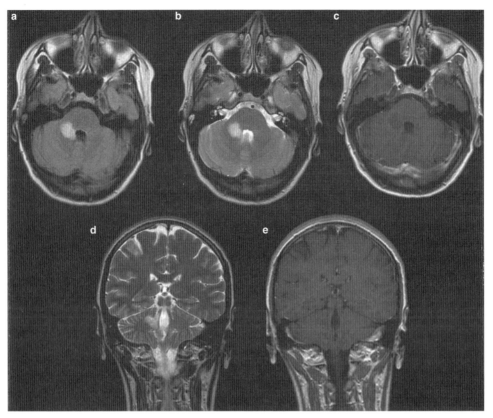

Figure 13.6 (a) Axial FLAIR, (b) T2-weighted, (c) post-contrast T1-weighted, (d) sagittal T2-weighted,and (e) post-contrast T1-weighted images of the brain from a patient with Behçet's disease. A lesion, hyperintense on FLAIR and T2-weighted images, is visible at the level of the right middle cerebellar peduncle, extending towards the pons and the right superior cerebellar peduncle. No enhancement is seen.

neurological symptoms. This typically occurs in the context of worsening of the systemic manifestations of Behçet's disease, and thus fever, oral, or genital ulceration, skin lesions, and uveitis can provide important clues to the diagnosis. Parenchymal Behçet's disease has a propensity to involve the brainstem and basal ganglia (Figure 13.6). Brainstem symptoms and signs including diplopia due to ophthalmoplegia, other cranial neuropathies, hemiparesis, and hemisensory disturbance with pyramidal signs are therefore common; surprisingly, given the frequency of basal ganglia involvement, extrapyramidal features are rare. Brainstem symptoms are often accompanied by headache, and behavioral change such as apathy or disinhibition is not unusual. The spinal cord is involved in a proportion of patients, who may report sphincter disturbance or have a paraparesis.

The MRI brain scan in acute parenchymal Behçet's disease is fairly stereotypical, with a large lesion in the upper brainstem extending into diencephalic structures, often with contrast enhancement and edema; bilateral changes occur in up to a third of cases.

Linear high signal in the internal capsule is also a characteristic feature. The cerebral cortex and cerebellum are usually spared. There may also be T2 high-signal abnormalities in the spinal cord, even in asymptomatic patients; longitudinally extensive signal change can occur. Another important clue to the diagnosis of Behçet's disease is the presence of a neutrophil-predominant pleocytosis in the CSF.

Primary CNS angiitis

Primary CNS angiitis is a rare disorder resulting in inflammation and destruction of CNS vessels without evidence of vasculitis outside the CNS. It can occur at any age, with a mean age at onset of around 50 years, though it is uncommon in the elderly. Men are twice as commonly affected as women. Although constitutional upset including fever, weight loss, and lethargy are rare, the majority of patients experience headache, which is usually chronic and progressive. Other neurological symptoms result predominantly from cerebral ischemia, which affects different

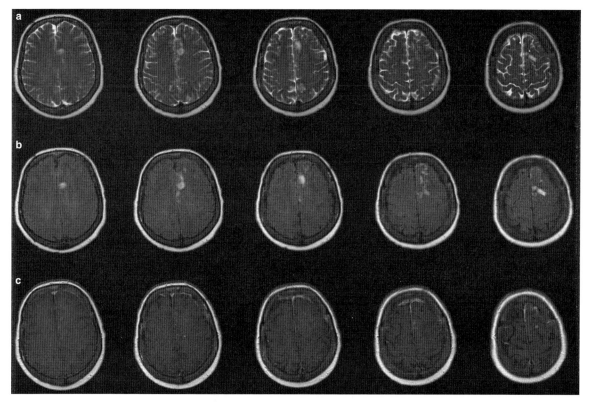

Figure 13.7 (a) Axial T2-weighted, (b) FLAIR, and (c) post-contrast T1-weighted images of the brain from a patient with primary CNS angiitis, who underwent brain biopsy. A subcortical lesion, involving the corpus callosum and cingulum, is visible in the left frontal lobe. Such a lesion appears as hyperintense on T2-weighted and FLAIR images and enhances after gadolinium administration.

vascular territories and can cause symptoms such as hemiparesis, aphasia, ataxia, visual-field defects, diplopia, and dysarthria. Insidious cognitive impairment is also a relatively common occurrence.

MRI abnormalities include T2 hyperintensities in subcortical white matter, deep gray matter, deep white matter, and the cortex (Figure 13.7). Multiple infarcts affecting different vascular territories are seen and microhemorrhages may be visible on gradient-echo sequences. Up to 10% of patients will have leptomeningeal enhancement and spinal cord involvement occurs in up to 15% of cases, usually simultaneously with brain involvement. Cerebral angiography may show beading of vessels, which typically occurs bilaterally. However, owing to frequent involvement of small- to medium-sized vessels, angiographic studies may be normal. Brain biopsy has a high diagnostic yield. Abnormal CSF findings occur in up to 90% of patients and usually consist of a moderate lymphocytic pleocytosis, moderately elevated protein, negative oligoclonal bands, and normal glucose levels.

Non-inflammatory vasculopathies and vascular causes

Susac's syndrome

Susac's syndrome is an immune-mediated endotheliopathy that affects the microvasculature of the brain, retina, and inner ear. It is most common in women aged 20 to 40 years. It is characterized by the clinical triad of encephalopathy, hearing loss, and branch retinal artery occlusion. Although it typically presents insidiously, more acute presentations can occur. Branch retinal artery occlusion may be subtle and asymptomatic or may cause unilateral or bilateral visual impairment. The hearing loss is commonly bilateral, though is often asymmetrical and may occur very suddenly; accompanying tinnitus can occur. The encephalopathy may present insidiously as headache, often migrainous, or may present with acute or subacute neuropsychiatric features. Brain MRI often shows multiple small cerebral white-matter lesions resembling

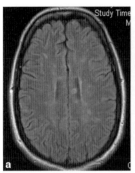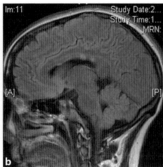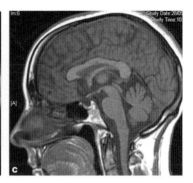

Figure 13.8 (a) Axial and (b) sagittal FLAIR and (c) sagittal T1-weighted images in Susac's syndrome demonstrating: (a) numerous small deep-white-matter hyperintensities and a central lesion within the corpus callosum and (b) multiple corpus callosal lesions. Some of the callosal lesions appear hypointense on the T1-weighted scan (c).

MS, which may enhance post-gadolinium. Central corpus callosal lesions, which may be very large (snow-ball lesions), are highly suggestive; such lesions are hypointense on T1-weighted images (Figure 13.8). Other MRI abnormalities that may occur include lesions in the deep gray nuclei and leptomeningeal enhancement. Cerebral angiography is normal as it is the small precapillary arterioles that are involved. Audiometry is helpful in demonstrating low-frequency hearing loss and formal ophthalmological assessment is essential if the diagnosis is suspected since branch retinal artery occlusion may be asymptomatic.

Posterior reversible encephalopathy syndrome

Posterior reversible encephalopathy syndrome (PRES) is a disorder of unknown cause, which can occur at any age and affects both genders equally. It has numerous triggers including acute hypertension, child birth, sepsis, renal failure, and immunosuppressant drugs. It is characterized by acute vasogenic edema, which has a predisposition for the parieto-occipital lobes. It presents acutely, usually over hours with acute neurological symptoms that usually occur alongside profound systemic hypertension. Seizures are the most frequent neurological symptom and are usually generalized tonic–clonic in nature; status epilepticus can occur. Headache, a degree of encephalopathy, and visual disturbance are also common; the latter may take the form of blurred vision, homonymous hemianopia, visual hallucinations, or cortical blindness. Less-frequent neurological manifestations include hemiparesis, brainstem symptoms such as diplopia, facial numbness and dysarthria, and ataxia. Brisk reflexes and upgoing plantar responses are not infrequent.

Although CT may show abnormalities in 50% of patients, MRI is the imaging modality of choice. This will show bilateral, often symmetrical, T2 high-signal lesions that occur predominantly in the parieto-occipital lobes, but which also commonly affect the frontal lobes and can also involve the basal ganglia, brainstem, and cerebellum. Although lesions are predominantly subcortical, cortical involvement may also be seen. Lesions tend not to enhance post contrast. In around 10 to 15% of patients, microhemorrhages or intraparechymal hematomas may also be seen. A hallmark of PRES is the diffusion-weighted MRI, which does not show hypointensity (restricted diffusion) on the apparent diffusion coefficient (ADC) map. This finding enables differentiation of PRES from posterior ischemia. MRA or catheter angiography may show vasoconstriction or vasodilation but are not necessary for a diagnosis to be made.

Cerebral autosomal dominant arteriopathy with subcortical infarcts and leukoencephalopathy

Cerebral autosomal dominant arteriopathy with subcortical infarcts and leukoencephalopathy (CADASIL) is a rare genetic disorder causing migraine, cognitive impairment, and multiple infarcts. Rarely, it can present acutely with multifocal infarcts, and is worth mentioning because of its characteristic MRI appearances. Diffuse T2 high-signal change is seen in the superior frontal lobes, anterior temporal lobes, and external capsule (Figure 13.9), and

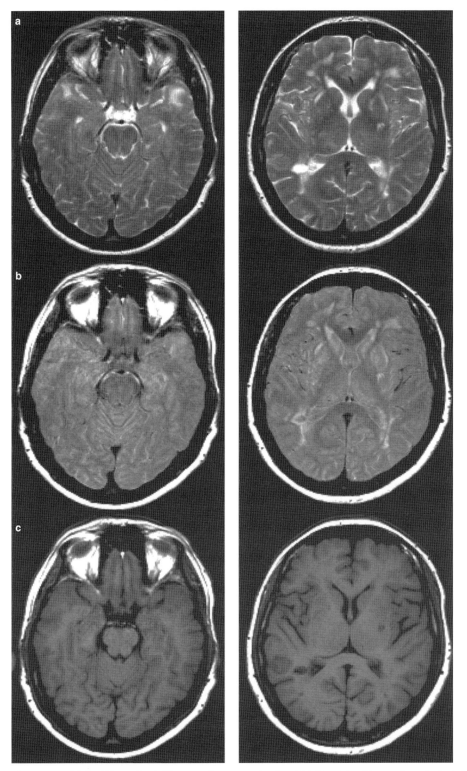

Figure 13.9 (a) Axial T2-weighted, (b) proton-density-weighted, and (c) T1-weighted images from the brain from a patient with CADASIL. Multiple T2 high-signal lesions are visible in the superior frontal lobes, anterior temporal lobes, and external capsule. Some of these lesions appear hypointense on the T1-weighted scan (c).

microhemorrhages are usually visible on gradient-echo sequences.

Thromboembolic disease

Embolic stroke can sometimes present with multifocal neurological symptoms if a shower of emboli occurs or if a single embolus fragments in the cerebral circulation. Although CT may be adequate for diagnosing large infarcts, it is less useful in the investigation of early acute and small embolic infarcts, particularly when the posterior circulation is affected. MRI remains the imaging modality of choice, where diffusion-weighted imaging will be positive in acute imaging, with characteristic restricted diffusion on ADC maps.

Miscellaneous causes of acute multifocal neurological symptoms

Infectious causes

Many infections can cause acute multifocal neurological symptoms and are a major differential diagnosis for CNS inflammatory disorders. These include syphilis, neuroborreliosis, toxoplasmosis, human immunodeficiency virus (HIV), and botulism. Many of these have been discussed in other chapters and will not be covered here.

Malignant causes

Malignancies, both primary and secondary, usually present insidiously but can occasionally cause acute or subacute neurological symptoms. Brain metastases, commonly from neoplasms of the breast or lung or from malignant melanoma are often multifocal. Primary neoplasms of the CNS, including lymphoma and gliomas, can also be multifocal. Lymphoma in particular can be difficult to differentiate from inflammatory causes because it may respond dramatically over the short term to corticosteroids. Intravascular lymphomas can cause multiple infarcts due to occlusion of small vessels by malignant cells. Neoplastic meningitis (carcinomatosis), occurring in patients with solid tumors, primary brain neoplasms, or hematological malignancies can also present with multifocal neurological symptoms. Neoplastic meningitis usually occurs in patients with evidence of disseminated malignancy and is often associated with intraparenchymal metastases. The most common clinical features are headache, cognitive disturbance, and cranial neuropathies. Spinal involvement can also occur, giving rise to radicular pain, sphincter disturbance, and limb weakness and paresthesia. MRI will show diffuse or focal leptomeningeal enhancement; involvement of the spinal cord is influenced by gravity and thus the cauda equina and caudal sac is frequently affected. Malignant cells can be detected in the CNS in up to 90% of patients.

Toxic and metabolic causes

Central pontine myelinolysis

Central pontine myelinolysis is a disorder that is usually seen in patients with chronic alcoholism. Acute demyelination occurs in the corticospinal and corticobulbar tracts in the pons. The condition presents subacutely with impaired consciousness, quadraparesis, pseudobulbar palsy, and extrapyramidal symptoms. MRI reveals T2 hyperintensity in the pons, which is usually central with peripheral sparing. Often there is also extra-pontine involvement including the deep-gray-matter nuclei, cerebellum, and, occasionally, the cortex.

Marchiafava–Bignami syndrome

Marchiafava–Bignami syndrome also usually occurs in alcoholics. Clinically, it presents with seizures, impaired consciousness, and pyramidal tract signs. Characteristically there is demyelination and necrosis of the corpus callosum, predominantly of the genu and splenium. Restricted diffusion may occur and other brain regions may be affected.

Drugs and toxins

Drugs and toxins can cause acute white-matter disorders of the CNS. These include methanol, ethylene glycol, and heroin and should be considered in the differential diagnosis of acute white-matter disorders when clinical suspicion is high.

Multifocal symptoms with normal imaging

Bickerstaff brainstem encephalitis

Bickerstaff brainstem encephalitis (BBE) refers to cases where the clinical triad of encephalopathy, ophthalmoplegia, and ataxia and an association with serum anti-GQ1b IgG antibodies is reported. There is overlap with the Miller Fisher syndrome (MFS) which also features areflexia and a higher incidence of anti-GQ1b IgG antibodies but without encephalopathic features. These two conditions appear to be on a spectrum with BBE having more central characteristics and MFS having more peripheral features (and indeed overlaps with Guillain–Barré syndrome). It can occur at any age, with a mean of 40 years, and has a slight male predominance. The vast majority of cases are preceded by an antecedent illness, usually a mild upper respiratory-tract infection, occurring between 1 and 30 days before the onset of neurological symptoms. Apart from the classic triad, other features include abnormal pupillary light reflexes, facial-nerve palsies, ptosis, bulbar palsy, extensor plantars, impaired proprioception, and mild limb weakness. GQ1b antibodies are positive in around 70% of cases and CSF protein is usually elevated. Brain MRI is normal in the majority of cases, although high-signal T2 abnormalities may be seen in the brainstem, cerebellum, or thalamus.

Functional neurological disorders

In patients presenting with multifocal neurological symptoms and a normal brain MRI, a functional neurological disorder should always be considered.

References

1. Krupp L, Banwell B, Tenembaum S (2007). Consensus definitions proposed for pediatric multiple sclerosis and related disorders. *Neurology* **68**: S7–S12.

2. Ketelslegers I, Visser I, Neuteboom R, *et al.* (2010). Disease course and outcome of acute disseminated encephalomyelitis is more severe in adults than in children. *Mult Scler* **17**: 441–448.

3. Miller D, Weinshenker B, Filippi M, *et al.* (2008). Differential diagnosis of suspected multiple sclerosis: a consensus approach. *Mult Scler* **14**: 1157–1174.

4. Schwarz S, Mohr A, Knauth M, *et al.* (2001). Acute disseminated encephalomyelitis. A follow up study of 40 adult patients. *Neurology* **56**: 1313–1318.

5. Callen D, Schroff M, Branson H, *et al.* (2009). Role of MRI in the differentiation of ADEM from MS in children. *Neurology* **72**: 968–973.

6. Inglese M, Salvi F, Iannucci G, *et al.* (2002). Magnetization transfer and diffusion tensor MR imaging of acute disseminated encephalomyelitis. *AJNR* **23**: 267–272.

7. Holtmannspötter M, Inglese M, Rovaris M, *et al.* (2003). A diffusion tensor MRI study of basal ganglia from patients with ADEM. *J Neurol Sci* **206**: 27–30.

8. Bizzi A, Uluğ AM, Crawford TO, *et al.* (2001). Quantitative proton MR spectroscopic imaging in acute disseminated encephalomyelitis. *AJNR* **22**: 1125–1130.

9. Balasubramanya KS, Kovoor JM, Jayakumar PN, *et al.* (2007). Diffusion-weighted imaging and proton MR spectroscopy in the characterization of acute disseminated encephalomyelitis. *Neuroradiology* **49**: 177–183.

10. Matthews L, Marasco R, Jenkinson M, *et al.* (2013). Distinction of seropositive NMO spectrum disorder and MS brain lesion distribution. *Neurology* **80**: 1330–1337.

11. Wingerchuk D, Lennon V, Pittock S, Lucchinetti C, Weinshenker B (2006). Revised diagnostic criteria for neuromyelitis optica. *Neurology* **66**: 1485–1489.

12. Filippi M, Rocca MA, Moiola L, *et al.* (1999). MRI and magnetization transfer imaging changes in the brain and cervical cord of patients with Devic's neuromyelitis optica. *Neurology* **53**: 1705–1710.

13. Benedetti B, Valsasina P, Judica E, *et al.* (2006). Grading cervical-cord damage in neuromyelitis optica and MS by diffusion tensor MRI. *Neurology* **67**: 161–163.

14. Rocca MA, Agosta F, Mezzapesa DM, *et al.* (2004). Magnetization transfer and diffusion tensor MRI show gray matter damage in neuromyelitis optica. *Neurology* **62**: 476–478.

15. Liu Y, Duan Y, He Y, *et al.* (2012). A tract-based diffusion study of cerebral white matter in neuromyelitis optica reveals widespread pathological alterations. *Mult Scler* **18**: 1013–1021.

16. Zhao DD, Zhou HY, Wu QZ, *et al.* (2012). Diffusion tensor imaging characterization of occult brain damage in relapsing neuromyelitis optica using 3.0 T magnetic resonance imaging techniques. *Neuroimage* **59**: 3173–3177.

Suggested further reading

ADEM

Alper G (2012). Acute disseminated encephalomyelitis. *J Child Neurol* **27**: 1408–1425.

Dale R, de Sousa C, Chong W, *et al.* (2000). Acute disseminated encephalomyelitis, multiphasic disseminated encephalomyelitis and multiple sclerosis in children. *Brain* **123**: 2407–2422.

Lin C-H, Jeng J-S, Hsieh S-T, Yip P-K, Wu R-M (2007). Acute disseminated encephalomyelitis: a follow-up study in Taiwan. *J Neurol Neurosurg Psychiatry* **78**: 162–167.

Palace J (2011). Acute disseminated encephalomyelitis and its place amongst other acute inflammatory demyelinating CNS disorders. *J Neurol Sci* **306**: 188–191.

Tenembaum S, Chamoles N, Fejerman N (2002). Acute disseminated encephalomyelitis. A long-term follow-up study of 84 pediatric patients. *Neurology* **59**: 1224–1231.

Tenembaum S, Chitnis T, Ness J, *et al.* (2007). Acute disseminated encephalomyelitis. *Neurology* **68**(suppl 2): S23–S36.

MS

Eckstein C, Saidha S, Levy M (2012). A differential diagnosis of central nervous system demyelination: beyond multiple sclerosis. *J Neurol* **259**: 801–816.

Filippi M, Rocca M (2011). MR imaging of multiple sclerosis. *Radiology* **259**: 659–681.

Giorgio A, Battaglini M, Assunta Rocca M, *et al.* (2013). Location of brain lesions predicts conversion of clinically isolated syndromes to multiple sclerosis. *Neurology* **80**: 234–241.

Miller D, Chard D, Ciccarelli O (2012). Clinically isolated syndromes. *Lancet Neurol* **11**: 157–169.

NMO

Cabrera-Gomez J, Kister I (2012). Conventional brain MRI in neuromyelitis optica. *Eur J Neurol* **19**: 812–819.

Calabrese M, Oh M, Favaretto M, *et al.* (2012). No MRI evidence of cortical lesions in neuromyelitis optica. *Neurology* **79**: 1671–1676.

Chan K, Tse C, Chung C, *et al.* (2011). Brain involvement in neuromyelitis optica spectrum disorders. *Arch Neurol* **68**: 1432–1439.

Jacob A, McKeon A, Nakashima I, *et al.* (2013). Current concept of neuromyelitis optica (NMO) and NMO spectrum disorders. *J Neurol Neurosurg Psychiatry* **84**: 922–930.

Krampla W, Aboul-Enein F, Jecel J, *et al.* (2009). Spinal cord lesions in patients with neuromyelitis optica: a retrospective long-term MRI follow-up study. *Eur Radiol* **19**: 2535–2543.

Lennon V, Kryzer T, Pittock S, Verkman A, Hinson S (2005). IgG marker of optic-spinal multiple sclerosis binds to the aquaporin-4 water channel. *J Exp Med* **202**: 473–477.

Nakamura M, Miyazawa I, Fujihara K, *et al.* (2008). Preferential spinal central gray matter involvement in neuromyelitis optica. An MRI study. *J Neurol* **255**: 163–170.

Pittock S, Weinshenker B, Lucchinetti C, *et al.* (2006). Neuromyelitis optica brain lesions localized at sites of high aquaporin 4 expression. *Arch Neurol* **63**: 964–968.

Wingerchuk D, Hogancamp W, O'Brien P, Weinshenker B (1999). The clinical course of neuromyelitis optica (Devic's syndrome). *Neurology* **53**: 1107–1114.

Wingerchuk D, Lennon V, Lucchinetti C, Pittock S, Weinshenker B (2007). The spectrum of neuromyelitis optica. *Lancet Neurol* **6**: 805–815.

Other

Akman-Demir G, Serdaroglu P, Tasci B, *et al.* (1999). Clinical patterns of neurological involvement in Behçet's disease: evaluation of 200 patients. *Brain* **122**: 2171–2181.

Akman-Demir G, Bahar S, Coban O, Tasci B, Serdaroglu P (2003). Cranial MRI in Behçet's disease: 134 examinations of 98 patients. *Neuroradiology* **45**: 851–859.

Al-Araji A, Kidd D (2009). Neuro-Behçet's disease: epidemiology, clinical characteristics, and management. *Lancet Neurol* **8**: 192–204.

Birnbaum J, Hellmann D (2009). Primary angiitis of the central nervous system. *Arch Neurol* **66**(6): 704–709.

Chai J, Logigian E (2010). Neurological manifestations of primary Sjögren's syndrome. *Curr Opin Neurol* **23**: 509–513.

Fugate J, Claasen D, Cloft H, *et al.* (2010). Posterior reversible encephalopathy syndrome: associated clinical and radiologic findings. *Mayo Clin Proc* **85**(5): 427–432.

Gleissner B, Chamberlain M (2006). Neoplastic meningitis. *Lancet Neurol* **5**: 443–452.

Gono T, Kawaguchi Y, Katsumata Y, *et al.* (2011). Clinical manifestations of neurological involvement in primary Sjögren's syndrome. *Clin Rheumatol* **30**: 485–490.

Hajj-Ali R, Singhai A, Benseler S, *et al.* (2011). Primary angiitis of the CNS. *Lancet Neurol* **10**: 561–572.

Hoitsma E, Faber C, Drent M, Sharma O (2004). Neurosarcoidosis: a clinical dilemma. *Lancet Neurol* **3**: 397–407.

Ideguchi H, Suda A, Takeno M, *et al.* (2010). Neurological manifestations of Behçet's disease in Japan: a study of 54 patients. *J Neurol* **257**: 1012–1020.

Ito M, Kuwabara S, Odaka M, *et al.* (2008). Bickerstaff's brainstem encephalitis and Fisher syndrome form a continuous spectrum. Clinical analysis of 581 cases. *J Neurol* **255**: 674–682.

Joseph F, Scolding N (2007). Sarcoidosis of the nervous system. *Pract Neurol* **7**: 234–244.

Joseph F, Scolding N (2010). Neurolupus. *Pract Neurol* **10**: 4–15.

Mori K, Iijima M, Koike H, *et al.* (2005). The wide spectrum of clinical manifestations in Sjögren's syndrome-associated neuropathy. *Brain* **128**: 2518–2534.

Odaka M, Yuki N, Yamada M, *et al.* (2003). Bickerstaff's brainstem encephalitis: clinical features of 62 cases and a subgroup associated with Guillain–Barré syndrome. *Brain* **126**: 2279–2290.

Pavlakis P, Alexopoulos H, Kosmidis M, *et al.* (2012). Peripheral neuropathies in Sjögren's syndrome: a critical update on clinical features and pathogenetic mechanisms. *J Autoimmun* **39**: 27–33.

Pula J, Eggenberger E (2008). Posterior reversible encephalopathy syndrome. *Curr Opin Ophthalmol* **19**: 479–484.

Roth C, Ferbert A (2011). The posterior reversible encephalopathy syndrome: what's certain, what's new? *Pract Neurol* **11**: 136–144.

Salvarani C, Brown RD Jr, Calamia K, *et al.* (2007). Primary central nervous system vasculitis: analysis of 101 patients. *Ann Neurol* **62**: 442–451.

Smith J, Matheus M, Castillo M (2004). Imaging findings of neurosarcoidosis. *AJR* **182**: 289–295.

Stern B, Krumholz A, Johns C, *et al.* (1985). Sarcoidosis and its neurological manifestations. *Arch Neurol* **42**: 909–917.

Yuki N (2009). Fisher syndrome and Bickerstaff brainstem encephalitis (Fisher–Bickerstaff syndrome). *J Neuroimmunol* **215**: 1–9.

Zajicek J, Scolding N, Foster O, *et al.* (1999). Central nervous system sarcoidosis – diagnosis and management. *QJM* **92**: 103–117.

Acute brain trauma

Carl D. Stevens and Jack H. Simon

Introduction

This chapter covers the clinical and imaging evaluation of closed head injuries. It focuses primarily on
the initial evaluation and management of mild to
moderate traumatic brain injury (TBI), as these injuries of lesser severity account for the vast majority of
patients confronted by the typical clinician practising
in civilian settings. The discussion centers on
deceleration-induced head injuries, those incurred
by patients in the setting of unintentional injuries
such as falls or motor-vehicle crashes in which the
head strikes a hard object with sudden deceleration
of the skull and its contents, or intentional injuries
in which the head is struck with a blunt object.
Penetrating brain injury is not discussed here, as
these less-common, generally devastating types of
head trauma require specialized imaging and interventions that lie beyond the scope of this book. The
discussion emphasizes injuries incurred in civilian
settings, and does not cover concussive blast injuries
and other combat-related traumatic brain injuries.
Newly identified entities such as "chronic traumatic
encephalopathy," which may result from repeated
minor brain injuries sustained in professional and
amateur sports such as football, hockey, and boxing
also lie beyond the scope of practice of the typical
clinician, require specialized evaluation and treatment, and are not covered here.

At least 1.7 million people seek medical attention
for a TBI each year in the United States. These injuries result in nearly 1.4 million emergency department (ED) visits, 275 000 hospitalizations, and 52 000
deaths. Approximately three -uarters of these injuries
constitute concussions, or other minor TBIs [1].
Worldwide estimates for TBI are about 10 million
people affected annually. Although falls account for a
majority of ED visits and hospitalizations, motor-
vehicle crashes cause the greatest number of fatal
TBIs. Falls predominate as the causes of brain injury
in children and the elderly, with motor-vehicle
crashes causing most brain injuries in working-aged
adults [2].

As might be expected given the complexity of the
organ itself, a vast, highly nuanced, and somewhat
daunting literature exists surrounding the optimal
management of brain trauma and the role of neuroimaging in particular. To appreciate the challenging
nature of even the most routine cases, consider the
following scenario: a toddler running through a
playground trips and strikes his forehead on the
jungle gym. He appears momentarily dazed, but
within seconds awakens and is crying loudly. When
brought to the local ED by a concerned parent, he is
noted to be fully alert and behaving normally, with a
small contusion and hematoma to his forehead. The
unenviable dilemma faced by the physician evaluating such patients is as follows: based on clinical
factors, the child has less than a 3% chance of having
any detectable intracranial injury, and the likelihood
of any lesion requiring surgery is extremely low –
but not zero. However, the consequences of missing
such a lesion would be medically devastating to the
child and legally catastrophic for the physician. Then
again, the lifetime attributable risk for death from
cancer due to radiation exposure from a single head
CT in an infant or very young child may reach
1:1000 [3]. Clearly, the clinicians have their work
cut out. This chapter seeks to summarize and distill
the literature on imaging of brain trauma into usable
guidelines and principles for generalist clinicians
and trainees. Reference material at the end of the
chapter directs readers to sources providing greater
detail or more precise evaluation and treatment
recommendations.

Imaging Acute Neurologic Disease, ed. Massimo Filippi and Jack H. Simon. Published by Cambridge University Press.

Clinical assessment

The chapter starts with three clinical-encounter-oriented sections concerned with the initial assessment of head trauma, with the goal of rapid identification of critical findings that require immediate action. This is followed by a broader discussion that is focused primarily upon the imaging evaluation utilized in the initial and early post-trauma interval, together constituting the comprehensive imaging assessment in the minutes, hours, and days following head trauma.

Clinical assessment is arranged in escalating order of injury severity. The Glasgow Coma Scale (GCS) developed by Teasdale and Jennett in the mid 1970s provides a systematic scoring of injury severity based on clinical parameters [4] (Table 14.1), and a convenient tool for clinicians to separate patients with head injuries into broad severity categories. GCS scores range from 3 (1–1–1) in comatose patients, to 15 (4–5–6) in alert, behaviorally intact individuals.

We begin with a discussion of minor head injury in adults and children (GCS 14–15). The focus of this section is the clinical evaluation of the patient and the application of validated decision rules to achieve selective use of imaging, without placing patients at undue risk of missed intracranial injuries requiring surgery. The next section discusses patients with moderate head injuries, GCS 9–13 at initial evaluation, indicating persistent deficits in eye-opening, verbalization, or motor function. All of these higher-risk patients require immediate imaging with non-contrast brain

computed tomography (CT) to exclude operable, primarily extra-axial hematomas. This section will include a discussion of imaging abnormalities that are often seen in this intermediate severity group of patients, which generally do not dictate specific treatment interventions but which, as markers of possible later deterioration, may indicate a need for more prolonged observation than is indicated for simple concussion. This is followed by a brief discussion of severe brain injury, patients with GCS 8 or less at initial evaluation who require immediate rapid sequence induction and endotracheal intubation prior to undergoing CT imaging to assess for operable blood collections. Many of these unfortunate patients will turn out to have extensive diffuse axonal injury (DAI), sometimes accompanied by parenchymal contusions, hematomas, and varying amounts of cerebral edema, with resulting compression of brain structures. Although craniectomy may be performed as a salvage procedure in some of these patients, these more severe diffuse injuries are not generally amenable to medical or surgical intervention to reverse brain injury and prevent long-term disability.

Throughout the chapter, two overarching principles apply across the injury severity spectrum, and therefore need not be restated within each section. (1) The immediate imaging modality of choice in acute trauma is non-contrast head CT. Magnetic resonance imaging (MRI) may replace CT at some point in the future; however, at present, considerations of

Table 14.1 Glasgow Coma Scale scoring in adults and children. Adapted from [5]. Reprinted with permission from EB Medicine, publisher of *Emergency Medicine Practice*, from: Haydel M. Management of mild traumatic brain injury in the emergency department. *Emerg Med Pract* 2012;14(9):1–24. www.ebmedicine.net.

Component	Adults	Score	Children	Score
Best eye opening	Spontaneous	4	Spontaneous	4
	To verbal stimuli	3	To verbal stimuli	3
	To painful stimuli	2	To painful stimuli	2
	No eye opening	1	No eye opening	1
Best verbal response	Oriented	5	Appropriate coo and cry	5
	Confused	4	Irritable cry	4
	Inappropriate words	3	Inconsolable crying	3
	Incomprehensible	2	Grunts	2
	No verbal response	1	No verbal response	1
Best motor response	Obeys commands	6	Normal, spontaneous movement	6
	Localizes pain	5	Withdraws to touch	5
	Withdraws to pain	4	Withdraws to pain	4
	Flexion to pain	3	Flexion to pain	3
	Extension to pain	2	Extension to pain	2
	No motor response	1	No motor response	1
	Total	–	Total	–

cost, accessibility, speed, and compatibility with ventilators and other equipment make CT the clear choice at most emergency care facilities. (2) Across the entire spectrum of head-injury severity, the first purpose of early CT imaging is to detect clinically significant hematomas, predominantly acute extra-axial (epidural or subdural) hematomas, to ensure that they can be surgically decompressed within the 30–60-minute timeframe before permanent neurologic injury occurs [1]. In other words, the pivotal, unifying principle across the severity spectrum in head-injury patients is that, unless clinical factors indicate that the patient is at extremely low risk, clinicians rapidly perform one test (non-contrast CT) to detect one injury type (operable hematoma). Keeping this principle in mind will make it easier to follow the discussion of the various brain-injury severity classes and the other imaging modalities and treatments that may come into play after the initial evaluation is completed, and the additional prognostic and treatment planning information that may be sought by the clinical team.

Minor head injury (GCS 14–15)

Clinical evaluation

History: Obtaining as detailed a description as possible of the injury-producing event from the patient, bystanders, and paramedics or ambulance personnel is critical to risk-stratification and evaluation of patients with closed head injury. Often, the available history will be incomplete and may well be inaccurate. The occurrence and duration of any loss of consciousness are important, but generally imprecise. It is important to remember that patients without loss of consciousness can still have significant, life-threatening intracranial injury. A history of seizure activity is important to elicit, both to aid in risk-stratification and as a possible cause of the injury-producing event. The patient and available observers should be questioned about vomiting, memory of events before and after the injury occurred, alcohol and drug ingestion, as well as past medical history and current medications, with a particular focus on anti-platelet (including aspirin) and anticoagulant use, as these medications increase the risk of intracranial hemorrhage and dictate more prolonged observation following even minor head injury [5].

Physical examination: Data to populate the GCS eye-opening, verbal response, and motor response subscales should be collected at the time of initial evaluation, and these should be compared with the paramedics' initial assessment scores if available. A focused examination of the head for external signs of trauma including scalp hematoma, lacerations, facial deformities, and evidence of hemotympanum, as well as a careful pupillary examination and assessment of extraocular eye movements should be recorded. A focused neurologic examination of cranial nerve, motor, sensory, and cognitive function, and balance, if the patient can ambulate, aid in the assessment of likelihood of intracranial injury, as do signs of concussion.

Laboratory: Routine laboratory studies are generally non-contributory, and could be limited to a point-of-care blood glucose measurement if there is a question of a syncopal fall. Patients taking anticoagulant medications should have coagulation studies, and those who appear intoxicated may benefit from serum alcohol and toxicology screening. Some may ultimately require contrast-enhanced CT; consequently, serum creatinine for estimated glomerular filtration rate (eGFR) calculation may be helpful if other blood samples are to be acquired.

Patients with minor-head-injury mechanisms by history who arrive in the ED or other care setting completely intact neurologically have an extremely low likelihood of a surgically treatable intracranial injury. Therefore, following a focused history and physical examination, the next priority is to decide on the need for neuroimaging to exclude the slight possibility of an operable hematoma. Numerous decision rules based on clinical factors have been developed and validated in a variety of settings to aid the clinician in deciding whether to obtain a head CT scan as part of the initial evaluation. Increasing concerns over both radiation exposure and cost make it important for the clinician to be aware of these decision rules and reflect their application in the medical record, regardless of what ultimate decision is made on imaging. In adults, two decision-rule sets have gained broadest use, the New Orleans criteria and the Canadian CT head rule (Table 14.2). CT scans should be obtained for patients meeting the criteria for either of the two decision rules [6]. Several decision rules specifically for the evaluation of children have also been published and validated. The Pediatric Emergency Care Applied Research Network (PECARN) clinical decision rule for children (Table 14.3) has received the broadest external validation and constitutes an appropriate approach for use in children [7].

Table 14.2 New Orleans criteria and Canadian CT head rule. Adapted from [5]. Reprinted with permission from EB Medicine, publisher of Emergency Medicine Practice, from: Haydel M. Management of mild traumatic brain injury in the emergency department. *Emerg Med Pract* 2012;14(9):1–24. www.ebmedicine.net.

	New Orleans criteria	Canadian CT head rules
CT if any criteria present	<ul><li>Headache</li><li>Vomiting (any)</li><li>Age > 60 years</li><li>Drug or alcohol intoxication</li><li>Seizure</li><li>Trauma visible above clavicles</li><li>Short-term memory deficits</li></ul>	<ul><li>Dangerous mechanism of injury*</li><li>Vomiting ≥ 2 times</li><li>Patient > 65 years</li><li>GCS score < 15.2 h postinjury</li><li>Any sign of basal skull fracture</li><li>Possible open or depressed skull fracture</li><li>Amnesia for events 30 min before injury</li></ul>
Need for neurosurgical intervention	Sensitivity: 99–100% Specificity: 10–20%	Sensitivity: 99–100% Specificity: 36–76%
Clinically significant intracranial injury	Sensitivity: 95–100% Specificity: 10–33%	Sensitivity: 80–100% Specificity: 35–50%

*Dangerous mechanisms of injury include ejection from a motor vehicle, a pedestrian struck by a motor vehicle, or a fall from a height of > 3 ft (0.9 m) or 5 steps.

Table 14.3 PECARN Clinical Decision Rule. Adapted from [5]. Reprinted with permission from EB Medicine, publisher of *Emergency Medicine Practice*, from: Haydel M. Management of mild traumatic brain injury in the emergency department. *Emerg Med Pract* 2012;14(9):1–24. www.ebmedicine.net.

CT if any high-risk variable present	CT or observe if any present
<ul><li>GCS score < 15</li><li>Altered mental status: agitation, somnolence, repetitive questioning, verbally slow to respond</li><li>Palpable skull fracture or suspected basilar skull fracture</li></ul>	<ul><li>Loss of consciousness</li><li>Severe headache</li><li>Vomiting</li><li>Non-frontal scalp hematoma age < 2 years</li><li>Not acting normal (per parent) age < 2 years</li><li>Severe mechanism of injury: MVC with ejection, death of passenger, rollover, being struck by vehicle, fall > 5 ft (1.5 m) (or > 3ft ([0.9 m]) if age < 2 years), head struck by high-impact object</li></ul>
Neurosurgical intervention	**Intracranial injury**
Sensitivity: 100% Specificity: 59%	Sensitivity: 97% Specificity: 58%

Note: In PECARN, *n* = 42 000.
Abbreviations: CT, computed tomography; GCS, Glasgow Coma Scale; MVC, motor vehicle crash; PECARN, Pediatric Emergency Care Applied Research Network.

Moderate head injury (GCS 9–13)

Although no strict criteria exist to distinguish between minor and moderate head injury, this intermediate designation generally applies to the group of patients who regain consciousness following an initial closed head injury, but arrive at the ED with persistent alterations in alertness or cognitive deficits (GCS 9–13). As is the case for the less severely injured, only a small percentage of these patients will have operable intracranial bleeding, but the incidence of treatable lesions is sufficiently high among this intermediate injury severity population to justify several differences in initial management. First, in urban or rural areas with designated trauma-receiving hospitals, pre-hospital care personnel (transport crew) should transport patients who remain confused or somnolent following a head injury to a trauma center staffed to provide immediate neurosurgical intervention at all times. Next, because of their altered alertness, occult unstable cervical spine injuries cannot be excluded in these patients based on clinical findings, therefore there should be immobilization of the cervical spine with an appropriately sized and applied rigid collar throughout transport to the hospital and through the initial imaging. Initial clinical evaluation must include a systematic examination of the entire patient to detect thoracic, abdominal, pelvic, and extremity injuries. A focused assessment with ultrasonography for trauma (FAST) may be indicated depending on the mechanism and physical examination evidence of injuries to the chest and abdomen. Long-bone fractures should be expeditiously splinted to prevent neurovascular damage, and external hemorrhage controlled with pressure dressings. Patients with facial fractures causing significant bleeding into the nasopharynx while immobilized supine on a backboard are at particular risk of aspiration, and must receive continuous suctioning and occasionally nasal packing to control the hemorrhage. However, none of these ancillary concerns should delay transport to the CT scanner for immediate brain and cervical spine imaging as soon as the patient's circulatory status, ventilation, and airway are secured.

Clinicians must approach the interpretation of the CT scan in this group of patients with intermediate injury severity with the awareness that the initial images often over- or underestimate the actual severity of underlying brain injury. Most importantly, some patients with severe, even fatal, DAI due to shearing forces applied to the brain at the moment of impact may show little evidence of these injuries on the initial CT scan. A frequent mistake is reassuring family members that because the initial CT scan looks normal, the patient is certain to make a full neurological recovery. Instead, the guarded prognosis of even intermediate brain injury should be explained to the patient and family members, with reassurance that the patient will not require immediate major neurosurgery and that substantial or complete recovery may be possible, though the time course varies greatly among patients.

By the same token, the initial CT scan may reveal findings that initially appear ominous, but in fact hold little clinical significance, require no specific therapeutic intervention, and generally have a benign prognosis. By far the most common of these non-actionable CT abnormalities is subarachnoid hemorrhage visible in the sulci over the anterior cerebral hemispheres. These hemorrhages, which presumably result from tears to small pial vessels, generally do not portend serious neurologic injury. A recent, large retrospective series followed 478 patients with mild TBI (GCS ≥ 13) and isolated traumatic subarachnoid hemorrhage found at initial imaging [8]. None of these patients experienced neurologic decline or required major neurosurgical procedures during the index hospitalization. A single patient was subsequently found to have

bilateral chronic subdural hematomas requiring drainage at 6-week follow-up. Therefore, while overnight observation in the hospital seems prudent in this group of patients, neither intensive-care admission nor immediate follow-up imaging is likely necessary as long as the neurologic status does not deteriorate. Similarly, small surface parenchymal contusions, most commonly seen in the temporal and frontal poles, generally carry a benign prognosis with low risk of neurologic deterioration, although they may signal a greater deceleration impact and therefore may represent a marker for diffuse injury not visible on initial CT imaging [9]. This has principally prognostic implications as discussed for post-concussive syndrome below. Linear, non-depressed skull fractures also carry relatively little prognostic significance unless they involve the skull base or cross major vessels, for example the middle meningeal artery. Patients with this specific injury are at high risk for delayed epidural hematoma and must receive intensive-care-level observation.

For clinicians managing this group of patients, a key consideration after initial imaging has excluded extra-axial hematomas or other severe brain injuries becomes making the patient and family members aware that, while an immediate life threat has been excluded, a majority of patients will experience some symptoms following a moderate head injury, and 5 to 20% of these patients will develop a range of bothersome, occasionally debilitating symptoms that collectively constitute the "post-concussive syndrome" [10–12]. Prominent symptoms of this poorly understood disorder include headache, dizziness, disequilibrium, irritability, difficulty concentrating, and fatigue. Specific difficulty with "multi-tasking" during the post-concussive period may limit the patient's return to work or school activities. The symptoms generally resolve in 7 to 10 days in most patients, but can persist for months in a small subset. In general, primary-care follow-up is sufficient following discharge from the ED following a moderate brain injury; however, patients and family members should be aware of the possible need for specialist referral to a neurologist should symptoms persist. Patients and responsible family members should receive a clearly printed and thoroughly explained set of discharge precautions at the time of discharge, listing concerning signs such as vomiting, increasing headache, or excessive sleepiness. Standard "head-injury precautions" discharge instructions are available in most EDs.

Severe head injury (GCS ≤8)

In addition to the 52 000 deaths caused annually by head injuries in the United States, a substantial proportion of the 275 000 patients hospitalized for head injury present initially with clinical evidence of severe brain injury (GCS ≤ 8) [2]. The clinical management of these patients is focused on rapid evaluation for surgically treatable lesions, while minimizing secondary brain injury from hypotension, hypoxia, hypo- or hyperglycemia, and, when indicated, controlling intracerebral pressure with ventriculostomy or, rarely, craniectomy. Nationally validated trauma guidelines call for immediate rapid sequence induction and endotracheal intubation of patients with a GCS < 8 on arrival at the trauma center. In addition to sedatives and paralytic agents, pre-treatment with lidocaine or other agents has been proposed to limit increases in intracranial pressure resulting from endotracheal intubation.

Excluding penetrating injuries, a subset of patients with severe brain injury may have focal injuries such as cortical lacerations, intraparenchymal hematomas, or intraventricular hemorrhage. However, the pathologic lesion underlying long-term disability or death in most patients with severe, deceleration-induced brain injury falls into the category of DAI, a result of widespread axonal stretch/shearing at the moment of impact, associated with a cascade of events including cerebral edema, neuronal degeneration, and ultimately ischemic brain injury [13]. Therefore, a thorough understanding of DAI is fundamental to diagnosis and management of patients with head injury across the severity spectrum, but especially in the most severely injured subset that experience long-term disability or even coma and persistent vegetative state.

The earliest description of a link between white-matter degeneration and neurocognitive disorders following head injury appeared in a pathologic series published by Strich and others in 1956 [14]. Over time, clinicians gained a deeper understanding of the relationship between linear and angular deceleration head injury, shear injury to axons between brain structures that differ in density and respond differently to compressive and torsional forces, and the observed spectrum of behavioral and cognitive outcomes seen in closed head injury. However, the mechanics of traumatic brain injury, as well as the downstream molecular consequences, are poorly understood and this remains an area of active research [15]. DAI seems to constitute a continuous variable without a known lower limit in deceleration-based brain injury. In other words, the clinical phenomenon of concussion, characterized by a brief loss of consciousness followed by full alertness but also often by objectively measurable post-concussive neurocognitive deficits, is thought to result from the lowest clinically distinguishable grade of DAI. At the opposite end of the spectrum are the unfortunate group of patients who after a single, severe blow to the head never regain consciousness, and either die from cerebral edema causing herniation of the brain, or remain in a persistent vegetative state. The key to understanding both the short-term imaging findings on initial CT, and the guarded prognosis of patients with severe injury who fail to recover clinically, is an appreciation that the extent of DAI is extremely difficult to determine at the time of injury, and that the resulting disabilities follow a highly variable course, the causes of which are not well understood.

TBI remains among the most important contributors to loss of life and productive life years in developed countries, especially impacting the very young, the very old through falls, and working-aged individuals through motor-vehicle crashes. Fortunately, most of these injuries are of low severity, and newly validated decision rules permit clinicians to selectively use CT imaging during initial evaluation to detect the few patients with occult, surgically treatable pathology. Patients who arrive comatose at the hospital following a severe blow to the head can awaken and recover completely, achieve partial recovery, remain in a vegetative state, or die from brain swelling, and reliably establishing prognosis can be extremely difficult based on clinical assessment and CT imaging at the time of injury. The advent of advanced MRI methods such as diffusion tensor imaging (DTI) brings us closer to the point where the severity and progression of axonal injury in living patients can be accurately assessed following head injury [16]. Early assessment with blood-sensitized MRI for microhemorrhage and DTI metrics may offer clinicians a way to distinguish between patients who are likely to recover and those with more severe injury with a lower likelihood of meaningful recovery [17]. Such imaging modalities may provide a platform for development of pharmacologic and other interventions that may ultimately alter the course of the pathophysiologic events including DAI that underlies severe TBI.

Imaging in the immediate and early post-traumatic interval

As discussed above, the initial imaging evaluation is designed to be efficient and, first and foremost, to detect actionable (surgical) pathology, most commonly extra-axial hematoma. Secondarily, this imaging provides a baseline for follow-up of neurologic deterioration and for subclinical expansion of hematoma or edema in the hours or days after trauma. The initial CT, particularly when acquired at high resolution, may provide direct evidence or clues to injury that require more intensive follow-up including specific skull base fractures that suggest the need for follow-up imaging (CT angiography (CTA)) or risk for intracranial infection or CSF leak. The approach outlined below is based on compartments – skull, extra-axial, brain parenchyma or ventricular, and vascular. MRI is discussed relative to CT in the initial evaluation of trauma, with consideration for early post-traumatic imaging as a problem-solving tool and for prognosis.

Skull fracture

Linear, or comminuted fracture of the skull and/or depressed skull fracture may be clinically inapparent even after careful inspection, although injury may be suspected. There are helpful but far from reliable signs for skull base fracture (e.g. Battle's, perimastoid hematoma, Raccoon eyes, peri-orbital hematoma). CT has replaced plain X-ray as the initial procedure of choice based on its sensitivity and far greater anatomical detail (Figure 14.1). As discussed above, skull fractures are not of equal importance. Subcategorizing these by type and anatomy is important. Depressed skull fractures, directly or transiently impacting the brain parenchyma, should be carefully documented, as these may indicate a need for surgical decompression, and may be associated with immediate or delayed clinical consequences including seizure. A rough guideline for surgical correction is displacement of the outer table beyond the inner table. Linear, non-depressed skull fractures, comminuted fractures, and even skull base fractures are not usually treated in

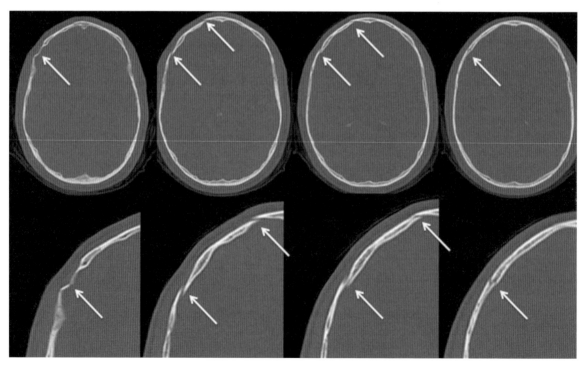

Figure 14.1 Depressed, comminuted, and linear skull fractures by CT (top row, consecutive sections). Bottom row shows magnified areas of interest, right frontal skull. The most depressed component (left panel) is focally depressed, and comminuted. A general guideline is that depressed skull fracture may require repair when the fracture extends beyond the adjacent inner cortical surface, or approximately one cortical thickness. This fracture was not repaired.

isolation, but may provide important clues to the overall severity of injury, and may direct attention to more critical associated injuries. Linear skull fracture along the course of the middle meningeal artery is associated with epidural hematoma. Skull base fracture extending to the carotid canal has been associated with carotid artery dissection, pseudoaneurysm, occlusion, or arteriovenous fistula. Skull fractures reaching the margins of the major dural veins are associated with venous sinus thrombus or occlusion [18, 19]. When identified, such fractures are indications for additional imaging by CTA or CT venography, and in some cases and practices may lead to formal catheter angiography.

Skull base fractures, with associated dural tears, are also associated with CSF leaks, which become evident as rhinorrhea with clear CSF oozing from the nose, for example from cribriform plate fracture; or otorrhea, with CSF passing a fracture through the tegmen tympani, entering the middle ear, and extending out through a ruptured tympanic membrane. CSF leak may also be evident by pneumocephalus with an air-fluid level, fluid extending into a paranasal sinus, or through the Eustachian tubes into the nasopharynx. Typically, CSF leak imaging is not required in the acute stages after trauma. These leaks often spontaneously resolve over hours or days, which is fortunate as establishing the source can be both challenging and technically demanding for both the patient and the imaging team. For persistent, unexplained CSF leaks, or for surgical planning, serial CT cisternography, MRI, or nuclear imaging may be required [20].

Fracture of the frontal, ethmoid, or sphenoid sinus or mastoid along the intracranial surfaces are important to note as these may permit intracranial entry of infectious agents and epidural or subdural empyema, meningitis, cerebritis, ventriculitis, or sigmoid sinus inflammation/infection and occlusion.

Intracranial hematoma

Intracranial hematoma is divided into extra-axial (outside brain) or intra-axial (parenchymal) compartments, including the ventricles. As discussed above, non-contrast CT is the procedure of choice for immediate imaging for hemorrhage. The technique is fast (seconds), therefore relatively resistant to the motion of disoriented and/or uncooperative patients, and with technical improvements usually provides adequate tissue contrast, fewer skull-associated reconstruction artifacts, and, if acquired using current helical multi-detector imaging, permits high-resolution imaging compatible with relatively seamless multiplanar or more complex image reconstruction. Multiplanar reconstruction is helpful in the detection, delineation, and characterization of findings, including subtle subarachnoid hemorrhage (SAH; Figure 14.2) or parenchymal blood collections along the brain surfaces [21].

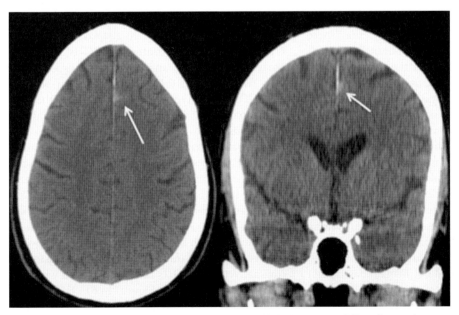

Figure 14.2 SAH. Small left parafalcine SAH (arrows) on axial helical acquisition (left), and coronal reconstruction (right).

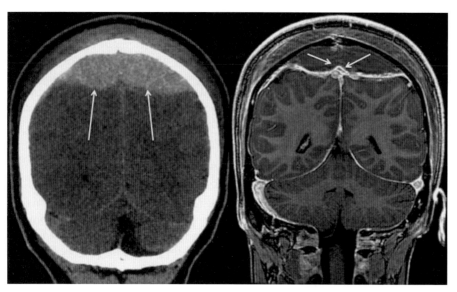

Figure 14.3 Acute bilateral epidural hematoma (EDH). Left image, non-contrast-CT. Arrows indicate brain surface, and dense acute blood. Right image from a contrast-enhanced T1-weighted MRI scan. The arrows indicate the displaced sagittal sinus and enhancing dura. The blood is hypointense on these early T1-weighted images. EDHs, unlike subdural hematomas, can extend across the midline external to the dura and, as shown here, external to the venous (sagittal) sinus. Case courtesy of P.-L. Westesson, University of Rochester Medical Center, Rochester NY, USA.

As discussed above, these most often do not impact immediate care, but their identification is important for medico-legal documentation, and they may contribute to other factors that determine the intensity and timing of follow-up care including additional imaging, or later clinical and/or neuropsychological evaluation.

Extra-axial hematoma is divided into three simple compartments, based on essentially three membranes. Epidural hematomas (EDHs) occupy the space between the thick dura mater (membrane) and periosteum lining the inner table of the skull; subdural hematomas occupy the potential space between dura and arachnoid membrane; and subarachnoid hematoma lies between the arachnoid membrane and the pia mater (pia-arachnoid), a loose space filled with arachnoid trabeculae extending between pia and the outer delimiting arachnoid membrane. EDHs tend to have inwardly convex (lenticular shape) surfaces as the adherent dura must be forcibly displaced by blood under pressure. Most frequently, EDHs are located along the temporal and temporoparietal skull, along the course of the middle meningeal artery, and are associated with fracture in the vast majority of adults, but less so in children. Epidural hematomas do not cross sutures, as the sutural dura is very tightly adherent, but EDHs do cross dural surfaces (Figure 14.3), for example across the midline past the sagittal sinus,

and across the tentorium [22]. A lucid interval has been described after the initial trauma resulting in EDHs, during which the patient may improve clinically, and the early CT scan may be initially unremarkable, followed by rapid neurological deterioration, at which time an immediate follow-up CT scan will be positive (Figure 14.4).

The subdural compartment is readily expandable with mild pressure. Acute subdural hematomas (SDHs) are typically crescent-shaped and dense on CT (Figure 14.5). In contrast to EDHs, SDHs can cross suture lines [22] and are not typically associated with fracture, with their source a tear in bridging veins. The SDHs typically are located over the cerebral convexities, the tentorium, along the midline interhemispheric fissures, and along the falx. Considerable mass effect, slow expansion, and immediate and delayed re-bleeding is common. Acute SDHs are typically homogeneous dense, more dense than the brain. But SDHs frequently appear as mixed density collections, indicative of re-bleed, or CSF and blood mixtures. Patients can sometimes present for the first time with minor signs and symptoms with a history of remote trauma or no recalled history of trauma, yet these SDHs can be associated with considerable mass effect (Figure 14.6). High-density SDHs convert to isodense to brain when imaged about 1–2 weeks after trauma. Consequently,

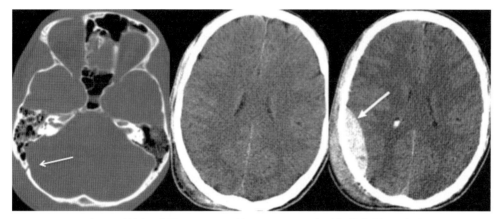

Figure 14.4 Lucid-interval (delayed) EDH. A 23-year-old construction worker fell off a ladder, hit his head, and had a brief loss of consciousness. He had a headache but was alert and oriented on arrival at the emergency room. The initial CT (left image) showed a right occipital fracture (arrow), a tiny subarachnoid hemorrhage (not shown), and a right scalp hematoma. The middle image shows scalp swelling and extracranial blood but is otherwise unremarkable. The following afternoon, due to persistent confusion, a repeat CT scan was acquired (right image) which showed development of a large right occipital EDH (arrow). Case courtesy of P.-L. Westesson, University of Rochester Medical Center, Rochester NY, USA.

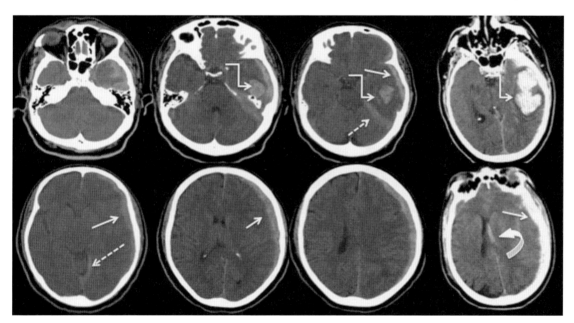

Figure 14.5 Rapidly expanding hematoma in a 61-year-old patient who had an observed fall and syncope after smoking crack cocaine. The patient had no recollection of the event. After walking into the emergency department, the initial GCS was 15. A CT (left six panels) showed a subdural hematoma over the left temporal-frontal-parietal surfaces (arrows), blood over the tentorium (dashed arrows), and a left temporal intraparenchymal hematoma (jagged arrow). There was a modest midline shift to the right, left ventricular and sulcal compression. The patient rapidly decompensated, GCS was 3, and required intubation in the emergency room. A CT scan within several hours of the initial CT (right panels) showed major expansion of the temporal-lobe hematomas (jagged arrow) and intraventricular hemorrhage (curved arrow). The patient was taken to the operating room immediately after the CT scan.

substantial SDHs can be missed without careful review. Rarely, acute SDHs may be isodense to brain as a result of anemia. Both SDHs and EDHs are frequently associated with mass effect as indicated by the distortion of brain cortical surfaces, obliteration of sulci, midline shift, compression of ventricles, asymmetric or obliterated cisternal spaces, and brain herniation.

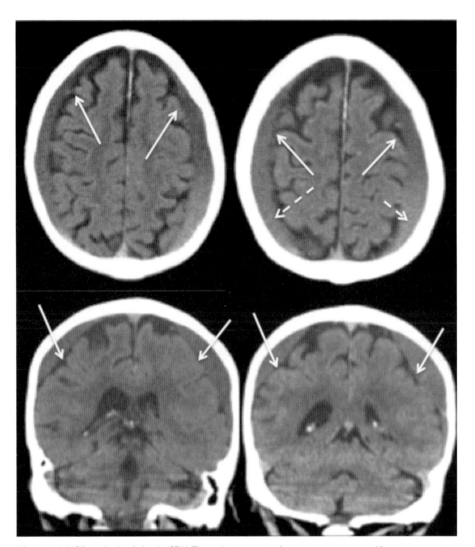

Figure 14.6 Bilateral mixed-density SDH. The patient came to the emergency room with vague symptoms and did not report a history of trauma. The top row shows axial helical CT acquisition. Arrows indicate cortical surfaces, beyond which is a hypodense SDH along the anterior surfaces (arrows), and hyperdense blood in the dependent regions inferiorly (dashed arrows). These mixed density subdural collections are suggestive of an acute SDH occurring additional to the pre-existing chronic or subacute SDH. The bottom row shows coronal reformatted images. Note that the coronal series shows to advantage that the cortical surfaces are mildly indented (arrows).

Traumatic SAH, from laceration of cortical vessels or from extension of parenchymal hemorrhage is not infrequently identified along with SDH or other CNS injury. While SAH alone does not require immediate surgical intervention, and when isolated in mild TBI without neurological decline may not require intensive follow-up [7], SAH nevertheless may be associated with a less favorable long-term outcome [23], and its identification may support medico-legal claims important to the patient.

Small SAHs are easily missed, but can be identified on CT scans as dense areas within the cerebral

sulci following the brain surface, or filling fissures or basal cisterns (Figure 14.2). It should be noted that SAHs in the setting of trauma may rarely be the consequence of pre-existing pathology such as berry aneurysm, with rupture or leakage resulting in impairment and secondary motor-vehicle or other accidents. Blood located in typical anatomic locations for aneurysmal SAHs (e.g. around the circle of Willis at the skull base, etc.) may suggest the correct diagnosis, with verification by CT angiography (CTA) or magnetic resonance angiography (MRA), or formal catheter angiography.

Intraventricular hemorrhage (IVH) is not uncommon in the setting of severe head trauma, but is found only rarely as isolated findings, as IVH is usually associated with multiple blood collections – adjacent bleeds (a potential source), superficial contusions, and SAHs [24]. The early morbidity of IVH is thought in large part to be related to the associated injury, although secondary hydrocephalus contributes to morbidity.

Brain parenchymal injury – with and without hemorrhage

From the imaging perspective, primary injury to the brain parenchyma can be categorized as focal and multifocal hemorrhagic contusion and non-hemorrhagic contusion, and as DAI. DAI based on the pattern of lesions may be non-hemorrhagic even with the most modern blood-sensitized MRI technique (see below), or may be suggested by classic locations – multifocal, small, petechial hemorrhages or diffusion abnormalities at gray–white-matter junctions, within the corpus callosum, anterior aspect of corona radiata, internal capsule, and more rarely visible but important within the brainstem.

With important exceptions, parenchymal hemorrhage, as compared to acute EDH and SDH, is less likely in many clinical practices to be an indication for immediate surgery after trauma. The rationale, in part, is that these often occur with additional, irreversible major injuries; they occupy regions of already irreversibly damaged tissue and, although surgery may decrease mortality, there are unanswered questions regarding improvement in quality of life. Large, symptomatic, isolated parenchymal hemorrhage with mass effect, and especially that in the cerebellum, is more likely to be approached surgically [25]. There are only limited outcome data for surgical treatment of post-traumatic parenchymal hemorrhage [25, 26]. However, the issue of optimal treatment including immediate surgery for parenchymal hemorrhage is under current investigation through randomized controlled trials [e.g. 26]. CT is sensitive to actionable acute parenchymal hemorrhage, and remains the initial imaging modality. CT can also adequately detect clinical and subclinically important expanding hematomas after the initial CT scan (Figure 14.6). While MRI has far greater sensitivity than CT to some acute blood collections (e.g. microhemorrhages), its value in depicting blood relevant to acute operative

management is limited. The sensitivity of MRI to blood does increase in the hours and certainly days after the traumatic event, particularly as blood passes through its evolution from oxy- to deoxyhemoglobin, then to the methemoglobin stage (hyperintense on T1-weighted MRI), followed by the hemosiderin stage (T2 hypointense, especially on T2* (pronounced T2 star)-weighted MRI [27]).

In the hours and days after hemorrhage is first identified by a CT evaluation, CT typically still remains the modality of choice for follow-up, as, relative to MRI, it is a quick test, requires less patient preparation, and there are fewer safety issues. There is some controversy regarding indications for follow-up imaging in the absence of neurological decline. The clarity of the literature is confounded, in part related to the variable patient populations and also the complexity of the initial pathology. Based on high reported rates of progressive hemorrhage, sometimes quoted as high as 30% of the population, or greater over short intervals (e.g. 8–12 hours), strong recommendations have been made for early follow-up and even routine serial imaging after hemorrhage is initially identified after trauma [28–30]. But other series [31] suggest low rates of progression for most ICH in the setting of mild TBI, with good clinical outcome, and recommend against repeat imaging in the absence of neurological decline, for example in the setting of convexity SAH, small convexity contusion, and small intraparenchymal hemorrhage.

TBI has been simplistically described as occurring through deceleration mechanisms with multiple directional and importantly rotational components, with rotational strain-shear. The older, classical terminology of coup/contre-coup injury remains descriptive of the frequently apparent group of injuries often detected by conventional CT and MRI, such as the blood collections followed later by encephalomalacia along the frontal and temporal surfaces, but such terminology is an oversimplification of trauma mechanisms and does not satisfactorily explain the important class of injury included within the current category of DAI [13, 15–17, 32, 33].

Although CT is the procedure of choice for immediate evaluation of head trauma, relative to MRI it lacks sensitivity to detect non-hemorrhagic cortical contusion, and is very insensitive to patterns of DAI and even hemorrhagic and certainly non-hemorrhagic clinically important brainstem injury. Cerebral edema can occur after head trauma in the absence of hemorrhage, and can be localized, diffuse, or both. Cerebral edema is broadly classified as vasogenic or cytotoxic. A third volume-gain process sometimes accompanied by imaging findings has been attributed to hyperemia. Vasogenic edema with expanded interstitial spaces is associated with abnormal leakage of water and solutes (protein, electrolytes) across the blood–brain barrier. Vasogenic edema can be recognized on CT scans as hypodense, sometimes obviously swollen areas, within sharply defined white-matter pathways. Cytotoxic edema, with expanded cellular volume, is related to cell-membrane pump failure, and abnormal intracellular osmolytes in neurons, astrocytes, and microglia, resulting in an overall expansion of cellular volume. Cytotoxic edema appears on CT scans as localized hypodense regions of round swelling, or loss of the normal gray–white-matter differentiation, the latter as the CT (Hounsfield unit) density of swollen gray matter decreases and approaches that of the white matter. When more extreme, cerebral edema results in obliteration of the sulci, ventricular compression or decreased, asymmetric, or absent cisternal compartments, or herniation. Cerebral hyperemia can also contribute to diffuse cerebral edema, based on abnormal autoregulation of blood flow and possibly increased blood volume, although the latter finding has been controversial. The imaging findings associated with generalized cerebral hyperemia include small sulci, cisternal spaces, and ventricles, with, however, the retention of gray–white-matter contrast, as the characteristic density changes in white and gray matter of vasogenic or cytotoxic edema are not observed [22].

Vascular injury assessment by CT

The cerebral vasculature can be injured or compromised in head and associated neck trauma by direct and indirect mechanical forces, secondarily to dissection and blood flow consequences, embolism, or delayed vasospasm. As many as 2–3% of trauma cases, or greater in some series [34], suffer cerebral infarction, with symptoms often delayed from hours to days. There is therefore an important window of opportunity for therapeutic intervention when vascular injury, compromise, or occlusion is recognized. Although duplex Doppler ultrasound is utilized in imaging the neck vessels, and provides flow information, it is not generally recommended for early assessment in blunt injury as anatomical coverage is limited, ultrasound is insensitive to high cervical injury, which would include most arterial dissections [35], and, not

unimportantly, the technique is highly operator-dependent. Although in some aspects imperfect against the "gold standard" of formal catheter angiography, CTA has replaced formal catheter angiography as the initial diagnostic test in many if not most practices [19], with some, but not all, studies suggesting near equivalency or equivalency. There are also major practical advantages for diagnostic CTA in acute trauma compared to catheter angiography, including speed, lower morbidity (e.g. vessel-wall injury and stroke with catheter angiography), and the additional anatomy outside the vessel lumen afforded by CT compared to catheter angiography. However, catheter angiography may still be required in select and equivocal cases, and is ultimately required for neuro-interventional procedures (e.g. stents, angioplasty, clot lysis or retrieval) when indicated.

Vascular injury is associated with specific skull fractures, including fracture reaching the carotid (artery) canal in the skull base, and fractures along the major venous sinuses or jugular bulb. In the cervical spine, facet or other cervical fractures, vertebral subluxations, or specific fractures of the foramen transversarium are associated with vascular injury [18, 19]. Vessel occlusion, dissection, pseudoaneurysm, and intramural hematomas are associated with post-traumatic cerebrovascular ischemia in from 10–60% of these cases. A scoring system has been proposed to guide decisions regarding inclusion of CTA after blunt craniocervical trauma [19].

MRI in acute head trauma

CT remains the standard modality for the immediate, first evaluation of head trauma, despite the far greater sensitivity of MRI to non-hemorrhagic contusions, some blood collections, and findings suggestive of DAI. Acquiring an MRI can potentially compromise care of the acutely ill trauma patient at risk due to the physical constraints of MRI (more restricted environment limiting monitoring of vital functions and neurologic status), the longer examination duration required for imaging, the risk of ferromagnetic projectiles in or around the strong magnet environment, and the risk of imaging a patient with contraindicated pacemakers, incompatible vascular (e.g. aneurysm clips), or electromechanical devices.

Head-to-head trials of MRI versus CT are limited, and some may be biased in favor of MRI (MRI is more likely to be delayed, or utilized with less severe injuries).

Despite the potential bias, at this time the literature still favors CT as the initial test of choice. In one prospective study, MRI detected minor findings that were not seen by CT in only 6 of 123 cases; the generally significant results overlapped on both modalities. The authors concluded that MRI did not affect management in the first 48 hours [36]. In a retrospective review, MRI was superior to CT specifically for detecting shear-like injury in the corpus callosum, but did not impact immediate care [37]. The MRI was noted to miss sub-arachnoid blood, and skull fracture [37].

In the specific evaluation of head trauma in suspected child abuse, CT is generally the initial imaging test. However, MRI may show blood collections of multiple ages [37, 38], increasing diagnostic certainty of findings suggestive of non-accidental trauma. For non-accidental trauma evaluation, improved detection of even "small" non-actionable injuries may be critically important in decisions affecting the infant or child's safety (i.e. return to an unsafe environment). Comprehensive assessment of injury associated with child abuse often includes MRI, with delayed MRI if not done initially.

Beyond the immediate evaluation of head trauma, there is unequivocal literature and consensus for the superiority of delayed MRI for specific indications, notably to detect findings associated with DAI, where CT is often unremarkable [see 32]. Delayed MRI is sometimes useful in problem solving, and guiding management and prognosis when CT does not provide sufficient information. MRI can depict multiple microhemorrhages in classic axonal shear patterns of DAI (Figure 14.7). MRI is unequivocally more sensitive to blood in the subacute interval (Figure 14.8), for small acute parenchymal blood collections, focal edema, brainstem injury (correlating with otherwise unexplained clinical signs), and findings (blood) within a vessel cross-section indicative of subacute arterial dissections. In a prospective study, early MRI, average ~ 12 days, combined with CT markers, improved predictive models for the 3-month clinical outcome after mild TBI. Twenty-seven percent of mild TBI patients with normal admission head CT studies had abnormal early brain MRI [23].

MRI in the identification of acute and subacute blood

Several blood-sensitive MRI pulse sequences have been developed and are in routine use (based on gradient-echo sequences) or under investigation but utilized in some practices (susceptibility-weighted imaging). These are generally feasible as blood or its degradation products, by virtue of iron content and its organization (magnetic susceptibility effects) disturb the magnetic field in their vicinity and result in signal loss emphasized by specific pulse sequences. Deoxyhemoglobin (acute deoxygenated blood quickly converted from oxyhemoglobin) and hemosiderin (late, chronic blood) are detected through this effect. The paramagnetic properties of methemoglobin (subacute blood) have T1-relaxation effects, and consequently high signal on standard T1-weighted images (Figure 14.8).

The magnetic-field inhomogeneity induced by deoxyhemoglobin and hemosiderin are best detected using MR pulse sequences that are especially sensitive to local field disturbance, as inhomogeneity contributes to proton spin dephasing, seen as signal loss and predictable signal patterns that can be analyzed with special post-processing algorithms. Gradient-echo ($T2^*$) sequences are a standard clinical basis for blood-sensitized imaging – local blood collections appear as signal-loss regions, often larger than the actual volume of blood (the "blooming" effect) (Figure 14.8). Gradient-echo sequences similarly detect temporally remote, chronic microhemorrhage, from hypertension or amyloid angiopathy, and hemosiderin staining of brain surfaces (hemosiderosis), an indication of a prior subarachnoid blood, for example from trauma, aneurysm rupture, amyloid angiopathy, and reversible vasoconstriction syndrome [39], among other causes.

Susceptibility-weighted imaging (SWI) is a technical step beyond standard gradient-echo imaging [40], where both the magnitude (standard) and additional phase information in the radiofrequency signal is collected and processed. SWI processing software is increasingly available on commercial MRI systems. As an indication of potential sensitivity, in one study SWI detected approximately four-fold more chronic microhemorrhages compared to conventional gradient-echo imaging [41]. In another series SWI increased sensitivity to microhemorrhages in children [42]. Microhemorrhage appears to be a parameter that can improve outcome prediction models after non-accidental trauma [43]. The blood sensitivity of MRI also increases with stronger main magnetic field strength, as $T2^*$ dephasing increases proportional to the field-square. Consequently, higher-field-strength

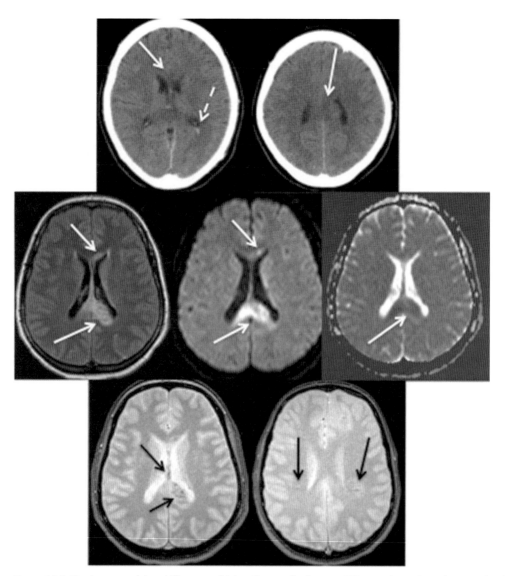

Figure 14.7 Classic pattern of shear (diffuse axonal) injury. Top row. On the acute CT images there is hypodensity within the left genu and body of corpus callosum (arrows) and a small left IVH (dashed arrow). Middle row. Follow-up FLAIR series (left), shows a swollen, hyperintense body and splenium of corpus callosum and a small lesion within the genu (arrows). Diffusion-weighted imaging (DWI) (middle) shows these areas as hyperintense (arrows); this hyperintensity can be T2-shine-through, or restricted diffusion. The apparent diffusion coefficient map (right image) shows the splenium of corpus callosum is hypointense (arrow), indicating restricted diffusion (a more stroke-like pattern). Bottom row. The T2* gradient-echo images show multiple focal areas of linear hypointensity typical of shear-injury-associated bleeds. Case courtesy of L. Riccelli, Oregon Health and Science University, Portland, Oregon, USA.

MRI instruments (e.g. 3 Tesla) tend to outperform 1.5 Tesla systems in clinical blood imaging [44], while research magnets (e.g. at 7 Tesla) show even greater sensitivity to local dephasing effects (Figure 14.9).

When MRI is used in the acute and early subacute interval, fluid attenuation inversion recovery (FLAIR) imaging may be sensitive to subarachnoid blood.

Unfortunately, in practice, FLAIR is associated with false-positive blood detection owing to various artifacts, for example from bulk CSF motion, and even from other sources such as administered oxygen. Consequently, FLAIR imaging for the accurate determination of subarachnoid blood has been controversial [45].

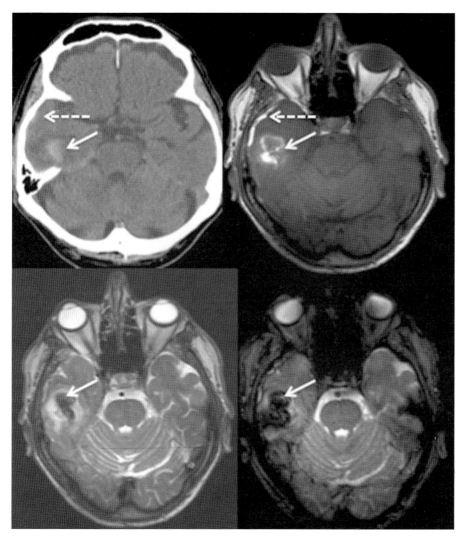

Figure 14.8 A 92-year-old patient admitted with confusion and amnesia. One day after admission, the CT series (upper left) was unchanged from baseline (not shown), and showed a right temporal lobe intraparenchymal hematoma (IPH) (arrow) with mild surrounding (hypodense) edema. Barely visible was a thin subdural hematoma (dashed arrow). A same-day T1-weighted MRI (upper right) shows both hemorrhages to advantage, based on methemoglobin (T1 hyperintense). A T2-weighted MRI scan (lower left) depicts the IPH as hypointense (arrow) surrounded by T2 hyperintensity from edema. On the T2* gradient-echo image (lower right), note the "stringy" appearing hypointense IPH (arrow). The lesion appears larger than its true volume (blooming effect) on the gradient-echo sequence, and is very conspicuous. The petrous temporal bones also artifactually bloom, mimicking blood.

Diffusion MRI in acute brain trauma, in subacute and later care

Although diffusion imaging sequences can add both sensitivity and specificity to the evaluation of acute injury of the brain (e.g. stroke detection), the indications for advanced diffusion methods (based on DTI) remain limited in the acute stages of trauma evaluation as referred to above. In special circumstances, for problem solving, the attributes of MRI can be used to great advantage. Routine proton density, T2-weighted, FLAIR MRI (based on suppressing the water signal by its prolonged T1, and detecting edema by its long T2) and diffusion-weighted imaging (DWI) have far greater sensitivity than CT to the non-specific water-space changes from trauma, including some of the multiple small areas of swelling and hemorrhage typical of post-traumatic shear injury (Figure 14.7).

Stroke results in diffusion restriction (a relative decrease in the apparent diffusion coefficient)

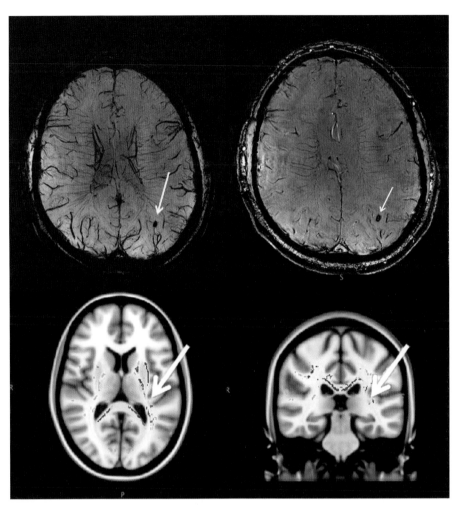

Figure 14.9 Advanced and research imaging applications in TBI. Top row. Images from a very high field (7 Tesla), heavily T2-weighted MRI series. Arrow points to the focal region of signal loss along the left gray–white-matter junction. This hypointensity on T2*-weighted imaging is not specific, but this is the typical appearance and common location for a post-traumatic microhemorrhage. Note the exquisite sensitivity to small blood vessels, afforded by the sequence and strong magnetic field effect. Bottom row. Images selected from a tract-based spatial statistics (TBSS) series in mild TBI. These statistical displays are based on pooled subject data, from a test (mild TBI) versus control group, rather than from an individual patient. Diffusion tensor imaging is used to generate fractional anisotropy (FA) data for each voxel, for analysis by the TBSS method. The display provides a statistical visual representation for abnormal white-matter tracts, with a pseudo-color scale reflecting statistical significance. Study at 7 Tesla in collaboration with W. Rooney, Advanced Imaging Research Center, Oregon Health and Sciences University; K. Powers (Portland VA Research Foundation) and E. Beaudreau, VA Medical Center, Portland, Oregon, USA.

within minutes of sufficient compromise, with characteristic signal loss on apparent diffusion coefficient maps. Clinical DWI sequences are very fast (50–100 millisecond per slice) and often routinely or easily acquired along with the standard set of brain MRI pulse sequences. Small regions of high signal on DWI have been described in TBI. More classic large or lobar or specific vascular territory stroke-findings with restricted diffusion on imaging in the setting of trauma may suggest the need for additional MRA sequences, and/or CTA or catheter angiography to detect treatable, very early infarction or ischemic tissue.

More sophisticated diffusion imaging is based on the diffusion tensor acquisition. DTI is based on applying a sufficient number of diffusion directional gradients to accurately sort out water diffusion and diffusion barriers, providing insight into the microscopic architecture of the structure of interest. In contrast to DWI (three gradient directions), DTI requires six or more gradient directions, necessitating longer scan time, and is often now applied with 32 or more gradient directions for optimized diffusion data quality. Once the elements of the diffusion tensor matrix are acquired, multiple diffusion parameters can be determined off line. For example, one popular measure is fractional anisotropy (FA), which scales from essentially 0 in water where diffusion is equal in all directions (isotropic diffusion), to a maximum of 1.0, when diffusion is only along one axis (anisotropic diffusion). Healthy white-matter tracts have high FA values, while white-matter pathology most often is characterized by a reduction in FA. Axial (parallel) and radial (perpendicular) diffusivity refer to water diffusion oriented with or transverse to the principal orientation of organized white matter. Early reduced axial diffusivity is thought to be associated with axonal degeneration. Consequently, there is interest in axial diffusivity as an imaging biomarker for DAI. However, complicating the interpretation of axial or other diffusion measures in human disease is the mixed and complex pathology. Directly equating abnormality on DTI specifically with axonal injury at this time in humans is premature and almost certainly incorrect. But these measures are nevertheless relevant and important as patients with trauma and a clinical history consistent with DAI frequently have abnormal diffusion values in anatomical regions associated with shear injury as previously established in the pathology literature. For example, injury in the corpus callosum, internal capsule, and centrum semiovale was detected in patients compared to control groups both in the early and later stages after mild TBI based on reduced FA [46]. Other population studies suggest various changes in axial diffusivity. The diffusion-based findings improve the predictive models for subsequent clinical or neuropsychological outcome [33].

In addition to their use as a measure of injury, FA or related measures from DTI can be used as the basis for generating diffusion tractography maps, through which white-matter tracts and organized fibers can be followed and graphically displayed in three dimensions. In one application, called tract-based spatial statistics (TBSS), diffusion data from groups of patients are referenced to a normal control group. The TBSS map is designed to show regions in the white matter that are abnormal based on statistical probability [47], and has become a popular methodology in TBI research (Figure 14.9) [e.g. 48].

Importantly, and unfortunately, the application of DTI in individual patients with mild injury is currently limited for technical reasons. In severe brain injury, in selected cases, the technique with metrics such as FA may provide additional interesting, if not relevant, information. Display of fiber-pathway disruption through diffusion tractography may be dramatic and provide potentially informative results in severe cases, but can also be potentially misleading [49] as apparent interruption of a white matter pathway may occur for technical reasons (local iron, possibly edema, complex fiber geometry, choice of technical parameters) rather than specifically from DAI or fiber discontinuity. Most post-traumatic lesions considered significant by imaging criteria do not result in disrupted tracts based on even high-quality tractography techniques [50]. Consequently, for these and other reasons, these advanced, quantitative DTI techniques are not considered a component of standard clinical care as yet in individual patients.

Conclusions

After head trauma, and the immediate clinical and neurologic evaluation of the patient, highly sensitive decision rule sets for imaging adult (New Orleans criteria and Canadian CT rules) and pediatric patients (PECARN Decision Rule) with minor head trauma are available. The approach to care after head trauma should be optimized for rapid stabilization and immediate evaluation of actionable intracranial hemorrhage, most often SDH and EDH, based on one test – non-contrast head CT (Figure 14.10). A comprehensive imaging assessment adds other clinically important findings that may be important in the hours and days after injury. Based on CT, clinical findings, and mechanism of injury, additional imaging (CTA or MRA) may be indicated in some patients, as there may be a window of opportunity for medical and/or more invasive intervention to prevent irreversible cerebral infarction. Early follow-up CT imaging may be utilized to evaluate expansion of extra-axial or parenchymal hemorrhages after their initial identification, and for evaluating delayed complications such as hydrocephalus. Delayed MRI provides additional sensitivity to small blood collections, non-hemorrhagic contusions, and blood collections of multiple ages that may be especially important in the evaluation of known or suspected non-accidental trauma in the pediatric population. Multiple microhemorrhages in classic locations may be indicative of shear injury in children and adults. More specialized MRI techniques such as SWI, particularly at higher field strength, can be utilized to identify

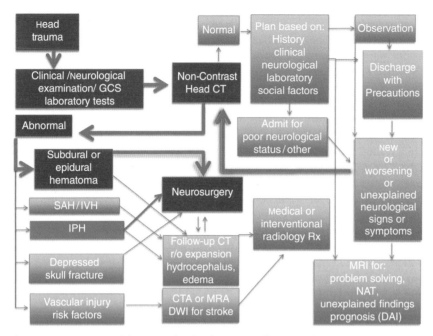

Figure 14.10 Summary of the approach to head trauma. Red boxes emphasize the immediate pathway to discovery and treatment of actionable pathology. Thick arrows emphasize more common pathways. Blue boxes represent some of the many additional considerations within the early hours and days after head trauma. Abbreviations: GCS = Glasgow Coma Scale; CT = computed tomography; SAH = subarachnoid hemorrhage; IVH = intraventricular hemorrhage; IPH = intraparenchymal hemorrhage; CTA = CT angiography; MRI = magnetic resonance imaging ; MRA = magnetic resonance angiography ; Rx = treatment; DWI= diffusion-weighted imaging; DAI = diffuse axonal injury; r/o = rule out

small hemorrhages with greater sensitivity compared to CT or even T2* gradient–echo MRI. DTI has become a standard research method for the evaluation of DAI, although the diffusion metrics are not necessarily specific to axonal injury. DTI is currently most applicable to statistical analyses based on groups of patients rather than individuals, and is a promising method for improving predictive models of late neurologic and neuropsychological deficit after TBI. Similarly, diffusion tractography maps, derived from DTI, are most informative in the statistical analyses of groups of patients. In individual patients, while the image findings may be dramatic, care must be exercised in their interpretation.

References

1. US Department of Health and Human Services, Centers for Disease Control and Prevention. See http://www.cdc.gov/traumaticbraininjury/pdf/BlueBook_factsheet-a.pdf, accessed April 11, 2013.

2. US Department of Health and Human Services, Centers for Disease Control and Prevention: See http://www.cdc.gov/traumaticbraininjury/pdf/tbi_blue_book_externalcause.pdf, accessed April 11, 2013.

3. Berrington de Gonzalez A, Mahesh M, Kim KP, *et al.* (2009). Projected cancer risks from computed tomographic scans performed in the United States in 2007. *Arch Internal Med* **169**: 2071–2077.

4. Teasdale G, Jennett B (1974). Assessment of coma and impaired consciousness. A practical scale. *Lancet* **2**: 81–84.

5. Haydel M (2012). Management of mild traumatic brain injury in the emergency department. *Emerg Med Pract.* **14**: 1–24.

6. Stiell IG, Clement CM, Rowe BH, *et al.* (2005). Comparison of the Canadian CT head rule and the New Orleans criteria in patients with minor head injury. *JAMA* **294**(12): 1511–1518.

7. Kuppermann N, Holmes JF, Dayan PS, *et al.* (2009). Identification of children at very low risk of clinically important brain injuries after head trauma: a prospective cohort study. *Lancet* **374**: 1160–1170.

8. Quigley MR, Chew BG, Swartz CE, Wilberger JE (2013). The clinical significance of isolated traumatic subarachnoid hemorrhage. *J Trauma Acute Care Surg* **74**(2): 581–584.

9. Ropper AH, Gorson KC (2007). Clinical practice. Concussion. *N Engl J Med.* **356**: 166–172.

10. Mott TF, McConnon ML, Rieger BP (2012). Subacute to chronic mild traumatic brain injury. *Am Fam Physician* **86**: 1045–1051.

11. Dischinger PC, Ryb GE, Kufera JA, Auman KM (2009). Early predictors of postconcussive syndrome in a population of trauma patients with mild traumatic brain injury. *J Trauma* **66**: 289–296; discussion 296–7.

12. Babcock L, Byczkowski T, Wade SL, et al. (2013). Predicting postconcussion syndrome after mild traumatic brain injury in children and adolescents who present to the emergency department. *JAMA Pediatr* **167**: 156–161.

13. Vos PE, Bigler ED (2011). White matter in traumatic brain injury: dis- or dysconnection? *Neurology* **77**: 810–811.

14. Strich SJ (1956). Diffuse degeneration of the cerebral white matter in severe dementia following head injury. *J Neurol Neurosurg Psychiatry* **19**: 163–185.

15. Andriessen TM, Jacobs B, Vos PE (2010). Clinical characteristics and pathophysiological mechanisms of focal and diffuse traumatic brain injury. *J Cell Mol Med* **14**: 2381–2392.

16. Wang JY, Bakhadirov K, Abdi H, et al. (2011). Longitudinal changes of structural connectivity in traumatic axonal injury. *Neurology* **77**: 818–826.

17. Gu L, Li J, Feng DF, et al. (2013). Detection of white-matter lesions in the acute stage of diffuse axonal injury predicts long-term cognitive impairments: a clinical diffusion tensor imaging study. *J Trauma Acute Care Surg* **74**: 242–247.

18. Delgado Almandoz JE, Kelly HR, Schaefer PW, et al. (2010). Prevalence of traumatic dural venous sinus thrombosis in high-risk acute blunt head trauma patients evaluated with multidetector CT venography. *Radiology* **255**: 570–577.

19. Delgado Almandoz JE, Schaefer PW, Kelly HR, et al. (2010). Multidetector CT angiography in the evaluation of acute blunt head and neck trauma: a proposed acute craniocervical trauma scoring system. *Radiology* **254**: 236–244.

20. Lloyd KM, Del Gaudio JM, Hudgins PA (2008). Imaging of skull base cerebrospinal fluid leaks in adults. *Radiology* **248**: 725–736.

21. Wei SC, Ulmer S, Lev MH, et al. (2010). Value of coronal reformations in the CT evaluation of acute head trauma. *AJNR* **31**: 334–339.

22. Kim JJ, Gean AD (2011). Imaging for the diagnosis and management of traumatic brain injury. *Neurotherapeutics* **8**: 39–53.

23. Yuh EL, Mukherjee P, Lingsma HF, et al. (2013). Magnetic resonance imaging improves 3-month outcome prediction in mild traumatic brain injury. *Ann Neurol* **73**: 224–235.

24. Atzema C, Mower WR, Hoffman JR, et al. (2006). Prevalence and prognosis of traumatic intraventricular hemorrhage in patients with blunt head trauma. *J Trauma Acute Care Surg* **60**: 1010–1017.

25. Bullock MR, Chesnut R, Gordon D, et al. (2006). Surgical management of traumatic parenchymal lesions. *Neurosurgery* **58**(suppl 2): 25–46.

26. Gregson BA, Rowan EN, Mitchell PM, et al. (2012). Surgical trial in traumatic intracerebral hemorrhage (STITCH(Trauma)): study protocol for a randomized controlled trial. *Trials* **13**: 193.

27. Atlas SW, Thulborn KR (2000). Intracranial hemorrhage. In SW Atlas, ed. *Magnetic Resonance Imaging of the Brain and Spine*, 4th edn. Philadelphia PA: Lippincott Williams and Wilkins, ch. 13, pp. 644–694.

28. Narayan RK, Maas AI, Servadei F, et al. (2008). Progression of traumatic intracerebral hemorrhage: a prospective observational study. *J Neurotrauma* **25**: 629–639.

29. Thorson CM, Van Haren RM, Otero CA, et al. (2013). Repeat head computed tomography after minimal brain injury identifies the need for craniotomy in the absence of neurologic change. *J Trauma Acute Care Surg* **74**: 967–975.

30. Tong WS, Zheng P, Xu JF, et al. (2011). Early CT signs of progressive hemorrhagic injury following acute traumatic brain injury. *Neuroradiology* **53**: 305–309.

31. Washington CW, Grubb RL Jr (2012). Are routine repeat imaging and intensive care unit admission necessary in mild traumatic brain injury? *J Neurosurg* **116**: 549–557.

32. Provenzale JM (2010). Imaging of traumatic brain injury: a review of the recent medical literature. *AJR* **194**: 16–19.

33. Shenton ME, Hamoda HM, Schneiderman JS, et al. (2012). A review of magnetic resonance imaging and diffusion tensor imaging findings in mild traumatic brain injury. *Brain Imaging Behav* **6**: 137–192.

34. Tawil I, Stein DM, Mirvis SE, Scalea TM (2008). Posttraumatic cerebral infarction: incidence, outcome, and risk factors. *J Trauma* **64**: 849–853.

35. Rodallec MH, Marteau V, Gerber S, Desmottes L, Zins M (2008). Craniocervical arterial dissection: spectrum of imaging findings and differential diagnosis. *Radiographics* **28**: 1711–1728.

36. Manolakaki D, Velmahos GC, Spaniolas K, de Moya M, Alam HB (2009). Early magnetic resonance imaging is unnecessary in patients with traumatic brain injury. *J Trauma Acute Care Surg* **66**: 1008–1014.

37. Fiser SM, Johnson SB, Fortune JB (1998). Resource utilization in traumatic brain injury: the role of magnetic resonance imaging. *Am Surg* **64**: 1088–1093.

247

38. Foerster BR, Petrou M, Lin D, *et al.* (2009). Neuroimaging evaluation of non-accidental head trauma with correlation to clinical outcomes: a review of 57 cases. *J Pediatr* **154**: 573–577.

39. Kumar S, Goddeau RP, Jr., Selim MH, *et al.* (2010). Atraumatic convexal subarachnoid hemorrhage: clinical presentation, imaging patterns, and etiologies. *Neurology* **74**: 893–899.

40. Haacke EM, Mittal S, Wu Z, Neelavalli J, Cheng YC (2009). Susceptibility-weighted imaging: technical aspects and clinical applications, part 1. *AJNR* **30**: 19–30.

41. Akiyama Y, Miyata K, Harada K, *et al.* (2009). Susceptibility-weighted magnetic resonance imaging for the detection of cerebral microhemorrhage in patients with traumatic brain injury. *Neurologia Medico-chirurgica* **49**: 97–99.

42. Tong KA, Ashwal S, Holshouser BA, *et al.* (2003). Hemorrhagic shearing lesions in children and adolescents with posttraumatic diffuse axonal injury: improved detection and initial results. *Radiology* **227**: 332–339.

43. Colbert CA, Holshouser BA, Aaen GS, *et al.* (2010). Value of cerebral microhemorrhages detected with susceptibility-weighted MR imaging for prediction of long-term outcome in children with nonaccidental trauma. *Radiology* **256**: 898–905.

44. Scheid R, Ott DV, Roth H, Schroeter ML, von Cramon DY (2007). Comparative magnetic resonance imaging at 1.5 and 3 Tesla for the evaluation of traumatic microbleeds. *J Neurotrauma* **24**: 1811–1816.

45. Stuckey SL, Goh TD, Heffernan T, Rowan D (2007). Hyperintensity in the subarachnoid space on FLAIR MRI. *AJR* **189**: 913–921.

46. Inglese M, Makani S, Johnson G, *et al.* (2005). Diffuse axonal injury in mild traumatic brain injury: a diffusion tensor imaging study. *J Neurosurg* **103**: 298–303.

47. Smith SM, Jenkinson M, Johansen-Berg H, *et al.* (2006). Tract-based spatial statistics: voxelwise analysis of multi-subject diffusion data. *NeuroImage* **31**: 1487–505.

48. Kinnunen KM, Greenwood R, Powell JH, *et al.* (2011). White matter damage and cognitive impairment after traumatic brain injury. *Brain* **134**(Pt 2): 449–463.

49. Grossman EJ, Inglese M, Bammer R (2010). Mild traumatic brain injury: is diffusion imaging ready for primetime in forensic medicine? *Topics MRI* **21**: 379–386.

50. Rutgers DR, Toulgoat F, Cazejust J, *et al.* (2008). White matter abnormalities in mild traumatic brain injury: a diffusion tensor imaging study. *AJNR* **29**: 514–519.

Chapter 15

Spinal cord trauma

Louis P. Riccelli, Michelle Cameron, Andrew G. Burke, and Rajarshi Mazumder

Introduction

This chapter discusses the clinical and radiologic examination and findings for patients with known or suspected acute spinal cord trauma. It does not cover injury to other structures of the spine, including the discs, ligaments, and vertebrae, except as these relate to acute spinal cord trauma.

The average estimated incidence of traumatic spinal cord injury (SCI) in the United States is 40 per million, which is higher than in the rest of the world [1]. In Western Europe, the median incidence of traumatic SCI is 16 per million, with reports ranging from 9.2 per million in Denmark to 33.6 per million in Greece [2]. In the United States, motor-vehicle crashes (MVCs) are the most common cause of SCI overall although, in people over 60, falls are the most common cause. In developed countries, the proportion of traumatic SCI due to MVCs tends to be stable or decreasing, likely due to safer cars and better infrastructure. In developing countries, the proportion of SCI caused by MVCs is increasing, likely because motor-vehicle use is increasing without standardized vehicle safety equipment or infrastructure. Injuries from falls in the elderly are also increasing in developed countries as the proportion of the population surviving to old age increases. In addition, SCI due to violence is more common in South Africa, the Middle East, Brazil, and the USA than in the rest of the world [2].

The mechanism and level of SCI also vary by age and gender. Rates are lowest in young children and highest in persons in their late teens or early twenties, with a possible secondary peak among the elderly [1]. SCI is three to four times more common in males than in females. In children younger than 8 years of age, SCI is more commonly due to MVCs, more commonly involves the upper cervical spine, and more commonly involves injury to the ligaments or spinal cord without necessarily involving the bones. In contrast, in children older than 8 years of age, SCI is most commonly sports-related, peaking at 13–15 years of age, is more common in males, and more often involves the lower cervical spine [3].

While this chapter focuses on traumatic SCI, it should be noted that the non-traumatic SCI is probably more common and is associated with a much poorer prognosis because such injuries are usually caused by a progressive underlying lesion.

General considerations for clinical examination

Clinical examination of the patient with spinal cord trauma begins with the standard measures for all potentially life-threatening medical conditions, and focuses on circulation, airway, and breathing. Once the patient has been medically stabilized, examination related specifically to spinal cord trauma is typically performed in rostro-caudal sequence, starting with findings associated with upper cervical cord levels and ending with the cauda equina.

Clinical findings associated with spinal cord trauma evolve over time. During the initial phase, the neural elements are affected by direct mechanical disruption or by displacement of adjoining support structures such as vertebral body, disc, or ligaments. Later, the injury evolves as a result of vascular dysfunction causing ischemia or edema, excitotoxicity, and inflammation, eventually resulting in cell death. Spinal shock (also known as areflexia) is common during the acute phase of spinal cord trauma. This phenomenon occurs immediately at the time of injury and lasts for days to weeks. Spinal shock is characterized by complete loss of motor, sensory, and autonomic function below the level of the spinal cord lesion. There is flaccid paralysis with hyporeflexia and reduced muscle tone. With resolution of spinal shock, deep tendon reflexes reappear and become hyperactive and muscle tone increases causing spasticity as is typically associated with upper-motor-neuron injury. However, at the level of injury where there is also lower-motor-neuron involvement, motor function remains flaccid even after resolution of spinal shock.

The International Standards for Neurological Classification of Spinal Cord Injury (ISNCSCI) published by the American Spinal Injury Association (ASIA) is a tool widely used to evaluate and classify neurological impairment associated with SCI [4]. The neurological examination required for this classification focuses on sensory and motor functions and is not comprehensive. The examination is performed in a supine position, except for the rectal examination, which can be performed in a lateral decubitus position.

Based on the functional findings of the neurological examination, ASIA grades the severity and the level of the injury. Injury severity ranges from normal to complete motor and sensory loss. Level of injury is defined as the most caudal segment of the spinal cord with intact bilateral motor and sensory function. According to the ISNCSCI guidelines for neurological examination, the sensory examination is performed by testing sensation to light touch and pin prick at 28 dermatomes from C2 to S4–S5 on both sides of the body. In addition, key muscle functions corresponding to 10 myotomes (C5–T1 and L2–S1) are tested to examine the motor system [4].

Craniocervical and high or mid-level cervical cord lesions may affect breathing and produce motor and sensory deficits below the neck. Mid and lower cervical injuries affect the upper and lower extremities. Thoracic and lumbar lesions affect the lower extremities and cauda equina lesions affect bowel and bladder function and perineal sensation. Clinical findings also vary depending on the completeness of the injury, which is related to the cross-sectional region of the cord affected. With complete cross-section injury there is complete loss of function below the level of the lesion. When only certain cross-sectional regions are damaged, only the functions impacted by these regions are affected. Examination should include testing of sensation and motor function associated with each spinal level to help ascertain the severity and level of injury and should be repeated over time to assess injury evolution.

Discussion of spinal cord injury is incomplete without the mention of the following well-recognized clinical syndromes: central cord syndrome, Brown–Séquard syndrome, anterior cord syndrome, posterior-cord syndrome, conus medullaris syndrome, and cauda equina syndrome.

As the name suggests, central cord syndrome is characterized by injury to the central portion of the cervical spinal cord with sparing of the peripheral spinal cord. Clinically, central cord syndrome presents with greater weakness of the upper extremities and lesser impairment or preservation of function in the lower extremities. Brown–Séquard syndrome is characterized by anterior to posterior hemisection of the spinal cord or localized damage to one side of the spinal cord. Clinically, this presents with ipsilateral loss of proprioception, vibration, and motor function and contralateral loss of sensitivity to light touch, pressure, pain, and temperature. Anterior cord syndrome results from isolated damage to the anterior portion of the cord's white and gray matter, with preservation of the dorsal columns. Clinically, this syndrome is characterized by complete loss of motor function and loss of pain and temperature sensation at and below the level of the injury. Posterior cord syndrome results from damage to the dorsal columns and relative sparing of the anterior cord. This clinically presents with loss of proprioception and vibration sensation and preservation of motor and other sensory functions. Conus medullaris syndrome results from injury to the terminal portion of the spinal cord, commonly due to thoraco-lumbar bony injury. Clinically, this presents with preserved sacral reflexes, including the bulbo cavernous reflex and anal wink, with spastic paralysis, hypertonia, and hyperreflexia of the lower extremities. Cauda equina syndrome is caused by damage to lumbosacral nerve roots after the spinal cord terminates at the L2 vertebral level. Clinically, this presents with flaccid paralysis and sensory loss in the lower extremities and bladder dysfunction.

General considerations for radiological examination

While magnetic resonance imaging (MRI) best characterizes the spinal cord and spinal-canal contents in patients with suspected SCI, in the setting of trauma computed tomography (CT) generally precedes MRI. CT is more available, quick, and can be used to rapidly assess for unstable fractures, major ligamentous disruption, and injuries in other areas including intracranial, intrathoracic, and intra-abdominal regions that might require immediate intervention.

When imaging the cervical spine after acute trauma, CT has replaced plain-film radiography in most cases because of its availability, higher sensitivity, and specificity for fractures compared to radiography, ability to consistently evaluate the entire cervical spine with infrequent need for repeat examination, and speed and convenience of imaging, especially when CT imaging of other body areas is needed [5]. CT has been shown to be cost effective in high and moderate risk groups [6]. In the rare situation that a patient cannot cooperate for CT examination, a lateral or full series of cervical radiographs may be used for gross assessment of alignment.

The most commonly used criteria for deciding if a patient with trauma requires CT imaging of the cervical spine are based on several large studies of plain-film imaging data. The National Emergency X-Radiography Utilization Study (NEXUS) [7], with over 34 000 patients, and Canadian C-spine rule (CCR) [8], developed from data from over 8 900 patients, provide imaging criteria with high sensitivities for identifying patients at risk for SCI. The NEXUS criteria have 99.6% sensitivity for imaging patients with a clinically significant injury. Patients are considered at low risk for cord injury and not requiring imaging if they meet all five criteria: no midline cervical spine tenderness, no focal neurological deficit, normal level of alertness, no intoxication, and no distracting injury. The CCR requires a fully alert patient with a Glasgow Coma Scale (GCS) score of 15. Three main questions are asked: (1) Are there high risk factors that would mandate imaging (age $\geq$ 65 years old, dangerous mechanism, or paresthesias)? (2) Is there at least one low risk factor that would allow safe assessment of range of motion (simple rear-end collision, sitting in the emergency department, ambulatory since injury, delayed onset of pain, or absence of midline cervical-spine tenderness)? (3) Is the patient able to actively rotate the neck 45° to the left and right? In the absence of high risk factors, the presence of a low risk factor, and the ability to actively rotate the neck in each direction, no imaging is needed. Dangerous mechanism includes a fall from more than 1 meter or five stairs, axial load to head, high speed MVC (>100 km/hr), rollover, ejection, motorized recreational vehicle, and bicycle collision.

Cervical spine CT imaging protocols generally consist of a thin helical acquisition of data from above the occipital condyles through the T1 vertebra, reconstructed in bone algorithms in axial, sagittal, and coronal planes with a reconstructed slice thickness of 1–2 mm. Soft-tissue algorithm images in at least one plane can be helpful for evaluating soft tissues, including intervertebral disks. Intravenous contrast is not needed for this examination unless there is concern for vascular injury, in which case a single arterial-phase helical scan can be obtained to then generate both CT angiogram (CTA) images and cervical-spine bone reconstructions from one acquisition, thereby reducing radiation exposure.

MRI is useful for evaluating ligamentous injury, the extent of spinal cord edema, the presence of intramedullary hemorrhage, the degree of spinal-cord compression, and the presence of transection or penetrating injury (Figure 15.1). A greater extent of soft tissue injury, a greater extent of spinal cord edema, the presence of intramedullary hemorrhage, and the severity of spinal cord compression have been correlated with worse prognosis [9]. MRI is also extremely sensitive for detecting soft-tissue edema near the spinal ligaments, even in stable injury patterns without major ligamentous disruption.

The role of MRI, if any, in "clearing" the cervical spine and in evaluating obtunded patients for ligamentous injury is debated. MRI is not generally recommended as a standard clearance test [7]. However, MRI has been suggested for specific scenarios such as clearance in obtunded patients who have a neurological deficit in the extremities.

MRI will not infrequently detect abnormality in the presence of a normal CT scan in patients with neurological deficit, perhaps in as many as 20% of cases. Although most findings will not prompt immediate surgical therapy or change in therapy, some centers advocate early MRI to take advantage of the potentially important immediate window of opportunity within the first 24 hours. However, the delay to intervention necessitated by adding MRI to the acute evaluation after injury must also be considered. The likelihood of a cervical MRI showing an abnormality after a normal CT in neurologically normal patients that would result in a change in surgical management has been estimated to be as low as 0.1% [8]. Rare spinal epidural hemorrhage and even more rare subdural hemorrhage have been described after major or minor trauma, especially in patients with hypocoagulable states. These hemorrhages may be large enough to compromise the spinal cord. While these could on

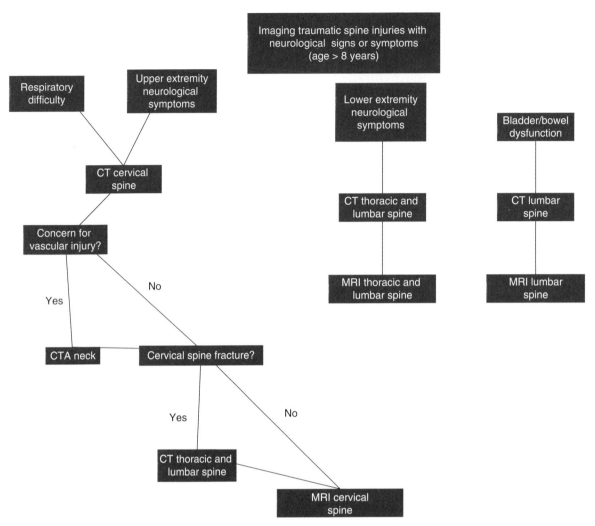

Figure 15.1 Imaging algorithm for patients 8 years of age or older with signs or symptoms of acute SCI.

occasion be detectable by CT based on their hyper-density, MRI offers far greater sensitivity, particularly in the early subacute stages as methemoglobin evolves (hyperintense to spinal cord on T1-weighted images).

MRI scanning protocols for cervical-spine trauma generally include routine T1- and T2-weighted sequences plus a fat-suppressed fluid weighted sequence such as fat-suppressed T2 or short tau inversion recovery (STIR). When MRI of the cervical spine is performed after trauma, axial fat-suppressed T2-weighted images should be extended through the craniocervical junction to evaluate the craniocervical junction ligaments. This is not typically done for routine cervical-spine MRI pro-tocols. A sagittal T2* gradient-echo (GRE) sequence should also be performed as this improves sensitivity for hemorrhage. Intravenous contrast is typically not

needed unless there is suspicion for underlying tumor or infection. If vascular injury is suspected and CTA has not been performed, axial fat-suppressed T1-weighted images and two-dimensional time-of-flight magnetic resonance angiogram (MRA) sequences of the neck can be added.

Compared to data regarding imaging for cervical SCI, there are fewer data regarding indications for thoracic and lumbar spine imaging. Based on a review of the literature, the American College of Radiology has established the following criteria for thoraco-lumbar imaging in trauma: back pain or midline tenderness, local signs of thoraco-lumbar injury, abnormal neurological signs, cervical-spine fracture, GCS score of less than 15, major distracting injury, and alcohol or drug intoxication [10]. CT of the

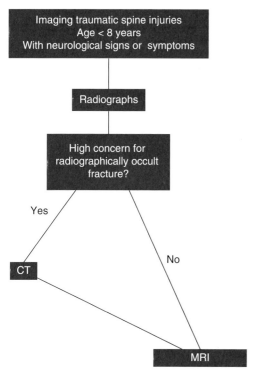

Figure 15.2 Imaging algorithm for patients younger than 8 years of age with signs or symptoms of acute SCI.

thoracic and lumbar spine is superior to radiographs, whether images are obtained as a dedicated CT spine protocol or reconstructed from the data obtained for a chest, abdomen, and pelvis CT [11], thereby obviating the need for an additional CT scan. With multi-detector CT, spine reconstructions can typically also be reformatted retrospectively from torso scan data even if spinal imaging was not ordered at the time of the initial scan.

Thoraco-lumbar (T-L) MRI is primarily used to further characterize myelopathy or known injury. Unstable thoracic or lumbar ligamentous injury in the setting of a normal CT is considered exceedingly rare or non-existent. Routine T-L spine imaging protocols can be used for myelopathy, to include a sagittal fat-suppressed T2-weighted sequence or STIR. A T2* GRE sequence can increase sensitivity for spinal canal or intramedullary spinal cord hemorrhage. As in the cervical spine, intravenous contrast is not needed unless there is concern for underlying tumor or infection.

Because of the different manifestations of injury in younger children, and concerns about radiation from CT, cervical (plain-film) radiography is often the initial method of imaging in children 8 years of age or younger. MRI is used for further evaluation for suspected ligamentous or SCI, and CT is used judiciously only when there is high suspicion for bony injury (Figure 15.2). The ideal role of CT versus radiographs in the initial evaluation of children remains unclear. When CT is utilized, lower-dose pediatric CT protocols should be utilized.

Breathing problems

Clinical presentation

Respiratory compromise after SCI is common, with reported incidence ranging from 36–83% [12, 13]. Respiratory complications such as bronchospasm, pulmonary edema, atelectasis, and pneumonia are the leading causes of morbidity and mortality associated with SCI. Without immediate respiratory support, complete SCI at or above the C3 level is incompatible with life because innervation to all the muscles of respiration is lost. With injury to the C3–C5 levels of the spinal cord, breathing is affected because these spinal nerves contribute to the phrenic nerve, which controls the diaphragm. In addition, nerves originating from the cervical and thoracic region of the spinal cord innervate muscles of respiration, such as the external intercostal muscles and the accessory muscles of respiration. Injury to these spinal levels can also compromise breathing by significantly decreasing tidal volume and vital capacity. Patients with respiratory compromise due to SCI often require ventilator support and pulmonary rehabilitation.

Thoracic SCI should be suspected in the presence of paradoxical breathing [12], where the soft tissues of the thorax cave in during inspiration. This occurs because negative intra-pleural pressure is produced by isolated diaphragmatic contraction when the chest wall is paralyzed by injury to the thoracic spinal cord.

Given the high rates of mortality and morbidity associated with respiratory complications in people with SCI, aggressive respiratory care must be provided and patients with spinal cord trauma need to be followed vigilantly to prevent or minimize these complications.

Case 1: fracture, intrinsic spinal cord hemorrhage, and edema

An 80-year-old man fell from a ladder and was found unresponsive with severe bradycardia, fixed and dilated pupils, and an initial GCS score of 3

253

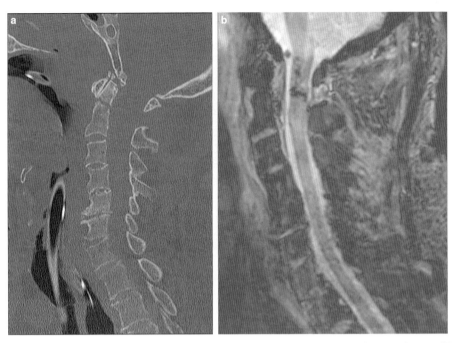

Figure 15.3 (a) Midline sagittal non-contrast CT scan shows an acute Type 2 odontoid process fracture. (b) Midline sagittal non-contrast T2* GRE MRI scan shows cord edema and hemorrhage and surrounding paraspinal edema.

with intubation of the patient. Cardio-pulmonary resuscitation was performed for 7 to 8 minutes and epinephrine and atropine were given in conjunction with transcutaneous pacing. A midline sagittal non-contrast CT image of the cervical spine (Figure 15.3a) shows an acute, minimally displaced fracture through the base of the C2 odontoid process (Type 2) and mild widening of the C1–C2 interspinous interval. A midline sagittal noncontrast T2* GRE MRI of the cervical spine (Figure 15.3b) showed extensive edema about the C1–C2 level and surrounding paraspinal soft tissues, edema within the upper cervical spinal cord, and multiple foci of susceptibility artifact within the cord at C1–C2 consistent with cord hemorrhage. Following imaging, the patient was found to have advanced directives for do not resuscitate (DNR) status and care was subsequently withdrawn, resulting in apnea and death.

Upper-extremity involvement

Clinical presentation

In addition to breathing compromise, injuries to the cervical spinal cord may lead to loss of sensation below the neck and loss of motor functions in muscle groups of the upper and lower extremities and the trunk. Tetraplegia or quadriplegia can result from injuries to the upper cervical cord (C1–C4). Along with motor and sensory impairment of the upper and lower extremities, these patients may also experience dysphagia and difficulty with coughing as well as bowel and bladder dysfunction. Lower cervical cord (C5–C8) injury leads to loss of function in the associated myotomes and dermatomes in the upper extremities. Depending on the completeness and level of the injury, patients will present with partial or complete paralysis of arms, hands, wrists, and lower extremities. A C5-spinal-level injury results in motor dysfunction of the biceps and brachialis, and consequent loss of elbow flexion. Injury to the C6 level affects wrist extension as a result of paralysis of the wrist-extensor muscle groups such as the extensor carpi radialis longus and brevis. Extension at the elbow is affected with injury at the C7 level and consequent motor dysfunction of the triceps. A C8-level injury disrupts finger flexion by affecting the flexor digitorum profundus muscles of the hand. Loss of fifth digit abduction due to dysfunction of the abductor digiti minimi indicates a T1-level spinal injury.

Case 2: ligamentous injury and spinal cord edema without fracture

A 30-year-old man sustained a hyperflexion injury of the neck while playing soccer resulting in diminished sensation from the chest down and paresthesias in the arms and legs. The patient regained motion of the legs after several minutes. On examination, there was decreased muscle strength at C5, C6, C8, T1, L2, and L3 motor levels. A midline sagittal non-contrast CT image of the cervical spine (Figure 15.4a) showed a flexion-distraction injury at C5–C6 with associated focal kyphosis, anterolisthesis of C5 on C6, and widening of the C5–C6 interspinous interval without evident fracture. A midline sagittal non-contrast STIR MR scan (Figure 15.4b) of the cervical spine showed the associated ligamentous injuries with disruption of the anterior and posterior longitudinal ligaments and ligamentum flavum with focal-cord spinal cord edema at C5–C6 and extensive paraspinal soft-tissue edema. The patient was treated surgically with C5–C6 anterior cervical fusion and placement in a hard collar, resulting in progressive improvement in hand strength and pain; he was able to perform activities of daily living without difficulty within 2 months.

Lower-extremity involvement

Clinical presentation – thoracic injury

Thoraco-lumbar SCIs affect trunk and lower-extremity function and spare respiratory and upper-extremity function. T1–T12 thoracic-level injuries produce loss of functions of muscle groups in the upper chest, mid-back, and abdominal muscles. Thoracic lesions affect the intercostal muscles and may affect trunk control. Injuries at the lower-thoracic level (T6–T12) may result in paraplegia due to loss of motor function of the trunk and the lower extremities.

Case 3: compression and edema of thoracic cord from retropulsed fracture fragment

A 29-year-old man involved in an all-terrain vehicle crash experienced immediate sensory and motor loss in the lower extremities bilaterally, confirmed on physical examination, with a sensory deficit beginning at the level of the xiphoid. A midline sagittal CT image of the thoracic spine (Figure 15.5a) reconstructed from a CT of the chest, abdomen, and pelvis with contrast showed an acute T7 vertebral body burst fracture with associated focal kyphosis and

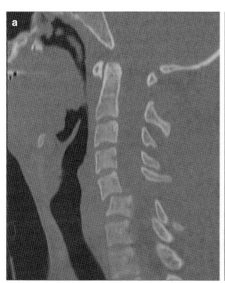
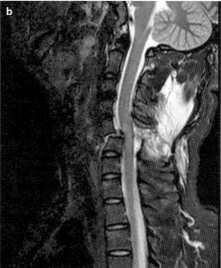

Figure 15.4 (a) Midline sagittal non-contrast CT scan shows a C5–C6 flexion-distraction injury without fracture. (b) Midline sagittal non-contrast STIR MRI scan shows anterior and posterior longitudinal ligament and ligamentum flavum disruption with focal cord edema at C5–C6.

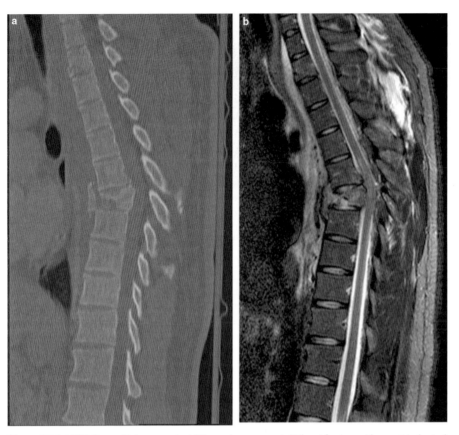

Figure 15.5 (a) Midline sagittal non-contrast CT scan shows an acute T7 burst fracture with associated spinal-canal stenosis and acute T2 and T6 vertebral body fractures without canal stenosis. (b) Midline sagittal non-contrast STIR MRI scan shows the T7 burst fracture with spinal cord edema at the T6 through T7 levels and extensive paraspinal edema.

retropulsion of the posterior cortex, resulting in spinal canal stenosis at the T7 level. Also present were minimally displaced acute fractures of the anterior, inferior T2, and posterior, inferior T6 vertebral bodies. A midline sagittal non-contrast STIR MRI scan (Figure 15.5b) of the thoracic spine showed the T7 burst fracture with associated cord edema at T6 and T7 and extensive anterior and posterior paraspinal edema. The patient was treated surgically with posterior decompression at T7 and fixation from T5 to T9 with no subsequent neurologic recovery.

Clinical presentation – lumbar injury

Injuries at the L1–L5 level lead to loss of motor function of the hip flexors and extensors, and the other lower extremity muscles. Specifically, injury at the L2 spinal level leads to a loss of iliopsoas muscle function and consequent hip-flexion weakness. Knee extension, powered by the quadriceps muscle group, is affected by injury at the L3 level. Ankle dorsiflexion, controlled primarily by the tibialis anterior, is disrupted by L4 spinal level injury and injury to the L5 spinal level causes loss of function of the extensor hallucis longus and consequent loss of great-toe extension. Ankle plantar flexion weakness is associated with loss of gastrocnemius and soleus muscle function due to injury at the S1 spinal level.

Since the spinal cord is shorter than the spinal canal and ends at around the L2 vertebral level, lower thoracic and lumbar cord levels are higher than their respective vertebral levels. As the spinal cord ends, it extends to form the cauda equina. Any injury rostral to this level will preserve the sacral reflex arc, but damage the upper motor neurons. This clinically presents with spastic paralysis, hypertonia, and hyperreflexia of the lower extremities. Injuries caudal to the beginning of the cauda equina will damage only the lower motor neurons, which results in flaccid paralysis, muscle atrophy, and areflexia of the lower extremities.

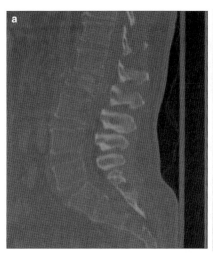
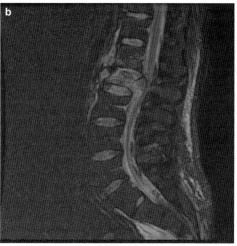

Figure 15.6 (a) Midline sagittal non-contrast CT scan shows an acute L2 burst fracture resulting in severe spinal canal stenosis. (b) Midline sagittal non-contrast STIR MRI scan shows the L2 burst fracture causing compression of the conus medullaris tip and cauda equina at the L2 level and a ventral epidural hematoma at L3 causing additional spinal canal stenosis below the fracture level.

Case 4: fracture, retropulsion, and epidural hematoma with conus tip and cauda equina compression

A 42-year-old man fell from a roof, and experienced immediate right lower-extremity weakness. The patient was intubated and sedated on presentation, so physical examination was limited, but it was clear that the patient had right lower extremity weakness. A midline sagittal CT image of the lumbar spine (Figure 15.6a) reconstructed from a CT of the chest, abdomen, and pelvis with contrast showed an acute L2 vertebral body burst fracture with retropulsion of the posterior cortex resulting in severe spinal canal stenosis. A midline sagittal non-contrast STIR MRI scan of the lumbar spine (Figure 15.6b) showed the burst fracture causing compression of the tip of the conus medullaris and nerve roots of the cauda equina at the L2 level and spinal canal stenosis at L3 secondary to an associated ventral epidural hematoma. At the time of surgical decompression, the patient was found to have a complex dural tear and several contused and lacerated nerve roots. Bowel and bladder function were normal. There was progressive recovery of right lower-extremity motor function.

Bowel and bladder dysfunction

Clinical presentation

Any lesion impacting the sacral S2–S4 spinal cord levels or above may result in neurogenic bowel or bladder. Neurogenic bladder may present with urinary retention and/or incontinence due to dysfunctional contraction of the detrusor or bladder sphincter muscles. Given the high risk for renal failure with untreated urinary retention, bladder function including assessment of post void residual urine volume should be performed as part of emergency evaluation of all patients with SCI. Long-term management of neurogenic bladder may require medications and ongoing catheterization.

Bowel dysfunction can be another distressing sequela of SCI. Depending on the level of the spinal cord lesion, different complications of neurogenic bowel may result. Cessation of gut peristalsis, gastric distention, and paralytic ileus can lead to severe morbidity and decline in quality of life. In the long term, patients may therefore need a bowel and bladder program after SCI.

Case 5: acute lumbar disk herniation with cauda equina compression

A 58-year-old man experienced acute lower-back pain, urinary hesitancy, pain radiating down his left leg, and bilateral lower-extremity weakness after lifting a heavy box. On examination, he was also found to have diminished plantarflexion and dorsiflexion strength, and diminished rectal tone. There was no sensory deficit. A midline sagittal non-contrast T2-weighted image of the lumbar spine showed an L4–L5 intervertebral disk extrusion causing severe spinal canal stenosis and compression of the nerve roots of the cauda equina (Figure 15.7). The patient was treated surgically with L4 and L5 laminectomies and L4–L5 diskectomy

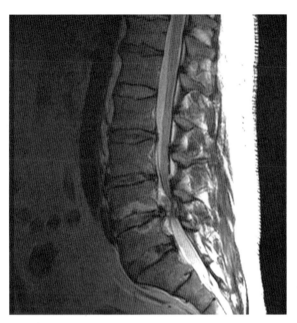

Figure 15.7 Midline sagittal non-contrast T2-weighted MRI scan shows an L4–L5 intervertebral disk extrusion causing severe spinal canal stenosis and compression of the cauda equina nerve roots.

with only mild residual lower-back pain and no residual neurologic deficit after 1 year.

Late-stage sequelae of SCI

Clinical presentation

The most common late-stage complications of SCI include pressure ulcers, pneumonia, and genitourinary issues. Other late-stage clinical sequalae may include spasticity, contractures, atrophy, immobility, and sensory loss. Pressure ulcers are tissue breakdown due to pressure, friction, and moisture. Pressure ulcers can be a significant late cause of morbidity and mortality in people with SCI.

By imaging, late or delayed pathology includes myelomalacia, with focal spinal cord atrophy evident as loss of cord thickness over a short segment, and/or loss of the normal spinal cord contour. Syringomyelia is usually detected and more optimally characterized by MRI compared to CT. Adhesions and tethering and entrapment of spinal cord in dural disruptions may require detailed anatomic imaging including CT myelography. Nerve root avulsion and pseudomeningocele may be visualized by CT/myelography or high-resolution heavily T2-weighted MRI. Wallerian degeneration, evident as vertically oriented T2-hyperintense signal following neuronal tracts may also become evident by MRI in follow-up series.

Chronic compression of the spinal cord may be associated with intrinsic cord hyperintensity on T2-weighted images, as not uncommonly observed in cervical degenerative and/or post-traumatic compression by disk and/or osteophytes. The etiology of the hyperintensity is reactive gliosis and/or edema.

Case 6: vertebral burst fracture with delayed syringomyelia

A 24-year-old man sustained a T7 burst fracture while skiing and was managed conservatively. One year after the initial injury, the patient had only mild residual pain and kyphoscoliosis but no neurologic deficits. A midline sagittal non-contrast T2 image of the thoracic spine obtained at the 1-year follow-up visit showed mild chronic vertebral height loss at T7 without residual spinal canal stenosis (Figure 15.8). A thin, post-traumatic syrinx is seen within the spinal cord from T5 through T8.

Advanced and experimental MRI

There is only a limited literature and some controversy surrounding the use of advanced MRI methods in the evaluation of acute spinal cord trauma, most notably methods based on diffusion imaging [14]. Nevertheless, there are considerable theoretical advantages and enthusiasm for using diffusion-weighted MRI for improved sensitivity to spinal cord infarction, and diffusion tensor imaging for detail regarding fiber pathway integrity. Blood products, the small size of the spinal cord, cerebral spinal fluid pulsations, and adjacent bony structures all contribute to technical limitations for the diffusion methodology as currently implemented. In the future, multiple quantitative MRI measures (e.g. magnetization transfer, proton magnetic resonance spectroscopy) will likely become important in monitoring neuroprotection and repair post spinal cord trauma.

Conclusions

It is important to assess patients with known or suspected SCI early to minimize the risk of avoidable complications. Clinical assessment focuses on the severity and level of injury. Early examination should pay particular attention to respiratory function. This is followed by assessment of bladder function and the myotomal and dermatomal distribution of the injury. Since SCI and its sequelae evolve over time, the examination should be repeated to assess for changes in function. In the setting of acute adult trauma, NEXUS and CCR criteria can guide the need for imaging in the

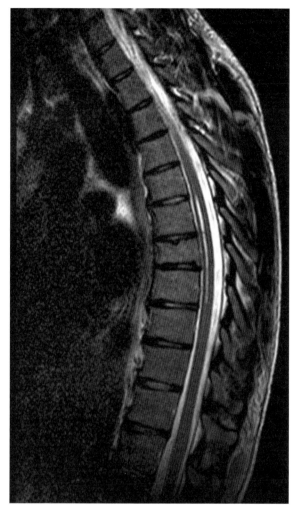

Figure 15.8 Midline sagittal non-contrast T2 MRI scan shows mild chronic T7 vertebral body height loss without spinal canal stenosis. A thin syrinx is present within the spinal cord from T5 through T8.

absence of neurological symptoms. CT is most often the initial method of imaging in trauma. MRI is useful for further evaluating suspected ligamentous injury and for evaluating acute neurological symptoms related to potential SCI. In the young pediatric population, there are fewer data to guide initial imaging in trauma, but radiographs may be used initially, with MRI used for further assessment of neurological symptoms or ligamentous injury, and CT used judiciously. With good early evaluation and long-term management, people with SCI have the potential to enjoy a high quality of life.

References

1. Devivo MJ (2012). Epidemiology of traumatic spinal cord injury: trends and future implications. *Spinal Cord* **50**: 365–372.

2. Lee BB, Cripps RA, Fitzharris M, Wing PC (2013). The global map for traumatic spinal cord injury epidemiology: update 2011, global incidence rate. *Spinal Cord* **52**: 110–116.

3. Platzer P, Jaindl M, Thalhammer G, *et al.* (2007). Cervical spine injuries in pediatric patients. *J Trauma* **62**: 389–396.

4. Kirshblum SC, Burns SP, Biering-Sorensen F, *et al.* (2011). International standards for neurological classification of spinal cord injury (revised 2011). *J Spinal Cord Med* **34**: 535–546.

5. Looby S, Flanders A (2011). Spine trauma. *Radiol Clin N Am* **49**: 129–163.

6. Blackmore CC, Ramsey SD, Mann FA, Deyo RA (1999). Cervical spine screening with CT in trauma patients: a cost-effectiveness analysis. *Radiology* **212**: 117–125.

7. Hoffman JR, Mower WR, Wolfson AB, Todd KH, Zucker MI (2000). Validity of a set of clinical criteria to rule out injury to the cervical spine in patients with blunt trauma. National Emergency X-Radiography Utilization Study Group. *N Engl J Med* **343**: 94–99.

8. Stiell IG, Wells GA, Vandemheen KL, *et al.* (2001). The Canadian C-spine rule for radiography in alert and stable trauma patients. *JAMA* **286**: 1841–1848.

9. Bozzo A, Marcoux J, Radhakrishna M, Pelletier J, Goulet B (2011). The role of magnetic resonance imaging in the management of acute spinal cord injury. *J Neurotrauma* **28**: 1401–1411.

10. American College of Radiology (2012). ACR appropriateness criteria. *Suspected Spine Trauma.* Available at: http://www.acr.org/Quality-Safety/Appropriateness-Criteria/Diagnostic, accessed March 9, 2012.

11. Sheridan R, Peralta R, Rhea J, Ptak T, Novelline R (2003). Reformatted visceral protocol helical computed tomographic scanning allows conventional radiographs of the thoracic and lumbar spine to be eliminated in the evaluation of blunt trauma patients. *J Trauma* **55**: 665–669.

12. Berlly M, Shem K (2007). Respiratory management during the first five days after spinal cord injury. *J Spinal Cord Med* **30**: 309–318.

13. Casha S, Christie S (2011) A systematic review of intensive cardiopulmonary management after spinal cord injury. *J Neurotrauma* **28**: 1479–1495.

14. Pouw MH, van der Vliet AM, van Kampen A, *et al.* (2012). Diffusion-weighted MR imaging within 24 h post-injury after traumatic spinal cord injury: a qualitative meta-analysis between T2-weighted imaging and diffusion-weighted MR imaging in 18 patients. *Spinal Cord* **50**: 426–431.

Chapter 16

Bladder, bowel, and sexual dysfunction

Firouz Daneshgari, Raj M. Paspulati, and Jack H. Simon

The main focus of this chapter is neurogenic bladder dysfunction, mostly referred to as neurogenic bladder (NGB), which is a dysfunction of the urinary bladder due to diseases of the central and/or peripheral nervous system that control bladder function [1]. The acute neurological disorders affecting bowel (e.g. neurogenic bowel) and sexual function (e.g. erectile dysfunction) are briefly considered within the context of associated dysfunctions as there are common and overlapping neurological pathways and pathologies affecting the three functional systems.

Common diseases of the nervous system that affect the bladder, bowel, and sexual function include multiple sclerosis (MS), spinal cord injury, spina bifida, and other congenital anomalies, Parkinson's disease, cerebrovascular events/stroke, and localized infectious/inflammatory disease affecting the spinal cord and nerve roots [2–5]. For MS alone, according to recent estimates, there are approximately 350 000 people in the USA with physician-diagnosed disease and worldwide estimates are on the order of 2.5 million people. The prevalence of NGB is more than 96% in patients with MS with duration longer than 10 years [2]. Long-term bladder, as well as bowel and sexual dysfunction contribute markedly to the morbidity and are major quality-of-life issues after spinal trauma, which also strikes individuals early in their lives.

It is not entirely understood how disturbances in neurological pathways result in NGB. However, studies have shown that patients with MS lesions, for example interrupting the neural pathways connecting the pontine micturition center to the sacral micturition center, develop a combination of storage and voiding problems, or a condition specific to neurogenic conditions termed detrusor sphincter dyssynergia (DSD) [6]. DSD is a clinical and urodynamic phenomenon in which the detrusor and urethral sphincters

contract simultaneously rather than reciprocally, thus leading to a functional outlet obstruction [7]. It is among the most difficult conditions to treat and may lead to other complications such as overflow incontinence, vesico-ureteral reflex, and ultimately renal failure. NGB is among the leading causes of morbidity and mortality in MS and other neurological conditions [8]. Similar to many other chronic diseases, such as diabetes, it is ultimately the multiple organ complications that lead to marked deterioration of quality of life and contribute to mortality.

Types of NGB

The bladder has two major and distinct functions: urine storage and urine disposal. A simplified categorization of bladder dysfunction into problems of storage or voiding has been widely accepted [9]. For instance, symptoms of urgency and urge incontinence often seen in idiopathic overactive bladder (OAB) are recognized as storage problems, whereas hesitancy and slow urine stream seen in patients with enlarged, yet atonic bladders, such as in diabetes and neurogenic conditions, are recognized as voiding problems. Urodynamic studies are often used to clarify the storage (e.g. sensory urgency and detrusor overactivity) or voiding (e.g. slow flow, high detrusor pressure and post-void residual) nature of the bladder dysfunction. Recently, associations of afferent and efferent innervation of the bladder with storage or voiding problems have been recognized [10].

NGB includes both storage problems (i.e. overactive bladder or OAB) and voiding problems (inability to empty, high residual volume), and DSD. In conditions such as bladder outlet obstruction [11] and diabetic bladder dysfunction the presence of both storage and voiding problems are indicative of compensatory and decompensatory stages, respectively, of bladder

Imaging Acute Neurologic Disease, ed. Massimo Filippi and Jack H. Simon. Published by Cambridge University Press.

dysfunction. While data to support this distinction in NGB are lacking, the presence of both storage and voiding problems may herald compensatory and decompensatory responses of the bladder in NGB. This distinction is very important clinically, because bladder remodeling may result in a permanent decompensatory stage of NGB that leaves patients suffering from NGB despite neurological remission (spontaneous) or recovery (with treatment).

Pathophysiology of NGB

Knowledge of the pathophysiology of NGB remains primitive. The majority of the published literature is focused on changes in the central and peripheral nervous systems, with the bladder often viewed as a bystander. Categorization of NGB by upper or lower motor-neuron lesions alone would be a reflection of that approach. For example, while bladder dysfunction is in large part related to the duration of MS and degree of pyramidal symptoms in the lower limbs [12], the neurology of the end organ should also be considered as multiple levels of disease contribute to the clinical impact. Underscoring this are the remarkable changes that are frequently observed in patients with NGB, including marked thickening of the bladder wall, formation of trabeculae, outpouchings of the wall called "cellulae formation," and an erythematous urothelium (Figure 16.1).

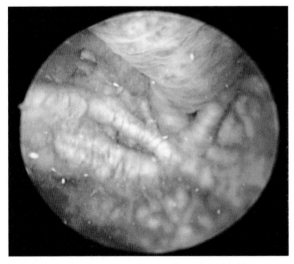

Figure 16.1 Trabeculation and remodeling of the bladder in NGB. Cystoscopic image from a patient with MS and NGB showing marked remodeling including trabeculation, outpouching of wall called "cellulae formation," and an erythematous urothelium.

Neuroanatomy

The neurological discussion of disorders of bladder, as well as bowel and sexual dysfunction, can be considered from a cranial to caudal neuroanatomic perspective, from cerebral cortex to peripheral nerves to the end organs (i.e. bladder, bowel, genitalia). Neurological localization has been discussed in detail in the comprehensive publications by Fowler [including 13, 14], and others. The simplified approach described below is derived from these major works, which should be consulted for more in-depth and highly informative reading. Table 16.1 from Fowler [13] summarizes the relationship between the level of neurological lesion and symptoms in pelvic organ dysfunction and corresponding symptoms in neurological systems.

As discussed above, bladder functions of storage and emptying (voiding) are controlled through pontine function, with suprapontine (voluntary) input. Intact connections are required between pons and cortex, and pons and sacral spinal cord/conus medullaris. Below the conus, the neurological pathway continues through the nerves in the cauda equina, and then the sacral plexus, with more peripheral innervation through the pelvic and pudendal nerves to the bladder and bladder sphincter. Because of the complex and physically long neurological pathways involved, urinary continence is considered a "severe" test of neurological integrity [13].

The functional imaging literature now provides support for the importance of focal pontine and other deep-brain centers, and regional cortical activation in humans, initially through positron emission tomography but increasingly based on functional magnetic resonance imaging (fMRI) studies as summarized in Fowler and Griffiths [15]. The role of frontal cortical pathways is also supported by clinical case series describing urgency, incontinence, and, more rarely, retention from frontal-lobe tumors, and from other types of frontal-lobe injury occurring as a result of rupture of cerebral aneurysm and in patients after frontal leukotomy [13]. Likewise, bladder dysfunction from stroke appears to be associated with the anteromedial frontal cortex, as well as its descending pathways and the basal ganglia [13, 16]. Posterior fossa including brainstem tumors and brainstem strokes are associated with voiding problems (retention) more so than incontinence in several series, with the pons and medulla involved typically rather than the midbrain. The frequent association of abnormalities of eye movements and voiding dysfunction is thought to be related to the

Table 16.1 Neurological level and corresponding pelvic organ/neurological symptoms. Adapted from [14].

Neurological lesion	Symptoms of pelvic organ dysfunction
Innervation within the pelvis	Bladder emptying difficulties Erectile dysfunction, sometimes female sexual dysfunction
Peripheral neuropathy	Erectile dysfunction (early) Bladder emptying difficulties (late) Diarrhea Postural hypotension
Cauda equina	Saddle sensory impairment Stress urinary incontinence Difficulty in initiation of micturition Urgency (occasionally) Sexual sensory loss Erectile dysfunction, female sexual dysfunction Constipation Fecal incontinence/difficulty in evacuation
Spinal	Somatic sensory level Urinary urgency Incomplete bladder emptying Erectile dysfunction, female sexual dysfunction Difficulty in bowel evacuation (in advanced disease)
Pontine (very rare)	Internuclear ophthalmoplegia Urinary retention
Extrapyramidal	Parkinsonism (advanced in idiopathic PD, minor in MSA) Erectile dysfunction (early in MSA) Urinary incontinence (early in MSA) Constipation
Frontal	Personality change Urinary urge incontinence Fecal incontinence (exceptional)

anatomic proximity of the presumed micturition centers of dorsal pons and the medial longitudinal fasciculus [13, 17].

Bowel and sexual-functional pathways

There is considerable neurological overlap between bladder, bowel, and sexual function. The colon has parasympathetic input from the vagus and pelvic nerves via S2 to S4. Sympathetic innervation includes thoraco-lumbar outflow (T5–L2), which influences the internal anal sphincter. The external sphincter is innervated by branches of the pudendal nerves, also from S2 to S4. Tension and stretch in the rectal wall and proximal anal canal are transmitted by pelvic nerves. Analogous to bladder control, cerebral cortex provides voluntary oversight of defecation through the medial frontal area and anterior cingulate [14, 18, 19].

Analogous to bladder and bowel pathways, intact sexual function, including arousal, sensation, erection, and vaginal lubrication are based on intact

pathways from cortex to end organ, with sacral loops from S2 to S4.

Clinical evaluation

The initial diagnosis of NGB in an acute setting starts with a detailed history of the acute event and its plausible association with bladder function. The storage problems usually present with an inability to hold on to urine, with symptoms such as frequency, urgency, and urinary incontinence. Most of the storage symptoms could easily be managed with pharmacological agents. However, the most acute neurological deficit would represent itself in the bladder with the inability to empty the bladder or urinary retention. After determination of symptoms, a thorough examination of the lower genitourinary system should be completed to assure the intact nature of the structures or determine the level of injuries. In the absence of gross anatomical injuries to the genitourinary system, this simple examination of the genitalia, and rectal examination, should allow a fairly accurate assessment of the lower

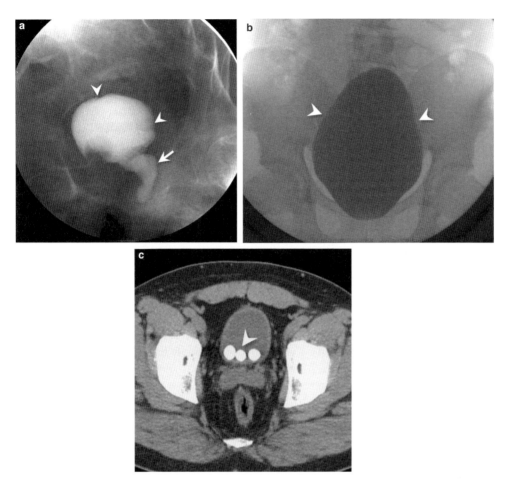

Figure 16.2 (a) Hypertonic-type NGB. Cystogram demonstrates prominent trabeculations (arrowheads) and a funnel-shaped, dilated, posterior urethra (arrow). (b) Atonic-type NGB. Cystogram demonstrates dilated bladder with smooth contour (arrowheads). (c) Bladder calculi. Unenhanced axial CT image of the pelvis demonstrates bladder calculi (arrowhead), a complication associated with long-standing NGB.

urinary tract. Assessment should include perianal sensation and tone [14]. The bulbocavernosis reflex can be tested through gentle tugging of the Foley catheter. An inability to urinate or urinary retention could be confirmed by a bladder ultrasound or catheterization of the bladder. Catheterization should be done only after assurance is obtained that no injury has interrupted the continuity of the urethra. In the absence of such assurance, catheterization could transform a minor interruption of the urethra to a complete interruption, thus causing further damage. In the majority of cases, the catheter has to be left in place until the patient's neurological status has improved.

Among the imaging modalities useful at this stage of evaluation, if the primary problem is thought to reside outside the neurological system, computed tomography (CT) is central. CT with intravenous contrast enhancement would provide assessment of the

status of the lower urinary system and, to an extent, the gastrointestinal system. Urography may be utilized to provide detail of the bladder (Figure 16.2), voiding, and reflux. Ultrasound determines bladder volume and post-void residual volume, and provides some detail of ureteral dilation/hydronephrosis, and kidney anatomy. Imaging evaluation for constipation or related symptoms may additionally require special manometric and imaging studies including defecography.

Common pathology affecting bladder, bowel, and sexual function

MS

As alluded to above, MS accounts for a large fraction of patients presenting with neurological related bladder symptoms, with the prevalence of the chronic bladder symptoms increasing with disease duration. Bladder presentations are also common in acute care clinics. The vast majority of patients with MS have spinal cord pathology, including in early stages of disease. A strong association between bladder symptoms and spinal cord findings (paraparesis, and upper-motor-neuron signs on examination of the lower extremities) has been observed [20]. Urgency is the most common symptom, related to detrusor hyperreflexia [13]. However, as a multicentric neurological disease, bladder dysfunction reflects multiple levels of central nervous system pathology, from the cortex through the conus, as well as secondary bladder pathology related to chronic dysfunction with obstruction, secondary to changes within the bladder, and bladder or other urinary tract infection.

Acute constipation as an early symptom in MS is less likely than bladder dysfunction, but bowel dysfunction including constipation and fecal incontinence become more common in established disease.

The characteristic imaging findings in the brain and spinal cord for MS and related diseases is included in detail in Chapter 13. Spinal MRI, which can be helpful in securing an early diagnosis of MS and, in cases of diagnostic uncertainty, is often utilized in the setting of MS to exclude additional, concurrent pathology, for example co-occurrence of significant intervertebral disk compression of spinal cord, cauda equina, or individual nerve roots. Spinal MRI would also reveal spinal stenosis, neoplasm, and infectious processes affecting the spinal cord, cauda equina, or leptomeninges.

Transverse myelitis including longitudinal extensive transverse myelitis

Transverse myelitis is characterized by acute or subacute spinal cord dysfunction. This typically results in weakness and a sensory level, but can also result in autonomic dysfunction involving bladder, bowel, and sexual impairment below the level of the lesion [21]. Diagnosis comes from history, physical and neurological examination, and laboratory findings. MRI supports the diagnosis when it shows vertically localized spinal cord T2 hyperintensity across much of the cross-section of the spinal cord on the axial views, and may show contrast enhancement. Overlapping presentations include acute disseminated encephalomyelitis (ADEM) with spinal cord involvement, neuromyelitis optica (NMO) spectrum disorders, sarcoidosis, Sjögren's

syndrome, and infectious diseases. This group of diseases can present as longitudinally extensive transverse myelitis (LETM) with paraparesis or tetraparesis, sensory disturbances, and gait, bladder, bowel, and/or sexual dysfunction. Spinal cord MRI shows characteristic intrinsic spinal cord T2 hyperintensity and cord swelling, typically over three or more vertebral segments in length (Figure 16.3). Longitudinally extensive primary spinal cord tumors may have a similar appearance and clinical presentation, although more typically they present by a more indolent clinical course.

Spinal cord trauma

While severe spinal cord injury from blunt or penetrating trauma is frequently associated with immediate and chronic bladder, bowel, and sexual dysfunction, it is interesting that bladder dysfunction in particular has been considered to have limited association with even severe compression of the cervical cord, for example by disk degenerative disease or tumor. However, bladder dysfunction may be under-appreciated with chronic compressive myelopathy [13, 22] (Figure 16.4). Associated neurological findings and MRI confirm the diagnosis. Acute spinal cord injury, while commonly associated with immediate bladder, bowel, and sexual dysfunction, is not usually a diagnostic dilemma, and these functional issues are of lesser immediate importance, although they become extremely important after stabilization of the patient [19].

Cauda equina syndromes

Cauda equina compression syndrome (CES) may be acute and rapidly progressive, or develop over days, weeks, or months. These are considered medical/surgical emergencies, requiring prompt evaluation, often including imaging, after the initial clinical assessment to preserve function, be it strength or bladder or other functional issue. CES presentations are variable, but are classically characterized by severe low-back pain; sciatica is often bilateral but may be unilateral, asymmetric, or absent. There is weakness and sensory loss affecting the lower limbs, and hyporeflexia [23]. Pathology of the cauda equina often also affects both the anterior and posterior sacral roots, containing the somatic and parasympathetic fibers [13]. The sacral roots lie closest to the midline in the cauda equina, and may therefore bear the brunt of the damage [23].

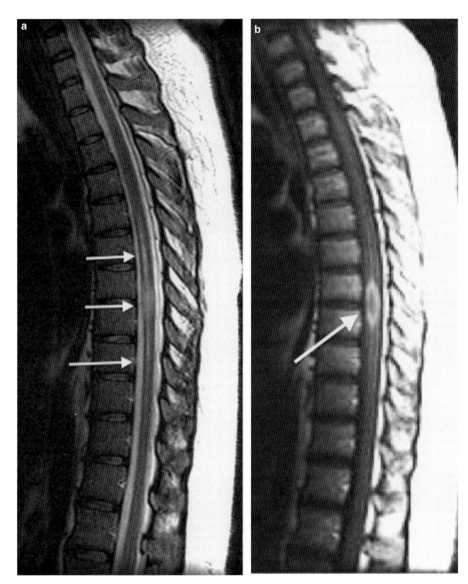

Figure 16.3 NMO with LETM. Multiple pathologies may present with clinical findings of LETM. Early bladder, bowel, and sexual dysfunction may occur, but most often the LETM is characterized by dramatic and rapidly progressive weakness. (a) Sagittal T2-weighted image shows multiple thoracic segments of intrinsic cord T2 hyperintensity (arrows). (b) Cavitary enhancement is seen on the corresponding sagittal post-contrast T1-weighted image (arrow).

There may be sensory loss in the perineum related to S2–S4 roots, loss of voluntary urethral and anal sphincter control, and sexual dysfunction [13]. The pattern of sensory loss restricted to the medial buttocks and perianal area is termed "saddle anesthesia" [23]. Findings include a patulous anal sphincter, and loss of the anal wink and bulbocavernosus reflexes. The patient may be aware of urinary retention or incontinence, or may not. Bladder ultrasound provides an objective measure.

Acute CES may occur from large central disk herniations, or vertebral body collapse with prolapse of tissue into the vertebral canal, typically from metastatic disease, or retropulsion of tissue into the spinal canal from severe trauma. More rarely, acute hemorrhage may cause a CES. CES also occurs from severe compression of the nerve roots by primary neoplasms, such as ependymoma and nerve-sheath tumors.

The CES is often compared to and contrasted with the conus medullaris syndrome, but there are

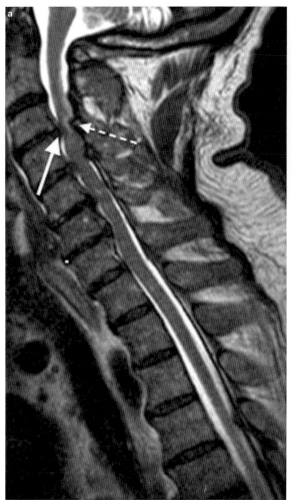
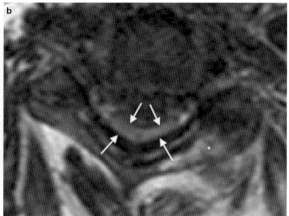

Figure 16.4 Severe cervical cord compression without bladder/bowel symptoms. Severe, chronic cervical cord compression in a 78-year-old man, with increasing weakness but without appreciable bladder/bowel symptoms. (a) The sagittal T2-weighted MRI shows multiple levels of cervical cord compression, but most severe at the C3–C4 level (arrows), where there is a large ventral-canal disk and/or osteophyte and dorsal ligamentum flavum hypertrophy. (b) The axial T2-weighted image shows severe compression and posterior displacement of the spinal cord; the spinal cord is abnormally hyperintense (arrows).

often overlapping characteristics and presentations. Associated upper-motor-neuron signs and symptoms suggest conus involvement.

Imaging for suspected cauda equina compression should always include some visualization of the conus medullaris, for example by T1- and T2-weighted sagittal acquisition, to exclude unanticipated conus-level pathology (Figure 16.5). When myelography or now most often CT myelography is utilized for low-back pain or cauda equina compression, additional CT-myelographic views should always be directed through the level of the conus medullaris. Additional examples

of cauda equina pathology with bladder dysfunction are illustrated by Case 5 in Chapter 15 (on spinal cord injury) and bladder involvement by cauda equina compression is presented in Chapter 5 (on backache, Figure 5.6).

Tethered cord syndrome

The tethered cord syndrome (TCS), well known in pediatrics, and often associated with spinal dysraphism, may present later in life, including in adults. In children, TCS usually presents with sensorimotor

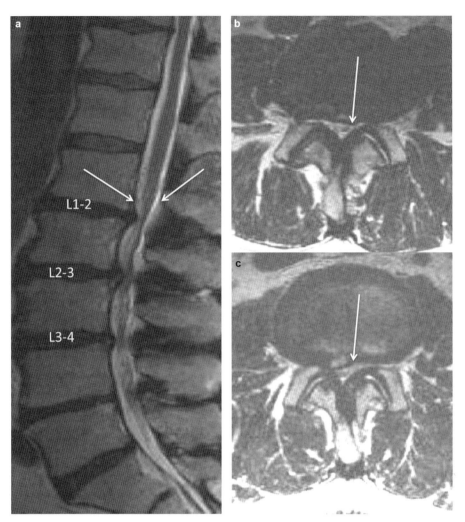

Figure 16.5 Cauda equina and conus medullaris compression from degenerative disk disease. (a) Sagittal T2-weighted image shows compression of the cauda equina at L3–L4, L2–L3, and compression of cauda equina/conus conus medullaris at L1–L2 (arrows). (b) Corresponding axial T2-weighted images show severe compression of the cauda equina (b) and the lower conus medullaris/cauda (c) with clustered rootlets and loss of cerebral spinal fluid signal intensity.

symptoms and signs, often in both legs, with bladder dysfunction. Some adults with TCS are apparently normal until symptoms and signs develop. The presentation can be confused with spinal stenosis. Patients with TCS characteristically have pain as the primary symptom, which has been described as localized to the anal, perineal, and gluteal areas, and sometimes radiating diffusely down the legs, while radicular-type pain is less common. Weakness and incontinence also occur, but with lower frequency [24]. Bladder dysfunction includes urinary urgency (hyperreflexic bladder), and sometimes is described in combination with sphincter weakness, contributing to incontinence. Distal spinal cord involvement

attributed to stretching may cause upper-motor-neuron signs, such as extensor plantar responses.

MRI or CT myelography are the imaging tests of choice, as they can show a low spinal cord, a thickened filum terminale, an associated lipoma, and other components of a spinal dysraphism.

Parkinson's disease

Early bladder dysfunction in Parkinson's disease is most frequently related to prostate pathology in men. In Parkinson's, urgency, frequency, and urge incontinence can occur with advanced disease, most frequently with a urodynamic abnormality related to detrusor hyperreflexia, from various causes. Obstructive and treatment-related (e.g. medication) causes should always be considered. In women, stress urinary incontinence also contributes, but neurological causes occur in relatively more advanced disease. Bladder dysfunction appears later than typical motor disorders [25, 26]. In more advanced disease, constipation and erectile dysfunction also occur.

Severe bladder symptoms with mild Parkinsonism should suggest the possibility of multiple system atrophy (MSA) [27], the urinary symptoms often preceding other neurological symptoms and the correct diagnosis by years. The same is true for erectile dysfunction, which often also precedes the diagnosis of MSA by years. While the literature describes electromyography (EMG) abnormalities of the sphincter and prolonged transit time in early Parkinson's, similar to bladder dysfunction, many of these patients may in fact have MSA [27].

Miscellaneous

Bladder and bowel dysfunction as a major symptom is relatively rare in chronic lumbar spinal stenosis, but does occur. Bladder dysfunction in individuals with spinal stenosis is statistically more likely the result of prostate hypertrophy or other prostate pathology (neoplasm). Characteristic imaging findings of lumbar stenosis are seen by MRI, or in patients with contraindications to MRI, by high-resolution CT or CT myelography.

Meningeal carcinomatosis presents with the triad of headache, cranial, and lumbosacral radiculopathies, but early in its course the predominant features are usually low-back pain radiating into the legs, leg weakness and numbness, and bladder dysfunction [23]. MRI without contrast enhancement is often ineffective in diagnosing meningeal carcinomatosis. Contrast-enhanced MRI increases the likelihood of detection of nodules or root enhancement, but cerebrospinal fluid analysis is both more sensitive and definitive for malignant cells.

Viral CES, particularly in immunocompromised patients, may be caused by cytomegalovirus or other agents. These may present with low-back pain and urinary disturbances as early symptoms [23]. Asymmetric leg weakness and sensory loss extending into the saddle area develop later, with progression to flaccid paraplegia, and bladder and bowel incontinence. Bladder symptoms in Guillian–Barré syndrome typically occurs after weakness is established.

Imaging of Guillain–Barré syndrome is discussed in Chapter 21.

Trauma from rectal, prostate, or uterine surgery may interrupt pelvic parasympathetic nerves

A condition of acute or slowly developing urinary retention or obstructed voiding in the absence of neurological symptoms in young woman, Fowlers syndrome [13], has been described that is associated with abnormal EMG findings localized to the urethral sphincter.

Other spinal cord pathology that may result in notable bladder and bowel symptoms and sexual dysfunction include syringomyelia, which may be associated with neoplasm or not, tabes dorsalis, tropical spastic paraparesis, arteriovenous or dural vascular malformations, and arteriovenous fistula. Diagnosis is based on history, clinical examination, laboratory, and characteristic imaging findings.

Conclusions

Acute bladder, bowel, and sexual dysfunction rarely present as isolated neurological disease, as the critical pathways, for example in the brain, spinal cord, or cauda equina, are anatomically related to other centers and pathways that produce early symptoms, for example abnormal visual tracking (pons) or weakness or pain (conus or cauda equina). There is considerable overlap of the neuroanatomy of bladder, bowel, and sexual dysfunction despite the differences in end organs. Neurologic imaging is based primarily on neurological localization, rather than symptoms alone.

References

1. Wein AJ (2007). Lower urinary tract dysfunction in neurologic injury and disease. In Wein AJ, Kavoussi LR, Novick AC, Partin AW, Peters CA, eds. *Campbell–Walsh Urology*, 9th edn. Philadelphia, PA: Saunders Elsevier.

2. Borello-France D, Leng W, O'Leary M, *et al.* (2004). Bladder and sexual function among women with multiple sclerosis. *Mult Scler* **10**: 455–461.

3. Manack A, Motsko SP, Haag-Molkenteller C, *et al.* (2011). Epidemiology and healthcare utilization of neurogenic bladder patients in a US claims database. *Neurourol Urodyn* **30**: 395–401.

4. Winge K, Fowler CJ (2006). Bladder dysfunction in parkinsonism: mechanisms, prevalence, symptoms, and management. *Mov Disord* **21**: 737–745.

5. Ersoz M, Tunc H, Akyuz M, Ozel S (2005). Bladder storage and emptying disorder frequencies in hemorrhagic and ischemic stroke patients with bladder dysfunction. *Cerebrovasc Dis* **20**: 395–399.

6. Litwiller SE, Frohman EM, Zimmern PE (1999). Multiple sclerosis and the urologist. *J Urol* **161**: 743–757.

7. Mamas MA, Reynard JM, Brading AF (2001). Augmentation of nitric oxide to treat detrusor external sphincter dyssynergia in spinal cord injury. *Lancet* **357**: 1964–1967.

8. de Seze M, Ruffion A, Denys P, Joseph PA, Perrouin-Verbe B (2007). The neurogenic bladder in multiple sclerosis: review of the literature and proposal of management guidelines. *Mult Scler* **13**: 915–928.

9. Zderic SA, Chacko S, Disanto ME, Wein AJ (2002). Voiding function: relevant anatomy, physiology, pharmacology, and molecular aspects. In Gillenwater JY, Grayhack JT, Howards SS, Mitchell ME, eds. *Adult and Pediatric Urology*. Philadelphia, PA: Lippincott Williams and Wilkins.

10. Birder L, de Groat W, Mills I, *et al.* (2010). Neural control of the lower urinary tract: peripheral and spinal mechanisms. *Neurourol Urodyn* **29**: 128–139.

11. Levin RM, Haugaard N, Levin SS, *et al.* (1995). Bladder function in experimental outlet obstruction: pharmacologic responses to alterations in innervation, energetics, calcium mobilization, and genetics. *Adv Exp Med Biol* **385**: 7–19; discussion 75–79.

12. Fowler CJ, Panicker JN, Drake M, *et al.* (2009). A UK consensus on the management of the bladder in multiple sclerosis. *J Neurol Neurosurg Psychiatry* **80**: 470–477.

13. Fowler CJ (1999). Neurological disorders of micturition and their treatment. *Brain* **122**: 1213–1231.

14. Fowler CJ (2001). A neurologist's clinical and investigative approach to patients with bladder, bowel and sexual dysfunction. In Munsat TL, ed. *Neurologic Bladder, Bowel and Sexual Dysfunction*. Amsterdam: Elsevier Science, pp. 1–6.

15. Fowler CJ, Griffiths DJ (2010). A decade of functional brain imaging applied to bladder control. *Neurourol Urodyn* **29**: 49–55.

16. Sakakibara R, Hattori T, Yasuda K, Yamanishi T (1996). Micturitional disturbance after acute hemispheric stroke: analysis of the lesion site by CT and MRI. *J Neurol Sci* **137**: 47–56.

17. Sakakibara R, Hattori T, Yasuda K, Yamanishi T (1996). Micturitional disturbance and the pontine tegmental lesion: urodynamic and MRI analyses of vascular cases. *J Neurol Sci* **141**: 105–110.

18. Winge K, Rasmussen D, Werdelin LM (2003). Constipation in neurological diseases. *J Neurol Neurosurg Psychiatry* **74**: 13–19.

19. Benevento BT, Sipski ML (2002). Neurogenic bladder, neurogenic bowel, and sexual dysfunction in people with spinal cord injury. *Phys Ther* **82**: 601–612.

20. Betts CD, D'Mellow MT, Fowler CJ (1993). Urinary symptoms and the neurological features of bladder dysfunction in multiple sclerosis. *J Neurol Neurosurg Psychiatry* **56**: 245–250.

21. Beh SC, Greenberg BM, Frohman T, Frohman EM (2013). Transverse myelitis. *Neurol Clin* **31**: 79–138.

22. Hattori T, Sakakibara R, Yasuda K, Murayama N, Hirayama K (1990). Micturitional disturbance in cervical spondylotic myelopathy. *J Spinal Disord* **3**: 16–18.

23. Stewart JD. Cauda equina disorders (2000). In Munsat TL, ed. *Neurologic Bladder, Bowel and Sexual Dysfunction*. Amsterdam: Elsevier Science, pp. 63–74.

24. Iskandar BJ, Fulmer BB, Hadley MN, Oakes WJ (2001). Congenital tethered spinal cord syndrome in adults. *Neurosurg Focus* **10**: e7.

25. Sakakibara R, Tateno F, Kishi M, *et al.* (2012). Pathophysiology of bladder dysfunction in Parkinson's disease. *Neurobiol Dis* **46**: 565–571.

26. Sakakibara R, Kishi M, Ogawa E, *et al.* (2011). Bladder, bowel, and sexual dysfunction in Parkinson's disease. *Parkinsons Dis*: 924605.

27. Beck RO, Betts CD, Fowler CJ (1994). Genitourinary dysfunction in multiple system atrophy: clinical features and treatment in 62 cases. *J Urol* **151**: 1336–41.

Vladimir S. Kostic, Federica Agosta, and Massimo Filippi

Introduction

Parkinsonism is a clinical syndrome characterized by a combination of six cardinal features: (1) bradykinesia, (2) rigidity, (3) tremor at rest, (4) postural instability, (5) flexed posture, and (6) freezing or motor blocks. Idiopathic Parkinson's disease (PD) is by far the most common cause of parkinsonism and should always be the diagnosis if a definite secondary cause cannot be identified (Table 17.1). Slow progression, unilateral presentation with asymmetrical signs, a pill-rolling rest tremor, and good sustained response to levodopa support the diagnosis [1] (Table 17.2). Other forms are broadly classified as atypical parkinsonian syndromes (multiple system atrophy parkinsonism (MSA-P), progressive supranuclear palsy (PSP), corticobasal syndrome (CBS)), heredodegenerative disorders associated with parkinsonism and secondary (symptomatic, acquired) parkinsonism (Table 17.1). Less frequently, patients who receive an initial clinical diagnosis of PD are found to have parkinsonian features as part of other diseases, such as dementia with Lewy bodies (DLB) or Alzheimer's disease (AD). The present chapter focuses on PD, PD with cognitive impairment, and DLB. Chapter 19 describes the most frequent causes of non-PD parkinsonism, both clinically and with respect to the neuroimaging characteristics.

The present diagnostic approach in PD

The definitive diagnosis of idiopathic PD requires a histological demonstration of intraneuronal Lewy body inclusions in the substantia nigra (SN) pars compacta [1]. In most cases, the diagnosis of probable PD can be made on clinical grounds and no ancillary investigations are needed. The most widely used clinical criteria for the diagnosis of PD are those introduced by the Queen Square Brain Bank (QSBB) [1]. These criteria are based on a three-step approach (Table 17.2): (1) signs that must be present, (2) signs that should not be present, and (3) supportive criteria. However, a number of pitfalls have been suggested: (a) some other forms of parkinsonism, including atypical ones, may also, albeit transiently, respond to dopamine replacement therapy and have prolonged disease course; (b) asymmetry may also occur in atypical parkinsonism; and (c) having more than one affected relative cannot exclude a diagnosis of PD. In practice, positive clinical criteria for PD-related parkinsonism (i.e. bradykinesia in combination with rigidity, tremor at rest, or postural instability) include the progressive character of the symptoms, the unilateral onset with persistent unilateral preponderance, and a persistent levodopa responsiveness. Clinicopathologic studies suggest that when an established PD is diagnosed according to QSBB criteria [1], there is a 90% concordance between expert clinical impression and the presence of nigral Lewy bodies [2].

However, in early PD the full triad of clinical symptoms and signs (bradykinesia, tremor at rest, and rigidity) may not yet be manifested [3]. In addition, even if made by a movement disorder expert, a PD diagnosis may change at follow-up for several reasons: development of atypical signs, insufficient response to dopaminergic treatment, or neuroimaging clues for an alternative diagnosis. The algorithm presented in Figure 17.1 summarizes the role of nuclear medicine techniques, conventional MRI, and transcranial sonography to support the clinical diagnosis in a patient suspected of having PD.

Table 17.1 Major causes of parkinsonism

A. Primary (idiopathic) parkinsonism.
  a. Parkinson's disease
B. Atypical parkinsonism (parkinsonism-plus)
  a. Progressive supranuclear palsy
  b. Multiple system atrophy
  c. Corticobasal degeneration
  d. Dementia with Lewy bodies
C. Heredodegenerative parkinsonism
D. Secondary (symptomatic) parkinsonism

  a. Drugs, toxins, vascular parkinsonism, trauma, infectious, others

Table 17.2 Queen Square Brain Bank clinical diagnostic criteria [1]

Step 1 Diagnosis of parkinsonian syndrome

Bradykinesia (slowness of initiation of voluntary movement with progressive reduction in speed and amplitude or repetitive actions)

And at least one of the following:
- Muscular rigidity
- 4–6 Hz rest tremor
- Postural instability not caused by primary visual, vestibular, cerebellar, or proprioceptive dysfunction

Step 2 Exclusion criteria for Parkinson's disease
- History of repeated strokes with stepwise progression of parkinsonian features
- History of repeated head injury
- History of definite encephalitis
- Oculogyric crises
- Neuroleptic treatment at onset of symptoms
- More than one affected relative
- Sustained remission
- Strictly unilateral features after 3 years
- Supranuclear gaze palsy
- Cerebellar signs
- Early severe autonomic involvement
- Early severe dementia with disturbances of memory, language, and praxis
- Babinski signs
- Presence of a cerebral tumor or communicating hydrocephalus on CT scan
- Negative response to large doses of levodopa (if malabsorption excluded)
- MPTP exposure

Step 3 Supportive prospective positive criteria of Parkinson's disease

Three or more required for diagnosis of definite Parkinson's disease:
- Unilateral onset
- Rest tremor present
- Progressive disorder
- Persistent asymmetry affecting the side onset most
- Excellent response (70–100%) to levodopa
- Severe levodopa-induced chorea
- levodopa response for 5 years or more
- Clinical course of 10 years or more
- Hyposmia
- Visual hallucination

Physical examination

The term bradykinesia, probably the most disabling symptom in PD, includes **akinesia** (absence or failure of most of the movements), **hypokinesia** (reduced frequency and amplitude of spontaneous movements, particularly noticeable in automatic movements), and **bradykinesia** (poverty and slowness when initiating and executing a single movement, including progressive reduction of its amplitude, sometimes up to a complete cessation during repetitive simple movements) (Table 17.3) [6]. Therefore, bradykinesia is not just a slowness of movements, but rather includes "*progressive fatiguing and decrement of repetitive alternating movements during finger or foot tapping*" [7]. "True" bradykinesia should be differentiated from slowness due to depression, pyramidal lesions, or other causes of muscle weakness. Bradykinesia can be clinically assessed: (a) by observation of spontaneous movements in different situations, or (b) by asking the patient to perform some repetitive movements as quickly and widely as possible (tapping thumb and index fingers, tapping foot on the ground, closing and opening the hand, etc.).

Rigidity is a continuous and uniform increase in the muscle tone, felt as a smooth resistance throughout the range of passive movements (i.e. **lead pipe rigidity**) or as a ratchet-like quality of resistance (**cogwheel rigidity**) of affected segments (neck and limbs). Unlike spasticity, it affects both flexor and extensor muscle groups and does not increase with the increased speed of passive movements during examination. In mild cases, rigidity can be unmasked by voluntary activation of the contralateral limb (Froment's sign).

Tremor in PD is classically defined as a 4–6 Hz rest tremor (affected body parts relaxed and supported by a surface, thus removing the action of gravitation) with or without postural/kinetic tremor in the limbs with distal predominance (i.e. "pill-rolling" tremor due to the simultaneous rubbing movements of thumb and index fingers against each other, but also in forms of abduction–adduction or finger flexion–extension). At least at the beginning of the disease, tremor can

271

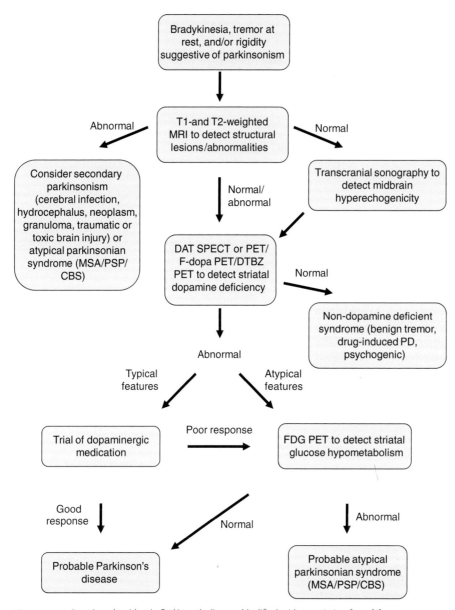

Figure 17.1 Imaging algorithm in Parkinson's disease. Modified with permission from [4].
Abbreviations: CBS, corticobasal syndrome; DAT-PET, dopamine transporter-PET; DAT-SPECT, dopamine transporter-SPECT; DTBZ-PET, dehydrotetrabenazine-PET; FDG-PET, ^{18}F-fluorodeoxyglucose PET; F-dopa PET, ^{18}F-3, 4-dehydroxyphenylalanine PET; MSA, multiple system atrophy; PSP, progressive supranuclear palsy

disappear with active movement. If only transient, it may be triggered with loading a mental task (i.e. serial "100–7" counting task). The jaw muscles and tongue can occasionally be affected in PD, but the presence of head and voice tremor is strongly suggestive of essential tremor. Rest tremor is the only tremor type included in the cardinal signs (Table 17.2) and is the strongest diagnostic predictor of PD after asymmetry of parkinsonian signs and levodopa responsiveness. However,

pure rest tremor is rare in PD; more common is the combination of rest and postural/kinetic tremors.

Postural instability rarely manifests before stage III of the Hoehn and Yahr classification [8] and is associated with a stooped posture. Posture and gait should be assessed in both an open space and while passing through narrow spaces (i.e. doorways) or between obstacles. The basic test is the "pull test": the examiner stands behind the patient, who is

Table 17.3 Signs of bradykinesia according to Paulson and Stern [5]

General
- Difficulty to initiate movement
- Slowed voluntary movements
- Amplitude diminution of voluntary movements
- Rapid fatigue with repetitive movements
- Difficulty executing simultaneous and/or sequential movements
- Decreased dexterity (brushing teeth, shaving, putting on make-up. . .)
- Loss of spontaneous movements such as gesturing
- Occasional arrests of movement execution

Specific
- Masked facies (hypomimia)
- Decreased frequency of blinking
- Hypometric saccades, impaired ocular convergence and upgaze
- Hypophonia with loss of inflection
- Dysarthria
- Sialorrhea due to decreased spontaneous swallowing
- Micrographia
- Difficulty with fast repetitive movement (i.e. pronation–supination)
- Difficulty rising from a chair
- Shuffling small-steps gait
- Decreased arm swing while walking

previously warned about the procedure, and suddenly applies a pull to the patient shoulders. The patient is allowed to make up to two steps back to recover balance: more steps for recovering or falls mean postural instability.

Finally, it is critical to note that in PD we are dealing with pure parkinsonism; the presence of other clinical signs, such as pyramidal, cerebellar, and sensory deficits, early dementia, lower-body parkinsonism, focal cortical symptoms, other dyskinesia (except tremor and dystonia), amyotrophy, neuropathy, and the other items mentioned in step 2 of the QSBB criteria (Table 17.2) exclude the diagnosis of idiopathic PD.

Present criteria (Table 17.2) focus on motor features. However, commonly levodopa-resistant non-motor features are also very important in PD and include cognitive and mood disorders, sleep disturbances, autonomic dysfunction, sensory problems, etc.

Laboratory tests

PD is a pure clinical diagnosis and no specific laboratory test exists that can establish such a diagnosis. In typical circumstances, a restricted number of investigations are helpful to exclude other causes mimicking parkinsonism (i.e. anemia and hypothyroid slowness). In appropriate circumstances (not routine) and on an individual basis (i.e. young age at onset and familial history), a diagnosis of PD can be achieved with genetic testing. However, less than 5% of all PD cases are secondary to known single-gene mutations and the results of testing do not guide treatment [3].

Olfactory testing reveals dysfunction in >80% of patients with PD, but it is not specific since olfaction is impaired in many disorders, including 30% of normal elderly subjects [9]. Recently, it has been concluded that olfactory testing may differentiate PD from atypical and secondary forms of parkinsonism, as well as from recessive forms of PD [7]. This test could be considered as a diagnostic screening procedure, but not as an indicator of disease progression in PD. In addition, olfactory testing is a sensitive, but not specific, screening test for premotor PD [7].

The diagnosis of PD was thought to be strongly substantiated by the significant clinical benefit gained from an acute challenge of oral levodopa or subcutaneous apomorphine (i.e. drug challenge test). However, there is an approximately 30% chance of a false negative and 20–30% chance of a false positive result [10]. Also, some patients respond only to chronic, high-dose levodopa treatment. As a consequence, recent EFNS/MDS-ES/ENS recommendations for the diagnosis of PD [7] do not recommend this challenge test for the diagnosis of *de novo* parkinsonian patients.

There is also no evidence for any diagnostic role of autonomic function assessment, neurophysiological evaluation, and neuropsychological tests. Finally, advances in genetic studies provided new ideas on potential markers, such as measurements of certain proteins in the cerebrospinal fluid (CSF; i.e. α-synuclein), but these studies are still in the investigational phase.

Imaging

Computed tomography and conventional MRI

Computed tomography (CT) scans can show nonspecific atrophy with enlarged ventricles and sulci. Conventional MRI at 1.5 T with visual assessment of T2-weighted and T1-weighted imaging does not reveal disease-specific abnormalities in PD and, particularly in the early phases, the MRI appears normal [11]. Its main clinical role is to exclude

273

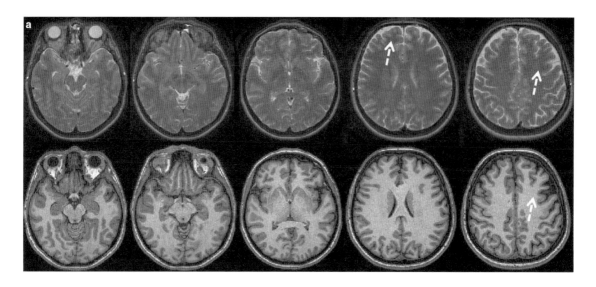

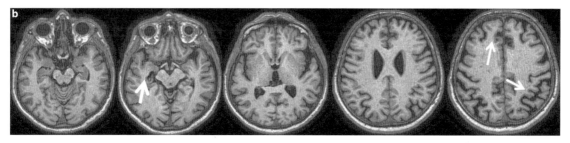

Figure 17.2 Conventional MRI findings in early Parkinson's disease (PD). (a) A 43-year-old patient with PD (disease duration= 6 months; Unified Parkinson Disease Rating Scale [UPDRS] III= 12; Mini-Mental State Examination [MMSE] = 30): axial T2- and T1-weighted images demonstrate a mild medial and dorsal prefrontal atrophy bilaterally (dashed arrows). (b) A 71-year-old patient with PD and mild cognitive impairment (disease duration= 2 years; UPDRS III= 17; MMSE = 23; Addenbrooke's Cognitive Examination Revised= 72): axial T1-weighted images show mild frontal and parietal cortical atrophy (arrows). Atrophy of the anterior temporal poles is also evident. Widening of the right temporal horn of lateral ventricle (bold arrow) is further evidence of temporal lobe atrophy. While atrophy may be a finding on conventional MRI in PD, it is neither sensitive nor specific.

subcortical vascular pathology, rare secondary causes of parkinsonism (e.g. tumors, granulomas, or calcification of basal ganglia; Wilson disease; normal-pressure hydrocephalus), and in discriminating atypical parkinsonian syndromes (see Chapter 19 for further details). With disease progression, findings remain non-specific, although a signal decrease in the SN on proton-density and T2-weighted images as well as mild frontal and hippocampal atrophy has been described [12], (Figure 17.2).

Imaging dopaminergic function

Presynaptic dopaminergic integrity can be assessed *in vivo* in three main ways [13] (Figure 17.3):

(a) Presynaptic dopamine uptake through the dopamine transporter (DAT) is the primary mechanism of dopamine removal from the striatal synaptic cleft. Striatal DAT availability provides a

measure of dopamine terminal function and can be assessed with a variety of single photon emission computed tomography (SPECT) and positron emission tomography (PET) tracers, such as ^{123}I-2β-carbomethoxy-3β-(4-iodophenyl)-N-(3-fluoropropyl)nortropane (^{123}I-FP-CIT; known commercially as the DaTSCAN™), ^{123}I-2β-carbomethoxy-3β-(4-iodophenyl)-N-(3-fluoropropyl)tropane (^{123}I-β-CIT), [2-{[2-({[3-(4-chlorophenyl)-8-methyl-8-azabicyclo]3.2.1}oct-2-yl)methyl](2-mercaptoethyl)amino}ethylamino] ethanethiolato(3-)-[N2, N20, S2, S20]oxo-[1R-(exo-exo)] (^{99m}Tc-TRODAT-1), ^{123}I-altropane SPECT tracers, and 2β-carbomethoxy-3β-(4-fluorophenyl)tropane (^{18}F/^{11}C-β-CFT), ^{18}F-FP-CIT, and ^{11}C-N-(2-fluoroethyl)-2b-carbomethoxy-3b-(4-iodophenyl)nortropane (^{11}C-FE-CIT) PET tracers;

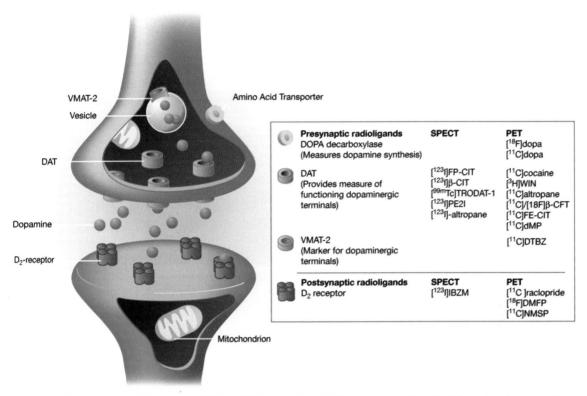

Figure 17.3 Dopaminergic radioligands for SPECT and PET. Abbreviations: β-CFT = 2b-carbomethoxy-3b-(4-fluorophenyl)tropane; DAT = dopamine transporter; dopa = dihydroxyphenylalanine; DMFP = desmethoxyfallypride; dMP = d-threo methylphenidate; DTBZ= dihydrotetrabenazine; FE-CIT= N-(2-fluoroethyl)-2b-carbomethoxy-3b-(4-iodophenyl)nortropane; IBZM = iodobenzamide; NMSP= 3-N-methylspiperone; PE2I= N-(3-iodoprop-(2E)-enyl)-2b-carboxymethoxy-3b-(4'-methylphenyl)nortropane; TRODAT-1= [2-{[2-({[3-(4-chlorophenyl)-8-methyl-8-azabicyclo]3.2.1}oct-2-yl)methyl](2-mercaptoethyl)amino}ethylamino]ethanethiolato(3–)-[N2, N20, S2, S20]oxo-[1R-(exo-exo)]; VMAT = vesicular monoamine transporter; WIN = WIN 55, 212–2 cannabinoid receptor agonist. Reproduced with permission from [13].

(b) ^{18}F-3, 4-dihydroxyphenylalanine (^{18}F-dopa) PET provides a marker of dopaminergic terminal dopa decarboxylase activity and dopamine turnover, since the tracer is taken up by L-aromatic amino acid dexarboxylase (AADC), converted to ^{18}F-fluorodopamine, and packaged in synaptic vesicles. However, ^{18}F-dopa uptake is not restricted to dopaminergic neurons, since AADC is also present in serotonergic and noradrenergic neurons;

(c) Vesicular monoamine transporter (VMAT2) availability in dopamine terminals can be examined with either ^{11}C- or ^{18}F-dihydrotetrabenazine (DTBZ) PET.

In PD, all the abovementioned tracers of presynaptic dopaminergic function show a characteristic pattern of asymmetric reduction of striatal uptake, more pronounced contralateral to the clinically more affected side of the body [13] (Figure 17.4). Typically, the nigrostriatal dopaminergic projections to the posterior (dorsal–caudal) putamen are affected earlier and more severely than those to the caudate nucleus. The caudal–rostral gradient is attributed to predominant degeneration of the ventrolateral portion of the SN that projects to the putamen, and relative preservation of the dorsomedial SN that projects to the caudate nucleus [14]. Reductions in striatal tracer uptake correlate with pathological measures (i.e. cell loss) and degree of motor disability, particularly bradykinesia and, to a lesser extent, rigidity; progression of the disease can be monitored using these tracers in longitudinal studies [4].

Bilateral reductions of putaminal uptake are observed even in the initial phases of PD, when only unilateral motor symptoms of parkinsonism are present (hemiparkinsonism) [4]. However, not all dopamine fibers are damaged in early PD, i.e., some

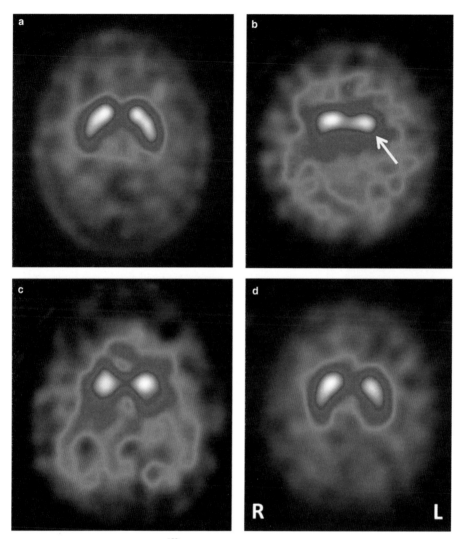

Figure 17.4 Dopaminergic imaging (^{123}I ioflupane DAT SPECT) in (a) a healthy control, (b) a patient with early PD (Hoehn and Yahr score I), (c) a patient with DLB, and (d) a patient with AD. Normal control and AD patient show normal, symmetric intense tracer uptake in striatum (both caudate nucleus and putamen). PD and DLB patients show bilaterally reduced uptake in the striatum, predominantly reduced in the putamen. Note the asymmetry (left reduced more than right) in the PD patient (arrow).

patients may increase dopamine turnover as an adaptive mechanism [4]. At the onset of brady-kinesia and rigidity, ^{18}F-dopa uptake in the globus pallidus pars interna can be found to be increased by up to 50% [15]. As the disease progresses, pallidal ^{18}F-dopa falls, eventually becoming slightly reduced [15].

Presynaptic dopaminergic imaging is clinically useful in differentiating PD from multiple other conditions that may overlap with features of PD, such as drug-induced parkinsonism, essential tremor, and psychogenic parkinsonism/tremor [13]. In 2011, the US Food and Drug Administration approved the

DaTSCAN^{TM} for evaluating parkinsonian syndromes and for distinguishing PD from essential tremor. However, it cannot differentiate PD from other forms of presynaptic parkinsonism, such as MSA-P, PSP, and CBS [13], although PD is associated with a rostro–caudal putamen gradient of dopamine dysfunction compared with the more uniform dysfunction detected in atypical parkinsonisms (see Chapter 19 for further details).

Up to 15% of patients suspected of having early PD have a normal DAT SPECT or PET scan (i.e. Subjects With Scans Without Evidence of Dopaminergic Deficit – SWEDD) [4]. While such a finding is still not fully understood, follow-up studies of SWEDD cases suggest that there is no disease progression, the response to dopaminergic medication is questionable [16], dopamine innervations remain intact, and the glucose metabolic pattern is normal [17]. These findings reinforce the viewpoint that normal dopaminergic imaging excludes the presence of a degenerative parkinsonian syndrome. A number of SWEDD patients may have adult-onset dystonic tremor, which may resemble unilateral parkinsonian resting arm tremor with impaired arm swing, but without typical decrement in the amplitude of repetitive movements (see Chapter 19 for further details).

Postsynaptic dopamine function can be assessed using PET or SPECT with ligands for D1 (D1, D5) and D2 (D2, D3, D4) receptors. Theoretically, abnormalities in ligand binding reflect either receptor density or affinity. Tracers with high affinity can be used to assess the availability of dopamine receptors in extrastriatal sites, while ligands with low affinity for the D2 receptor (e.g. ^{11}C-raclopride) compete with endogenous dopamine and can be used to estimate dopamine release (i.e. alterations of synaptic dopamine concentrations) in response to a variety of pharmacological, physical, and behavioral interventions [15]. In early, untreated PD patients, striatal D2 receptor binding is increased (probably due to receptor upregulation) and returns to normal or slightly reduced levels once dopamine replacement treatment is started [18]. Again, the initial increase of striatal binding is higher in putamen (posterior > anterior) than in the caudate nucleus. In contrast, striatal D2 binding is reduced in MSA-P, PSP, and CBS. Striatal D1 receptor density is unchanged in PD compared to controls [19].

Recent EFNS/MDS-ES/ENS guidelines for the diagnosis of PD recommended DAT SPECT "for the differential diagnosis between degenerative parkinsonism and essential tremor" [7]. More specifically, "DAT SPECT is indicated in the presence of significant diagnostic uncertainty and particularly in patients presenting atypical tremor manifestations" [7]. Although PET has better spatial resolution and higher sensitivity than SPECT (e.g. the resolution in SPECT limits the separation of putamen and caudate), EFNS/MDS–ES/ENS guidelines did not make "any formal recommendation for the routine use of PET studies in the diagnostic work-up of PD," since "none of the reviewed studies has been performed according to the regulatory standards" [7].

Glucose metabolism and regional cerebral blood flow

In PD, ^{18}F-fluorodeoxyglucose (FDG) PET reveals a characteristic profile characterized by increased metabolism in the putamen/globus pallidus, thalamus, cerebellum, pons, and sensorimotor cortex, and reduced metabolism in the lateral frontal, paracentral, and parieto-occipital areas [20] (Figure 17.5). The PD-related covariance pattern (PDRP) linearly correlates with clinical motor ratings (mainly with bradykinesia and rigidity, rather than tremor) and increases with disease progression. PDRP can be normalized by successful levodopa treatment or deep brain stimulation. Abnormal PDRP activity was shown to precede motor symptoms by 2 years [21].

^{18}F-FDG PET can be helpful for separating PD from atypical parkinsonian syndromes since glucose metabolism of the lentiform nucleus is preserved or raised in PD, whereas it is reduced in most atypical cases (see Chapter 19 for further details).

Transcranial sonography

Transcranial sonography detects bilaterally increased echogenicity in the lateral midbrain of patients with PD, which is likely to reflect SN iron deposition (Figure 17.6). Guidelines for the assessment of SN echogenicity have been published [22, 23], and for an accurate examination a qualified investigator is requested. The differentiation into normal or abnormal SN echogenicity is based on cut-off values derived from percentile ranks obtained in healthy subjects (i.e., these values must be established for each laboratory and ultrasound system): **marked** hyperechogenicity refers to hyperechogenicity above the 90th percentile, while **moderate** values are between the 75th and 90th percentiles obtained in the healthy population [22, 23]. EFNS/MDS-ES/ENS guidelines recommend two standardized scanning planes to be used [7]: (a) the mesencephalic scanning plane in which SN, red nucleus, and the hyperechogenic brainstem midline raphe structures are visible, and (b) the third ventricular plane, which visualizes the ventricular system and the normally hypoechogenic basal ganglia. Whereas 90% of subjects have a suitable preauricular acoustic bone window, in 10% no echoes can be detected [22, 23].

An initial study showed that about 90% of patients with PD show SN hyperechogenicity [24]. SN hyperechogenicity can be present in the prediagnostic stages of PD and most studies were not able to show a correlation between its extent and disease progression,

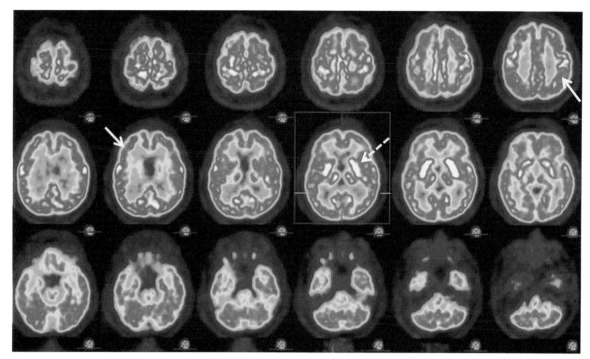

Figure 17.5 ^{18}F-FDG PET in a patient with Parkinson's disease showing an increased metabolism in the striatum (dashed arrows) and a slightly reduced glucose metabolism in the dorsolateral and medial prefrontal and parietal cortex (arrows).

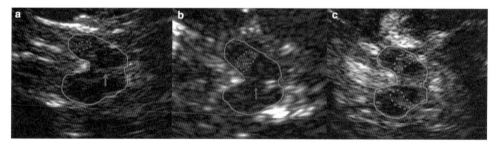

Figure 17.6 Transcranial sonography depicts the midbrain (encircled) of a healthy subject with normal echogenicity of the substantia nigra (SN) (a) of patients with Parkinson's disease (PD), and unilateral (b) or bilateral (c) enlargement of the area of hyperechogenicity of the SN (encircled with dotted line). Arrow shows normal, highly echogenic brainstem raphe in the healthy subject and reduced raphe echogenicity, thought to reflect alteration of the serotonergic system, in the PD patient. The butterfly-shaped midbrain is encircled for better visualization.

suggesting that midbrain hyperechogenicity is a trait rather than a state marker for susceptibility to parkinsonism [22]. However, increased midbrain echogenicity has also been reported in 17% of patients with essential tremor, 40% of depressed patients without parkinsonism, and 10% of healthy subjects [22], suggesting that the specificity of this technique is suboptimal. Also, interpretation of the images in patients with severe tremor and associated movement artifacts may not be reliable.

The EFNS/MDS-ES/ENS recommendations for the diagnosis of PD [7] suggested the utility of transcranial sonography in conjunction with other screening tests for an early diagnosis of PD in clinically unclear cases, for the detection of subjects at risk for PD, including asymptomatic mutation carriers for monogenic forms of PD, and for the differential diagnosis of PD from atypical parkinsonisms and secondary parkinsonian syndromes (e.g. vascular parkinsonism, hydrocephalus, trace-metal accumulation, and calcification of the basal ganglia). A recent study reported that a combined assessment of motor asymmetry, hyposmia, and SN hyperechogenicity improves diagnostic specificity and allows an early diagnosis of PD [25]. Transcranial sonography may be particularly useful to distinguish PD patients from patients with SWEDD and suspected parkinsonism (SN hyperechogenicity reported in only 9% of SWEDD patients) [26]. Studies with patients that have already been diagnosed with PSP and MSA-P revealed SN hyperechogenicity only rarely in MSA-P and in up to a third of patients with PSP of the Richardson type. In contrast, hyperechogenicity of the lentiform nucleus was not frequently seen in PD (10–25%), but present in 70% and 80% of patients with MSA-P and PSP, respectively. The combination of the SN hyperechogenicity and normal echogenicity of the lentiform nuclei has a positive predictive value of 0.91 for PD; a combination of normal SN echogenicity and hyperechogenicity of the basal ganglia has a positive predictive value of at least 0.96 for MSA-P and PSP [22].

Cardiac imaging

[123]I-metaiodobenzylguanidine (MIBG) SPECT imaging is useful for visualizing catecholaminergic terminals *in vivo* and hence is useful in detecting cardiac sympathetic denervation. In PD, there is significant loss of ^{123}I-MIBG binding in the heart, whereas in vascular parkinsonism and atypical parkinsonian syndromes there is only a mild reduction of cardiac sympathetic innervations [27]. The main drawback of ^{123}I-MIBG imaging is a low specificity (37%), while its sensitivity is relatively high (88%) [28]. Cardiac ^{123}I-MIBG SPECT may assist in the differential diagnosis between PD and vascular/atypical parkinsonisms [7].

The future landscape of imaging biomarkers of PD diagnosis

Imaging nigral structural abnormalities using high and ultra-high-field MRI

Volumetric T1-weighted MRI studies at 1.5 T have failed to detect a reduction in SN volume in PD, possibly because of difficulties in accurately delineating the border of the SN pars compacta [29]. Advanced MRI techniques, particularly those implemented on 3.0 T and 7.0 T systems, are promising for a better SN visualization [30, 31]. At present, however, these

techniques are still being evaluated and are not used in clinical practice.

A potential advance in the field is the use of diffusion tensor (DT) MRI at 3.0 T to assess fractional anisotropy of the SN [32]. SN fractional anisotropy values were found to be reduced in PD patients compared with controls [32]. The greatest difference between the two groups was observed in the caudal part of the SN and this distinguished PD patients from healthy subjects with 100% sensitivity and specificity [32]. Another study using fractional anisotropy and R2* changes in the SN showed 95% global accuracy in distinguishing PD patients from controls [33]. If confirmed in larger studies, these findings suggest that DT MRI at 3.0 T could be valuable for supporting a PD diagnosis.

Depigmentation of the SN pars compacta is a key pathological feature of the PD brain. This is because of loss of neuromelanin, a black pigment in dopaminergic SN neurons that accounts for the characteristic (and name-giving) dark appearance of the SN. Neuromelanin, a byproduct of catecholamine synthesis, can be found in neurons in several brain regions and in abundance in the dopamine-producing neurons of the SN and noradrenergic neurons of the locus coeruleus. Because of its iron-chelating capacity, neuromelanin is involved in intra-neuronal iron homeostasis and it is considered neuroprotective. In PD, decreased neuromelanin or decreased iron-binding capacity has the potential to increase oxidative cell damage. Iron overload or extracellular neuromelanin likely contribute to neurodegeneration in PD. Similar to melanin, neuromelanin has paramagnetic properties resulting in signal increase on high-resolution short-echo T1-weighted scans obtained at 3.0 T, the so-called "neuromelanin-sensitive" MRI sequence. The neuromelanin-sensitive technique is able to visualize neuromelanin-containing nuclei (SN and locus ceruleus) as distinct high-intensity areas compared with the surrounding brain tissue. This technique showed signal attenuation in the SN and locus coeruleus in PD patients compared to healthy controls [34, 35], reporting sensitivities and specificities in discriminating early PD patients from controls of 73% and 87%, respectively, in lateral SN and 82% and 90% in locus coeruleus [36].

Several 3.0 T MRI studies have reported decreased T2 and T2* relaxation times, and increased relaxation rates (R2 and R2*) in the SN of PD patients compared with controls [33, 37, 38]. The transverse relaxation time

(T2) reflects effects including dipolar–dipolar interactions and chemical exchange. T2* additionally reflects the effect of local magnetic susceptibility. T2 and T2* and R2 and R2* abnormalities have been interpreted as reflecting increased iron content in the SN of PD patients [33, 37, 38]. Measurement of iron content in the SN may provide an indication of the pathologic severity of the disease. Further studies in larger groups of patients are warranted to assess the reproducibility of results and their usefulness in clinical practice.

MRI signal changes as a consequence of brain iron deposition can also be utilized in characterizing anatomical alterations associated with PD using ultra-high-field MRI, given that the T2* effect is significantly greater at 7.0 T than 1.5 T or 3.0 T. High-resolution two-dimensional T2*-weighted gradient-echo sequences obtained at 7.0 T permit improved delineation of the shapes and boundaries of the SN. In healthy controls, the boundaries between the SN and crus cerebri appear smooth [39]. In contrast, these smooth and clean arch-like boundaries are lost in PD subjects [39]. Based on three-dimenional T2*-weighted gradient-echo sequences at 7.0 T [40], undulation in the lateral surface of the SN appeared more intense in the side contralateral to that with more severe symptoms, and was more prominent at the rostral level of the SN than at the intermediate or caudal levels. In addition to the lateral surface, there was a striking difference in the dorsomedial aspects of the SN between PD and control subjects [40]. In control subjects, a brighter signal region was observed along the dorsomedial surface of the lateral portion of the SN, whereas in PD subjects this region appeared as a dark region with a hypointense signal on T2*-weighted images.

Imaging premotor stages of PD

Classical motor symptoms in PD do not become manifest until about 50% of the SN dopaminergic neurons and approximately 80% of striatal dopamine content have been lost, suggesting the existence of significant compensatory mechanisms. The magnitude of degeneration in the premotor phase of PD is large enough to be detected with dopaminergic PET and SPECT. Subclinical dopamine deficiency has been documented using both ^{18}F-dopa and DAT imaging in subjects with an increased risk of developing PD, such as carriers of genetic mutations associated with parkinsonism (e.g. Parkin) [41], asymptomatic relatives

of familial PD cases [42], elderly patients with hyposmia [43], or rapid-eye-movement (REM) sleep behavior disorders [44, 45]. A prospective study of non-parkinsonian subjects with a positive family history of PD showed that 10% of those with hyposmia and reduced DAT SPECT binding at baseline developed PD over a 2-year follow-up [43]. Increased midbrain echogenicity has been reported in asymptomatic Parkin gene carriers [46], idiopathic hyposmic subjects [47], and patients with idiopathic REM sleep behavior disorder [45].

Cognitive disturbances and dementia in PD

Clinical findings

Prevalence of dementia in the course of PD is about 30%, with a cumulative risk of up to 80% in those who survive 20 years: this means that patients with PD have three- to six-fold increased risk of developing dementia when compared to non-PD elderly [48]. Dementia in PD (PDD) has both subcortical (bradyphrenia, impaired working memory, and poor performance on visuospatial and executive tasks) and cortical (mainly memory and language problems) features, and is associated with behavioral/neuropsychiatric symptoms, such as apathy, anxiety, depression, hallucinations, delusions, and excessive daytime sleepiness. Risk factors include older age at onset, early mild cognitive impairment (MCI), severe gait disturbances, depression, early-onset hallucinations, and lack of adequate response to levodopa. Some patients develop dementia only a few years after the diagnosis of PD, while others may remain non-demented for decades. However, the mean time to diagnosis of dementia in PD is 6.2 years [49].

According to the model proposed by Kehagia *et al.* [50], subcortical cognitive deterioration is most probably associated with dopaminergic deficits and consequent disruption of frontostriatal circuits, causing mainly executive dysfunction. Impairment of the cholinergic system in PDD was found to be associated with an impairment in working memory, attention, and visuoconstructional deficits [51]. Cholinergic dysfunction provides a rationale for treating PDD with cholinesterase inhibitors, while only preliminary data support the efficacy of memantine, an NMDA antagonist [7].

Before the development of overt dementia, early MCI occurs in PD patients with no effect on social or occupational functioning [48]. The prevalence of MCI is slightly lower than that of dementia (26.7%), and MCI may be present even in 15–20% of de novo, drug-naive patients with PD [52]. Patients with PD and MCI are more likely to develop dementia compared with cognitively normal patients [48]. There is a substantial heterogeneity in the range of cognitive deficits in patients with PD, some developing impairment in only one domain of cognition, while others have deficits in multiple domains. The predictive value of such a heterogeneity is far from being clear, but deficits involving posterior cortical regions seem to be more predictive than frontal-executive deficits for future development of PDD [53].

Neuropsychological testing

PDD is characterized by an insidious and slowly progressive cognitive deterioration in at least two of the following four cognitive domains: attention (which may fluctuate), executive function, visuospatial function, and free recall memory (which usually improves with cueing). This is severe enough to impact on daily life performance independently of motor or autonomic features [54]. The crucial point is that dementia develops in the context of an established PD [48]. It is also particularly important to rule out DLB; the main difference is that in DLB the onset of dementia precedes or coincides with presentation of motor symptoms of parkinsonism, while in PDD the dementia presents ≥1 year after a diagnosis of PD. In comparison to AD, executive dysfunction (in particular verbal fluency) is more pronounced in PDD, while episodic memory and orientation performance are worse in AD than in PDD, where they are considerably spared until the late stages [51]. Patients with AD have deficits in the encoding and consolidation of information, while patients with PD mainly have an impaired information retrieval. In the task of recall of three words after a short time period (also part of the Mini-Mental State Examination (MMSE)), patients with PD and cognitive impairment (but not those with AD) can recall the second and/or third word, if reminded of the first word. PD patients sometimes exhibit a "tip of the tongue" phenomenon (effort and slowness in finding the right word or answer).

Recently, criteria for the diagnosis of MCI in PD and guidelines for diagnostic procedures have been published [52]. Briefly, the clinical prerequisite is a gradual cognitive decline reported by the patient or an informant or observed by the clinician in the context of established PD. The guidelines offer (a) an abbreviated approach, with the use of a cognitive screening scale or a few cognitive tests, or (b) a comprehensive approach with at least two neuropsychological tests for each of the following five cognitive domains: attention, executive functions, visuospatial functions, memory, and language. MCI has been defined as one to two standard deviations below appropriate norms, or as a significant decline demonstrated by longitudinal cognitive testing or compared with an estimated premorbid level. For making a diagnosis of MCI in PD, a patient should be impaired in at least two tests of one domain or at least one test of two or more domains. In this case, cognitive deficits do not interfere with daily life performance, except for subtle difficulties with the execution of complex tasks. Patients should be classified with a single- or multiple-domain MCI, with specification of the impaired domains.

Neuroimaging

Dopaminergic and cholinergic imaging

Significant correlation between ^{123}I-FP-CIT binding and global cognition in PDD patients supports the hypothesis of the role, albeit not exclusively, of striatal dopaminergic loss in cognitive decline in PD [55]. Patients with PD without cognitive impairment have relatively selective putaminal loss of DAT binding and subsequent caudate–putamen gradient. Conversely, PDD patients, as well as those with DLB but not AD, show a more uniform striatal decline of ^{123}I-FP-CIT uptake, with a reduced caudate–putamen gradient [13] (Figure 17.4). A diminished frontal ^{18}F-dopa uptake has been reported in PD patients impaired on tests of verbal fluency, verbal recall, and digit span [56]. In a longitudinal, 1-year follow-up study, striatal binding decreased from baseline in PDD and DLB patients (posterior and anterior putamen in both disorders, and caudate decrease only in those with PDD), while no changes were observed in cognitively normal PD cases [57].

Molecular imaging studies also demonstrated a widespread cholinergic dysfunction in PD, more pronounced and extensive in those with PDD. ^{123}I-iodobenzovesamicol SPECT is a marker of acetylcholine vesicle transporter binding in cholinergic nerve terminals. A reduced ^{123}I-iodobenzovesamicol

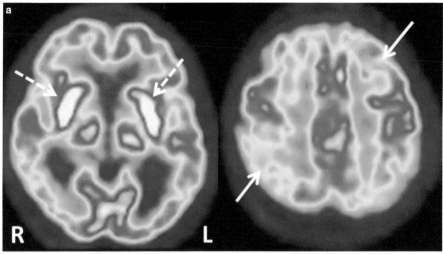

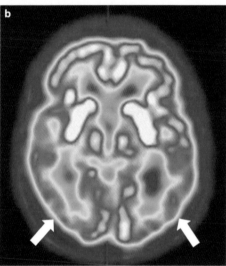

Figure 17.7 ^{18}F-FDG PET in (a) a patient with PDD showing multiple areas of cortical hypometabolism in parietal, parietotemporal, dorsolateral prefrontal and occipital cortices (arrows), and (b) a patient with DLB with a parietotemporo-occipital pattern of hypometabolism bilaterally (wide arrows).

binding has been found only in the parietal and occipital cortices of cognitively unimpaired PD patients, while it involves all cortical regions in PDD [58]. Another biomarker of cholinergic function is the level of acetylcholinsterase activity, which can be assessed with 1-^{11}C-methylpiperidin-4-yl acetate (^{11}C-PMP) PET. Cortical binding of ^{11}C-PMP was found to be reduced in PDD when compared to PD patients with no cognitive impairment [59].

Glucose metabolism and regional cerebral blood flow

Resting brain metabolism and perfusion studies using PET and SPECT showed decreased tracer uptake in the temporal and parietal lobes in PDD (Figure 17.7), which is similar to AD [13]. Additionally, PDD patients also had involvement of the basal ganglia, and frontal and occipital lobes [4]. Patients with PD-MCI have hypometabolism in the same areas when compared to PD subjects without cognitive impairment [60]. A longitudinal study found that early metabolic changes in the visual association cortex and posterior cingulate cortex could be useful biomarkers of incident dementia in PD [61].

The cognitive-related network pattern of PD (PDCP) defined by ^{18}F-FDG PET involves metabolic reduction in the frontal and parietal association areas, in parallel with relative increases in the cerebellar hemispheres and dentate nuclei [62]. Values of PDCP correlated with cognitive function in multiple cohorts of cognitively normal PD patients, and increased stepwise depending on the extent of cognitive dysfunction (cognitively unimpaired PD patients < PD patients with single-domain MCI < PD patients with multiple domain MCI < PD patients with dementia) [63].

Amyloid imaging

Limbic and neocortical Lewy body pathology has been claimed to be the main determinant of the development of cognitive impairment in PD, while cortical β-amyloid deposition seems to determine the rate of progression to dementia [64]. Therefore, of particular interest is the potential of PET amyloid imaging (currently just a research tool). Both ^{11}C and ^{18}F ligands are available.

While the majority of DLB patients showed an increased ^{11}C-Pittsburgh compound B (PIB) binding in associative cortical regions (see below), some degree of amyloid deposition is observed only in a minority of PDD cases (from 17 to 33%) and it is more rarely present in PD patients without dementia (from 0 to 23%) [65]. Such a different pattern of amyloid imaging between PDD and DLB is intriguing since distinction between the two disorders is primarily based on the relative timing of the onset of dementia and parkinsonism. In a prospective study of cognitively normal PD patients, amyloid was found to contribute to cognitive, but not motor, decline over up to 5 years of follow-up, although amyloid burden did not distinguish PD-MCI from cognitively unimpaired PD patients at baseline [66]. In this study, PD patients had generally modest PIB retention, well below the values observed in the majority of AD cases [66]. A cross-sectional study of 40 PD patients at risk of developing dementia (with MCI or other known dementia risk factors) had an increased cerebral PIB retention at levels seen in AD in only six patients; a significant correlation was found between cortical binding values and measures of cognitive impairment in this cohort [67]. These findings suggest that low levels of amyloid are likely to be necessary to cause dementia in synucleinopathies [66].

Structural neuroimaging

In established PDD, cortical atrophy involves the frontal, temporal, and occipital lobes, with a relative

sparing of parietal lobes [4, 11] (Figure 17.8). Although less severe than in AD, and not a universal finding [68, 69], hippocampal atrophy is reported in PDD [70–73]. Limbic structures that are atrophic in PDD, but not in cognitively unimpaired PD, include the entorhinal cortex, amygdala, and anterior cingulate cortex. Atrophy of the caudate nucleus, putamen, and thalamus has been reported in PDD [68, 74]. Enlargement of the lateral ventricles, possibly reflecting both gray- and white-matter loss, was observed in PDD patients [75].

In patients with PD-MCI, a mild gray-matter atrophy of the frontal, temporal, and parietal cortices has been detected [73, 76–78] (Figure 17.2). Prefrontal atrophy has been correlated with increased reaction times, and volume reduction of the orbitofrontal cortex with an impaired decision-making performance. A number of studies, however, failed to find significant atrophy in PD-MCI relative to cognitively normal PD patients [79].

DT MRI may prove useful for investigation of hippocampal connections, frontostriatal circuits, and possibly brainstem connections, that are all relevant for cognitive decline in PD [79]. DT MRI studies of cognitively normal, early, idiopathic PD patients showed subtle white-matter alterations [80], which were found to be associated with executive [81, 82] and color-discrimination deficits [83]. A large study of idiopathic non-demented PD cases at different disease stages showed that white-matter damage is more marked with increasing PD severity and is associated with the degree of global cognitive impairment [84]. So far, only a few studies have used DT MRI to explore white-matter tract abnormalities in PD-MCI patients, showing an involvement of the corpus callosum, cingulum, and major-association white-matter tracts [85–87].

Dementia with Lewy bodies

Clinical findings

DLB is probably the second or third largest group of elderly patients with dementia (mean age at onset 68 years) after AD [88]. Disease progression in DLB is faster than in AD. The core clinical features of DLB include fluctuating attention, recurrent visual hallucinations, and spontaneous parkinsonism, as well as cognitive impairment characterized by deficits of attention, executive functions (such as planning deficits), and complex visual abilities (Table 17.4)

283

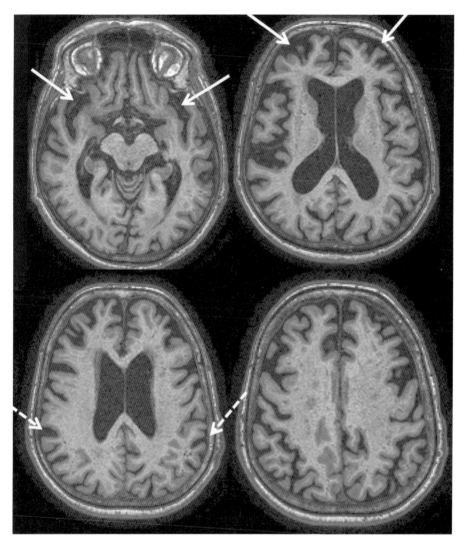

Figure 17.8 MRI findings in an advanced PDD patient: axial T1-weighted images showing severe atrophy of the temporal and frontal lobes (arrows), a mild involvement of the parietal cortex (dashed arrows), and significant ventricular enlargement.

[89]. Memory deficits are not inevitably present, particularly in the early stages. Fluctuations of cognitive function over minutes, hours, or days are a core feature and affect mainly the level of arousal. The examiner may be puzzled by the relatively high scores on the MMSE in the morning, but very poor performance in the evening, particularly since such fluctuations are not necessarily linked to corresponding changes in motor and behavioral symptoms.

The clinical profile of patients with DLB overlaps with PDD and no major differences in cognitive profile have been observed between them. Therefore, PDD and DLB are often considered not to be distinct entities, but rather parts of the same disease spectrum (synucleinopathies). One of the most useful features for the diagnosis of DLB is the occurrence of complex visual hallucinations, which generally present early in the course of the disease [51]. Parkinsonism is not a *sine qua non* for the diagnosis of DLB. However, at present, the most important criteria for differentiating DLB from PDD are the temporal sequence of appearance of cognitive deterioration and parkinsonian symptoms. In comparison with PD, parkinsonism in DLB is more frequently characterized by bilateral bradykinesia, axial rigidity, and masked facies, while resting tremor seems to be less common [88]. There are claims that parkinsonism in DLB is poorly responsive to levodopa [88].

Table 17.4 Consensus criteria for DLB [89]

1. Central feature (essential for a diagnosis of possible or probable DLB)
   a. Dementia defined as progressive cognitive decline of sufficient magnitude to interfere with normal social or occupational function
   b. Prominent or persistent memory impairment may not necessarily occur in the early stages, but is usually evident with progression
   c. Deficits on tests of attention, executive function, and visuospatial ability may be especially prominent
2. Core features (two core features are sufficient for a diagnosis of probable DLB; one for possible DLB)
   a. Fluctuating cognition with pronounced variations in attention and alertness
   b. Recurrent visual hallucinations that are typically well formed and detailed
   c. Spontaneous features of parkinsonism
3. Suggestive features (one or more of these in the presence of one or more core features is sufficient for a diagnosis of probable DLB; one or more suggestive features is sufficient for a diagnosis of possible DLB; probable DLB should not be diagnosed on the basis of suggestive features alone)
   a. REM sleep behavior disorder
   b. Severe neuroleptic sensitivity
   c. Low dopamine transporter uptake in basal ganglia demonstrated by SPECT or PET imaging
4. Supportive features (commonly present but proven to have diagnostic specificity)
   a. Repeated falls and syncope
   b. Transient, unexplained loss of consciousness
   c. Severe autonomic dysfunction
   d. Hallucinations in other modalities
   e. Systematized delusions
   f. Depression
   g. Relative preservation of mesial temporal lobe structures on CT/MRI
   h. Low-uptake MIBG myocardial scintigraphy
   i. Prominent slow wave activity on electroencephalogram (EEG) with temporal-lobe transient sharp waves

Neuroimaging

Dopaminergic imaging

DLB is characterized by nigrostriatal dopaminergic neurodegeneration, making dopaminergic imaging a potentially useful diagnostic tool in the differential diagnosis with AD [13] (Figure 17.4). In a multicenter phase III trial of ^{123}I-FP-CIT SPECT performed in 326 patients with a diagnosis of probable or possible DLB or non-DLB dementia [90], the mean sensitivity of ^{123}I-FP-CIT SPECT for a diagnosis of probable DLB was 78%, and the mean specificity for excluding non-DLB dementia (which was predominantly due to AD) was 90%, giving an overall diagnostic accuracy of 86%. Follow-up clinical diagnosis at 12 months, when

diagnosis had become clear in nearly 60% of patients, confirmed the ability of ^{123}I-FP-CIT SPECT to discriminate DLB from non-DLB dementia [91]. Of 44 patients with a clinical diagnosis of possible DLB at baseline, the diagnosis at follow-up remained as possible DLB in 18; however, diagnosis was changed to probable DLB in 19, 12 of whom had an abnormal SPECT scan at baseline, and to non-DLB dementia in seven, all of whom had a normal baseline scan [91]. ^{123}I-FP-CIT SPECT has demonstrated higher sensitivity and specificity for differentiating DLB from non-DLB than clinical diagnosis in a series of 20 patients who had post-mortem brain examination [92]. In this study, the sensitivity of an initial clinical diagnosis of DLB against autopsy diagnosis was 75% and specificity was 42%, in comparison with 88% sensitivity and 100% specificity with ^{123}I-FP-CIT SPECT imaging [92]. These results suggest that an abnormal dopaminergic imaging scan in individuals with possible DLB strongly supports such a diagnosis. As a consequence, low DAT uptake in the basal ganglia demonstrated by SPECT or PET has been included as a suggestive feature in the diagnostic criteria for DLB (one suggestive feature plus one core feature being sufficient to allow a diagnosis of probable DLB) [89]. On the contrary, its negativity does not exclude a clinical diagnosis of probable DLB, as about 20% of probable DLB cases have a normal or inconclusive scan [91].

Dopaminergic imaging cannot distinguish DLB from alternative nigrostriatal disorders, such as PDD [55, 57, 58, 93], MSA-P, PSP, CBS, vascular parkinsonism with dementia, or frontotemporal dementia with parkinsonism, as all are associated with presynaptic dopaminergic deficiency.

Glucose metabolism and regional cerebral blood flow

Numerous studies reported predominant medial occipital cortex hypoperfusion or hypometabolism in DLB patients compared with AD, with a parietotemporal reduction common to both the diseases [94–96]. Occipital lobe hypometabolism differentiated patients with DLB from AD in both clinically diagnosed [96–98], and autopsy confirmed [95, 99] cohorts. One study comparing ^{18}F-FDG PET findings with autopsy results found that occipital hypometabolism, particularly in the primary visual cortex, distinguished DLB from AD with 90% sensitivity and 80% specificity [95]. Furthermore, the sensitivity in discriminating DLB and AD using ^{18}F-FDG PET was greater than that with clinical diagnostic criteria applied retrospectively to the data from medical charts [95]. However, on individual SPECT and PET scans, the patterns of abnormalities in DLB and AD cases can be identical. Moreover, occipital hypometabolism is not a specific marker for DLB, and can occasionally be associated with AD. In the light of these findings, the consensus diagnostic criteria [89] consider a generalized low uptake on SPECT/PET with a reduced occipital activity as a supportive feature in the diagnostic criteria for DLB.

Amyloid imaging

Small case series using amyloid imaging reveal that DLB patients often have an increased cortical amyloid deposition (from 33 up to 87% of cases) similar to that observed in AD [65]. The regional pattern of ^{11}C-PIB retention in patients with DLB who were ^{11}C-PIB-positive reflects the pattern typically seen in patients with AD, involving the frontal, parietal, and superior temporal-lobe association cortices. Increased striatal ^{11}C-PIB retention has been reported in patients with DLB [100]. Amyloid imaging with ^{18}F-florbetaben showed cortical binding in 29% of DLB cases [101].

Structural neuroimaging

No clear signature pattern of cerebral atrophy associated with DLB has been established so far. Similar to AD, a diffuse pattern of global gray-matter atrophy including temporal, parietal, frontal, and insular cortices may occur in DLB [102–104], but at the same time a pattern of cortical gray-matter loss restricted to frontal and parietal lobes has also been reported [105, 106]. On the whole, several volumetric studies have not found significant or disproportionate occipital atrophy in DLB [104, 105, 107].

A relatively robust MRI finding in DLB is that of a relative preservation of the medial temporal lobe when compared with AD of similar clinical severity [68, 103, 105]. This finding is supported by a prospective MRI study with pathological verification, which found that medial temporal-lobe atrophy on MRI has a robust discriminatory power for distinguishing AD from DLB (sensitivity of 91% and specificity of 94%) [103]. Thus, a relative preservation of medial temporal-lobe structures on CT or MRI supports a diagnosis of DLB in the consensus diagnostic criteria [89].

Subcortical structural alterations in terms of putamen atrophy have been described in some cases of DLB relative to AD [108], while no significant atrophy was detected in the caudate nucleus [73, 108, 109]. A pattern

of relatively focused atrophy of the midbrain, hypothalamus, and substantia innominata, with a relative sparing of the hippocampus and temporoparietal cortex has been found in DLB compared to AD cases [105]. Whether these findings can contribute to an early diagnosis remains unknown. Furthermore, a substantial overlap between DLB and AD with regard to atrophy in these regions detracts from the usefulness of these markers in individual cases.

Conclusions

Although the clinical diagnosis of PD may be straightforward in cases with classic presentations, accurate distinction among variants of parkinsonism may be difficult, particularly in the early disease stages. Conventional MRI demonstrates findings in symptomatic and atypical causes of parkinsonism. However, it does not show specific findings in PD. Modern neuroimaging biomarkers, especially at ultra-high-field strengths, hold a substantial promise for early diagnosis. Nuclear medicine techniques including PET and SPECT allow confirmation of the clinical suspicion of PD by demonstrating presynaptic loss of the DAT. The clinical use of DAT imaging may be limited in some practices, however, because of the high cost. Functional changes are measureable also using functional MRI (fMRI), which can measure neuronal activity at rest or, alternatively, during the performance of specific tasks, but it is too early to determine the utility of fMRI as a biomarker in the diagnosis of PD. Transcranial ultrasound has been shown to detect increased echogenicity in the SN in PD, with a relatively high accuracy. This technique is somewhat limited by the requirement of a good temporal bone window and still lacks validation against other diseases. Blood and CSF markers of neurodegenerative parkinsonism (e.g. α-synuclein) are still in the early phase of development.

References

1. Gibb WR, Lees AJ (1988). The relevance of the Lewy body to the pathogenesis of idiopathic Parkinson's disease. *J Neurol Neurosurg Psychiatry* **51**: 745–752.

2. Hughes AJ, Daniel SE, *et al.* (2001). Improved accuracy of clinical diagnosis of Lewy body Parkinson's disease. *Neurology* **57**: 1497–1499.

3. Massano J, Bhatia KP (2012). Clinical approach to Parkinson's disease: features, diagnosis, and principles of management. *Cold Spring Harb Perspect Med* **2**: a008870.

4. Brooks DJ (2010). Imaging approaches to Parkinson disease. *J Nucl Med* **51**: 596–609.

5. Paulson H, Stern M (2004). Clinical manifestations of Parkinson's disease. In Watts RL, Koller WC, eds. *Movement Disorders: Neurologic Principles and Practive*. 2nd edn. New York: McGraw-Hill, pp. 233–246.

6. Rodriguez-Oroz MC, Jahanshahi M, *et al.* (2009). Initial clinical manifestations of Parkinson's disease: features and pathophysiological mechanisms. *Lancet Neurol* **8**: 1128–1139.

7. Berardelli A, Wenning GK, *et al.* (2013). EFNS/MDS-ES/ENS [corrected] recommendations for the diagnosis of Parkinson's disease. *Eur J Neurol* **20**: 16–34.

8. Hoehn MM, Yahr MD (1967). Parkinsonism: onset, progression and mortality. *Neurology* **17**: 427–442.

9. Berg D, Lang AE, *et al.* (2013). Changing the research criteria for the diagnosis of Parkinson's disease: obstacles and opportunities. *Lancet Neurol* **12**: 514–524.

10. Pahwa R, Lyons KE (2010). Early diagnosis of Parkinson's disease: recommendations from diagnostic clinical guidelines. *Am J Manag Care* **16** (suppl): S94–99.

11. Seppi K, Poewe W (2010). Brain magnetic resonance imaging techniques in the diagnosis of parkinsonian syndromes. *Neuroimaging Clin N Am* **20**: 29–55.

12. Zarei M, Ibarretxe-Bilbao N, *et al.* (2013). Cortical thinning is associated with disease stages and dementia in Parkinson's disease. *J Neurol Neurosurg Psychiatry* **84**: 875–881.

13. Cummings JL, Henchcliffe C, *et al.* (2011). The role of dopaminergic imaging in patients with symptoms of dopaminergic system neurodegeneration. *Brain* **134**: 3146–3166.

14. Goto S, Hirano A, *et al.* (1989). Subdivisional involvement of nigrostriatal loop in idiopathic Parkinson's disease and striatonigral degeneration. *Ann Neurol* **26**: 766–770.

15. Whone AL, Moore RY, *et al.* (2003). Plasticity of the nigropallidal pathway in Parkinson's disease. *Ann Neurol* **53**: 206–213.

16. Marshall VL, Patterson J, *et al.* (2006). Two-year follow-up in 150 consecutive cases with normal dopamine transporter imaging. *Nucl Med Commun* **27**: 933–937.

17. Eckert T, Feigin A, *et al.* (2007). Regional metabolic changes in parkinsonian patients with normal dopaminergic imaging. *Mov Disord* **22**: 167–173.

18. Antonini A, Schwarz J, *et al.* (1997). Long-term changes of striatal dopamine D2 receptors in patients with Parkinson's disease: a study with positron emission tomography and [11C]raclopride. *Mov Disord* **12**: 33–38.

19. Shinotoh H, Inoue O, *et al.* (1993). Dopamine D1 receptors in Parkinson's disease and striatonigral degeneration: a positron emission tomography study. *J Neurol Neurosurg Psychiatry* **56**: 467–472.

20. Eidelberg D, Moeller JR, *et al.* (1990). The metabolic anatomy of Parkinson's disease: complementary [^{18}F]fluorodeoxyglucose and [^{18}F]fluorodopa positron emission tomographic studies. *Mov Disord* **5**: 203–213.

21. Tang CC, Poston KL, *et al.* (2010). Abnormalities in metabolic network activity precede the onset of motor symptoms in Parkinson's disease. *J Neurosci* **30**: 1049–1056.

22. Berg D, Godau J, *et al.* (2008). Transcranial sonography in movement disorders. *Lancet Neurol* **7**: 1044–1055.

23. Walter U, Behnke S, *et al.* (2007). Transcranial brain parenchyma sonography in movement disorders: state of the art. *Ultrasound Med Biol* **33**: 15–25.

24. Becker G, Seufert J, *et al.* (1995). Degeneration of substantia nigra in chronic Parkinson's disease visualized by transcranial color-coded real-time sonography. *Neurology* **45**: 182–184.

25. Busse K, Heilmann R, *et al.* (2012). Value of combined midbrain sonography, olfactory and motor function assessment in the differential diagnosis of early Parkinson's disease. *J Neurol Neurosurg Psychiatry* **83**: 441–447.

26. Stockner H, Schwingenschuh P, *et al.* (2012). Is transcranial sonography useful to distinguish scans without evidence of dopaminergic deficit patients from Parkinson's disease? *Mov Disord* **27**: 1182–1185.

27. Courbon F, Brefel-Courbon C, *et al.* (2003). Cardiac MIBG scintigraphy is a sensitive tool for detecting cardiac sympathetic denervation in Parkinson's disease. *Mov Disord* **18**: 890–897.

28. Nagayama H, Hamamoto M, *et al.* (2005). Reliability of MIBG myocardial scintigraphy in the diagnosis of Parkinson's disease. *J Neurol Neurosurg Psychiatry* **76**: 249–251.

29. Geng DY, Li YX, *et al.* (2006). Magnetic resonance imaging-based volumetric analysis of basal ganglia nuclei and substantia nigra in patients with Parkinson's disease. *Neurosurgery* **58**: 256–262.

30. Lehericy S, Sharman MA, *et al.* (2012). Magnetic resonance imaging of the substantia nigra in Parkinson's disease. *Mov Disord* **27**: 822–830.

31. Stoessl AJ, Martin WW, *et al.* (2011). Advances in imaging in Parkinson's disease. *Lancet Neurol* **10**: 987–1001.

32. Vaillancourt DE, Spraker MB, *et al.* (2009). High-resolution diffusion tensor imaging in the substantia nigra of de novo Parkinson disease. *Neurology* **72**: 1378–1384.

287

33. Peran P, Cherubini A, *et al.* (2010). Magnetic resonance imaging markers of Parkinson's disease nigrostriatal signature. *Brain* 133: 3423–3433.

34. Sasaki M, Shibata E, *et al.* (2006). Neuromelanin magnetic resonance imaging of locus ceruleus and substantia nigra in Parkinson's disease. *Neuroreport* 17: 1215–1218.

35. Schwarz ST, Rittman T, *et al.* (2011). T1-weighted MRI shows stage-dependent substantia nigra signal loss in Parkinson's disease. *Mov Disord* 26: 1633–1638.

36. Ohtsuka C, Sasaki M, *et al.* (2013). Changes in substantia nigra and locus coeruleus in patients with early-stage Parkinson's disease using neuromelanin-sensitive MR imaging. *Neurosci Lett* 541: 93–98.

37. Martin WR, Wieler M, *et al.* (2008). Midbrain iron content in early Parkinson disease: a potential biomarker of disease status. *Neurology* 70: 1411–1417.

38. Ordidge RJ, Gorell JM, *et al.* (1994). Assessment of relative brain iron concentrations using T2-weighted and T2*-weighted MRI at 3 Tesla. *Magn Reson Med* 32: 335–341.

39. Cho ZH, Oh SH, *et al.* (2011). Direct visualization of Parkinson's disease by in vivo human brain imaging using 7.0 T magnetic resonance imaging. *Mov Disord* 26: 713–718.

40. Kwon DH, Kim JM, *et al.* (2012). Seven-Tesla magnetic resonance images of the substantia nigra in Parkinson disease. *Ann Neurol* 71: 267–277.

41. Khan NL, Scherfler C, *et al.* (2005). Dopaminergic dysfunction in unrelated, asymptomatic carriers of a single Parkin mutation. *Neurology* 64: 134–136.

42. Piccini P, Morrish PK, *et al.* (1997). Dopaminergic function in familial Parkinson's disease: a clinical and ^{18}F-dopa positron emission tomography study. *Ann Neurol* 41: 222–229.

43. Ponsen MM, Stoffers D, *et al.* (2004). Idiopathic hyposmia as a preclinical sign of Parkinson's disease. *Ann Neurol* 56: 173–181.

44. Eisensehr I, Linke R, *et al.* (2000). Reduced striatal dopamine transporters in idiopathic rapid eye movement sleep behaviour disorder. Comparison with Parkinson's disease and controls. *Brain* 123: 1155–1160.

45. Iranzo A, Lomena F, *et al.* (2010). Decreased striatal dopamine transporter uptake and substantia nigra hyperechogenicity as risk markers of synucleinopathy in patients with idiopathic rapid-eye-movement sleep behaviour disorder: a prospective study [corrected]. *Lancet Neurol* 9: 1070–1077.

46. Walter U, Klein C, *et al.* (2004). Brain parenchyma sonography detects preclinical parkinsonism. *Mov Disord* 19: 1445–1449.

47. Sommer U, Hummel T, *et al.* (2004). Detection of presymptomatic Parkinson's disease: combining smell tests, transcranial sonography, and SPECT. *Mov Disord* 19: 1196–1202.

48. Svenningsson P, Westman E, *et al.* (2012). Cognitive impairment in patients with Parkinson's disease: diagnosis, biomarkers, and treatment. *Lancet Neurol* 11: 697–707.

49. Evans JR, Mason SL, *et al.* (2011). The natural history of treated Parkinson's disease in an incident, community based cohort. *J Neurol Neurosurg Psychiatry* 82: 1112–1118.

50. Kehagia AA, Barker RA, *et al.* (2010). Neuropsychological and clinical heterogeneity of cognitive impairment and dementia in patients with Parkinson's disease. *Lancet Neurol* 9: 1200–1213.

51. Liepelt-Scarfone I, Graber S, *et al.* (2012). Cognitive profiles in Parkinson's disease and their relation to dementia: a data-driven approach. *Int J Alzheimers Dis*: 910757.

52. Litvan I, Goldman JG, *et al.* (2012). Diagnostic criteria for mild cognitive impairment in Parkinson's disease: Movement Disorder Society Task Force guidelines. *Mov Disord* 27: 349–356.

53. Christopher L, Strafella AP (2013). Neuroimaging of brain changes associated with cognitive impairment in Parkinson's disease. *J Neuropsychol* 7: 225–240.

54. Emre M, Aarsland D, *et al.* (2007). Clinical diagnostic criteria for dementia associated with Parkinson's disease. *Mov Disord* 22: 1689–1707.

55. O'Brien JT, Colloby S, *et al.* (2004). Dopamine transporter loss visualized with FP-CIT SPECT in the differential diagnosis of dementia with Lewy bodies. *Arch Neurol* 61: 919–925.

56. Rinne JO, Portin R, *et al.* (2000). Cognitive impairment and the brain dopaminergic system in Parkinson disease: [18F]fluorodopa positron emission tomographic study. *Arch Neurol* 57: 470–475.

57. Colloby SJ, Williams ED, *et al.* (2005). Progression of dopaminergic degeneration in dementia with Lewy bodies and Parkinson's disease with and without dementia assessed using ^{123}I-FP-CIT SPECT. *Eur J Nucl Med Mol Imaging* 32: 1176–1185.

58. Kuhl DE, Minoshima S, *et al.* (1996). In vivo mapping of cholinergic terminals in normal aging, Alzheimer's disease, and Parkinson's disease. *Ann Neurol* 40: 399–410.

59. Hilker R, Thomas AV, *et al.* (2005). Dementia in Parkinson disease: functional imaging of cholinergic and dopaminergic pathways. *Neurology* 65: 1716–1722.

60. Pappata S, Santangelo G, *et al.* (2011). Mild cognitive impairment in drug-naive patients with PD is associated with cerebral hypometabolism. *Neurology* 77: 1357–1362.

61. Bohnen NI, Koeppe RA, *et al.* (2011). Cerebral glucose metabolic features of Parkinson disease and incident dementia: longitudinal study. *J Nucl Med* **52**: 848–855.

62. Huang C, Mattis P, *et al.* (2007). Metabolic brain networks associated with cognitive function in Parkinson's disease. *Neuroimage* **34**: 714–723.

63. Hirano S, Shinotoh H, *et al.* (2012). Functional brain imaging of cognitive dysfunction in Parkinson's disease. *J Neurol Neurosurg Psychiatry* **83**: 963–969.

64. Compta Y, Parkkinen L, *et al.* (2011). Lewy- and Alzheimer-type pathologies in Parkinson's disease dementia: which is more important? *Brain* **134**: 1493–1505.

65. Brooks DJ (2009). Imaging amyloid in Parkinson's disease dementia and dementia with Lewy bodies with positron emission tomography. *Mov Disord* **24** (suppl 2): S742–747.

66. Gomperts SN, Locascio JJ, *et al.* (2013). Amyloid is linked to cognitive decline in patients with Parkinson disease without dementia. *Neurology* **80**: 85–91.

67. Petrou M, Bohnen NI, *et al.* (2012). A beta-amyloid deposition in patients with Parkinson disease at risk for development of dementia. *Neurology* **79**: 1161–1167.

68. Burton EJ, McKeith IG, *et al.* (2004). Cerebral atrophy in Parkinson's disease with and without dementia: a comparison with Alzheimer's disease, dementia with Lewy bodies and controls. *Brain* **127**: 791–800.

69. Apostolova LG, Beyer M, *et al.* (2010). Hippocampal, caudate, and ventricular changes in Parkinson's disease with and without dementia. *Mov Disord* **25**: 687–695.

70. Nagano-Saito A, Washimi Y, *et al.* (2005). Cerebral atrophy and its relation to cognitive impairment in Parkinson disease. *Neurology* **64**: 224–229.

71. Summerfield C, Junque C, *et al.* (2005). Structural brain changes in Parkinson disease with dementia: a voxel-based morphometry study. *Arch Neurol* **62**: 281–285.

72. Tam CW, Burton EJ, *et al.* (2005). Temporal lobe atrophy on MRI in Parkinson disease with dementia: a comparison with Alzheimer disease and dementia with Lewy bodies. *Neurology* **64**: 861–865.

73. Beyer MK, Janvin CC, *et al.* (2007). A magnetic resonance imaging study of patients with Parkinson's disease with mild cognitive impairment and dementia using voxel-based morphometry. *J Neurol Neurosurg Psychiatry* **78**: 254–259.

74. Almeida OP, Burton EJ, *et al.* (2003). MRI study of caudate nucleus volume in Parkinson's disease with and without dementia with Lewy bodies and Alzheimer's disease. *Dement Geriatr Cogn Disord* **16**: 57–63.

75. Camicioli R, Sabino J, *et al.* (2011). Ventricular dilatation and brain atrophy in patients with Parkinson's disease with incipient dementia. *Mov Disord* **26**: 1443–1450.

76. Lee JE, Park HJ, *et al.* (2010). Neuroanatomic basis of amnestic MCI differs in patients with and without Parkinson disease. *Neurology* **75**: 2009–2016.

77. Song SK, Lee JE, *et al.* (2011). The pattern of cortical atrophy in patients with Parkinson's disease according to cognitive status. *Mov Disord* **26**: 289–296.

78. Melzer TR, Watts R, *et al.* (2012). Grey matter atrophy in cognitively impaired Parkinson's disease. *J Neurol Neurosurg Psychiatry* **83**: 188–194.

79. Duncan GW, Firbank MJ, *et al.* (2013). Magnetic resonance imaging: a biomarker for cognitive impairment in Parkinson's disease? *Mov Disord* **28**: 425–438.

80. Karagulle Kendi AT, Lehericy S, *et al.* (2008). Altered diffusion in the frontal lobe in Parkinson disease. *AJNR* **29**: 501–505.

81. Matsui H, Nishinaka K, *et al.* (2007). Wisconsin Card Sorting Test in Parkinson's disease: diffusion tensor imaging. *Acta Neurol Scand* **116**: 108–112.

82. Rae CL, Correia MM, *et al.* (2012). White matter pathology in Parkinson's disease: the effect of imaging protocol differences and relevance to executive function. *Neuroimage* **62**: 1675–1684.

83. Bertrand JA, Bedetti C, *et al.* (2010). Color discrimination deficits in Parkinson's disease are related to cognitive impairment and white-matter alterations. *Mov Disord* **27**: 1781–1788.

84. Agosta F, Canu E, *et al.* (2013).The topography of brain damage at different stages of Parkinson's disease. *Hum Brain Mapp* **34**: 2798–2807.

85. Hattori T, Orimo S, *et al.* (2012). Cognitive status correlates with white matter alteration in Parkinson's disease. *Hum Brain Mapp* **33**: 727–739.

86. Deng B, Zhang Y, *et al.* (2013). Diffusion tensor imaging reveals white matter changes associated with cognitive status in patients with Parkinson's disease. *Am J Alzheimers Dis Other Demen* **28**: 154–164.

87. Agosta F, Canu E, *et al.* (2013). Mild cognitive impairment in PD is associated with a distributed pattern of brain white matter damage. *Hum Brain Mapp*: Epub ahead of print, doi: 10.1002/hbm.22302.

88. McKeith I, Mintzer J, *et al.* (2004). Dementia with Lewy bodies. *Lancet Neurol* **3**: 19–28.

89. McKeith IG, Dickson DW, *et al.* (2005). Diagnosis and management of dementia with Lewy bodies: third report of the DLB Consortium. *Neurology* **65**: 1863–1872.

90. McKeith I, O'Brien J, *et al.* (2007). Sensitivity and specificity of dopamine transporter imaging with

^{123}I-FP-CIT SPECT in dementia with Lewy bodies: a phase III, multicentre study. *Lancet Neurol* **6**: 305–313.

91. O'Brien JT, McKeith IG, *et al.* (2009). Diagnostic accuracy of ^{123}I-FP-CIT SPECT in possible dementia with Lewy bodies. *Br J Psychiatry* **194**: 34–39.

92. Walker Z, Jaros E, *et al.* (2007). Dementia with Lewy bodies: a comparison of clinical diagnosis, FP-CIT single photon emission computed tomography imaging and autopsy. *J Neurol Neurosurg Psychiatry* **78**: 1176–1181.

93. Klein JC, Eggers C, *et al.* (2010). Neurotransmitter changes in dementia with Lewy bodies and Parkinson disease dementia in vivo. *Neurology* **74**: 885–892.

94. Ishii K, Soma T, *et al.* (2007). Comparison of regional brain volume and glucose metabolism between patients with mild dementia with Lewy bodies and those with mild Alzheimer's disease. *J Nucl Med* **48**: 704–711.

95. Minoshima S, Foster NL, *et al.* (2001). Alzheimer's disease versus dementia with Lewy bodies: cerebral metabolic distinction with autopsy confirmation. *Ann Neurol* **50**: 358–365.

96. Mosconi L, Tsui WH, *et al.* (2008). Multicenter standardized ^{18}F-FDG PET diagnosis of mild cognitive impairment, Alzheimer's disease, and other dementias. *J Nucl Med* **49**: 390–398.

97. Ishii K, Imamura T, *et al.* (1998). Regional cerebral glucose metabolism in dementia with Lewy bodies and Alzheimer's disease. *Neurology* **51**: 125–130.

98. Teune LK, Bartels AL, *et al.* (2010). Typical cerebral metabolic patterns in neurodegenerative brain diseases. *Mov Disord* **25**: 2395–2404.

99. Higuchi M, Tashiro M, *et al.* (2000). Glucose hypometabolism and neuropathological correlates in brains of dementia with Lewy bodies. *Exp Neurol* **162**: 247–256.

100. Edison P, Rowe CC, *et al.* (2008). Amyloid load in Parkinson's disease dementia and Lewy body dementia measured with [^{11}C]PIB positron emission tomography. *J Neurol Neurosurg Psychiatry* **79**: 1331–1338.

101. Villemagne VL, Ong K, *et al.* (2011). Amyloid imaging with (18)F-florbetaben in Alzheimer disease and other dementias. *J Nucl Med* **52**: 1210–1217.

102. Beyer MK, Larsen JP, *et al.* (2007). Gray matter atrophy in Parkinson disease with dementia and dementia with Lewy bodies. *Neurology* **69**: 747–754.

103. Burton EJ, Barber R, *et al.* (2009). Medial temporal lobe atrophy on MRI differentiates Alzheimer's disease from dementia with Lewy bodies and vascular cognitive impairment: a prospective study with pathological verification of diagnosis. *Brain* **132**: 195–203.

104. Burton EJ, Karas G, *et al.* (2002). Patterns of cerebral atrophy in dementia with Lewy bodies using voxel-based morphometry. *Neuroimage* **17**: 618–630.

105. Whitwell JL, Weigand SD, *et al.* (2007). Focal atrophy in dementia with Lewy bodies on MRI: a distinct pattern from Alzheimer's disease. *Brain* **130**: 708–719.

106. Ballmaier M, O'Brien JT, *et al.* (2004). Comparing gray matter loss profiles between dementia with Lewy bodies and Alzheimer's disease using cortical pattern matching: diagnosis and gender effects. *Neuroimage* **23**: 325–335.

107. Middelkoop HA, van der Flier WM, *et al.* (2001). Dementia with Lewy bodies and AD are not associated with occipital lobe atrophy on MRI. *Neurology* **57**: 2117–2120.

108. Cousins DA, Burton EJ, *et al.* (2003). Atrophy of the putamen in dementia with Lewy bodies but not Alzheimer's disease: an MRI study. *Neurology* **61**: 1191–1195.

109. Barber R, McKeith I, *et al.* (2002). Volumetric MRI study of the caudate nucleus in patients with dementia with Lewy bodies, Alzheimer's disease, and vascular dementia. *J Neurol Neurosurg Psychiatry* **72**: 406–407.

Chapter 18

Hyperkinesia, dystonia, and tics

Antonio E. Elia, Gaëtan Garraux, and Alberto Albanese

Introduction

Movement disorders can be classified into two broad categories of akinetic/rigid and hyperkinetic disorders. Hyperkinetic movement disorders (hyperkinesias) are manifested by abnormal, uncontrollable, and unwanted movements. Hyperkinesias include different phenotypic categories, which can appear in isolation or in variable combinations [1]. Some conditions combine hypokinetic and hyperkinetic features, as exemplified by the coexistence of bradykinesia and tremor in Parkinson's disease (PD) or levodopa-induced dyskinesia in patients with PD and chorea or dystonia in patients with Huntington's disease, many of whom have an underlying hypokinesia. The crucial role of the basal ganglia is increasingly recognized, not only in hyperkinetic movement disorders, but also in motor control, muscle tone, posture, behavior, and cognition.

Although at first sight involuntary movements resemble each other, each hyperkinetic disorder has a specific phenomenology (signature) that can be identified by direct observation of the patient or videotaped examination. Duration, rhythmicity, topography, and other features must be carefully analyzed and noted in order to make a specific phenomenological diagnosis. The hallmark features and phenomenology of the main hyperkinetic disorders are reported in Table 18.1, and a detailed review can be found in [1].

Phenotypic categories of hyperkinesia

As previously mentioned, the main phenotypic categories of hyperkinesias are: tremor, chorea, tics, myoclonus, dystonia, and stereotypies. In addition to these six categories there are other abnormalities of motor control that are also included within the field of movement disorders, such as akathisia, amputation stumps, ataxia, athetosis, ballism, hyperekplexia, mannerisms, myorhythmia, restlessness, and spasticity. The term "dyskinesia" is commonly used to indicate any or a combination of abnormal involuntary movements, such as tardive or paroxysmal dyskinesias or levodopa-induced dyskinesia, but more specific phenomenological categorization should be used whenever possible.

Tremor is an involuntary, rhythmic, oscillation of a body region about a joint axis. It is usually produced by alternating or synchronous contractions of reciprocally innervated agonistic and antagonistic muscles that generate a relatively symmetric velocity in both directions about a midpoint of the movement [2, 3]. Chorea is an irregular, unpredictable, involuntary random-appearing sequence of one or more, discrete, involuntary jerk-like movements or movement fragments. Movements appear random due to the variability in timing, duration, direction, or anatomic location; they may, therefore, appear to flow randomly from one muscle group to another [1]. Ballism is characterized by high amplitude, almost violent, movements that mainly involve the proximal limb joints. It is considered an extreme phenomenological expression of the spectrum of chorea that affects proximal joints such as shoulder or hip [1]. Tics are repeated, individually recognizable, intermittent movements or movement fragments that are almost always briefly suppressible and are usually associated with the awareness of an urge to perform the movement, the so-called "premonitory sensation" [4]. Athetosis is a slow, continuous, involuntary writhing movement that prevents the maintenance of a stable posture, involves continuous smooth movements that appear to be random and are not composed of recognizable movement fragments and typically involves the distal extremities [1]. Myoclonus consists of repeated, often non-rhythmic,

Table 18.1 Distinctive features of main hyperkinetic disorders (modified from [1])

Hyperkinetic disorder	Clinical pattern	Typical features	Associated features
Tremor	Rhythmic oscillation of a body part around one or more joints	Regular, oscillatory	Cog-wheeling (postural tremor)
Chorea	Brief purposeless and quick movements that often progress from proximal to distal segments (fluency)	Random, arrhythmic, rapid, occasionally suppressible	Hypotonia Motor impersistence
Ballism	Violent flinging (usually unilateral) movements involving one limb and the shoulder in a coordinated way	Arrhythmic, rapid, non-suppressible	Hypotonia
Tics	Stereotyped intermittent movements (motor tics) or sounds (phonic tics) with abrupt onset	Arrhythmic, rapid, suppressible	Temporarily suppressible by will
Athetosis	Slow writhing movement or sequence of postures involving the fingers, hand, and wrist	Arrhythmic, slow, sustained, non-suppressible	
Myoclonus	Sudden brief muscle jerks (positive myoclonus) or releases (negative myoclonus) of one or more motor units	Arrhythmic, rapid, non-suppressible	
Dystonia	Sustained patterned repetitive movements, often torsional, occasionally rhythmic, associated with abnormal postures	Arrhythmic, sustained, patterned, non-suppressible	Gestes antagonistes Mirroring
Stereotypies	Patterned, coordinated, repetitive, non-reflexive movements that are typically rhythmic and occur in the same fashion with each repetition	Rhythmic, intermittent, continuous, prolonged	

brief shock-like jerks due to the sudden involuntary contraction or relaxation of one or more muscles. These "lightning-like" movements differ from epileptic myoclonus and do not affect consciousness [5]. In dystonia, involuntary sustained or intermittent muscle contractions cause twisting and repetitive movements, abnormal postures, or both. The combination of postures and dystonic movements is typical of dystonia [6]. Stereotypies are involuntary or "unvoluntary" (in response to or induced by inner sensory stimulus or unwanted feeling), coordinated, patterned, repetitive, rhythmic, seemingly purposeless movements or utterances [7].

Dystonia

Dystonia is a movement disorder characterized by sustained or intermittent muscle contractions causing abnormal, often repetitive, movements, postures, or both. Dystonic movements are typically patterned, twisting, and may be tremulous. Dystonia is often initiated or worsened by voluntary action and associated with overflow muscle activation [6].

Following David Marsden's seminal observation [8], it is commonly accepted that dystonia encompasses a combination of movements and postures to generate sustained muscle contractions, repetitive twisting movements, and abnormal postures (torsion dystonia). Dystonia may occur at rest, during activity, or only during a specific motor movement or posture, so-called task- or position-specific dystonia. The most common adult-onset upper limb task-specific dystonia is writer's cramp [9]. Musician's cramp occurs while playing a musical instrument [10]. Embouchure dystonia affects the control of the lip, jaw, and tongue muscles, and may be seen in woodwind and brass players [11].

Dystonic movements may vary in terms of speed, amplitude, rhythmicity, forcefulness, and distribution in the body, but the same muscles are usually involved; hence the term "patterned" movement disorder. They have specific features that can be recognized by clinical examination: speed of contractions may be slow or rapid, but at the peak of movement are sustained; movements almost always have a consistent directional or posture-assuming character. Dystonic movements may be regular, appearing as tremor (so-called dystonic tremor) [12]. When fast and jerky, they may resemble myoclonus. Dystonic tremor may precede clear abnormal posturing, thus raising doubts about the actual diagnosis. A tremor similar to essential tremor may occur in dystonia and can be mistaken for non-dystonic tremor, particularly when isolated [6].

Dystonic postures can precede the occurrence of dystonic movements and in rare cases can persist without appearance of the latter (so-called fixed dystonia) [13]. Dystonic postures are repeated. Particular patterns or postures are characteristic of each patient at a given point in time. Similar dystonic postures may occur in different patients. Postures can be sustained, particularly at the peak of dystonic movements, or may occur during very brief intervals. Dystonic postures are often triggered by attempts at voluntary movement or voluntary posture, and in some cases they are triggered only in particular body positions or by particular movements as may occur in task-specific dystonia. Relaxation may be impaired so that the dystonic posture may be maintained well beyond the end of the attempted voluntary movement that triggered it. There may be multiple dystonic postures in the same patient, so that different dystonic postures may be combined. The term "fixed dystonia" is used to indicate persistent, abnormal posture, without a dynamic component. When present but untreated for weeks or longer, fixed dystonia may lead to painful contractures, as in post-traumatic, chronic regional pain syndrome [14].

Dystonia has some unique activation/deactivation features that can be recognized when looked for and these can serve as a basis for the diagnosis: gestes antagonistes (or sensory tricks), mirroring, and overflow. Criteria for identifying these features, when present, have been recently published [6, 15]. The diagnosis of dystonia can be missed or delayed in a number of patients with task- and position-specific tremors, particularly primary writing tremor, occupational tremors, or isolated voice tremor, as typical features of dystonia may develop only many years after onset. Head or voice tremors observed in tremulous forms of cervical dystonia can be very hard to distinguish from essential tremor. In some cases, family history suggests the correct diagnosis, particularly if family members are ascertained to have dystonia.

Classification

A new classification of dystonia has been recently proposed [6]. This two-axis classification distinguishes the clinical features (axis I) and the etiology (axis II) of dystonia. The combination of these two sets of descriptors provides meaningful information for any dystonia patient and serves as a basis for the development of research and treatment strategies (Table 18.2).

Table 18.2 Classification of dystonia (from [6])

Axis I. Clinical characteristics

Clinical characteristics of dystonia

- Age at onset
  - Infancy (birth to 2 years)
  - Childhood (3–12 years)
  - Adolescence (13–20 years)
  - Early adulthood (21–40 years)
  - Late adulthood (>40 years)

- Body distribution
  - Focal
  - Segmental
  - Multifocal
  - Generalized (with or without leg involvement)
  - Hemidystonia

- Temporal pattern
  - Disease course
    - Static
    - Progressive
  - Variability
    - Persistent
    - Action-specific
    - Diurnal
    - Paroxysmal

Associated features

- Isolated dystonia or combined with another movement disorder
- Occurrence of other neurological or systemic manifestations
  - Isolated dystonia
  - Combined dystonia
  - List of co-occurring neurological manifestations

Axis II. Etiology

- Nervous-system pathology
  - Evidence of degeneration
  - Evidence of structural (often static) lesions
  - No evidence of degeneration or structural lesion

- Inherited or acquired
  - Inherited
    - Autosomal dominant
    - Autosomal recessive
    - X-linked recessive
    - Mitochondrial
  - Acquired
    - Perinatal brain injury
    - Infection
    - Drug
    - Toxic
    - Vascular
    - Neoplastic
    - Brain injury
    - Psychogenic
  - Idiopathic
    - Sporadic
    - Familial

Axis I: clinical features

The clinical characteristics describe the phenomenology of dystonia in a given patient. Five descriptors are utilized to specify clinical characteristics: age at onset, body distribution, temporal pattern, coexistence of other movement disorders, and other neurological manifestations. This structure is also useful for prognostic purposes and for identifying management strategies.

Dystonia may occur in isolation or in combination with other movement disorders. The resulting syndromes may give rise to recognizable associations, such as isolated dystonia or dystonia with myoclonus, parkinsonism, or other movement disorders (Figure 18.1). In isolated dystonia, dystonia is the only motor feature, with the exception of tremor; in combined dystonia, dystonia is combined with other movement disorders (such as myoclonus, parkinsonism, etc.). Isolated dystonia encompasses many cases previously described as "pure" or "primary", whereas most patients previously classified under "dystonia plus" or "heredodegenerative" would now be classified as having combined dystonia. Unlike previous classifications, in the new classification the term isolated or combined refers to the phenomenology, and does not carry implications about the underlying etiology. In combined forms, dystonia does not necessarily have to be the predominant movement disorder and may not be the prominent motor phenomenology (e.g. foot dystonia in PD, mild dystonic features in myoclonus dystonia).

In addition to movement disorders, the presence of other neurologic or systemic features may be associated with dystonia. Non-motor features have been recently described in cases of dystonia with different etiologies [16]. Cognitive decline is typically observed in degenerative or progressive dystonia syndromes. Wilson disease is a disorder where dystonia is typically combined with other neurological or psychiatric symptoms and liver disease [17].

Axis II: Etiology

Autopsy studies of what previously was called "primary dystonia" have indicated that there are no obvious degenerative changes or other structural defects. However, these studies are not as yet sufficient to exclude subtle cell loss or minor structural defects. Human neuroimaging studies have consistently revealed subtle abnormalities in several brain regions in syndromes of isolated dystonia involving the basal ganglia, cerebellum, cortex, brainstem, and thalamus. These studies reveal changes in the volume or integrity of both gray and white matter and suggest that some underlying structural defect may exist. Furthermore, autopsy studies of isolated generalized DYT1 gene-linked dystonia have indicated some of such changes: one autopsy study described inclusion bodies in the brainstem, while another described enlarged dopamine neurons in the midbrain [18].

These findings raise questions regarding the criteria used to define neuropathological defects, which may not require frank neuronal degeneration, but instead may involve dystrophic cells, axonal or dendritic loss, synapse loss, pathological inclusions, or merely alteration of axonal or dendritic branch

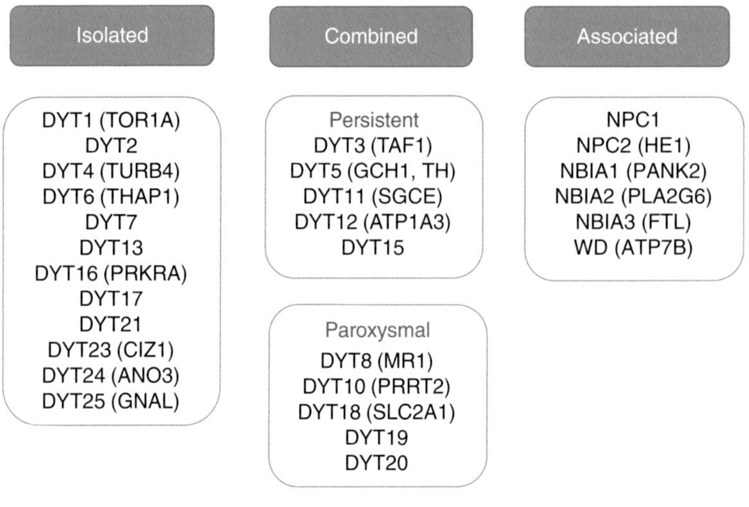

Figure 18.1 Monogenic dystonias: prevalent phenotype. The name of the genes is shown in parentheses. Abbreviations: NPC1, Niemann-Pick type C1; NPC2, Niemann-Pick type C2; NB1A1, Neurodegeneration with brain iron accumulation type 1; NB1A2, Neurodegeneration with brain iron accumulation type 2; NB1A3, Neurodegeneration with brain iron accumulation type 3; WD, Wilson disease.

Isolated	Combined	Associated
DYT1 (TOR1A)	Persistent	NPC1
DYT2	DYT3 (TAF1)	NPC2 (HE1)
DYT4 (TURB4)	DYT5 (GCH1, TH)	NBIA1 (PANK2)
DYT6 (THAP1)	DYT11 (SGCE)	NBIA2 (PLA2G6)
DYT7	DYT12 (ATP1A3)	NBIA3 (FTL)
DYT13	DYT15	WD (ATP7B)
DYT16 (PRKRA)		
DYT17		
DYT21	Paroxysmal	
DYT23 (CIZ1)	DYT8 (MR1)	
DYT24 (ANO3)	DYT10 (PRRT2)	
DYT25 (GNAL)	DYT18 (SLC2A1)	
	DYT19	
	DYT20	

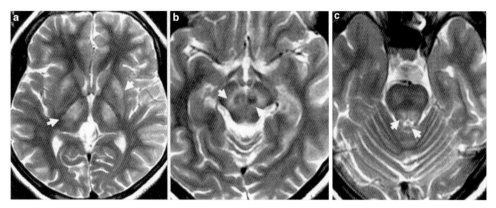

Figure 18.2 Wilson disease. Wilson disease from copper accumulation in multiple organs is diagnosed based on characteristic clinical, biochemical, and genetic testing and is often accompanied by neurological findings including dystonia. T2-weighted axial MRI demonstrates (a) symmetric hyperintense signals in the putamen, posterior internal capsule, and thalami (arrows), (b) "face of the giant panda" in the midbrain with high signal in tegmentum and normal red nuclei (arrows), and (c) "face of the panda cub" in the pons with hypointensity of central tegmental tracts with hyperintensity of aqueductal opening to the fourth ventricle (arrows). From [19].

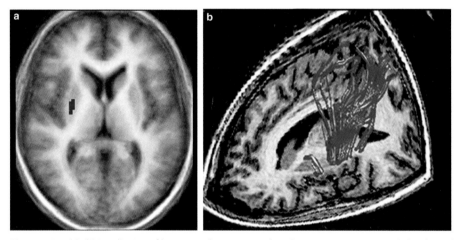

Figure 18.3 (a), (b) Localization of lesions resulting in secondary dystonia in 14 patients with basal ganglia infarct. Lesions were manually segmented on three-dimensional T1-weighted images. The area of overlap of all lesions was determined after normalization in the Montreal Neurological Institute (MNI) space. The overlap area (in blue) is superimposed to the mean normalized anatomical images of the patients. The overlap was located in the posterior sensorimotor part of the putamen (Delmaire C *et al.*, unpublished data). Diffusion-based tractography using this overlap area as the seed region showed that this region was connected to the primary sensorimotor and premotor cortex. Adapted from [20].

structure and complexity. Evidence of degeneration, either at the gross, microscopic, or molecular level, provides a useful means to discriminate subgroups of dystonia into degenerative and non-degenerative forms. Dystonic syndrome may be characterized by degeneration (progressive structural abnormality, such as neuronal loss; Figure 18.2), static lesions (non-progressive neurodevelopmental anomalies or acquired lesions, Figures 18.3, 18.4), or by the absence of evidence of degeneration or structural lesion.

Acute dystonia

Hyperkinetic disorders usually have a slow progressive onset with stabilization and occasional worsening (or remissions). Acute onset is rare and characteristic of few hyperkinetic conditions. Acute dystonic reaction is most commonly seen after exposure to dopamine receptor blockers, both neuroleptics and anti-emetics [22]. Acute dystonic reactions are more common in young men [23], while tardive dyskinesia and drug-induced parkinsonism are more common in

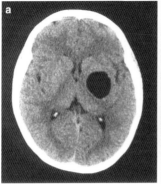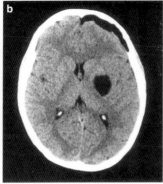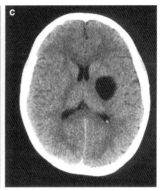

Figure 18.4 Patient with movement disorders affected by neuroepithelial cysts in the basal ganglia. 1: Sequential CT. (a) Pre-operative basal ganglia cyst at the time of the acute symptomatic presentation. (b) Immediate post-operative imaging demonstrating reduction of cyst size and creation of its wall. This corresponded to symptomatic improvement. (c) Delayed re-accumulation of cyst fluid corresponding to symptomatic worsening. From [21].

elderly individuals. Clinical manifestations are diverse, usually affecting the head and neck. Laryngeal dystonia, blepharospasm, cervical dystonia, oculogyric crisis, and focal limb dystonia have all been reported. Dystonia begins within 24 hours of exposure, and usually occurs within 5 days [24]. Acute dystonic reactions affect approximately 6% of patients exposed to "typical" neuroleptics and 1–2% of those exposed to "atypical" neuroleptics [25].

Acute non-traumatic torticollis occurs more commonly in children than adults and should be considered a medical emergency. Conditions that can determine acute torticollis in children include posterior fossa tumors, cervical cord tumors, and infection [22]. Acute torticollis in children should be differentiated from Grisel syndrome that is a pseudodystonia due to atlantoaxial rotatory subluxation. Physical examination may reveal painful, fixed torticollis following an infection or recent surgical procedure in the head and neck area [26]. Another cervical pseudodystonia in children is Sandifer syndrome, which is characterized by acute/subacute abnormal posturing secondary to gastroesophageal reflux [27].

Tics

Tic disorders start in childhood and are characterized by multiple sudden, rapid, recurrent, and non-rhythmic movements (motor tics) or utterances (vocal tics), or both. The best studied chronic tic disorder is Tourette syndrome, which has a prevalence of 0.3–1% in the general pediatric population. The syndrome is characterized by multiple motor tics as well as one or more vocal tics over a period of more than 1 year [28]. Broad expression of Tourette syndrome is manifested not only by motor and phonic tics but by a variety of behavioral comorbidities (such as attention deficit with hyperactivity, obsessive-compulsive disorder, and impulsivity) [1]. The European Clinical Guidelines for Tourette syndrome and other tic disorders were recently compiled and published by the European Society for the Study of Tourette Syndrome [29–33]. The take-home message of these guidelines is that tic disorders are common and complex neuropsychiatric conditions.

Motor tics often result in either a simple jerk-like movement such as a blink, facial grimace, head jerk, or shoulder shrug, or more complex, stereotyped, semi-voluntary, intermittent movements. Tics are usually abrupt in onset, fast and brief (clonic tics), slow and sustained (dystonic tics), or manifested by sudden cessation of movement because of isometric muscle contractions (tonic tics), or inhibition of voluntary movement (blocking tics). The duration of each tic movement is characteristic of that tic, and the duration does not generally vary between different repetitions [4].

The movements can appear purposeful, such as touching, throwing, hitting, jumping, and kicking, or non-purposeful, such as head-shaking or trunk-bending. Characteristic features include predictability of both the nature of the movement and its onset, suggestibility, exacerbation during excitement or stress and also after stress (rebound), and brief voluntary suppressibility. Complex motor tics may resemble normal motor acts or gestures, but are generally inappropriately intense and timed [4]. Occasionally, tics can be so severe as to cause neurological sequels, with reports of compressive cervical myelopathy resulting from recurrent head thrusting and violent neck hyper-extension tics [34]. Complex motor tics can also include copropraxia (grabbing or exposing one's genitals) or echopraxia (imitating gestures).

Motor tics are almost invariably accompanied by vocal or phonic tics and many experts view motor and phonic tics as having the same pathophysiological mechanism. Simple phonic tics can involve brief occurrences of sniffing, throat clearing, grunting, screaming, coughing, blowing, or sucking sounds. Pathological laughter has also been reported as a manifestation of a simple phonic tic [35]. In contrast, complex phonic tics are semantically meaningful utterances and include coprolalia, or shouting of obscenities, profanities, or other insults. Other complex phonic tics include echolalia (repeating someone else's words or phrases) and palilalia (repeating one's own utterances, particularly the last syllable, word, or phrase in a sentence).

Acute tics

Even though it is rare for tics to present with acute onset they can exacerbate and lead to neurologic compromise. Tic disorders wax and wane and some factors lead to marked exacerbation of tic severity including fatigue, stress (physical or emotional), infection, and medications. When this occurs, the dramatic increase in severity (amplitude, violence, or frequency) may be quite alarming to patients and their families. Medications used to treat attention-deficit/hyperactivity disorder or obsessive-compulsive disorder, such as stimulants and antidepressants, are often reported to exacerbate tics [36, 37], although a controlled trial did not confirm this [38]. Rarely, tics may be continuous and disabling, resulting in a so-called "tic status" [39] or in severe, self-injurious, even life-threatening behaviors, so called "malignant Tourette syndrome" [40].

In the emergency department, tics should be diagnosed, and potential exacerbating factors including psychiatric ones should be identified and removed. Pharmacologic treatment, if needed, can be initiated. Initial treatment for debilitating tics uses a neuroleptic or a dopamine-depleting agent. Patients with focal tics may benefit from botulinum toxin injections [41]. Neurologic compromise secondary to tics is uncommon; however, severe tics can cause both compressive neuropathies and cervical myelopathy [34, 42].

Imaging

A large number of neuroimaging studies have been performed in patients with hyperkinetic movement disorders. The high spatial resolution combined with the high contrast-to-noise ratio of MRI enables in vivo demonstration of lesions of central nervous system (CNS) structures. However, the pattern of abnormal MRI findings is rarely pathognomonic of a specific type of hyperkinetic movement disorder (Table 18.3). Imaging studies do not point to a single dominant anatomic brain region for a given disorder. This is in agreement with network models of movement disorders, suggesting that a given disorder can be associated with a dysfunction in one or several node(s) of a distributed circuit that may include multiple interconnected areas within the CNS [44]. Furthermore, a dysfunction in one node can cause a combination of different movement disorders in the same patient. An example of this is the combination of chorea, athetosis, and dystonia after thalamic stroke [43].

Brain imaging techniques beyond structural MRI have been exploited in the diagnostic work-up of hyperkinetic movement disorders, including functional MRI, positron emission tomography, or single photon emission computed tomography (CT), but these modalities are not routinely performed in an emergency setting. The pathophysiology of these disorders has also been studied by advanced imaging approaches in groups of patients compared to normal control populations, but these studies have not proven useful as yet for diagnostic purposes at the individual level.

Nevertheless, imaging is an integral part of the diagnostic work-up of dystonia and provides the basis for the morphological classification on Axis II. Acquired dystonia syndromes often have abnormal imaging, such as the MRI lesions observed in dystonia following perinatal brain injury, vascular pathology, or brain trauma. In familial dystonias, imaging may show usually more subtle abnormalities that indicate morphological changes detected in genetically determined forms. Wilson disease, pantothenate-kinase-associated neurodegeneration (PKAN), and other familial dystonias combined with other movement disorders or associated with other neurological features typically display relevant neuroimaging abnormalities. More subtle white-matter abnormalities have also been reported in myoclonus dystonia associated to mutations in the DYT11 gene [45] and even in isolated dystonia associated to DYT1 gene mutations [46].

Table 18.3 Summary of focal lesions of the CNS or supplying arteries associated with hyperkinetic movement disorders (modified from [43])

Dystonia	Lenticular nucleus
	Thalamus
	Brainstem (midbrain/pons)
	Cerebellum
	Cerebral lobes (parietal)
	Cervical cord
Tics	Striatum
	Cerebral lobes (frontal/parietal)
	Limbic circuit
	Midbrain
Chorea	Striatum
	Pallidum
	Thalamus
	Subthalamic nucleus
	Cerebral lobes (frontal/temporal)
	Vascular abnormality (e.g. Moya-moya disease)
Ballism	Striatum
	Thalamus
	Subthalamic nucleus
	Cerebral lobes (parietal)
Cerebellar outflow tremor	Thalamus
	Cerebellum and dentatorubrothalamic tract
	Striatum
	Cerebral lobes (frontal/parietal)
Holmes tremor	Midbrain
	Cerebellum
	Mesencephalo-thalamic region
The bobble head doll syndrome	Third ventricle
	Suprasellar region
	Sylvius aqueduct stenosis
	Dandy Walker syndrome
Myoclonus	Brainstem (midbrain/pons)
	Thalamus
	Striatum
Exaggerated startle syndromes	Brainstem (pons)
Asterixis	Thalamus
	Striatum
	Cerebral lobes (frontal/parietal)
	Brainstem
	Cerebellum
Transcient dyskinesia	High-grade stenosis or occlusion of the internal carotid artery/vertebrobasilar arteries
Stereotypies	Thalamus
	Striatum
	Cerebral lobes (frontal/parietal)
	Cerebellum
Akathisia	Posterior thalamus

Although there are rare case reports of association of tics and structural brain lesions, for example after trauma, or associated with brain tumors, and infection, structural imaging is not likely to reveal an etiology. CT and/or MRI may be beneficial when there are unexpected associated clinical/neurological findings, or for unusual presentations, principally to exclude treatable pathology. Mechanistic studies in groups of patients such as by functional MRI include evaluation of the cortico-striato-thalamo-cortical circuits [47], adaptive control mechanisms [48], and functional connectivity [49], but these are not as yet relevant to clinical evaluation of the individual patient presenting with a tic disorder.

References

1. Albanese A, Jankovic J (2012). Distinguishing clinical features of hyperkinetic disorders. In Albanese A, Jankovic J, eds. *Hyperkinetic Movement Disorders*, 1st edn. Oxford: Wiley-Blackwell, pp. 3–14.

2. Deuschl G, Bain P, Brin M (1998). Consensus statement of the Movement Disorder Society on Tremor. Ad Hoc Scientific Committee. *Mov Disord* **13** (Suppl 3): 2–23.

3. Hallett M (1991). Classification and treatment of tremor. *JAMA* **266**: 1115–1117.

4. Jankovic J (1997). Tourette syndrome. phenomenology and classification of tics. *Neurol Clin* **15**: 267–275.

5. Halliday AM (1967). The electrophysiological study of myoclonus in man. *Brain* **90**: 241–284.

6. Albanese A, Bhatia K, Bressman SB, *et al.* (2013). Phenomenology and classification of dystonia: a consensus update. *Mov Disord* **28**: 863–873.

7. Fahn S, Jankovic J, Hallett M (2013). *Principles and Practice of Movement Disorders*, 2nd edn. Philadelphia, PA: Elsevier Saunders.

8. Marsden CD (1976). Dystonia: the spectrum of the disease. *Res Publ Assoc Res Nerv Ment Dis* **55**: 351–367.

9. Sheehy MP, Marsden CD (1982). Writers' cramp – a focal dystonia. *Brain* **105**: 461–480.

10. Altenmuller E, Jabusch HC (2010). Focal dystonia in musicians: phenomenology, pathophysiology and triggering factors. *Eur J Neurol* **17** (suppl 1): 31–36.

11. Frucht SJ, Fahn S, Greene PE, *et al.* (2001). The natural history of embouchure dystonia. *Mov Disord* **16**: 899–906.

12. Lalli S, Albanese A (2010). The diagnostic challenge of primary dystonia: evidence from misdiagnosis. *Mov Disord* **25**: 1619–1626.

13. Albanese A, Barnes MP, Bhatia KP, *et al.* (2006). A systematic review on the diagnosis and treatment of primary (idiopathic) dystonia and dystonia plus syndromes: report of an EFNS/MDS-ES Task Force. *Eur J Neurol* **13**: 433–444.

14. Schrag A, Trimble M, Quinn N, Bhatia K (2004). The syndrome of fixed dystonia: an evaluation of 103 patients. *Brain* **127**: 2360–2372.

15. Albanese A, Lalli S (2009). Is this dystonia? *Mov Disord* **24**: 1725–1731.

16. Stamelou M, Edwards MJ, Hallett M, Bhatia KP (2012). The non-motor syndrome of primary dystonia: clinical and pathophysiological implications. *Brain* **135**: 1668–1681.

17. Pfeiffer RF (2011). Wilson's disease. *Handb Clin Neurol* **100**: 681–709.

18. McNaught KS, Kapustin A, Jackson T, *et al.* (2004). Brainstem pathology in DYT1 primary torsion dystonia. *Ann Neurol* **56**: 540–547.

19. Shivakumar R, Thomas SV (2009). Teaching neuroimages: face of the giant panda and her cub: MRI correlates of Wilson disease. *Neurology* **72**: e50.

20. Lehericy S, Tijssen MA, Vidailhet M, Kaji R, Meunier S (2013). The anatomical basis of dystonia: current view using neuroimaging. *Mov Disord* **28**: 944–957.

21. Heran NS, Berk C, Constantoyannis C, Honey CR (2003). Neuroepithelial cysts presenting with movement disorders: two cases. *Can J Neurol Sci* **30**: 393–396.

22. Robottom BJ, Factor SA, Weiner WJ (2011). Movement disorders emergencies Part 2: hyperkinetic disorders. *Arch Neurol* **68**: 719–724.

23. van Harten PN, Hoek HW, Kahn RS (1999). Acute dystonia induced by drug treatment. *BMJ* **319**: 623–626.

24. Diederich NJ, Goetz CG (1998). Drug-induced movement disorders. *Neurol Clin* **16**: 125–139.

25. Pierre JM (2005). Extrapyramidal symptoms with atypical antipsychotics: incidence, prevention and management. *Drug Saf* **28**: 191–208.

26. Yu KK, White DR, Weissler MC, Pillsbury HC (2003). Nontraumatic atlantoaxial subluxation (Grisel syndrome): a rare complication of otolaryngological procedures. *Laryngoscope* **113**: 1047–1049.

27. Kabakus N, Kurt A (2006). Sandifer syndrome: a continuing problem of misdiagnosis. *Pediatr Int* **48**: 622–625.

28. Robertson MM, Eapen V, Cavanna AE (2009). The international prevalence, epidemiology, and clinical phenomenology of Tourette syndrome: a cross-cultural perspective. *J Psychosom Res* **67**: 475–483.

29. Roessner V, Rothenberger A, Rickards H, Hoekstra PJ (2011). European clinical guidelines for Tourette syndrome and other tic disorders. *Eur Child Adolesc Psychiatry* **20**: 153–154.

30. Cath DC, Hedderly T, Ludolph AG, *et al.* (2011). European clinical guidelines for Tourette syndrome and other tic disorders. Part I: assessment. *Eur Child Adolesc Psychiatry* **20**:155–171.

31. Roessner V, Plessen KJ, Rothenberger A, *et al.* (2011). European clinical guidelines for Tourette syndrome and other tic disorders. Part II: pharmacological treatment. *Eur Child Adolesc Psychiatry* **20**: 173–196.

32. Verdellen C, van de Griendt J, Hartmann A, Murphy T (2011). European clinical guidelines for Tourette syndrome and other tic disorders. Part III: behavioural and psychosocial interventions. *Eur Child Adolesc Psychiatry* **20**: 197–207.

33. Muller-Vahl KR, Cath DC, Cavanna AE, *et al.* (2011). European clinical guidelines for Tourette syndrome and other tic disorders. Part IV: deep brain stimulation. *Eur Child Adolesc Psychiatry* **20**: 209–217.

34. Krauss JK, Jankovic J (1996). Severe motor tics causing cervical myelopathy in Tourette's syndrome. *Mov Disord* **11**: 563–566.

35. Cavanna AE, Ali F, Leckman JF, Robertson MM (2010). Pathological laughter in Gilles de la Tourette syndrome: an unusual phonic tic. *Mov Disord* **25**: 2233–2239.

36. Erenberg G, Cruse RP, Rothner AD (1985). Gilles de la Tourette's syndrome: effects of stimulant drugs. *Neurology* **35**: 1346–1348.

37. Gatto E, Pikielny R, Micheli F (1994). Fluoxetine in Tourette's syndrome. *Am J Psychiatry* **151**: 946–947.

38. Tourette's Syndrome Study Group (2002). Treatment of ADHD in children with tics: a randomized controlled trial. *Neurology* **58**: 527–536.

39. Collicott NJ, Stern JS, Williams D, *et al.* (2013). Tic attacks in Tourette syndrome. *J Neurol Neurosurg Psychiatry* **84**: e2.

40. Cheung MY, Shahed J, Jankovic J (2007). Malignant Tourette syndrome. *Mov Disord* **22**: 1743–1750.

41. Marras C, Andrews D, Sime E, Lang AE (2001). Botulinum toxin for simple motor tics: a randomized, double-blind, controlled clinical trial. *Neurology* **56**: 605–610.

42. Goetz CG, Klawans HL (1980). Gilles de la Tourette syndrome and compressive neuropathies. *Ann Neurol* **8**: 453.

43. Mehanna R, Jankovic J (2013). Movement disorders in cerebrovascular disease. *Lancet Neurol* **12**: 597–608.

44. Blood AJ (2013). Imaging studies in focal dystonias: a systems level approach to studying a systems level disorder. *Curr Neuropharmacol* **11**: 3–15.

45. van der Meer JN, Beukers RJ, van der Salm SM, *et al.* (2012). White matter abnormalities in gene-positive myoclonus-dystonia. *Mov Disord* **27**: 1666–1672.

46. Vo A, Eidelberg D, Ulug AM (2013). White matter changes in primary dystonia determined by 2D distribution analysis of diffusion tensor images. *J Magn Reson Imaging* **37**: 59–66.

47. Wang Z, Maia TV, Marsh R, *et al.* (2011)The neural circuits that generate tics in Tourette's syndrome. *Am J Psychiatry* **168**: 1326–1337.

48. Eichele H, Plessen KJ (2013). Neural plasticity in functional and anatomical MRI studies of children with Tourette syndrome. *Behav Neurol* **27**: 33–45.

49. Worbe Y, Malherbe C, Hartmann A, *et al.* (2012). Functional immaturity of cortico-basal ganglia networks in Gilles de la Tourette syndrome. *Brain* **135**: 1937–1946.

Chapter 19

Non-Parkinson's disease tremor

Richard Salazar-Montero and Jan Kassubek together with
William J. Weiner (deceased December 2012)

Introduction

The diagnostics of tremor syndromes are complex and are mainly based on clinical features of the tremor itself and accompanying neurological symptoms, both in Parkinson's disease (PD) tremor and in non-PD tremor. Neuroimaging both with MRI and nuclear medicine techniques has the role to analyze certain brain signs on the one hand and to exclude pathologies on the other hand. In the following, the different types of non-PD tremor are described both clinically and with respect to the neuroimaging characteristics.

Resting tremor

Vascular parkinsonism

Definition

The concept of vascular parkinsonism (VP) was introduced in 1929 by Critchley. The clinical presentation of what Critchley termed arteriosclerotic parkinsonism included rigidity, fixed faces, and short stepping gait as the main clinical signs. A relationship between parkinsonism and cerebrovascular disease is defined as: acute or delayed progressive onset of parkinsonism (within 1 year) after stroke with evidence of infarcts in or near areas that increase basal ganglia motor output or decrease the thalamo-cortical drive directly, or an insidious onset of parkinsonism with extensive subcortical white-matter lesions, bilateral symptoms at the onset, and the presence of early shuffling gait or early cognitive dysfunction.

Clinical presentation

Patients with VP often present with prominent gait difficulties. As reviewed by Demirkiran *et al.* [1], tremor is not a main feature of VP in comparison to PD, but postural tremor is more prevalent in VP.

Hypokinesia or bradykinesia tend to be less frequent in VP than PD. Patients with PD are described as more rigid than patients with VP, while postural instability, falls, dementia, pyramidal signs, pseudobulbar palsy, and incontinence are more common in VP. The only clinicopathological study comparing patients with VP and patients with PD found pyramidal signs in 63% of patients with VP and none in PD. VP showed more prominent and severe features in the lower limbs [1].

Demirkiran *et al.*[1] defined an acute onset subgroup of VP, which accounted for 25–26% of the VP study. Here, the onset of parkinsonism occurred soon after hypertensive encephalopathy or brainstem stroke. The remainder of patients with VP had a progressive symptom onset. Several studies reported significantly poorer levodopa response in VP than in PD, with response rates in VP ranging from 20 to 38% versus 74 to 100% in PD [1].

Neuroimaging

Brain structural neuroimaging

Patients with VP are more likely to have abnormal imaging, varying from 90 to 100% compared with patients with PD, varying from 12 to 43%. The main abnormalities include infarction in multiple territories (96% in VP versus 22% in PD), periventricular and subcortical white-matter lesions (75–90% in VP versus 7–16% in PD), and ischemic lesions in the basal ganglia (38–44% in VP versus 4.6–8% in PD) [1].

A study comparing 15 VP, 15 PD, and 10 hypertensive age-matched controls [2] found more subcortical lesions in patients with progressive VP compared with PD or hypertensive patients. In the acute-onset VP subgroup, lesion load was greater than patients with PD, but not different from the hypertensive controls. Neither the lesion volume nor the location of the lesions correlated with disease severity [2].

Imaging Acute Neurologic Disease, ed. Massimo Filippi and Jack H. Simon. Published by Cambridge University Press.
© Cambridge University Press 2014.

Presynaptic striatal dopamine transporter functional imaging

Three studies compared presynaptic striatal dopamine transporter (DAT) single photon emission computed tomography (SPECT) between VP and PD [3–5]. In two of these, there was a significant reduction in striatal uptake ratios in PD but not in VP [3, 4], whereas the remaining study showed that only the mean asymmetry index was significantly lower in patients with VP compared with those with PD at group level [5].

Atypical parkinsonism

Definition

Atypical parkinsonism can be caused by different neurodegenerative syndromes such as multiple system atrophy (MSA), progressive supranuclear palsy (PSP), and corticobasal syndrome (CBS), which are frequently accompanied by denervation of both pre- and postsynaptic dopaminergic pathways and are usually levodopa-resistant.

Clinical manifestations

Parkinsonian syndromes are characterized by slowness of initiation (akinesia), movement (bradykinesia), and thought (bradyphrenia), tremor at rest (3–5 Hz) and on posture (4–8 Hz), and extrapyramidal rigidity. It is now recognized that a number of diverse pathologies can manifest with these signs, making clinical diagnosis complex, especially in early disease.

MSA is characterized clinically by symptoms that can be subdivided into pyramidal, extrapyramidal, cerebellar, and autonomic categories [6] or, in other words, includes within its spectrum striatonigral degeneration (MSA of parkinsonian type, MSA-P), olivopontocerebellar atrophy (MSA of cerebellar type, MSA-C), and isolated autonomic failure. The diagnosis of probable MSA requires the presence of urinary dysfunction or orthostatic hypotension with a decrease in blood pressure of at least 30 mm Hg systolic and 15 mm Hg diastolic within 3 minutes after standing up, as well as a motor syndrome, which includes parkinsonism with a poor response to levodopa, or a cerebellar syndrome [7]. The diagnostic criteria derived from the Neuroprotection and Natural History in Parkinson Plus Syndromes (NNIPPS) study showed for both PSP and MSA excellent convergent validity with the investigators' assessment of diagnostic probability and excellent predictive validity against histopathology [8].

The presence of non-motor features (e.g. erectile dysfunction, urgency, nocturia, postural dizziness, rapid-eye-movement (REM) behavioral disorders (RBD), or stridor) at presentation or first neurological visit, in the absence of ataxia and parkinsonism, should be regarded as suggestive of MSA. Up to half of patients later diagnosed with the disorder do not have motor symptoms at first presentation, and these patients are sometimes initially classified as having pure autonomic failure. Jecmenica-Lukic et al. [9] proposed that, in MSA, non-motor symptoms that precede the classic motor features show a distinctive pattern of early genitourinary dysfunction followed by orthostatic hypotension in association with sleep disorders such as RBD, sleep apnea, excessive snoring, and stridor (Figure 19.1).

PSP presents as a symmetrical rather than asymmetrical akinetic–rigid syndrome in contrast to PD. It initially targets the trunk and neck rather than the limbs, causing early postural and gait instability with falls and a dystonic posture where the trunk is flexed but the neck extended. Later, limb rigidity and bradykinesia develop in a symmetrical fashion but rest tremor is uncommon. Voluntary gaze problems are pathognomonic but may be a late feature or may be absent. In PSP the optokinetic reflex is lost early with a sustained deviation of the eyes rather than saccades. Early bulbar impairment with spastic dysarthria and hypophonia is common and dysphagia follows. Impairment of frontal executive functions is frequent in PSP associated with dementia of a frontal type.

Although the classic PSP syndrome presents with clear clinical signs in its later stages, several clinical variants have recently been identified that are less distinctive [10]. The classic clinical picture of PSP is termed Richardson's syndrome. The commonest of the variants is PSP-parkinsonism (PSP-P) and it has been shown that the associated tau pathology is less severe and presents in a more restricted distribution than the tau pathology seen in patients with Richardson's syndrome. Some patients present with early gait disturbance, micrographia, and hypophonia, with eventual gait freezing. This variant has been labeled PSP-pure akinesia with gait freezing (PAGF). Patients with PAGF have severe atrophy and neuronal loss restricted to the globus pallidus, substantia nigra (SN), and subthalamic nucleus. Other groups of patients present with progressive, asymmetric dystonia, apraxia, and cortical sensory loss (PSP-corticobasal syndrome (PSP-CBS)) or apraxia of speech (PSP-progressive non-fluent aphasia (PSP-PNFA)) and have

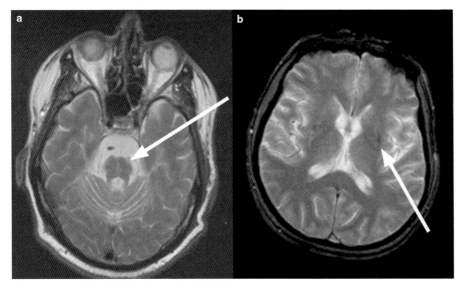

Figure 19.1 Imaging findings in MSA-P. (a) A 61-year-old patient with MSA: axial T2-weighted MRI demonstrates the "hot-cross-bun" sign of the pons (arrow), with prominent hyperintensity of transverse pontine fibers, and atrophy. There is also atrophy of the cerebellum. (b) A 48-year-old patient with MSA: axial T2* weighted MRI demonstrates a hypointense signal ("rim") in the dorsolateral putamen (arrow).

more severe cortical tau pathology than the patients with PSP-P.

In a current publication, corticobasal degeneration was differentiated in four phenotypes: CBS, frontal behavioral-spatial syndrome (FBS), non-fluent/agrammatic variant of primary progressive aphasia (naPPA), and progressive supranuclear palsy syndrome (PSPS) [11]. Clinical manifestations of CBS include movement disorders (akinesia, rigidity, limb dystonia, focal reflex myoclonus, postural/action tremor, postural instability), cerebral cortical features (cortical sensory loss, apraxia, alien limb, frontal release signs, dementia, and dysphasia), and other features (corticospinal tract signs, oculomotor dysfunction, eyelid motor dysfunction, dysarthria, and dysphagia) [12]. In neuropathologically studied cases, a "CBS" was observed in PSP, Pick disease, Alzheimer's disease (AD), frontotemporal dementia with parkinsonism, and frontotemporal lobar degeneration with ubiquitin-positive inclusions. In other neuropathologic studies, CBS pathology was found to be associated with several clinical syndromes, e.g. primary progressive aphasia, frontal lobe dementia, dementia/ apraxia/ parkinsonism, speech apraxia, and Balint syndrome (Figure 19.2).

Neuroimaging

Brain structural neuroimaging

Brain MRI can aid in this classification of patients, and several radiologic signs have been described for

differentiating the atypical parkinsonism syndromes from PD.

A number of findings have been described as suggestive of MSA. These include atrophy and signal intensity alterations (particularly at 1.5 T) in the putamen, including a hyperintense rim, and hypointensity especially in the dorsolateral part of the putamen on T2-weighted images. Infratentorial findings include pontine atrophy, the "hot-cross-bun" sign in the pons, atrophy of the cerebellum, and T2 hyperintensity and reduced width of the middle cerebellar peduncle (< 8mm) [13]. However, at higher magnetic field strengths (3 T and above), some of these signal intensity patterns can also be found in healthy elderly subjects and their utility is, therefore, currently debatable. Specificity of the above-mentioned abnormalities for MSA compared to PD and healthy controls is considered quite high, in contrast to sensitivity, which seems to be insufficient especially in the early stages of disease. Sensitivity to early findings may be improved using higher-resolution imaging and sequences with greater sensitivity to signal loss (T2*), combined with post-processing algorithms (susceptibility-weighted imaging). Specific brain MRI findings associated with PSP include midbrain atrophy with enlargement of the third ventricle and tegmental atrophy, signal increase in the midbrain and in the inferior olives, as well as frontal- and temporal-lobe atrophy [13]. Midbrain atrophy can be indicated

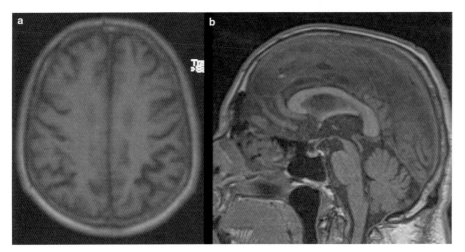

Figure 19.2 Imaging findings in CBS. (a) Asymmetrical cortical atrophy in axial T1-weighted MRI. (b) The overlap of the tauopathies with PSP, which can be found in several CBS cases, has a morphological correlate in midbrain atrophy in the same patient.

by reduced anteroposterior (AP) diameter (< 14 mm) and by its abnormal superior contour (flat or concave) [13]. Furthermore, visual assessment of atrophy of the superior cerebellar peduncle has been shown to distinguish patients with PSP from controls and from patients with other parkinsonian disorders including MSA and PD with a sensitivity of 74% and a specificity of 94%. In the NNIPPS study in MSA and PSP, 627 MRI data sets were evaluated (PSP, 297; MSA, 330) [14]. Four meaningful clusters of covarying parameters with respect to regional volume or signal alterations were defined (i.e. brainstem and cerebellum, midbrain, putamen, other basal ganglia) with good to excellent internal consistency and moderate to excellent reliability. The total score significantly discriminated for disease severity or diagnosis and was considered to be a reliable and consistent measure of MRI abnormalities in PSP and MSA.

Some patients with PSP have increased signal changes in the superior cerebellar peduncle on fluid-attenuated inversion recovery (FLAIR) images, which seem to be absent in PD and MSA [14]. In addition, region-of-interest analyses (SN and globus pallidus internus) of T2-weighted scans performed in 70 subjects with PD, 170 age- and gender-matched controls, and 38 patients with an atypical form of neurodegenerative parkinsonian syndrome ($N = 11$ MSA, $N = 22$ PSP, $N = 5$ CBS) demonstrated that, in patients with PD, significant changes in signal intensities within the SN were observed compared to controls. Signal changes in the globus pallidus internus could be used to differentiate PSP patients from controls [15].

Only a few conventional MRI studies have been concerned with CBS, although several findings have been described. These include cortical – especially frontoparietal – atrophy, which as a characteristic feature is strictly asymmetric; putaminal hypointensity and hyperintense signal changes in the motor cortex or subcortical white matter on T2-weighted images [13]. Unfortunately, none of these MRI abnormalities is considered to be of clearly diagnostic or even pathognomonic relevance for CBS.

All these radiologic signs are based on standard MRI acquisitions. Several advanced quantitative MRI methods have been used to scrutinize the anatomic involvement and dynamics of the pathologic processes in patients with PD and/or atypical parkinsonism syndromes. The clinically most relevant finding resulted from R2* relaxometry measurements, thought to be related to the higher sensitivity of the technique to iron deposition between patients with PD and MSA, where there was good predictive power (area under the curve = 0.96) in the putamen and partial predictive power in the globus pallidum. Based on a right putaminal region of interest, a sensitivity of 77.8% could be achieved. By aiming for 100% sensitivity, the resulting specificity would be 72.7% [14]. These results at 1.5 T are superior to what has been found in previous, qualitative MRI studies.

The more informative pattern of quantitative MRI changes in PSP is different from that in the MSA group. In PSP the most striking feature is based on diffusion tensor imaging (DTI), where an increase in mean diffusivity is seen for the SN compared with controls and (to a lesser extent) with patients with PD and MSA-type parkinsonism [16]. Mean diffusivity (MD) values were also higher in the globus pallidus compared with both controls and patients with PD. Volumetric MRI confirms the profound volume loss in the brainstem [17].

The value of quantitative MRI in differentiating atypical parkinsonism syndromes is yet to be established with neuropathologic confirmation or long-term follow-up. From the data available [14], R2* mapping seems to be the most promising candidate at this time for patients with MSA, and DTI for patients with PSP. The role of susceptibility-weighted imaging (SWI) in a clinical setting remains to be determined [18].

By another quantitative post-processing approach, voxel-based morphometry (VBM), patients with pathology-confirmed CBS [19] showed gray-matter loss in preferential locations, including the bilateral frontal cortex, supplementary motor area, dorsolateral prefrontal cortex, and pre- and postcentral gyrus, striatum, and brainstem. In CBS patients, atrophy was found primarily in bilateral perirolandic cortex and striatum, whereas in PNFA-CBS patients atrophy was primarily left-sided in these regions. Behavioral variant FTD-CBS patients showed the most widespread atrophy, extending beyond the perirolandic cortex and striatum into the orbitofrontal, dorsomedial, and dorsolateral prefrontal cortex. Common regions of atrophy across the three main clinical syndromes of CBS included left perirolandic cortex and striatum. PCA-CBS atrophy included regions of temporal and occipital cortex, bilateral fusiform gyrus, and left hippocampus.

By means of DTI in 14 CBS patients, a significantly increased MD and decreased fractional anisotropy (FA) was observed in the posterior portion of the corpus callosum in CBS patients compared to PD, but not in PD patients compared to controls, postulated to reflect atrophy and degraded transcallosal connectivity in the corpus callosum in CBS [20].

Pre- and postsynaptic striatal DAT functional imaging

The development of specific ligands for SPECT and positron emission tomography (PET) allows in-vivo evaluation of both pre- and postsynaptic parts of the dopaminergic system. SPECT imaging with [123]I- iodobenzamide (IBZM) and other D2 receptor ligands such as ^{123}I-IBF and ^{123}I-epipride has been shown

to be useful for the differentiation of PD from MSA and PSP [21] since the postsynaptic component of the dopaminergic system is not affected in patients with PD except in advanced disease stages.

It has been shown that DAT SPECT is sensitive in detecting presynaptic nigrostriatal degeneration in PD and atypical PD [22]. The amount and pattern of reduced striatal DAT binding in MSA have been shown to be in the range of PD with a more pronounced loss of DAT binding in the posterior putamen compared with the caudate to be typical for both. Asymmetry of DAT binding loss tends to be more pronounced in PD [22], even if disease progression is faster in MSA compared with PD. DAT SPECT studies have shown that even clinically pure forms of MSA-C have some decrease in DAT binding but less compared with MSA-P or PD. DAT SPECT is also of limited value in the differential diagnostics between PD and PSP, although PSP seems to have a more symmetrical and profound DAT loss in the whole striatum, whereas in PD the posterior part of the putamen shows more loss of DAT density compared with the anterior part and the caudate [23]. DAT loss in CBS is in the same range as it is in PD and atypical PD [22] although DAT loss is much more asymmetrical and less pronounced than that seen in MSA and PSP [23]. In conclusion, DAT SPECT imaging does not help to differentiate between the neurodegenerative parkinsonian disorders.

SPECT with ^{123}I-IBZM and other D2 receptor ligands such as ^{123}I-IBF and ^{123}I-epipride has been shown to be useful for the differentiation of PD from MSA and PSP. However, D2 receptor binding imaging methods are influenced by dopaminergic therapy. Plotkin et al. [24] reported D2 receptor deficiency in patients with MSA-P and only in one-fifth of patients with MSA-C. The majority of patients with CBS in that study had a preserved D2 receptor binding. In PSP, a clear reduction of DAT receptor binding was found in seven out of eight patients and D2 receptor loss in six out of eight patients. One patient with PSP who initially had a normal IBZM SPECT was investigated 2 years later and re-examination demonstrated severely decreased D2 receptor binding, accompanied by further reduction of DAT. This case demonstrates that the presynaptic nerve terminals may be affected in some patients earlier than postsynaptic D2 receptors.

When comparing the performance of IBZM SPECT excluding the CBD group, the diagnostic accuracy was 87% (sensitivity 62%, specificity 100%) for the differentiation of levodopa-non-responsive parkinsonism from PD and dementia with Lewy bodies (DLB), which was comparable with published results varying from 80 to 90% [25]. The negative predictive value for the diagnosis of atypical PD in the studied patient population was low (62.5%). Consequently, a negative finding of IBZM SPECT cannot exclude atypical parkinsonisms. In contrast, a positive IBZM scan is highly specific for it (positive predictive value 100%). IBZM SPECT was normal in all patients with normal findings on SPECT with ^{123}I-2β-carbomethoxy-3β-(4-iodophenyl)-N-(3-fluoropropyl)nortropane (^{123}I-FP-CIT), which should be reserved for cases with reduced DAT.

Miscellaneous

PET studies may contribute in the differential diagnosis of these entities. Striatal metabolic studies using fluorodeoxyglucose (FDG) are of value in the differential diagnosis of atypical parkinsonism with hypometabolism in the dorsolateral putamen in PD, bilateral hypometabolism in the putamen in MSA, and hypometabolism of the brainstem and the middle frontal cortex in PSP [26]. In CBS, unlike PSP or PD, unilateral balanced (caudate/putamen) reduction in tracer uptake has been observed [27].

Meta-iodobenzylguanidine (MIBG) scintigraphy is an accurate test for PD detection and differential diagnosis between PD and MSA. A recent meta-analysis reported a pooled sensitivity of MIBG scintigraphy to detect PD of 89% (95% confidence interval (CI): 86–91%) a pooled specificity of MIBG scintigraphy to discriminate between PD and MSA of 77% (95% CI: 68–84%). Nevertheless, possible causes of false positive and false negative results of this scintigraphic method should be considered when interpreting the scintigraphic results as it is well known that various heart diseases and diabetes may damage the postganglionic sympathetic neurons [28].

Midbrain (Holmes) tremor

Definition

In 1904, Gordon Holmes described a tremor syndrome arising as a consequence of lesions in the upper brainstem and cerebral peduncles [29].

Clinical manifestations

The tremor has a rest, intention, and postural component. It can be irregular and is of low frequency (less than 4.5 Hz). Variable delay (4 weeks to 2 years)

between the inciting lesion and onset of tremor is typical as well as its secondary etiology due to different types of brain lesions: stroke, vascular malformation, tumor, multiple sclerosis, trauma, infection, and hyperglycemia. Associated signs and symptoms depend on the underlying lesion and may include ataxia, nystagmus and ophthalmoplegia, bradykinesia, emotional lability, depression, and apathy.

Neuroimaging

MRI studies of patients with Holmes tremor showed lesions of the superior and external part of the red nucleus, rubrothalamic pathways, thalamus, the central tegmental tract, deep nuclei of the cerebellum or their outflow tracts (the superior cerebellar peduncles), and the SN [30]. Both clinical and neuroimaging observations suggest that Holmes tremor requires the interruption of both cerebellorubrothalamic and nigrostriatal pathways. Additionally, there have been a few cases describing T2 signal changes diagnostic of hypertrophic olivary degeneration resulting in the development of Holmes tremor followed by the onset of palatal tremor, sometime after the appearance of Holmes tremor [31] (Figure 19.3).

A PET study performed in six Holmes tremor patients with lesions confined to the cerebellar peduncle showed significant asymmetry in ^{18}F-fluorodopa uptake with intact postsynaptic D2 receptor binding of [^{76}Br]bromolisuride [32]. Almost all of those patients reported improvement after levodopa treatment. Some studies have revealed severe unilateral dopaminergic striatal denervation (^{123}I- FP-CIT SPECT) [29, 32] in subjects clinically diagnosed with Holmes tremor. However, Gajos et al. [33] reported six patients lacking asymmetry in radiotracer uptake on ^{123}I- FP-CIT SPECT. All these patients were nonresponsive to dopaminergic therapy. Therefore, it may be concluded that the dopaminergic deficit revealed by ^{123}I- FP-CIT SPECT may serve as a predictor of levodopa responsiveness.

Palatal tremor

Definition

Palatal tremor (PT) consists of brief, rhythmic involuntary movement of the soft palate that comprises two different nosological entities: essential palatal tremor (EPT) and symptomatic palatal tremor (SPT). The site of the abnormality in EPT is unknown, whereas SPT is

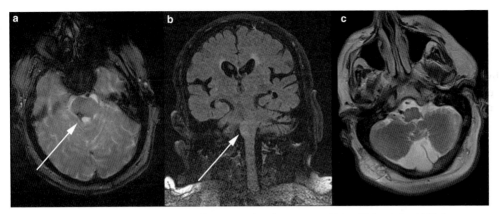

Figure 19.3 Imaging findings in a 62-year-old patient with Holmes tremor: (a) Axial T2*-weighted MRI shows an area of T2 shortening (hemosiderin appearance) in the right dorsal pons indicative of a remote pontine hemorrhage (3 years before) as the causative lesion. (b) Hypertrophic olivary degeneration is seen on coronal FLAIR MRI (arrow). (c) Axial T2-weighted MRI demonstrates that the hypertrophic olivary degeneration is asymmetric but bilateral.

believed to arise from a lesion of the brainstem or cerebellum (within the Guillain–Mollaret triangle).

Clinical manifestations

PT is characterized by rhythmic movements of the soft palate and sometimes other muscles innervated by cranial or spinal nerves. Frequently, PT is due to a localized lesion within the brainstem or the upper cerebellar peduncle and is known as SPT. In about a quarter of the patients with PT, no cause can be found and the condition is diagnosed as EPT. The presenting complaint in EPT is usually the earclick produced by contraction of the tensor veli palatini muscle. Patients with EPT have normal cerebellar function, and there are no pathology findings reported in EPT. Patients with SPT show clinical signs of cerebellar dysfunction (nystagmus, ataxia, dysarthria). The palatal movements are consistent with activation of the tensor veli palatini muscle in EPT and of the levator veli palatini muscle in SPT. During sleep, EPT stops, whereas SPT continues with only slight variations in the tremor rate.

Patients with SPT usually have hypertrophic degeneration of the inferior olives. Hypertrophy develops approximately 3 weeks after the lesion, and SPT begins after a variable time delay from 2 to 49 months after a cerebral event [34].

Neuroimaging

MRI of the brainstem with proton density or T2-weighted imaging may show a hyperintense signal in the region of the inferior olive and, additionally, an enlargement of the inferior olive. These MRI abnormalities are typical of SPT. A single case with MRI–

autopsy correlation confirmed that the olivary MRI features are equivalent to hypertrophic degeneration according to histologic criteria. In contrast, MRI scans in patients with EPT were normal. A meta-analysis of MRI findings in approximately 45 published cases demonstrated that abnormal olivary features appear 1 month after the origin of the lesion and persist for at least 3 to 4 years, but most likely are lifelong [35]. Olivary hypertrophy develops within 6 months after the acute event and resolves by 3 to 4 years [35]. The condition may change into olivary atrophy.

Functional MRI (fMRI) has been used to identify neuronal activation associated with PT, although it is of limited use in the clinical context. Abnormality within the Guillain–Mollaret triangle has been previously associated with PT [36]. In one case of PT neuronal activation was localized to the putamen bilaterally, potentially related to loss of the normal inhibition of the Guillain–Mollaret triangle on the basal ganglia [37]. Consistent with this model, the Guillain–Mollaret triangle itself showed no focal activation. This fMRI study does not contradict, but complements, previous anatomic/pathologic studies and implies that disinhibition of the putamen bilaterally is an essential component of EPT.

Postural tremor

Essential tremor

Definition

Essential tremor (ET) is one of the most common movement disorders, with prevalence of 0.4–6% in the general population and is characterized by a 4–12 Hz postural and kinetic limb tremor that worsens with movement.

Clinical manifestations

ET was defined by the Movement Disorder Society Consensus Statement on Tremor (1998) as a bilateral, largely symmetric postural or kinetic tremor involving hands and forearms. Additional or isolated tremor of the head may occur but in the absence of abnormal posture. Between 50 and 70% of ET patients report a positive family history. Duration is more than 5 years and the neurological examination is normal. In the last years, ET has been postulated to be of two different phenotypes. First, ET as a monosymptomatic disorder and second, as a heterogenous disorder. ET can be classified with both motor and non-motor elements. Tremor may occur in the legs, feet, trunk, jaw, chin, tongue, and voice. Although postural and kinetic tremors are the main features of ET, tremor at rest may also occur in some patients. Other motor features described in patients with ET are gait ataxia, postural instability, and eye-motion abnormalities. Non-motor features include cognitive (memory and executive problems and dementia), psychiatric (anxiety, depression, and social phobia), and sensory abnormalities (olfactory deficits, hearing loss) [38].

Neuroimaging

Brain structural neuroimaging

Although conventional MRI does not reliably differentiate between ET and PD, DTI found changes in FA and MD in the superior cerebellar peduncle and dentate nucleus in a series of 25 familial ET patients compared with 15 PD patients and 15 healthy controls [39]. In a study using midbrain sonography, hyperechogenicity in the area of the SN, considered a marker of nigral degeneration, was seen more frequently in ET patients than in controls [40]. A VBM study in 27 patients with ET [41] found no substantial decrease in regional gray-matter volumes including the cerebellum.

Presynaptic striatal DAT functional imaging

DAT SPECT as a marker for nigrostriatal neuronal degeneration has proven useful and feasible in the differential diagnosis of PD and ET in numerous studies, with a sensitivity of up to 97% and a specificity of 100% [42].

Previous neuroimaging studies in ET and PD patients reported contradictory data. A recent study by Antonini et al. [43] specifically sought to determine if the striatal DAT deficit as measured by DAT imaging with ^{123}I-ioflupane SPECT was demonstrable in familial and non-familial ET cases when compared to PD patients and controls. Low putaminal DAT values were found in a significant proportion of ET cases, but more commonly in those with familial ET. The authors concluded that "abnormalities are frequent in the dopaminergic system of ET patients particularly in those individuals presenting with positive family history" and that "these subjects may be at risk for future development of parkinsonism". The DAT loss in some ET individuals was marked, involving both caudate nucleus and putamen, but less severely than PD.

Schwartz et al. [44] studied 10 ET patients who failed visuo-motor coordination testing, a finding that is more typical of patients with PD. On striatal ^{123}I-FP-CIT SPECT studies, eight of these subjects demonstrated reduced striatal binding volumes. In a reflection of the possible association between ET and tremor-dominant PD, the pattern of DAT loss in ET and tremor-dominant PD is predominantly in the caudate or in both caudate/putamen unlike the akinetic–rigid PD with more involvement in the posterior putamen [45]. Furthermore, Isaias et al. [46] performed two sequential N-omega-fluoropropyl-2b-carbomethoxy-3b-(4-iodophenyl)tropane SPECT scans in 20 subjects with ET, 13 with PD, and 23 healthy controls and found that although PD and ET show different patterns of dopaminergic loss over time, both disorders exhibit the impairment of DAT in the caudate nucleus, providing support for overlap between the two disorders. However, not all patients with ET have evidence of nigrostriatal deficit.

The same study revealed that in ET there was no annual loss of ^{123}I-FP-CIT in any of the brain regions investigated. In contrast, uptake values were significantly decreased in PD, with a 5.6% per year change in the contralateral caudate, 6.4% per year in the ipsilateral caudate, 7.3% per year in the contralateral putamen, and 6.6% per year in the ipsilateral putamen.

More recently, Sixel-Döring et al. [47] performed a retrospective case analysis of 125 patients with diagnostically uncertain parkinsonian or non-parkinsonian tremor syndromes with clinical assessments and ^{123}I FP-CIT SPECT. They concluded that there was no evidence of a decrease in DAT binding in the majority of patients with postural and/or kinetic tremor. Furthermore, the striatal asymmetry index was a further helpful tool for differentiating PD from non-PD tremor syndromes.

In conclusion, PD and ET do not share a common dopaminergic decline over time. However, mild dopaminergic nerve terminal loss in the caudate nucleus may prompt tremor onset in some patients with ET.

Dystonic tremor and tremor associated with dystonia

Definition

The Movement Disorder Society consensus criteria for dystonic tremor include a low-frequency (usually less than 7 Hz) and low-amplitude irregular position or task-specific tremor in an extremity or body part that is affected by dystonia. A more heterogeneous entity is tremor associated with dystonia, which is defined as tremor in a body part not affected by dystonia, but dystonia is present elsewhere.

Clinical manifestations

It should be recognized that patients with dystonic tremor often have a rest tremor, sometimes even with classical pill-rolling, jaw tremor, hypomimia, and impaired arm swing in the affected arm – all features that may suggest PD to the unwary[48]. In addition, some dystonia patients have increased limb tone. This does not necessarily equate with parkinsonian rigidity but may be difficult to distinguish. However, these patients do not have true akinesia, as defined by progressive fatiguing and decrement of alternating repetitive movements. Uni- or bilateral position/action tremor of the hands is a common feature, for example, in patients with cervical dystonia.

Neuroimaging

Patients with dystonic tremor or tremor associated with dystonia have normal DAT SPECT, and normal structural imaging. Dystonic tremor can sometimes mimic PD as scans without evidence for dopaminergic deficit (SWEDDs) [48]. Diagnosis on clinical grounds alone can be very difficult. Normal DAT SPECT is the clue for accurate diagnosis and treatment.

Orthostatic tremor

Definition

Orthostatic tremor (OT), first described by Heilman in 1984, is a rare condition characterized by unsteadiness on standing accompanied by a rapid 13 to 18 Hz tremor of the legs. The symptoms characteristically decrease markedly on sitting or walking.

Clinical manifestations

OT is generally considered to be a distinct and mostly "idiopathic" disorder, as brain imaging and other investigations are usually normal. However, there have been rare reports of patients in whom OT was associated with other features, for instance postural tremor of the arms and PD [49]. Also, OT has rarely been described in patients with pontine lesions, cerebellar degeneration, or after head trauma. These cases might be considered forms of symptomatic OT. OT was initially classified as a variant of ET, because of the presence of a postural arm tremor resembling ET in some cases.

Gerschlager et al. [50] reported that 10 of 41 (25%) cases in their study had additional neurological features, and they defined this group as having "OT plus" syndrome. Of these 10, six had parkinsonism; four of these had typical PD, one had vascular and one had drug-induced parkinsonism. Among the remaining four patients, two had restless legs syndrome (RLS), one had tardive dyskinesia, and one orofacial dyskinesias of uncertain etiology.

Neuroimaging

Recently, a ^{123}I-FP-CIT SPECT study [51] showed no dopaminergic deficit in a group of patients with OT, whereas another study of similar patients based on the same technique showed such a deficit [52]. Trocello et al. suggested that high-frequency OT may be divided into three different subtypes: type A corresponds to primary OT without dopaminergic loss; type B consists of OT with mild dopaminergic loss but no parkinsonian symptoms (corresponding to some previously reported patients) [52], and type C is associated with PD [51].

The fact that some cases of OT are associated with mild dopaminergic loss (some of them subsequently progressing to PD) [52] and that OT may precede the onset of PD [51] suggest that a subtype of OT might be a "soft sign" heralding the onset of PD. A new role may thus emerge for ^{123}I-FP-CIT SPECT in the management of OT. Indeed, ^{123}I-FP-CIT SPECT may be helpful in distinguishing patients who are potentially at risk of PD from those who will continue to have "primary OT."

The fragile X-associated tremor/ataxia syndrome

Definition

Fragile X-associated tremor/ataxia syndrome (FXTAS) is a neurodegenerative disorder caused by a CGG repeat expansion in the premutation range (55–200) in the fragile X mental retardation 1 gene. Men are principally affected.

Clinical manifestations

Kinetic tremor and cerebellar ataxia form the core features of FXTAS. Associated features include parkinsonism, neuropsychiatric and frontal executive dysfunction, autonomic dysfunction, and peripheral neuropathy. Affected women have less severe disease, less cognitive decline, and some symptoms that are different from that of men (e.g. muscle pain).

Neuroimaging

Imaging in FXTAS is useful because it typically shows atrophy, white-matter changes, and a distinctive abnormality of the middle cerebellar peduncles. These finding are more severe in affected men than women [53]. MRI reveals atrophy of the cerebrum, cerebellar cortex, corpus callosum, and pons. Cerebral and cerebellar white matter demonstrates increased T2 and decreased T1 signal intensity. These white-matter changes resemble those seen in microvascular ischemia, except that they are often juxtacortical and patchy. The middle cerebellar peduncles show increased T2 signal in about 60% of affected men and 13% of affected women [54]. This is called the "middle cerebellar peduncle sign" and is relatively specific for FXTAS, although it has also been reported in MSA, acquired hepatocerebral degeneration, and recessive ataxia. Brainstem volume was described to be significantly smaller in unaffected male carriers compared to controls (Figure 19.4).

With regard to the integrity of the nigrostriatal dopaminergic pathway, small-scale studies provide contradictory data. In support of a postsynaptic process is the data from Ceravolo *et al.* [54] which reported normal presynaptic nigrostriatal function using ^{123}I FP-CIT SPECT in four patients with FXTAS-associated parkinsonism. Other studies show pre- and postsynaptic abnormality in similarly small cohorts of patients [55]. Larger-scale studies are required to clarify the extent and nature of dopaminergic abnormalities in FXTAS-associated parkinsonism.

Kinetic tremor

Cerebellar tremor

Definition

Cerebellar tremor is defined as a proximal 3–5 Hz action tremor in the extremity ipsilateral to

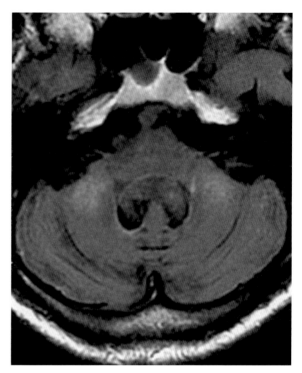

Figure 19.4 T2 FLAIR MRI demonstrates a hyperintense region in the bilateral middle cerebellar peduncles (MCP sign) in a patient with FXTAS.

lesions of the deep cerebellar nuclei or the outflow tracts of these nuclei in the superior cerebellar peduncle. Classically, the tremor amplitude of cerebellar tremor increases as the limb is visually guided to the target, and thus termed "kinetic tremor." There may be a postural component to the tremor.

Causes

Multiple sclerosis

Tremor has been reported in 25–50% of patients with multiple sclerosis (MS). The two most prevalent types of tremor in these patients are postural and kinetic tremors. Tremor typically involves the upper limbs, although the legs, head, and trunk may also be affected.

Neuroimaging

MRI is the test of choice. While cerebellar disease is believed to be the factor underlying tremor in MS, there are no specific findings in this population associated with tremor.

Wilson disease

Definition

Wilson disease (WD), also known as hepatolenticular degeneration, is an autosomal recessive disorder of copper transport that results in accumulation of copper primarily in the liver, the brain, and the cornea. Mutations in the ATP7B gene cause failure of copper excretion into the bile and a defective incorporation of copper into ceruloplasmin.

Clinical manifestations

The most common presenting neurologic feature is symmetrical tremor, occurring in approximately half of individuals with WD. The tremor is variable and may be predominantly resting, postural, or kinetic. Frequent early symptoms include difficulty speaking, excessive salivation, ataxia, masklike facies, clumsiness of the hands, and personality changes. Late manifestations include dystonia, spasticity, seizures, rigidity, and flexion contractures.

Psychiatric features include emotional lability, impulsiveness, disinhibition, and self-injurious behavior. The reported percentage of patients with psychiatric symptoms as the presenting clinical feature is 10–20%.

WD is described in four distinct diagnostic categories based on patients' major neurologic findings, as follows: the parkinsonian group (45%); the pseudosclerotic group (24%) – tremor resembling MS; the dystonic group (15%); and the choreic group (11%) – predominantly characterized by choreoathetoid abnormal movements associated with dystonia.

Neuroimaging

(a) *Brain structural neuroimaging*. WD may show fairly characteristic but not pathognomonic late findings on CT, as bilateral symmetric hypodensity of the putamen, and atrophy with enlarged frontal horns. MRI is far more sensitive to the pathology, characteristic findings increase as disease advances, and may recede with effective therapy. While MRI may suggest the diagnosis, it is also not pathognomonic.

On MRI, lesions of the bilateral putamen, caudate, globus pallidus, and thalamus tend to be symmetric, and typically T2 hyperintense with smaller areas of T2 shortening thought to be associated with copper or other cations (iron). Additionally, T2-hyperintense lesions are common in the claustrum, midbrain, pons, vermis, and dentate nucleus. White-matter lesions tend to be relatively asymmetric. The symmetric hyperintense signal changes on T2-weighted imaging may reflect reactive gliosis. T2 hyperintensity is seen in the dentatorubrothalamic, corticospinal, and pontocerebellar tracts, and there is atrophy of the white and gray matter [56]. Though infrequently noted, the finding of the "face of giant panda" is considered to be pathognomonic of untreated WD, based on diffuse hyperintense midbrain signal changes, which spare the red nucleus and substantia nigra [57]. The most common pattern reported in the literature is the bilateral lateral nuclear involvement of the thalamus [58].

A study by Kishibayashi *et al.* [58] dealt with DTI in cases of WD. They studied four patients and noted that there were abnormal high signals in some areas of the basal ganglia in each case (on heavily diffusion-weighted images).

Various proton magnetic resonance spectroscopy (^{1}H-MRS) studies suggest neuronal injury in the basal ganglia and pons of WD patients based on decreased N-acetilaspartate (NAA) ratios [59]. Alternations of the NAA/Cr ratio in neurologically impaired patients and mI/Cr and Glx/Cr in patients with liver failure could be a sensitive marker of the clinical recovery and deterioration [60].

(b) *Pre- and Postsynaptic striatal DAT functional imaging*. Applying SPECT and PET, several authors have reported on the alteration of the postsynaptic dopamine D2 receptors in patients with WD [61]. In addition, preliminary findings of a presynaptic dopaminergic deficit in WD have been reported [62]. Barthel *et al.* [61] found concordant pre- and postsynaptic dopaminergic deficits in patients with neurologic WD, with a strong intercorrelation between the severity of the deficits in the pre- and the postsynaptic compartments (Figure 19.5).

Miscellaneous

Psychogenic tremor

Definition

The *Diagnostic and Statistical Manual of Mental Disorders*, 4th edition (*DSM-IV*) defined psychogenic tremor as a movement disorder that cannot be explained by organic damage to the nervous system; and is thought to have a psychological origin.

Clinical manifestations

Psychogenic movement disorders can present with a whole variety of movements seen in movement

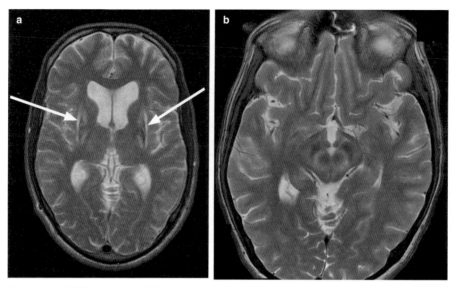

Figure 19.5 MRI from a 35-year-old patient with confirmed WD: (a) Axial T2*-weighted image shows mixed hypo-/hyperintense signals in the putamen and globus pallidus (arrows), and mildly hyperintense signals in the head of the caudate. The expanded frontal horn of lateral ventricles is indicative of brain atrophy. (b) The T2-weighted MRI shows diffuse hyperintense midbrain signal changes, which spare the red nucleus and substantia nigra ("giant panda sign").

disorders of organic origin (tremor, dystonia, chorea, bradykinesia, myoclonus, tics, athetosis, ballism, incoordination) and can affect speech and gait. The estimated frequency of psychogenic tremor in movement disorder clinics is 2–3% or even higher. In an analysis of 88 patients with psychogenic movement disorders [63], abnormal gait was the most common phenomenon and present in 60% of the patients, followed by action tremor (48%), and resting tremor (39%). Psychogenic parkinsonism (PsyP) is a rare syndrome, accounting for 0.17–0.5% of all parkinsonism cases. The clinical characteristics of PsyP are atypical variable tremor, which lessens with distraction or concentration, in contrast with the usual enhancement seen in typical parkinsonian tremor. In addition, extremely slow movements ("deliberate slowness of movement") often accompanied by grimacing, sighing, or whole-body movements when patients do simple motor tasks may be observed. Onset is usually abrupt with a precipitating event, and the progression to maximum symptom severity and disability is usually fast. Although it is possible to identify a patient with PsyP, it can sometimes be difficult to rule out organic parkinsonism. Psychogenic movement disorders can coexist with an underlying organic parkinsonism.

Neuroimaging

^{18}F-fluorodopa PET imaging [63] has been used to differentiate psychogenic movement disorders from organic etiologies. Fahn and co-workers [64] reported all of the patients with a clinically established degree of diagnostic certainty for PsyP had normal imaging, and among the four patients with a probable degree of certainty, imaging was normal in three and abnormal in one, who turned out to have Parkin gene-related parkinsonism. In other studies of patients with suspected PsyP, DAT SPECT was also normal [65]. Although data are limited, normal DAT SPECT in PsyP is the rule, whereas decreased striatal tracer uptake strongly suggests degenerative parkinsonism.

Drug-induced tremor

Definition

Drug-induced tremor and specifically parkinsonism (DIP) may develop in individuals treated with dopamine-receptor blocking agents (DRBAs). Parkinsonism regresses in 60–70% of patients within 2 months after medication withdrawal, while in the remaining cases motor symptoms persist or even worsen, suggesting the development of degenerative parkinsonism.

Clinical manifestations

Clinically, the symptoms are typically indistinguishable from those of PD. Symmetry of symptoms and signs, together with the absence of tremor, has been considered typical of DIP. Asymmetry may occur, however, in about 30–40% of patients or even more, and the presence of tremor has been reported in 44–50% of patients with DIP [66]. Probably, the most common distinctive feature of DIP is its association with other drug-induced complications such as tardive dyskinesias, e.g. buccolinguo-masticatory, which occur in 25–40% of patients.

Neuroimaging

Tinazzi et al. [67] assessed ^{123}I-FP-CIT SPECT in 32 consecutive patients treated with neuroleptic drugs who had developed DIP. They observed normal putamen ^{123}I-FP-CIT DAT binding in 18 patients (group I) and reduced binding in the remaining 14 (group II). They suggested that significant putaminal DAT binding abnormalities may be present in some DIP patients, consistent with the loss of dopamine nerve terminals. A second study was designed to reassess clinical features and DAT scan imaging in the same patients after a 19–39 month follow-up [68]. In group I patients, ^{123}I-FP-CIT uptake was still normal in all patients at follow-up; DAT binding values of the putamen did not differ from baseline values. In group II patients, ^{123}I-FP-CIT binding was still abnormal at follow-up; putamen DAT binding values were significantly reduced compared to baseline.

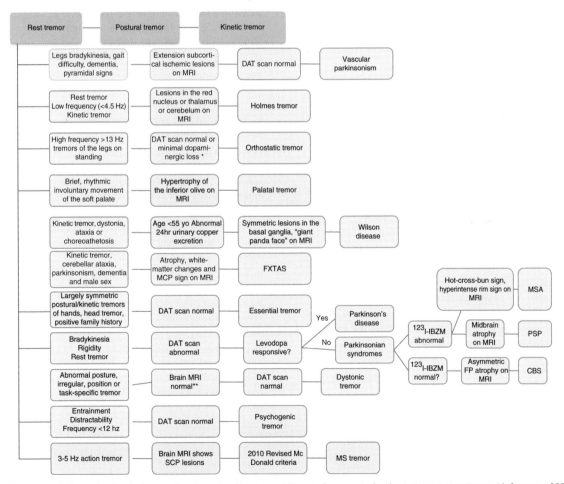

Figure 19.6 Synopsis of main features for atypical parkinsonism. (*Few studies reported orthostatic tremor patients with features of PD. ** There is some evidence of post-traumatic basal ganglia injuries resulting in hemidystonia.).

Burn and Brooks [69] reported that only four of 13 DIP patients showed reduced putamen PET ^{18}F-fluorolevodopa uptake. After drug withdrawal, patients with normal PET followed for about 2 years showed an improvement of motor symptoms, while in three out of four patients with abnormal PET, parkinsonism worsened. Recently, Tinazzi et al. [70] reported neuroimaging abnormalities in 41 of 97 patients who underwent ^{123}I-FP-CIT SPECT (42%). It is postulated that in patients with DIP, the presence of SPECT abnormalities is highly predictive of continuing or worsening of motor symptoms in the context of a progressive degenerative parkinsonism, while DIP induced only by DRBAs is associated with normal DAT. In other words, in DIP patients with SPECT abnormalities, DRBAs might aggravate a pre-existing subclinical nigrostriatal defect, thus resulting in clinical manifestations, while in DIP patients with normal DAT, parkinsonism is caused only by a D2 receptor blockade induced by DRBAs.

Acute parkinsonism

Definition

Development of parkinsonism over a period of days to weeks as a result of a secondary cause.

Diagnostic approach

The acute or subacute onset of parkinsonism has a broad differential diagnosis. Parkinsonism as part of a primary neurodegenerative disease is insidious in onset and slowly progressive. However, when parkinsonism develops over a period of days to weeks, a secondary cause must be considered [71]. In this situation, a review of the medication list and examination for pathognomonic findings are important. An investigation for a structural lesion should ensue with imaging studies including MRI.

A chart with a synopsis of main features for atypical parkinsonism and tremor is given in Figure 19.6.

References

1. Demirkiran M, Bozdemir H, Sarica Y (2001). Vascular parkinsonism: a distinct, heterogeneous clinical entity. *Acta Neurol Scand* **104**: 63–67.

2. Zijlmans JC, Thijssen HO, Vogels OJ, et al. (1995). MRI in patients with suspected vascular parkinsonism. *Neurology* **45**: 2183–2188.

3. Tzen KY, Lu CS, Yen TC, et al. (2001). Differential diagnosis of Parkinson's disease and vascular parkinsonism by (99m)Tc-TRODAT-1. *J Nucl Med* **42**: 408–413.

4. Gerschlager W, Bencsits G, Pirker W, et al. (2002). [123I]beta-CIT SPECT distinguishes vascular parkinsonism from Parkinson's disease. *Mov Disord* **17**: 518–523.

5. Zijlmans J, Evans A, Fontes F, et al. (2007). [(123)I] FP-CIT spect study in vascular parkinsonism and Parkinson's disease. *Mov Disord* **22**: 1278–1285.

6. Ubhi K, Low P, Masliah E (2011). Multiple system atrophy: a clinical and neuropathological perspective. *Trends Neurosci* **34**: 581–590.

7. Stefanova N, Bücke P, Duerr S, et al. (2009). Multiple system atrophy: an update. *Lancet Neurol.* **8**: 1172–1178.

8. Bensimon G, Ludolph A, Agid Y, et al.(2009). NNIPPS Study Group. Riluzole treatment, survival and diagnostic criteria in Parkinson plus disorders: the NNIPPS study. *Brain* **132**: 156–171.

9. Jecmenica-Lukic M, Poewe W, Tolosa E, et al. (2012). Premotor signs and symptoms of multiple system atrophy. *Lancet Neurol* **11**: 361–368.

10. Williams DR, Lees AJ (2009). Progressive supranuclear palsy: clinicopathological concepts and diagnostic challenges. *Lancet Neurol* **8**: 270–279.

11. Armstrong MJ, Litvan I, Lang AE, et al. (2013). Criteria for the diagnosis of corticobasal degeneration. *Neurology* **80**: 496–503.

12. Ludolph AC, Kassubek J, Landwehrmeyer BG, et al. (2009). Tauopathies with parkinsonism: clinical spectrum, neuropathologic basis, biological markers, and treatmentoptions. *Eur J Neurol* **16**: 297–309.

13. Seppi K (2007). MRI for the differential diagnosis of neurodegenerative parkinsonism in clinical practice. *Parkinsonism Relat Disord.* **13** (suppl 3): S400–405.

14. Rolland Y, Vérin M, Payan CA, et al. (2011). NNIPPS Study Group. A new MRI rating scale for progressive supranuclear palsy and multiple system atrophy: validity and reliability. *J Neurol Neurosurg Psychiatry* **82**: 1025–1032.

15. Jesse S, Kassubek J, Müller HP, Ludolph AC, Unrath A (2012). Signal alterations of the basal ganglia in the differential diagnosis of Parkinson's disease: a retrospective case-controlled MRI data bank analysis. *BMC Neurol* **12**: 163.

16. Focke NK, Helms G, Pantel PM, et al. (2011). Differentiation of typical and atypical Parkinson syndromes by quantitative MR imaging. *AJNR* **32**: 2087–2092.

17. Focke N, Helms G, Scheewe S, et al. (2011). Individual voxel-based subtype prediction can differentiate progressive supranuclear palsy from idiopathic

Parkinson syndrome and healthy controls. *Hum Brain Mapp* **32**: 1905–1915.

18. Wang Y, Butros SR, Shuai X, *et al*. Different iron-deposition patterns of multiple system atrophy with predominant parkinsonism and idiopathic Parkinson diseases demonstrated by phase-corrected susceptibility-weighted imaging. *AJNR* 2012; **33**: 266–273.]

19. Lee SE, Rabinovici GD, Mayo MC, *et al*. (2011). Clinicopathological correlations in corticobasal degeneration. *Ann Neurol* **70**: 327–340.

20. Boelmans K, Bodammer NC, Suchorska B, *et al*. (2010). Diffusion tensor imaging of the corpus callosum differentiates corticobasal syndrome from Parkinson's disease. *Parkinsonism Relat Disord* **16**: 498–502.

21. Varrone A, Innis RB, Marek K, *et al*. (1998). Evaluation of patients with parkinsonism with [123]IBF and b-CIT SPECT. *J Nucl Med* **39**: 14.

22. Pirker W, Asenbaum S, Bencsits G, *et al*. (2000). [123I] beta-CIT SPECT in multiple system atrophy, progressive supranuclear palsy, and corticobasal degeneration. *Mov Disord* **15**: 1158–1167.

23. Antonini A, Benti R, De Notaris R, *et al*. (2003). 123I-Ioflupane/SPECT binding to striatal dopamine transporter (DAT) uptake in patients with Parkinson's disease, multiple system atrophy, and progressive supranuclear palsy. *Neurol Sci* **24**: 149–150.

24. Plotkin M, Amthauer H, Klaffke S, *et al*. (. 2005). Combined 123I-FP-CIT and 123I-IBZM SPECT for the diagnosis of parkinsonian syndromes: study on 72 patients. *J Neural Transm* **112**: 677–692.

25. Larisch R, Klimke A (1998). On the clinical impact of cerebral dopamine D2 receptor scintigraphy. *Nuklearmedizin* **37**: 245–250.

26. Eckert T, Barnes A, Dhawan V, *et al*. (2005). FDG PET in the differential diagnosis of parkinsonian disorders. *NeuroImage* **26**: 912–921.

27. Sawle GV, Brooks DJ, Marsden CD, *et al*. (1991). Corticobasal degeneration: a unique pattern of regional cortical oxygen hypometabolism and striatal fluorodopa uptake demonstrated by positron emission tomography. *Brain* **114**: 541–556.

28. Treglia G, Stefanelli A, Cason E, *et al*. (2011). Diagnostic performance of iodine-123-metaiodobenzylguanidine scintigraphy in differential diagnosis between Parkinson's disease and multiple-system atrophy: a systematic review and a meta-analysis. *Clin Neurol Neurosurg* **113**: 823–829.

29. Holmes G (1904). On certain tremors in organic cerebral lesions. *Brain* **27**: 325–375.

30. Paviour DC, Jäger HR, Wilkinson L, *et al*. (2006). Holmes tremor: application of modern neuroimaging technique. *Mov Disord* **21**: 2260–2662.

31. Rieder CR, Rebouças RG, Ferreira MP (2003). Holmes tremor in association with bilateral hypertrophic olivary degeneration and palatal tremor: chronological considerations. Case report. *ArqNeuropsiquiatr* **61**: 473–477.

32. Remy P, de Recondo A, Defer G, *et al*. (1995). Peduncular rubral tremor and dopaminergic denervation: a PET study. *Neurology* **45**: 472–477.

33. Gajos A, Bogucki A, Schinwelski M, *et al*. (2010). The clinical and neuroimaging studies in Holmes tremor. *Acta Neurol Scand* **122**: 360–366.

34. Matsuo F, Ajax ET (1979). Palatal myoclonus, and denervation supersensitivity in the central nervous system. *Ann Neurol* **5**: 72–88.

35. Goyal M, Versnick E, Tuite P, *et al*. (2000). Hypertrophic olivary degeneration: metaanalysis of the temporal evolution of MR findings. *AJNR* **21**: 1073–1077.

36. Haller S, Winkler DT, Gobbi C, *et al*. (2006). Prominent activation of the putamen during essential palatal tremor: a functional MR imaging case study. *AJNR* **27**: 1272–1274.

37. Nitschke MF, Kruger G, Bruhn H, *et al*. (2001). Voluntary palatal tremor is associated with hyperactivation of the inferior olive: a functional magnetic resonance imaging study. *Mov Disord* **16**: 1193–1195.

38. Louis ED, Okun MS (2011). It is time to remove the "benign" from the essential tremor label. *Parkinsonism Relat Disord* **17**: 516–520.

39. Nicoletti G, Manners D, Novellino F, *et al*. (2010). Diffusion tensor MRI changes in cerebellar structures of patients with familial essential tremor. *Neurology* **74**: 988–994.

40. Budisic M, Trkanjec Z, Bosnjak J, *et al*. (2009). Distinguishing Parkinson's disease and essential tremor with transcranial sonography. *Acta Neurol Scand* **119**: 17–21.

41. Daniels C, Peller M, Wolff S, *et al*. (2006). Voxel-based morphometry shows no decreases in cerebellar gray matter volume in essential tremor. *Neurology* **67**: 1452–1456.

42. Benamer TS, Patterson J, Grosset DG, *et al*. (2000). Accurate differentiation of parkinsonism and essential tremor using visual assessment of [123I]-FP-CIT SPECT imaging: the [123I]-FP-CIT study group. *Mov Disord* **15**: 503–510

43. Antonini A, Isaias IU, Cilia R, *et al*. (2005). Striatal dopamine transporter (DAT) abnormalities in patients with sporadic and familial essential tremor (ET): a comparative study with (123I)ioflupane-SPECT. *Mov Disord* **20**: S172.

44. Schwartz M, Groshar D, Inzelberg R, *et al*. (2004). Dopamine transporter imaging and visuo-motor

testing in essential tremor, practical possibilities for detection of early stage Parkinson's disease. *Parkinsonism Relat Disord* **10**: 385–389.

45. Isaias IU, Benti R, Cilia R, *et al.* (2007). [^{123}I]FP-CIT striatal binding in early Parkinson's disease patients with tremor vs. akinetic–rigid onset. *Neuroreport* **18**: 1499–1502.

46. Isaias IU, Marotta G, Hirano S, *et al.* (2010). Imaging essential tremor. *Mov Disord* **25**: 679–686.

47. Sixel-Döring F, Liepe K, Mollenhauer B, *et al.* (2011). The role of ^{123}I-FP-CIT-SPECT in the differential diagnosis of Parkinson and tremor syndromes: a critical assessment of 125 cases. *J Neurol* **258**: 2147–2154.

48. Schneider SA, Edwards MJ, Mir P, *et al.* (2007). Patients with adult-onset dystonic tremor resembling parkinsonian tremor have scans without evidence of dopaminergic deficit (SWEDDs). *Mov Disord* **22**: 2210–2215.

49. Apartis E, Tison F, Arne P, *et al.* (2001). Fast orthostatic tremor in Parkinson's disease mimicking primary orthostatic tremor. *Mov Disord* **16**: 1133–1136

50. Gerschlager W, Munchau A, Katzenschlager R, *et al.* (2004). Natural history and syndromic associations of orthostatic tremor: a review of 41 patients. *Mov Disord* **19**: 788–795.

51. Trocello JM, Zanotti-Fregonara P, Roze E, *et al.* (2008). Dopaminergic deficit is not the rule in orthostatic tremor. *Mov Disord* **23**: 1733–1738.

52. Katzenschlager R, Costa D, Gerschlager W, *et al.* (2003). [^{123}I]-FP-CIT-SPECT demonstrates dopaminergic deficit in orthostatic tremor. *Ann Neurol* **53**: 489–496.

53. Adams JS, Adams PE, Nguyen D, *et al.* (2007). Volumetric brain changes in females with fragile X-associated tremor/ataxia syndrome (FXTAS). *Neurology* **69**: 851–859.

54. Ceravolo R, Antonini A, Volterrani D, *et al.* (2005). Dopamine transporter imaging study in parkinsonism occurring in fragile X premutation carriers. *Neurology* **65**: 1971–3.

55. Scaglione C, Ginestroni A, Vella A, *et al.* (2008). MRI and SPECT of midbrain and striatal degeneration in fragile X-associated tremor/ataxia syndrome. *J Neurol* **255**: 144–146.

56. Mascalchi M, Vella A, Ceravolo R (2012). Movement disorders: role of imaging in diagnosis. *J Magn Reson Imaging* **35**: 239–256

57. Sinha S, Taly AB, Ravishankar S, *et al.* (2006). Wilson's disease: cranial MRI observations and clinical correlation. *Neuroradiology* **48**: 613–621.

58. Kishibayashi J, Segawa F, Kamada K, *et al.* (1993). Study of diffusion weighted magnetic resonance imaging in Wilson's disease [in Japanese]. *Rinsho Shinkeigaku* **33**: 1086–1089.

59. Algin O, Taskapilioglu O, Hakyemez B, *et al.* (2010). Structural and neurochemical evaluation of the brain and pons in patients with Wilson's disease. *Jpn J Radiol* **28**: 663–671.

60. Tarnacka B, Szeszkowski W, Golebiowski M, *et al.* (2008). MR spectroscopy in monitoring the treatment of Wilson's disease patients. *Mov Disord* **23**: 1560–1566.

61. Barthel H, Hermann W, Kluge R, *et al.* (2003). Concordant pre- and postsynaptic deficits of dopaminergic neurotransmission in neurologic Wilson disease. *AJNR* **24**: 234–238.

62. Jeon B, Kim J, Jeong JM, *et al.* (1998). Dopamine transporter imaging with [^{123}I]-CIT demonstrates presynaptic nigrostriatal dopaminergic damage in Wilson's disease. *J Neurol Neurosurg Psych* **65**: 60–64.

63. Hinson VK, Cubo E, Comella C, *et al.* (2005). Rating scale for psychogenic movement disorders: scale development and clinimetric testing. *Mov Disord* **20**: 1592–1597.

64. Lang AE, Koller WC, Fahn S (1995). Psychogenic Parkinsonism. *Arch Neurol* **52**: 802–810.

65. Gaig C, Marti MJ, Tolosa E, *et al.* (2006). ^{123}I-Ioflupane SPECT in the diagnosis of suspected psychogenic Parkinsonism. *Mov Disord* **21**: 1994–1998.

66. Hassin-Baer S, Sirota P, Korczyn AD, *et al.* (2001). Clinical characteristics of neuroleptic-induced parkinsonism. *J Neural Transm* **108**: 1299–1308.

67. Tinazzi M, Ottaviani S, Isaias IU, *et al.* (2008). [^{123}I] FP-CIT SPET imaging in drug induced parkinsonism. *Mov Disord* **23**: 1825–1829.

68. Tinazzi M, Antonini A, Bovi TT, *et al.* (2009). Clinical and [^{123}I]FP-CIT SPET imaging follow-up in patients with drug-induced parkinsonism. *J Neurol* **256**: 910–915.

69. Burn DJ, Brooks DJ (1993). Nigral dysfunction in drug-induced parkinsonism: an ^{18}F-dopa PET study. *Neurology* **43**: 552–556.

70. Tinazzi M, Cipriani A, Matinella A, *et al.* (2012). [^{123}I] FP-CIT single photon emission computed tomography findings in drug-induced Parkinsonism. *Schizophr Res* **139**: 40–45.

71. Robottom BJ, Weiner WJ, Factor SA (2011). Movement disorders emergencies. Part 1: hypokinetic disorders. *Arch Neurol* **68**: 567–572.

Chapter

20

Neuromuscular weakness

Angelo Quattrini, Nilo Riva, Federica Agosta,
Massimo Filippi, and Marianne de Visser

Introduction

Weakness is defined as a reduced strength in skeletal muscles and it is the most common complaint in patients with neuromuscular disorders, often resulting in disability. Neuromuscular disease is a very broad term that encompasses many different conditions that either directly, via intrinsic muscle pathology, or indirectly, via motor neuron cells, motor nerve, or neuromuscular junction pathology, impair the function of the skeletal muscles. Muscular weakness is therefore the denominator of all neuromuscular diseases in which the motor system is involved. Patients may use the word "weakness" with different meanings. Therefore, such a complaint should be probed unless there is clinical evidence of loss of muscle strength. The terms **paralysis** or **plegia** indicate total loss of muscle contractility, whereas **paresis** refers to mild or moderate weakness. Patients usually do not complain about muscle weakness, but experience diminished function, e.g. difficulty in getting up from a chair, inability to walk on tiptoes, difficulty with washing one's hair, impaired swallowing, or respiratory insufficiency. Weakness should be distinguished from **fatigue**. Fatigue, defined as a subjective feeling of excess tiredness or lack of energy, is a common initial complaint in patients with amyotrophic lateral sclerosis (ALS), Pompe disease, and myotonic dystrophy (DM). Fatigue may be a late or residual symptom in patients with postpoliomyelitis syndrome, Guillain–Barré syndrome (GBS), and myositis. If fatigue is the predominant feature, without weakness or elevated serum creatine kinase (CK) activity, a neuromuscular disease is very unlikely. Chronic fatigue syndrome is not a neuromuscular disease.

In neuromuscular junction disorders the hallmark of the disease is the fluctuating character of the muscle weakness. If weakness is associated with sensory abnormalities there is likely to be a (poly)neuropathy.

However, there exists also a pure motor type of neuropathy, i.e. multifocal motor neuropathy (MMN) which is a treatable condition.

Clinical approach to the weak patient

There are many other potential causes of weakness than neuromuscular, including metabolic (may result from a variety of conditions, including Addison's disease, low sodium or potassium serum levels, hyperparathyroidism, thyrotoxicosis, or hypothyroidism), as well as more general neurologic and toxic disorders (e.g. botulism and organophosphate poisoning). However, in this chapter, we confine ourselves to weakness associated with neuromuscular disorders, caused by involvement of the upper motor neurons, lower motor neurons, or both, neuromuscular junction, and the muscle. Diagnosis of neuromuscular diseases has often been considered difficult, but the clinical semiology, i.e. the careful gathering and interpretation of data from taking a (family) history and examining patients, is the cornerstone of the diagnosis. The first step for the differential diagnosis of a weak patient is to determine the distribution of weakness (Table 20.1), in order to define the localization of the underlying lesion. The most common convention for grading muscle strength is the Medical Research Council (MRC) scale (0 to 5). The patient should be investigated for evidence of atrophy, hypertrophy, contractures, spasticity, and clonus. Fasciculations, myokymia, myotonia polyminimyoclonus, tremor, or rippling of muscles should also be noted.

Various laboratory tests may aid in the diagnostic work-up of patients with neuromuscular weakness. If an axonal motor-sensory polyneuropathy is considered to be present, complete blood count, glucose level, liver and kidney functions, sedimentation rate, serum protein electrophoresis in search of a monoclonal

Table 20.1 Patterns of weakness

	Distribution	Tone	Atrophy	Fasciculations	Reflexes	Extensor plantar response
Upper motor neuron	Pyramidal (also (pseudo) bulbar muscles)	Spastic	None	None	Hyperactive – clonus	Present
Lower motor neuron	Distal-segmental (also generalized, including bulbar and respiratory muscles), often asymmetric	Decreased	Severe	Common	Hypoactive–absent	Absent
Neuromuscular-junction	Proximal and extraocular (also bulbar, distal, respiratory muscles), often asymmetric	Normal-decreased	Uncommon, but tongue atrophy in anti-MuSK MG	None	Normal–hypoactive	Absent
Myopathic	Proximal (also trunk, distal, facial, bulbar muscles, diaphragm, external ophthalmoplegia), mostly symmetric	Normal-decreased	Mild	None	Normal–hypoactive	Absent

MuSK = muscle-specific kinase; MG = myasthenia gravis

gammopathy, thyroid stimulating hormone, vitamin B1 (alcohol abuse), B6 (both intoxication and deficiency), B12 level, and folic acid may be useful laboratory tests for peripheral neuropathy screening. If pain is a predominant feature, human immunodeficiency virus (HIV) status and vasculitis serology should be considered. Subacute-onset sensory neuropathy may be consistent with a paraneoplastic disorder and frequently anti-Hu antibodies can be found. Serum creatine kinase (CK) may be helpful for the diagnosis of a muscle disease, especially if it is more than 10 times the upper limit of normal. CK is usually markedly elevated in Kennedy's disease (bulbospinal muscular atrophy), and rarely in spinal muscular atrophy type III and ALS. If myasthenia gravis (MG) is in the differential diagnosis, antibodies against acetylcholine receptors or muscle-specific kinase should be performed. Antibodies against voltage-gated calcium channels are consistent with a diagnosis of Lambert–Eaton syndrome (LEMS). In the latter, weakness is also exercise-related, but not as prominent as in MG. In LEMS, muscle weakness is often associated with autonomic symptoms such as a dry mouth. In 50% of the patients LEMS is associated with small-cell lung cancer.

In all neuromuscular disorders, electromyography (EMG) and nerve conduction studies (NCS) are extremely helpful, identifying signs of damage of muscle and nerves. Needle EMG may distinguish neurogenic from myogenic lesions and in the former it is essential to be informed about acute versus chronic damage.

Other diagnostic tests that may be helpful include lumbar puncture, muscle imaging by ultrasound, magnetic resonance imaging (MRI), or computed tomography (CT) (although this is less often used because of ionizing radiation), and muscle and, less frequently, nerve biopsies. The indications for nerve biopsy have changed over the years and therefore currently a nerve biopsy is virtually only indicated in selected cases, such as when nerve vasculitis is suspected.

Motor neuron diseases

ALS is the most common and severe form of progressive motor neuron disease (MND), leading to death 3–4 years after symptom onset [1]. The pathologic hallmark of ALS is degeneration of both lower and upper motor neurons. However, other diseases may involve only a particular subtype of motor neurons and many conditions may mimic ALS. Therefore, a careful diagnostic evaluation is needed.

The first step is the clinical identification of an upper or lower motor neuron syndrome (Table 20.1). **ALS** may present with focal upper or lower motor neuron involvement, but ultimately there is progressive loss of both categories of motor neurons. Examples of diseases presenting with an **upper motor neuron syndrome** include primary lateral sclerosis (PLS), including pseudobulbar palsy, and hereditary spastic paraplegia (HSP). HSP may also in turn be distinguished into "pure" and "complicated" forms, and therefore, careful family history and sometimes examination of the relatives should be performed in order to appropriately characterize the patient [2]. The presentation with a **lower motor neuron syndrome** implies a wide spectrum of differential diagnostic considerations. It is very important to distinguish between diseases of the lower motor neuron and mimic syndromes, such as MMN with distinctive electrophysiological characteristics on NCS, namely, conduction blocks outside the typical locations of compression neuropathies [3]. In contrast with ALS and other MNDs, this neuropathy may respond dramatically to intravenous immunoglobulin therapy. Other forms of lower MND should be appropriately identified. These include X-linked spinobulbar muscular atrophy (Kennedy's disease), spinal muscular atrophy (SMA), Fazio–Londe syndrome, and Brown–Vialetto–Van Laere disease. In a proportion of the latter two diseases, mutations in the SLC52A3 gene, which encodes the intestinal (hRFT2) riboflavin transporter, are found [4]. In these patients riboflavin deficiency is the cause and supplementation with riboflavin is a life-saving treatment. Kennedy's disease, caused by mutation in the androgen receptor gene is a late-onset disease [5]. The SMA family follows an autosomal recessive trait and includes four subtypes. Infantile SMA (SMA I, Werdnig–Hoffmann disease), with onset in the first 3 months of life, is a lethal disease with a life expectancy of about 7 months. Childhood SMA (SMA II) begins later in childhood and the children will never be able to walk. Juvenile SMA (SMA III, Kugelberg–Welander disease) manifests during late childhood and runs a slow, indolent course [6]. These three types are invariably caused by mutations in the survival motor neuron (SMN1) gene. There is also a very rare adult-onset SMA type IV, sometimes caused by SMN1 mutation.

The diagnosis of MND remains clinical, and implies the exclusion of other diseases that may mimic disorders of the motor unit. Therefore, extensive laboratory, neurophysiological, and MRI studies should be performed (see below). In selected cases, a motor nerve biopsy could be considered in order to reach a final diagnosis [7]. ALS has been categorized into various levels of certainty for research purposes depending on the presence and on the progressive spread of upper and lower motor neuron signs (El Escorial criteria [2]). Establishing a diagnosis of ALS is generally considered fairly simple, but may be less certain in patients presenting with sporadic progressive disease of lower motor neurons. Notably, the reported percentage of misdiagnosis is 19% for progressive muscular atrophy [8], and up to 10% for ALS (1% rediagnosed as neuropathy) [9, 10]. Electrodiagnostic testing provides a recognized support in the diagnosis of MND. In ALS, the current criteria require contemporary signs of both spontaneous muscle fiber activity, such as fibrillation potentials, positive sharp waves or fasciculations, and chronic collateral partial reinnervation, as defined by enlarged, frequently unstable motor units of increased duration in more than one region (cervical, thoracic, or lumbosacral). Once all mimic syndromes are excluded, the clinician should determine the specific diagnosis within the spectrum of MND. Familial ALS, commonly with an autosomal-dominant inheritance, is rare (5–10% of the cases), but hexanucleotide repeat expansions in the C9ORF72 gene are found in up to 60% of the familial cases, with a marked regional variation, and are found in less than 10% of sporadic ALS patients [11]. Currently, much attention is being given to the associated cognitive and behavioral disturbances in familial ALS leading to frank frontotemporal dementia in 5% of the cases [12].

Peripheral neuropathies

The clinician approaching a patient suspected of a peripheral neuropathy is faced with two problems. First, establishing the existence of a disease of the peripheral nerve and, subsequently, ascertaining its nature and the possibility of treatment. The first step is generally obtained through a history, neurologic examination, and electrophysiological assessment. Peripheral nerves are composed of sensory, motor, and autonomic fibers. Nerve fibers can be anatomically distinguished into unmyelinated and myelinated fibers; motor axons are usually large myelinated fibers that conduct rapidly. The clinical manifestations of neuropathies depend on the subtype as well as the severity and distribution of fibers affected. Once identified as a disease of the peripheral nerve, a stepwise, systematic approach will help identify the correct diagnosis, although it is important to consider that up to 30% of peripheral neuropathies may remain categorized as idiopathic [13, 14]. The following characteristics of presentation should be determined:

- **Distribution and patterns of involvement**. The term **mononeuropathy** indicates a focal lesion of a single peripheral nerve. Common causes are entrapment (e.g. median nerve in the carpal tunnel or ulnar nerve at the elbow), focal compression, and trauma [15]. Mononeuropathia multiplex (multiple mononeuropathy) is defined by the involvement of multiple separate non-contiguous nerves either serially or simultaneously. This pattern of presentation is important to recognize, as the differential diagnosis includes treatable forms of neuropathy (such as vasculitis, leprosy, lymphoma, sarcoidosis, amyloidosis, Lyme disease, HIV, cryoglobulinemia, asymmetric variants of chronic inflammatory polyradiculoneuropathy (CIDP) and MMN). Moreover, hereditary neuropathy with liability to pressure palsies (HNNP, associated with a PMP22 gene deletion) has to be considered. In more than 50% of the HNPP cases a pes cavus is present. The most common variety of polyneuropathy is **distal symmetrical polyneuropathy**, in which distal limb segments are affected first (stocking/glove distribution). After diabetes mellitus, idiopathic polyneuropathy, hereditary polyneuropathy (Charcot–Marie–Tooth disease (CMT)), inflammatory polyneuropathy, and polyneuropathy due to alcohol abuse or medication are the most frequent causes of polyneuropathy [16].
- **Nerve-fiber-type involvement**. Signs and symptoms are determined by which fiber types are affected (motor, sensory, autonomic). In most cases there is an overlap; however, the identification of a preferential fiber-type involvement can narrow the differential diagnosis (Table 20.2) [17].
- **Time course/temporal profile**. Determining the temporal evolution of the neuropathy is helpful for the diagnosis and directs the acuity of investigations

and treatment. The time from onset to nadir has to be defined as being acute (days to 4 weeks in GBS), subacute (4 weeks to 6 months in CIDP), or chronic (6 months to years in MMN) [18]. The course should be determined as being monophasic, progressive (uniform or stepwise), or relapsing remitting. Acute sensory-motor neuropathies include acute inflammatory demyelinating neuropathy (AIDP), the classical presentation of GBS, acute sensory motor axonal neuropathy (AMSAN), vasculitis, and arsenic toxicity. Common etiologies of acute motor neuropathies include acute motor axonal neuropathy (AMAN), porphyria, dapsone and vincristine toxicity, and critical illness neuropathy (CRIME), while examples of acute sensory neuropathy are paraneoplastic and inflammatory sensory ganglionopathy, acute pyridoxine and cisplatin toxicity, and Miller–Fisher syndrome [19].

- **Hereditary/acquired**. The unique clinical circumstance of the patient should be determined, considering family and past medical history, current and past medications, and social history (including vocational and recreational history and risk factor for exposure to toxic agents). Inherited neuropathies characteristically present with deformities of the foot (pes cavus) and have little or no positive symptoms, such as pain or paresthesia. Medical history should further include inquiries about diabetes mellitus, connective tissue disease, malignancies, hematologic disorders, infection, malnutrition, vitamin deficiencies/toxicity, and exposure to drugs, alcohol, or toxins. Laboratory tests should be performed accordingly in order to rule out that the neuropathy might be the presenting symptom of a yet unknown systemic disorder. Genetic tests can be done in hereditary neuropathies (e.g. CMT) [20].
- **Determination of the primary pathology**. The neuropathy should be characterized as being primarily axonal or demyelinating. In most cases, electrodiagnostic (EDX) studies clarify the underlying pathophysiology. Primarily axonal neuropathies usually detected by NCS are characterized by a reduction of the motor action potentials amplitude with relatively preserved (up to 30% reduction) conduction velocities, distal latencies, and late potentials; on needle examination, signs of active denervation can be observed. Primary demyelinating neuropathy

Table 20.2 Differential diagnosis of peripheral neuropathy based on clinical presentation

Motor (-sensory)	Small-fiber (painful neuropathies and dissociated sensory loss)	Large-fiber (ataxic neuropathies)	Autonomic
Symptoms			
Cramps Weakness Twitching (sensory and autonomic symptoms may be associated)	Pain: burning, shock-like, stabbing, prickling, shooting, lancinating Allodynia	Numbness Tingling Ataxia	Decreased or increased sweating Dry eyes, mouth Erectile dysfunction Gastroparesis/diarrhea Faintness, light-headedness
Signs			
Reduced – strength – reflexes – muscle size Fasciculations (sensory features)	Decreased – pin prick – temperature sensation	Decreased – vibration sense – joint-position sense – reflexes	Orthostasis Unequal pupil size
Common etiology			
Inflammatory demyelinating neuropathies (AMAN, GBS, CIDP, MMN) Hereditary motor-sensory neuropathies (usually predominantly motor symptoms) Brachial neuritis (mostly motor) Diabetic lumbosacral plexus neuropathy (diabetic amyotrophy) (mostly motor) Dapsone, vincristine toxicity Critical illness polyneuropathy Acute intermittent porphyria Diphtheritic neuropathy Lead neuropathy	Lepromatous leprosy Diabetic (includes glucose intolerance) small-fiber neuropathy Hereditary sensory neuropathies Amyloidosis Tangier disease Fabry's disease (pain predominates) Alcohol Dysautonomia (Riley–Day syndrome) HIV and antiretroviral therapy neuropathy	Paraneuroplastic sensory neuropathy Sjögren's syndrome – Miller–Fisher syndrome Vitamin B12 neuropathy (from dorsal column involvement) Cisplatin neuropathy Pyridoxine toxicity Friedreich's ataxia Hereditary sensory neuropathies (recessive and dominant)	Acute: Acute pandysautonomic neuropathy, botulism, porphyria, GBS, amiodarone, vincristine Chronic: Amyloid, diabetes, Sjögren's syndrome, HSAN I and III (Riley–Day), Chagas, paraneoplastic

shows relatively preserved sensory action amplitudes, slow conduction velocities, prolonged distal latencies and late potentials, and no active denervation on needle examination. Non-uniform slowing of conduction velocity, conduction block, or temporal dispersion further suggest an acquired demyelinating neuropathy (e.g. GBS or CIDP) as opposed to a hereditary demyelinating neuropathy (e.g. CMT type 1). EDX studies further complement the neurologic examination providing information regarding distribution, fiber selectivity, and temporal profile of the neuropathy [21].

At this point, the clinician should have made an adequate characterization of the neuropathy. Guided by the clinical hypothesis, further investigations can be performed in order to reach a final causative diagnosis, including MRI studies (e.g. in CIDP or MMN) and lumbar puncture. In selected cases, a **nerve biopsy** can be considered, particularly when amyloid neuropathy or vasculitis is suspected [22]. The most common site of biopsy is the sural (sensory) nerve; however, motor (obturator or peroneal) nerve biopsy may also be performed, particularly when a differential diagnosis between MND and motor neuropathy is needed [7].

Neuromuscular junction and muscle disease

The prototypical clinical presentation of most myopathies includes symmetric proximal limb weakness (limb girdle syndrome) with preserved sensation and reflexes. There are two other common phenotypes, i.e. distal myopathy and floppy infant syndrome. The clinician should systematically define the following characteristics [23]:

(1) **The age at onset and rate of progression** are important clues for the diagnosis. Onset can be at birth, in (early) childhood, adolescence, or (early) adulthood, or there can be a late onset. The floppy-infant syndrome only occurs in neonates [24]. Typical childhood-onset diseases are the muscular dystrophies. Examples of late-onset diseases are oculopharyngeal muscular dystrophy, myofibrillar myopathy, and sporadic inclusion body myositis [25]. Several disorders can occur at any age, such as acid maltase deficiency or Pompe disease, DM type 1, and mitochondrial myopathy. Acute onset suggests a toxic or metabolic disturbance. Rhabdomyolysis, which occurs acutely, is a serious and potentially life-threatening condition. It is defined by an elevation of serum CK activity of at least 10 times the upper limit of normal followed by a fast decrease of the serum CK to (near) normal values. The clinical presentation can vary widely. Classical features are myalgia, weakness, and myoglobinuria. However, this classic triad is seen in less than 10% of patients. A subacute onset is often found in inflammatory myopathies, whereas hereditary myopathies and disorders with an endocrinologic or degenerative cause, such as inclusion body myositis, have a chronic course [26]. It is important to inquire about associated symptoms that may suggest cardiac involvement or imminent respiratory insufficiency. One should also ask for exercise-related weakness of muscles, impaired relaxation, as in myotonia, rippling of muscles, and the use of medication. In infants and children, prenatal and perinatal events and rate of acquisition of motor milestones should be determined. Since many myopathies have a hereditary basis, family history is extremely important; the clinical examination of the proband's parents and relatives can be helpful.

(2) **Evaluation of muscle weakness**. The first step is to distinguish between persistent and intermittent muscle weakness. Disorders causing intermittent weakness include neuromuscular junction disorders (characterized by muscle fatigability), electrolyte disturbances (periodic paralyses), and myotonic disorders caused by mutation in

ion-channel genes, such as congenital myotonia or paramyotonia congenita [27]. Rhabdomyolysis, which causes transient muscle weakness, can be caused by hereditary disease including deficiencies of fatty-acid utilization (carnitine palmitoyltransferase 2 deficiency) or distal glycolysis disorders (myophosphorylase deficiency is the most frequent hereditary cause), and by some mitochondrial myopathies [28]. In 75% of patients a first episode of rhabdomyolysis is provoked by an acquired cause. The most common acquired causes are: substance abuse (34%), medication (11%), trauma (9%), and epileptic seizures (7%) [29].

Reduction of weakness with a series of voluntary contractions – without myotonia – is characteristic of the inverse myasthenic (Lambert–Eaton) syndrome, and is also observed in botulism [30]. Most muscle disorders, however, cause persistent weakness. In all these cases, the patterns of muscle involvement and distribution of weakness should be determined through systematic examination of the main groups of muscles from forehead to toe. While in most myopathies, including most types of muscular dystrophy and inflammatory myopathies, proximal muscles are preferentially involved (**limb-girdle distribution**); other patterns of weakness may suggest alternative diagnoses (Table 20.3) [25]. Moreover, muscle weakness may result in abnormalities of posture, alteration of functional tests and gait dynamics, and secondary joint and spine changes (scoliosis, rigid spine, contractures). Neurological examination should also include inspection for atrophy or muscle hypertrophy, and muscle hyperactivity such as myotonia and rippling of muscles.

(3) **Associated symptoms and signs:**

(a) **Myotonia** is a painless, prolonged failure of relaxation associated with abnormal repetitive depolarization of muscle fibers. Myotonia may follow voluntary muscle activation (action myotonia), or be elicited by mechanical stimulation (percussion myotonia) of the muscle. The myotonic phenomenon is typical of myotonia congenita (a chloride channel disorder) and of DM type 1 (DM1), and type 2 (DM2), associated with distal- and proximal-limb muscle weakness, respectively [31]. In **paradoxical myotonia** (paramyotonia), the

Table 20.3 Patterns of muscle weakness and differential diagnosis in disorders of the skeletal muscle and the neuromuscular junction

Distribution of muscle weakness	Symptoms/signs	Most common muscular causes
Extraocular muscles and m. levator palpebrae	Diplopia Ptosis Strabismus	Myasthenia gravis Chronic progressive external ophthalmoplegia Oculopharyngeal muscular dystrophy Exophthalmic (hyperthyroid) ophthalmopathy Kearns–Sayre syndrome and other mitochondrial myopathies Congenital myotubular/centronuclear myopathy and Möbius syndrome Myotonic dystrophy type 1 (mainly ptosis)
Facial muscles	Inability to smile, expose the teeth, close the eyes, whistle, inflate a balloon	Myasthenia gravis Myotonic dystrophy Facioscapulohumeral dystrophy (sometimes asymmetric) Congenital facies myopathica (centronuclear, nemaline, RYR1-related myopathies) Möbius syndrome Sporadic inclusion body myositis (advanced stage)
Bulbar muscles	Dysarthria Dysphagia Dysphonia	Myasthenia gravis/anti-MuSK MG Mitochondrial myopathies, Inflammatory myopathies (polymyositis, dermatomyositis inclusion body myositis) Myotonic dystrophy Botulism Oculopharyngeal muscular dystrophy, Pompe disease
Cervical and thoracic muscles	Dropped head Camptocormia (bent spine)	Myasthenia gravis/anti-MuSK MG Polymyositis and inclusion body myositis Nemaline myopathy (late-onset) Hyperparathyroidism Focal myositis Acid maltase deficiency/Pompe disease Idiopathic axial myopathy
Respiratory and trunk muscles	Dyspnea Orthopnea Nocturnal dyspnea Sleep apnea Respiratory arrest	Myasthenia gravis Congenital myasthenic syndrome Glycogen storage disease Subacute inflammatory myopathies Hereditary myopathy with early respiratory involvement Congenital myotonic dystrophy Congenital myopathies: nemaline myopathy, myotubular myopathy, Bethlem myopathy Juvenile or adult-onset acid maltase deficiency/Pompe disease
Limb-girdle muscles	Inability to raise the arms Inability to arise from a squatting, kneeling, or sitting position Lumbar lordosis and protuberant abdomen Waddling gait Gowers' sign Winging of the scapulae	Inflammatory myopathies (polymyositis, dermatomyositis, inclusion body myositis) Duchenne and Becker muscular dystrophies LGMDs Facioscapulohumeral dystrophy Metabolic myopathies Congenital myopathies (central core, nemaline, myotubular, etc.) Myotonic dystrophy type II (DM2) Acid maltase deficiency/Pompe disease Myofibrillar myopathies Hypothyroidism Steroid myopathy
Distal limb muscles	Inability to walk on heels and tiptoes Difficulties in manipulating objects	Distal forms of muscular dystrophies (e.g. Miyoshi(-like) myopathy caused by mutations in the dysferlin or actonamine-5 gene) Myotonic dystrophy type Inclusion body myositis (forearm flexors and lower leg muscles) Hereditary inclusion body myopathy (caused by GNE mutations) Myofibrillar myopathies

myotonia worsens with repetitive activity, in contrast to myotonia in which the myotonic phenomenon is eased by repetitive activity [27].

(b) **Muscle contracture**. True muscular contracture is due to failure of the metabolic mechanisms necessary for relaxation; EMG remains relatively silent, in contrast to the high-voltage, rapid discharges observed with cramp, tetanus, and tetany [31]. Contractures occur in metabolic myopathies associated with defects of glycolysis or glycogen metabolism such as McArdle disease (phosphorylase deficiency). **Pseudocontracture** (or fibrous contracture) refers to muscle and tendon shortening (fixed contracture) because of fibrosis. This may result from immobility and is seen in well-advanced cases of muscular dystrophy, but it is also typically found in early stage Emery–Dreifuss muscular dystrophy and Bethlem myopathy.

(c) **Muscle stiffness**: there is no precise and generally accepted definition of muscle stiffness; therefore, this term can refer to different conditions. The term is often used to describe spontaneously occurring muscle contractions that may be accompanied by muscle cramps. Stiffness can occur in disorders associated with continuous muscle fiber activity, such as **stiff-person syndrome, neuromyotonia** (Isaac's syndrome), and tetanus [32, 33].

(d) **Cramps** are involuntary movements characterized by painful shortening of muscle, and high-amplitude, high-frequency motor unit discharges at EMG [34]. Few diseases manifest with cramps without muscular weakness. Some patients with Becker muscular dystrophy may complain in early childhood about exercise-related muscle cramps.

(e) **Myalgia** is seldom due to primary muscle disease, while hypothyroidism and drug use are frequent causes. Primary myopathies that may present with exertion myalgia include DM2, inflammatory myopathies, carnitine palmitoyl transferase 2 deficiency (CPT2), very long-chain acylcoenzyme A dehydrogenase deficiency (VLCAD), limb-girdle muscular dystrophy (LGMD) 2B and 2I, ryanodine receptor 1 (RYR1) core myopathy, and McArdle disease [25, 26, 34, 35].

(f) **Rippling** of muscles is a sign of spontaneous and continuous muscle hyperactivity. Differentiation from generalized peripheral nerve hyperexcitability can be achieved with EDX studies. Patients with rippling muscle disease have percussion-induced rapid muscle contractions that are extremely slow (0.6 m/s; i.e., 10 times slower than normal muscle contraction). These contractions are associated with electrical silence on needle EMG [36, 37].

(g) **Non-muscular involvement**. Heart involvement is very frequent in myopathies, including Duchenne and Becker muscular dystrophy (cardiomyopathy), DM (conduction disturbances and arrhythmia), sarcoglycanopathies, LGMD 2I (cardiomyopathy), LGMD 1B and autosomal and X-linked recessive Emery–Dreifuss muscular dystrophies (both cardiomyopathy and conduction disturbances). In mitochondrial myopathies cardiac involvement (dilated or hypertrophic cardiomyopathy, conduction disease, or left ventricular non compaction) is common and may occur as the principal clinical manifestation or part of multisystem disease [38]. In many muscular dystrophies (e.g. Duchenne and Becker muscular dystrophy, merosin (laminin α2-chain) muscular dystrophy, Fukuyama muscular dystrophy, and myotonic dystrophies), the central nervous system (CNS) may be impaired, and mental retardation may be present [39]. Mitochondrial myopathies often present with a simultaneous involvement of the retina, cerebellum, and other parts of the CNS [40]. Dysmorphic features (such as arched palate, long face, protruding jaw, and dental malocclusion) may suggest specific conditions (e.g. nemaline myopathy, congenital DM, and myotubular myopathy). Characteristic skin abnormalities are the hallmark of dermatomyositis [26].

After careful characterization of the patient, including history and neurological examination, further investigations should be performed to reach a final causative diagnosis. Blood tests should at least include serum CK activity. If McArdle disease is in the differential diagnosis an exercise forearm test can be helpful to detect the absence of an increase of the serum lactate. In Pompe disease, acid maltase is usually dramatically low in leukocytes or fibroblasts. In patients suspected of mitochondrial (encephalo)myopathy, lactate in serum and cerebrospinal fluid (CSF) may be elevated.

EDX studies should include NCS, needle examination, and repetitive nerve stimulation. NCS are often normal, but in some cases a reduction of compound muscle action potential (cMAP) amplitudes may be seen. At needle EMG the typical feature is the presence of short-duration, small-amplitude, polyphasic motor-unit action potentials (MUAPs), with early recruitment of motor units. Associated signs of spontaneous muscle fiber activity suggest a necrotizing myopathy (inflammatory or toxic), but can also be found in Becker muscular dystrophy and Pompe disease. The finding of myotonic discharges narrows the differential diagnosis [31, 41].

In many cases, **DNA analysis** can be performed without muscle biopsy, e.g. childhood-onset SMA, facioscapulohumeral dystrophy, Bethlem myopathy, oculopharyngeal muscular dystrophy, etc. However, there are a number of limitations in currently available molecular diagnostics and **muscle biopsy** remains an important tool for the diagnosis of a suspected myopathy [42].

Role of neuroimaging in neuromuscular diseases

Motor neuron diseases

Although a detailed clinical assessment remains the basis of the evaluation of patients suspected of having MND, current international diagnostic criteria [43] and European guidelines [44] recommend that "all patients suspected of having a MND, where a plausible alternative unifying neuroanatomical explanation exists, should undergo an MRI of either or both the brain and spinal cord depending on the clinical presentation". The greatest contribution of neuroimaging is the exclusion of several MND mimic syndromes, including cerebral lesions (e.g. MS and cerebrovascular disease), skull base lesions, cervical spondylotic myelopathy, other myelopathy (e.g. foramen magnum lesions, intrinsic and extrinsic tumors, and syringomyelia), conus lesions, and brachial or thoraco-lumbar-sacral radiculopathy [45].

In ALS patients, a low signal intensity (hypointense rim) can be found in the precentral cortex on T2-weighted images [46]. This so called "ribbon-like"

hypointensity is sharply contrasted by the hyperintense signal of CSF in the adjacent sulci.

Corticospinal tract (CST) hyperintensities on T2-weighted, proton-density-weighted, and fluid-attenuated inversion recovery (FLAIR) images are frequently found in ALS patients (Figure 20.1) [46]. CST hyperintensities, which are best followed on coronal scans, have been reported mostly bilaterally and are most frequently seen in the caudal portion of the posterior limb of the internal capsule. They typically extend downward to the ventral portion of the brainstem, and less consistently upward through the corona radiata. Such lesions may occur more often in younger patients with greater disability. Nevertheless, there is a wide range in reported frequency of conventional MRI abnormalities in ALS, from 15% to 76%. More importantly, increased CST signal intensity has also been described in healthy individuals and, strikingly, in patients with other conditions, such as Krabbe disease, X-linked CMT, adrenomyeloneuropathy, and after hepatic transplantation. Therefore, a primary search for these abnormalities for the purpose of making a diagnosis of ALS is not usually recommended [44].

Conventional brain MRI is usually normal in patients with pure HSP and with PLS, which may mimic HSP. Exceptions include variable degrees of cerebellar atrophy in patients with SPG7 mutations, thin corpus callosum, and mental impairment in HSP caused by SPG11 and SPG15 mutations (Figure 20.2).

Over the past 10 years, there has been significant progress in the identification of the advanced neuroimaging patterns in MND. As in other neurodegenerative conditions (e.g. Alzheimer's disease), future criteria should acknowledge the value of these (supportive) features in the clinical diagnosis of MND. Significant cortical thinning of the precentral gyrus, damage to the CST and corpus callosum assessed using diffusion tensor (DT) MRI, and altered N-acetylaspartate levels in the primary motor cortex and CST hold particular promise as markers for grading upper motor neuron injury [47]. In particular, extra-motor damage was demonstrated in all MND phenotypes (ALS, PLS, and PMA) in several MRI studies [48, 49]. Importantly, DT MRI measures of the CST are likely to have a prognostic value in ALS patients [50]. Furthermore, patterns of brain damage are emerging to identify patients prone to develop dementia (Figure 20.1) or rapid progression. Functional neuroimaging techniques, such as positron

325

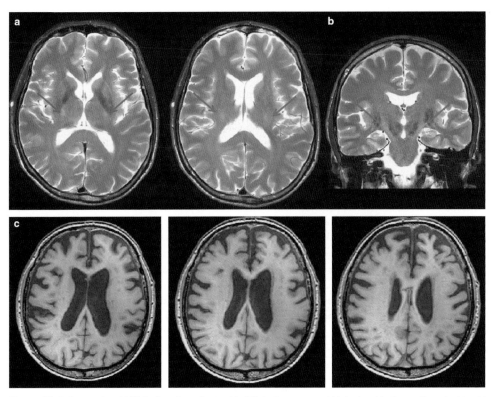

Figure 20.1 Conventional MRI findings in patients with ALS. In the top panel high signal in the corticospinal tract is seen on axial (a) and coronal (b) T2-weighted fast spin-echo images. The bottom panel (c) shows moderate frontotemporal atrophy in an ALS patient with cognitive impairment on a series of axial T1-weighted images.

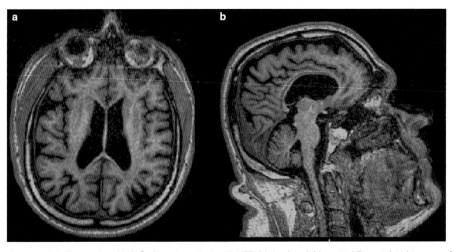

Figure 20.2 Conventional MRI findings in patient with HSP. (a) Axial and (b) sagittal T1-weighted images of an SPG11 patient show the thin corpus callosum and global cortical atrophy.

emission tomography and functional MRI provide a more complete picture of extra-motor involvement, and can disclose how functional changes interact with structural damage to determine the clinical outcome [51].

Peripheral neuropathies

Imaging is increasingly utilized for evaluation of peripheral nerves, as described elsewhere in this book (Chapter 21). It is noteworthy to mention here the role

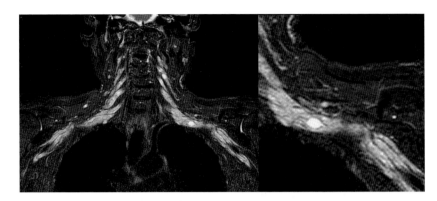

Figure 20.3 Coronal 3-mm-thick short tau inversion recovery (STIR) images at the level of emergency roots and brachial plexus: bilateral hypertrophy of brachial plexuses in CIDP. All nervous structures in CIDP are highly hyperintense on the STIR images, characterized by notable hypertrophy and conspicuity of the internal fascicular structure (note the enlarged image). Courtesy of Dr. S. Gerevini, Head and Neck Department, Neuroradiology Department, Ospedale San Raffaele.

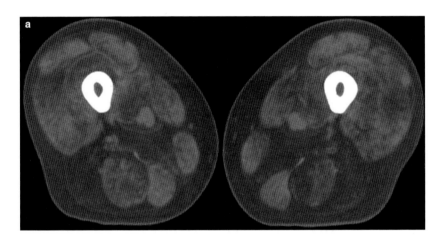

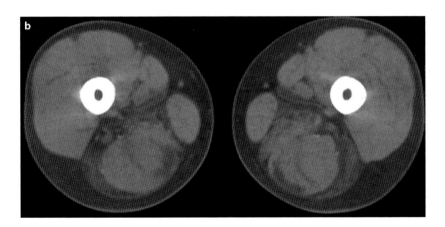

Figure 20.4 (a) CT scan shows areas of lower attenuation in all upper leg muscles, indicating fatty replacement of muscle tissue, despite the absence of weakness on clinical examination in a patient with LGMD type 2I (caused by mutations in the fukutin-related protein). At the thigh level the adductor magnus, semitendinosus, and biceps femoris muscles show areas of lower attenuation. (b) Areas of lower attenuation in the biceps femoris muscles and the adductor longus muscles with compensatory hypertrophy of the gracilis muscles in this patient with Becker muscular dystrophy.

of MRI studies for the diagnosis of CIDP (Figure 20.3) or MMN, both treatable disorders. In most cases, clinical, EDX and, in CIDP, CSF examination findings allow for the diagnosis [3, 18]. However, in order to improve the accuracy of diagnostic criteria, MRI findings, together with sural nerve biopsy and treatment response are included as supportive criteria for diagnosis [52]. In CIDP and GBS, MRI studies can show hyperintensity, gadolinium enhancement, and/ or hypertrophy of the cauda equina, lumbosacral or cervical nerve roots, or the brachial or lumbosacral plexuses (Figure 20.3) [53, 54].

Myopathies

Muscle imaging (MRI, CT, or ultrasound) can be helpful in myopathies [55]; first, as a guide in muscle biopsy as it clearly distinguishes muscle tissue from adipose tissue; second, to show which muscles are affected or preserved and which show compensatory hypertrophy. Frequently, muscle imaging reveals that many more muscles are involved than can be determined by the clinical examination (Figure 20.4). MRI

or CT are usually not helpful in differentiating the LGMDs from each other [56]. In a few disorders there is a characteristic pattern, such as in Bethlem mypathy [57, 58], Becker muscular dystrophy (Figure 20.4) [59], and ryonadine receptor-1 related congenital myopathies [60].

In inflammatory myopathies (Table 20.4) hyperintensity is observed in affected muscles [61]. Muscle MRI, used as a triage test or in conjunction with muscle biopsy, can decrease the false negative diagnostic rate of 10–20% that is known to occur in myositis [62].

Table 20.4 Clinical features of inflammatory myopathies

	Age of onset	Time course of onset	Distribution of muscle weakness	Rash	Muscle biopsy	Response to immunosuppressive treatment and prognosis	Other organ involvement and associated conditions
Polymyositis	> 18 years	Weeks to months	Proximal > distal, neck flexors, dysphagia	No	Inflammation: endomysial (CD8+ T cells, macrophages) or perimysial and perivascular inflammation	A monocyclic disease course was seen in 15–48% of patients	Connective tissue disease, interstitial lung disease
Necrotising myopathy	> 18 years	Weeks to months	Proximal > distal, neck flexors, dysphagia	No	Necrotic myopathy, sparse inflammation	High dosages of steroids required, usually also second-line treatment	Connective tissue disorders, malignancy, statin use
Dermatomyositis	Childhood and adult	Weeks to months (in children sometimes days)	Proximal > distal, neck flexors, dysphagia	Yes	Inflammation: perymysial and perivascular (CD4+ T cells, B cells) perifascicular atrophy (mostly in the childhood form and usually in advanced disease)	A monocyclic disease course was seen in 15–48% of patients. In childhood form low mortality rate, in adults 10% mortality rate mostly due to concomitant malignancy	Malignancy, connective tissue disease, myocarditis, vasculitis, interstitial lung disease
Inclusion body myositis	> 50 years	Months to years	Proximal (quadriceps more than iliopsoas) dysphagia, finger flexors and lower leg muscles, facial muscles in 40%	No	Inflammation: endomysial (CD8+ T cells) rimmed vacuoles	None. Disabling disorder with normal or lightly reduced life expectancy	Autoimmune disorders, in particular Sjögren's disease and rheumatoid arthritis; no other organ involvement

References

1. Turner MR, Hardiman O, Benatar M, *et al.* (2013). Controversies and priorities in amyotrophic lateral sclerosis. *Lancet Neurol* **123**: 310–322.

2. Schule R, Schols L (2011). Genetics of hereditary spastic paraplegias. *Semin Neurol* **315**: 484–493.

3. Vlam L, van der Pol WL, Cats EA, *et al.* (2012). Multifocal motor neuropathy: diagnosis, pathogenesis and treatment strategies. *Nature Rev Neurol* **81**: 48–58.

4. Spagnoli C, De Sousa C (2012). Brown–Vialetto–Van Laere syndrome and Fazio–Londe disease – treatable motor neuron diseases of childhood. *Developmental Med Child Neurol* **544**: 292–293.

5. Banno H, Katsuno M, Suzuki K, Tanaka F, Sobue G (2012). Pathogenesis and molecular targeted therapy of spinal and bulbar muscular atrophy (SBMA). *Cell Tissue Res* **3491**: 313–320.

6. Mercuri E, Bertini E, Iannaccone ST (2012). Childhood spinal muscular atrophy: controversies and challenges. *Lancet Neurol* **115**: 443–452.

7. Riva N, Iannaccone S, Corbo M, *et al.* (2011). Motor nerve biopsy: clinical usefulness and histopathological criteria. *Ann Neurol* **691**: 197–201.

8. Visser J, van den Berg-Vos RM, Franssen H, *et al.* (2002). Mimic syndromes in sporadic cases of progressive spinal muscular atrophy. *Neurology* **5811**: 1593–1596.

9. Davenport RJ, Swingler RJ, Chancellor AM, Warlow CP (1996). Avoiding false positive diagnoses of motor neuron disease: lessons from the Scottish Motor Neuron Disease Register. *J Neurol Neurosurg Psychiatry* **602**: 147–151.

10. Traynor BJ, Codd MB, Corr B, *et al.* (2000.Clinical features of amyotrophic lateral sclerosis according to the El Escorial and Airlie House diagnostic criteria: a population-based study. *Arch Neurol* **578**: 1171–1176.

11. Renton AE, Majounie E, Waite A, *et al.* (2011). A hexanucleotide repeat expansion in C9ORF72 is the cause of chromosome 9p21-linked ALS-FTD. *Neuron* **722**: 257–268.

12. Dobson-Stone C, Luty AA, Thompson EM, *et al.* (2013). Frontotemporal dementia–amyotrophic lateral sclerosis syndrome locus on chromosome 16p12.1-q12.2: genetic, clinical and neuropathological analysis. *Acta Neuropathologica* **1254**: 5235–33.

13. Burns TM, Mauermann ML (2011). The evaluation of polyneuropathies. *Neurology* **767** (suppl 2): S6–13.

14. Chaundry V. Peripheral neuropathy (2008). In: Fauci AS, Braunwald E, Kasper DL, Hauser S, eds. *Harrison's Principles of Internal Medicine*, 17th edn. New York: McGraw-Hill, pp. 2651–2667.

15. England JD (1999). Entrapment neuropathies. *Current Opin Neurol* **125**: 597–602.

16. Mygland A, Monstad P (2001). Chronic polyneuropathies in Vest-Agder, Norway. *Eur J Neurology* **82**: 157–165.

17. Thompson PD, Thomas PK (2005). Clinical patterns of peripheral neuropathy. In PJ Dyck, PK Thomas, eds. *Peripheral Neuropathy*. Philadelphia, PA: Elsevier Saunders, pp. 1137–1361.

18. Yuki N, Hartung HP (2012). Guillain–Barré syndrome. *New Engl J Med* **36624**: 2294–2304.

19. Bai HX, Wang ZL, Tan LM, *et al.* (2013). The effectiveness of immunomodulating treatment on Miller–Fisher syndrome: a retrospective analysis of 65 Chinese patients. *J Peripheral Nerv System* **182**: 195–196.

20. Murphy SM, Laura M, Fawcett K, *et al.* (2012). Charcot–Marie–Tooth disease: frequency of genetic subtypes and guidelines for genetic testing. *J Neurol Neurosurg Psychiatry* **837**: 706–710.

21. England JD, Gronseth GS, Franklin G, *et al.* (2009). Practice parameter: the evaluation of distal symmetric polyneuropathy: the role of autonomic testing, nerve biopsy, and skin biopsy (an evidence-based review). Report of the American Academy of Neurology, the American Association of Neuromuscular and Electrodiagnostic Medicine, and the American Academy of Physical Medicine and Rehabilitation. *Neurology* **72**: 177–184.

22. Said G (2002). Indications and usefulness of nerve biopsy. *Arch Neurol* **5910**: 1532–1535.

23. Banwell BL, Gomez, MR (2004). The clinical examination. In Engel AG, Franzini-Armstrong C., eds. *Myology*. New York: McGraw-Hill, pp. 599–617.

24. Prasad AN, Prasad C (2003). The floppy infant: contribution of genetic and metabolic disorders. *Brain Devel* **257**: 457–476.

25. Mercuri E, Muntoni F (2013). Muscular dystrophies. *Lancet* **381**: 845–860.

26. Ernste FC, Reed AM (2013). Idiopathic inflammatory myopathies: current trends in pathogenesis, clinical features, and up-to-date treatment recommendations. *Mayo Clinic Proceed* **881**: 83–105.

27. Heatwole CR, Statland JM, Logigian EL (2013). The diagnosis and treatment of myotonic disorders. *Muscle Nerve* **475**: 632–648.

28. Landau ME, Kenney K, Deuster P, Campbell W (2012). Exertional rhabdomyolysis: a clinical review with a focus on genetic influences. *J Clin Neuromusc Dis* **133**: 122–136.

29. Melli G, Chaudhry V, Cornblath DR (2005). Rhabdomyolysis: an evaluation of 475 hospitalized patients. *Medicine* **846**: 377–385.

329

30. Titulaer MJ, Lang B, Verschuuren JJ (2011). Lambert–Eaton myasthenic syndrome: from clinical characteristics to therapeutic strategies. *Lancet Neurol* **1012**: 1098–1107.

31. Hehir MK, Logigian EL (2013). Electrodiagnosis of myotonic disorders. *Phys Med Rehabil Clinics North Am* **241**: 209–220.

32. Serratrice G, Serratrice J (2011). Continuous muscle activity, Morvan's syndrome and limbic encephalitis: ionic or non ionic disorders? *Acta Myologica: Myopath Cardiomyopath* **301**: 32–33.

33. Hadavi S, Noyce AJ, Leslie RD, Giovannoni G (2011). Stiff person syndrome. *Practical Neurol* **115**: 272–282.

34. Miller TM, Layzer RB (2005). Muscle cramps. *Muscle Nerve* **324**: 431–442.

35. Parekh R, Care DA, Tainter CR (2012). Rhabdomyolysis: advances in diagnosis and treatment. *Emerg Med Pract* **143**: 1–15.

36. Schulte-Mattler WJ, Kley RA, Rothenfusser-Korber E, *et al.* (2005). Immune-mediated rippling muscle disease. *Neurology* **642**: 364–367.

37. Gazzerro E, Sotgia F, Bruno C, Lisanti MP, Minetti C (2010). Caveolinopathies: from the biology of caveolin-3 to human diseases. *Eur J Human Genet* **182**: 137–145.

38. Hermans MC, Pinto YM, Merkies IS, *et al.* (2010). Hereditary muscular dystrophies and the heart. *Neuromusc Disord* **208**: 479–492.

39. Nardes F, Araujo AP, Ribeiro MG (2012). Mental retardation in Duchenne muscular dystrophy. *Jornal de pediatria* **881**: 6–16.

40. Pfeffer G, Chinnery PF (2013). Diagnosis and treatment of mitochondrial myopathies. *Annals Med* **451**: 4–16.

41. Lacomis D (2012). Electrodiagnostic approach to the patient with suspected myopathy. *Neurologic Clinics* **302**: 641–660.

42. Joyce NC, Oskarsson B, Jin LW (2012). Muscle biopsy evaluation in neuromuscular disorders. *Phys Med Rehabil Clinics N Am* **233**: 609–631.

43. Brooks BR, Miller RG, Swash M, Munsat TL, World Federation of Neurology Research Group on Motor Neuron D (2000). El Escorial revisited: revised criteria for the diagnosis of amyotrophic lateral sclerosis. *Amyotrophic Lat Scler Other Motor Neuron Disord* **15**: 293–299.

44. Filippi M, Agosta F, Abrahams S, *et al.* (2010). EFNS guidelines on the use of neuroimaging in the management of motor neuron diseases. *Eur J Neurol.* **174**: 526–e20.

45. Traynor BJ, Codd MB, Corr B, *et al.* (2000). Amyotrophic lateral sclerosis mimic syndromes: a population-based study. *Arch Neurol* **571**: 109–113.

46. Hecht MJ, Fellner F, Fellner C, *et al.* (2002). Hyperintense and hypointense MRI signals of the precentral gyrus and corticospinal tract in ALS: a follow-up examination including FLAIR images. *J Neurological Sci* **1991–2**: 59–65.

47. Agosta F, Valsasina P, Riva N, *et al.* (2012). The cortical signature of amyotrophic lateral sclerosis. *PLoS One* **78**: e42816.

48. van der Graaff MM, Sage CA, Caan MW, *et al.* (2011). Upper and extra-motoneuron involvement in early motoneuron disease: a diffusion tensor imaging study. *Brain* **134**: 1211–1228.

49. Turner MR, Agosta F, Bede P, *et al.* (2012). Neuroimaging in amyotrophic lateral sclerosis. *Biomarkers Med* **63**: 319–337.

50. Menke RA, Abraham I, Thiel CS, *et al.* (2012). Fractional anisotropy in the posterior limb of the internal capsule and prognosis in amyotrophic lateral sclerosis. *Arch Neurol* **6911**: 1493–1499.

51. Agosta F, Valsasina P, Absinta M, *et al.* (2011). Sensorimotor functional connectivity changes in amyotrophic lateral sclerosis. *Cerebral Cortex* **2110**: 2291–2298.

52. Joint Task Force of the European Federation of Neurological Societies/Peripheral Nerve Society (2010). Guideline on management of chronic inflammatory demyelinating polyradiculoneuropathy: report of a joint task force of the European Federation of Neurological Societies and the Peripheral Nerve Society – First Revision. *J Peripheral Nerv System* **151**: 1–9.

53. Beydoun SR, Muir J, Apelian RG, Go JL, Lin FP (2012). Clinical and imaging findings in three patients with advanced inflammatory demyelinating polyradiculoneuropathy associated with nerve root hypertrophy. *J Clin Neuromusc Dis* **133**: 105–112.

54. Tanaka K, Mori N, Yokota Y, Suenaga T (2013). MRI of the cervical nerve roots in the diagnosis of chronic inflammatory demyelinating polyradiculoneuropathy: a single-institution, retrospective case-control study. *BMJ Open* **38**: e003443.

55. Costa AF, Di Primio GA, Schweitzer ME (2012). Magnetic resonance imaging of muscle disease: a pattern-based approach. *Muscle Nerve* **464**: 465–481.

56. ten Dam L, van der Kooi AJ, van Wattingen M, de Haan RJ, de Visser M (2012). Reliability and accuracy of skeletal muscle imaging in limb-girdle muscular dystrophies. *Neurology* **7916**: 1716–1723.

57. Mercuri E, Clements E, Offiah A, *et al.* (2010). Muscle magnetic resonance imaging involvement in muscular dystrophies with rigidity of the spine. *Annals Neurol* **672**: 201–208.

58. Morrow JM, Pitceathly RD, Quinlivan RM, Yousry TA (2013). Muscle MRI in Bethlem myopathy. *BMJ Case Rep*: doi 10.1136/bcr-2013-008596.

59. Tasca G, Iannaccone E, Monforte M, *et al.* (2012). Muscle MRI in Becker muscular dystrophy. *Neuromusc Disord* **22** (suppl 2): S100–106.

60. Klein A, Jungbluth H, Clement E, *et al.* (2011). Muscle magnetic resonance imaging in congenital myopathies due to ryanodine receptor type 1 gene mutations. *Arch Neurol* **689**: 1171–1179.

61. Del Grande F, Carrino JA, Del Grande M, Mammen AL, Christopher Stine L (2011). Magnetic resonance imaging of inflammatory myopathies. *Topics Magn Reson Imaging* **222**: 39–43.

62. Tomasova Studynkova J, Charvat F, Jarosova K, Vencovsky J (2007). The role of MRI in the assessment of polymyositis and dermatomyositis. *Rheumatology* **467**: 1174–1179.

Chapter 21

Paresthesias and dysesthesias

Priyesh Mehta, Christopher A. Potter, Joseph H. Feinberg,
Jack H. Simon, and Ken R. Maravilla

Introduction

Paresthesias are abnormal sensations in the absence of specific stimuli typically characterized as tingling, prickling, pins and needles, or burning sensations. The symptoms may be transient or persistent and can involve any portion of the body, but most commonly involve the hands, arms, legs, and feet [1]. Paresthesias differ from dysesthesias, which are abnormal interpretations of appropriate stimuli. Dysesthesias often present as a painful sensation and can involve any bodily tissue most commonly the mouth, scalp, skin, or legs [2]. Paresthesias can be caused by a dysfunction or abnormality affecting any level of the somatosensory pathway, with the most common causes affecting peripheral sensory nerves.

The somatosensory pathway encompasses multiple types of sensation from the body including light touch, pain, pressure, temperature, and proprioception. However, these modalities are grouped into three different pathways in the spinal cord and have different targets in the brain. Paresthesias represent abnormal impulses from an ectopic focus and can originate from anywhere along the sensory pathway, from the peripheral nerves to the sensory cortex. Any disruption in this pathway can result in altered nerve function and a clinical response [3].

Etiology

Paresthesias can be caused by central or peripheral nervous system abnormalities. Disruption can occur in the somatosensory pathway at the level of the peripheral nerve, dorsal root ganglion, dorsal sensory nerve roots, spinal cord or brain. Central nervous system (CNS)-induced paresthesias are most commonly caused by infectious or inflammatory processes, ischemia, structural causes (including tumor

or trauma) or degenerative processes (Table 21.1). Peripheral nerve-related paresthesias may be due to a wide variety of etiologies, including entrapment syndromes, traumatic nerve stretch or compression injuries, metabolic disturbances, connective-tissue disorders, autoimmune diseases, vasculitic or inflammatory disorders, toxins, hereditary conditions, malignancy, infections, and nutritional deficiencies (Table 21.2). The focus of this chapter will be on peripheral nerve causes of paresthesias.

Nerve compression and focal entrapment can lead to paresthesias in the distribution of the involved peripheral nerve. The most common site of nerve entrapment is compression of the median nerve at the wrist causing carpal tunnel syndrome. Other common peripheral nerve-entrapment syndromes include ulnar neuropathy due to entrapment in the cubital tunnel, fibular neuropathy caused by peroneal nerve compression, and tarsal nerve entrapment [4]. In addition, nerve compression can involve the brachial plexus at any one of three points, resulting in thoracic outlet syndrome. Thus, compression can occur at the root, trunk, division, cord, or branch level as seen in idiopathic brachial neuritis such as Parsonage–Turner syndrome, often due to traumatic injury or inflammatory injury to the brachial plexus [5]. Radiculopathies caused by compression of the dorsal spinal nerve roots in cervical, thoracic, and lumbosacral regions by foraminal stenosis or intervertebral disk herniation can cause the burning, tingling, pins and needles sensation seen in paresthesias. Traumatic brachial plexopathies are relatively uncommon but when they occur will frequently cause paresthesias and dysesthesias. Atraumatic plexopathies from primary and metastatic cancer, radiation, and viral syndromes can also result in these types of symptoms.

Imaging Acute Neurologic Disease, ed. Massimo Filippi and Jack H. Simon. Published by Cambridge University Press.
© Cambridge University Press 2014.

Table 21.1 Central causes of paresthesias

Infections:
- Brain abscess
- Encephalitis
- Neurosyphilis

Inflammatory:
- Multiple sclerosis
- Systemic lupus erythematosus
- Acute disseminated encephalomyelitis

Ischemic:
- Cerebrovascular event
- Transient ischemic attack

Structural:
- Tumor
- Trauma
- Degenerative process

Table 21.2 Peripheral causes of paresthesia

Nerve entrapment:
- Median neuropathy
- Ulnar neuropathy
- Fibular neuropathy
- Tibial neuropathy
- Lateral femoral cutaneous nerve of the thigh
- Radiculopathy
- Parsonage–Turner syndrome

Metabolic:
- Diabetes
- Uremia
- Hypocalcemia
- Hypothyroidism

Connective tissue/autoimmune disorders:
- Systemic lupus erythematosus
- Rheumatoid arthritis
- Guillain–Barré syndrome

Vasculitic disorders:
- Polyarteritis nodosa
- Churg–Strauss syndrome
- Wegener's granulomatosis
- Microscopic polyangitis
- Sjögren's syndrome
- Neuro-Behçet disease

Drug/toxin:
- Alcohol
- Chemotherapy drugs (cisplatin, cincristine, cytosine arabinoside, thalidomide, paclitaxel)
- Antibiotics (metronidazole, nitrofurantoin)
- Antiretroviral agents (zidovudine, staudine, lamivudine)
- Antiepileptic (phenytoin)
- Heavy metals (lead, arsenic, mercury, thallium)
- Radiation treatment

Hereditary conditions:
- Charcot–Marie–Tooth disease
- Tangier disease
- Fabry disease
- Krabbe disease
- Friedrich ataxia
- Spinocerebellar ataxia
- Niemann–Pick disease

Malignancy:
- Tumor compression
- Paraneoplastic syndromes
- Lymphomas
- Multiple myeloma
- Waldenstroms macroglobulinema

Infectious:
- HIV
- CMV
- Herpes zoster infection (shingles)
- Leprosy
- Lyme disease

Nutritional:
- Vitamin B12 deficiency
- Vitamin B6 deficiency or excess
- Vitamin B1 deficiency
- Vitamin E deficiency
- Copper deficiency

Metabolic causes of paresthesias include diabetes in which hyperglycemia causes nerve damage affecting peripheral nerve fibers and Schwann cells [6]. Uremia can result in accumulation of toxic substances resulting in generalized peripheral neuropathy. Hypocalcemia and hypothyroid disorders also play a role in nerve damage, affecting neural function with significant imbalances in calcium levels and thyroid hormone levels, respectively. Connective-tissue disorders such as rheumatoid arthritis and systemic lupus erythematosus (SLE) and vasculitic inflammatory diseases such as polyarteritis nodosa, Sjögren's syndrome, and Wegener's granulomatosis can cause autoantibody immune-mediated nerve inflammation or monoclonal protein depositions resulting in disruption in peripheral nerves. These often result in a more painful clinical response [7].

Toxin exposure to heavy metals including lead, arsenic, and mercury can cause sensory polyneuropathy as a result of environmental or occupational exposures [8]. More commonly, chronic alcohol use produces a polyneuropathy secondary to direct alcohol effects as well as nutritional deficiencies that result from long-term alcohol use [9]. Pharmacologic agents such as chemotherapeutic drugs, antibiotics, and anti-seizure medications can result in drug induced paresthesias. In addition, radiation therapy for cancer treatment can result in radiation-induced brachial plexopathy or lumbosacral plexopathy when these specific nerves are in the field of radiation [10].

Genetic mutations that alter the structure of nerve fibers occur in inherited disorders such as Charcot–Marie–Tooth disease and can lead to peripheral neuropathy or plexopathy due to altered myelin structure resulting in demyelination or defects in axon formation [11]. Charcot–Marie–Tooth disease and related disorders often cause hypertrophic neuropathic changes that are readily discernible on specialized, high resolution forms of MRI such as magnetic resonance (MR) neurography (see below).Tumors, in particular benign nerve-sheath tumors, can cause direct compression on the underlying peripheral nerve that can result in significant paresthesias due to compression, metabolic derangements, and/or nutritional deficiencies. Paraneoplastic syndromes related to tumors can cause direct anti-neuronal antibody involvement [12]. Infections such as human immunodeficiency virus (HIV) can cause direct injury to the dorsal root ganglion producing a peripheral neuropathy and, in addition, associated HIV-related infections such as cytomegalovirus (CMV) can produce an inflammatory neuritis in the immune-compromised host. Herpes zoster infections due to viral dissemination to regional lymph nodes, spinal intercostal, or peripheral nerves may cause severe pain and paresthesias in a dermatome distribution generally associated with a characteristic rash [13]. Common nutritional deficiencies such as vitamin B12 and thiamine that are important in neural function can cause paresthesias if deficient [14].

There are limited indications for emergent or urgent MRI evaluation of peripheral nerves in acute trauma since the edema and inflammation that occurs from associated tissue damage hides the relatively subtle changes that occur in the small peripheral nerves. Urgent evaluation is required when patients present with paresthesias of central origin such as cerebrovascular injury, seizures, spinal cord compression, and in central demyelinating diseases such as multiple sclerosis (MS). These are discussed elsewhere in this volume. Urgent evaluation is also necessary in patients with paresthesias of peripheral origin seen in Guillain–Barré syndrome (GBS) where paresthesias are a result of immune-mediated attack to the myelin sheath. The symptoms typically start from the toes and may rapidly progress proximally over hours to days. These patients require early diagnosis and treatment since they are at high risk of developing respiratory muscle fatigue resulting in respiratory depression as well as acute dysautonomia that can cause significant fluctuations in blood pressure and heart rate [15].

In most cases, specific neurologic findings can provide the physician with a framework for diagnosis. Often, appropriate laboratory and nerve conduction studies (NCS) are essential for confirming the etiology. Imaging with MR neurography is utilized in selective cases presenting with paresthesia or dysethesia, when it can be supportive of a diagnosis or exclude clinically overlapping presentations. MR neurography is also used for specific indications such as when it can provide a definitive diagnosis and when it is used to guide early therapy as described below.

Diagnostic approach

Paresthesias can be due to a variety of conditions affecting both the peripheral and central nervous systems. Most patients with paresthesias will have peripheral neuropathy as the etiology; however, other causes need to be considered and ruled out. An effective history and physical examination can narrow the differential diagnosis and can guide the physician to further testing such as laboratory, imaging, or electromyography.

History

When gathering the history from the patient it is important to characterize the paresthesia using their own words. Some common descriptions of paresthesias include burning pain that is commonly associated with neuropathy affecting small unmyelinated fibers, or stabbing pain that suggests an inflammatory etiology or vasculitis. Shooting pains, on the other hand, more commonly characterizes nerve entrapment or compression syndromes. The rapidity of onset of symptoms (seconds, minutes, hours, days, or weeks) can also help the physician narrow the differential diagnosis. It is essential to determine the duration and severity of symptoms and to note any symptom progression. Any associated muscle pain, weakness, or atrophy can be correlated with a more advanced disease or a longer duration of disease [16]. Localization of symptoms and an understanding of sensory spinal root distribution (Figure 21.1) and cutaneous nerve distribution are important in diagnosing many common paresthesias (Figure 21.2). A specific dermatome-type pattern can suggest a radiculopathy while patterns including specific single nerves or multiple nerves can indicate a peripheral nerve compression or more complex disease, respectively.

Information regarding the patient's past medical history, medications, and possible illicit drug history, as well as dietary habits, should be documented. A

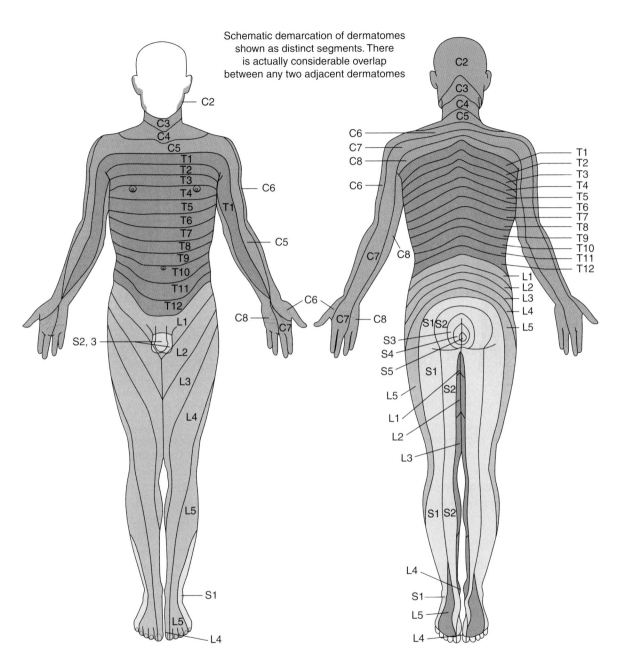

Schematic demarcation of dermatomes shown as distinct segments. There is actually considerable overlap between any two adjacent dermatomes

Levels of principal dermatomes

C5	Clavicles	**T10**	Level of umbilicus
C5, 6, 7	Lateral parts of upper limbs	**T12**	Inguinal or groin regions
C8, T1	Medial sides of upper limbs	**L1, 2, 3, 4**	Anterior and inner surfaces of lower limbs
C6	Thumb	**L4, 5, S1**	Foot
C6, 7, 8	Hand	**L4**	Medial side of great toe
C8	Ring and little fingers	**S1, 2, L5**	Posterior and outer surfaces of lower limbs
T4	Level of nipples	**S1**	Lateral margin of foot and little toe
		S2, 3, 4	Perineum

Figure 21.1 Sensory dermatomes

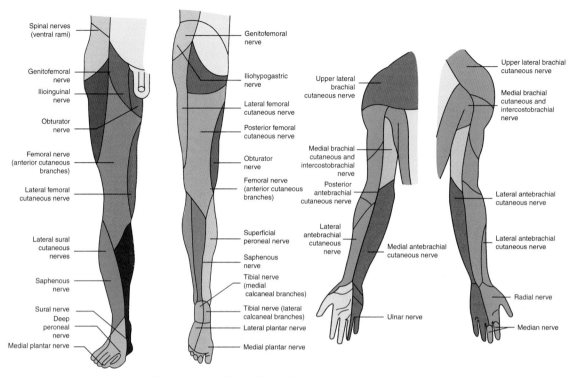

Figure 21.2 Cutaneous nerve distribution of upper limb and lower limb

positive family history of paresthesias may indicate an inherited neuropathy or metabolic disorder. An occupational and environmental history of exposure to toxic substances as well as the immunization history is significant to rule out other etiologies [16].

Physical examination

Patients presenting with complaints of paresthesias and dysesthesias should receive a complete general physical and neurological exam. The neurological examination should focus on the area corresponding to the patient's symptoms, but a general neurological examination should be performed to identify any other diagnostic clues. The sensory examination should test response to light touch using a cotton swab; temperature, using thermal stimulus; pinprick with a pin and needle; vibration with a tuning fork; and proprioception by testing patients' sense of joint position. Sensory loss in the distribution of a single peripheral nerve indicates a mononeuropathy. Paresthesia elicited through provocative tests such as Tinel sign, indicates a possible nerve-entrapment syndrome. Loss of sensation in the distribution of multiple nerves may signify polyneuropathy or plexopathy,

while sensory loss in a dermatome distribution indicates a radiculopathy. The motor system evaluation is performed to look for muscle weakness or atrophy. Abnormalities may suggest a specific nerve, nerve root, or spinal cord lesion. Decreased reflexes suggest a spinal-nerve-segment dysfunction or a peripheral nerve injury, while hyperreflexia indicates an upper motor neuron or central neurologic cause. Gait abnormalities such as a wide based gait, ataxia, or foot drop and difficulty walking are important to note. Cerebellar function with finger-to-nose and heel-to-shin maneuvers as well as the integrity of cranial nerves helps detect CNS causes of paresthesias or a possible paraneoplastic etiology [16].

Laboratory

Laboratory examination is often used to support the findings on physical examination, as well as to confirm a likely diagnosis. Most initial laboratory evaluations for paresthesisas consist of a complete blood-cell count, serum chemistry profile, and a urinalysis. Metabolic or endocrine tests including hemoglobin A1C (HgbA1C) to detect glycemic control in diabetics as a cause of peripheral neuropathy, serum calcium, vitamin D, parathyroid hormone levels if hypocalcemia is suspected, and thyroid studies including serum thyroid stimulating hormone (TSH) and free T4 to rule out hypothyroidism. Blood and urine toxin levels, as well as heavy-metal screening should also be ordered to rule out a drug-induced paresthesia. Serum analysis for infection or inflammation, such as herpes simplex virus (HSV), HIV, and Lyme disease, erythrocyte sedimentation rate (ESR), and C-reactive protein (CRP) levels, can also be helpful in identifying an infectious or vasculitic disorder. Autoantibody testing is indicated when trying to rule out autoimmune disorders such as rheumatoid arthritis and SLE. An autoimmune panel consisting of rheumatoid factor and anti-cyclic citrullinated peptides (anti-CCP) can identify rheumatoid arthritis. Antinuclear antibodies (ANA), anti-phospholipid antibodies, anti-smith antibodies, and antibodies to double-stranded DNA can be ordered to diagnose SLE. Lumbar puncture can be performed in patients with unusual presentations of radiculopathy. The cerebrospinal fluid (CSF) should be examined for evidence of inflammation (including elevated CSF protein and mononuclear cells) and serologic testing performed for Lyme disease, syphilis, and CMV [16].

Nerve studies

Electrodiagnostic (EDX) studies including electromyography (EMG) and NCS are often the most useful tests for evaluating a patient with peripheral neuropathy. EMG includes needle examination of selected muscles and NCS include the stimulation and recording of electrical activity from individual peripheral nerves. Both studies should be directed at nerves and muscles whose involvement is suspected based on the clinical examination. They can confirm the presence of a neuropathy and help to rule out a polyneuropathy (genetic and acquired), compression neuropathy, myopathy (genetic and acquired), plexopathy (traumatic and atraumatic), radiculopathies, and motor neuron disease. This study provides information as to the type of fibers involved (motor, sensory, or both), the pathophysiology (axonal loss versus demyelination), and a symmetric versus asymmetric or multifocal pattern of involvement. However, a normal EMG/NCS test does not preclude a peripheral nerve etiology for paresthesias [17].

EDX nerve studies remain the cornerstone in the diagnosis as well as management of nerve injuries. NCS help identify focal slowing of conduction and

conduction block that are caused by myelin disruption as well as conduction failure as a result of axonal loss. EDX studies are specifically helpful in distinguishing preganglionic versus postganglionic injuries particularly in the setting of trauma (i.e. traumatic brachial plexopathies). For example, in traumatic brachial plexopathies leading to root avulsions, the sensory nerve action potentials (SNAPs) are normal because injury within the spinal canal proximal to the dorsal root ganglion (DRG) leaves the postganglionic sensory fibers and the cell bodies intact. In addition, needle EMG findings of fibrillation potentials (spontaneous action potentials generated by denervated muscle fibers) in the paraspinal muscles suggest a more proximal lesion or radiculopathy because these muscles are innervated by the posterior primary rami that leave the spinal roots soon after the intervertebral foramina [18]. Involvement of the serratus anterior or rhomboids suggests a more proximal plexus injury because of their proximal takeoff from the plexus but does not guarantee preganglionic localization. This type of anatomic localization is necessary not only for making a diagnosis but also for prognosticating outcome, deciding on the role of nerve reconstruction, and on the timing of intervention.

Compression neuropathies such as median neuropathy of the hand seen in carpal tunnel syndrome are commonly diagnosed with EDX nerve studies. The study aims to confirm the diagnosis by assessing the status of the median sensory and motor fibers across the carpal tunnel as well as ruling out other possible causes such as cervical radiculopathy. The hallmark of this syndrome is primary demyelinating injury resulting in focal slowing of conduction across the wrist; therefore, on NCS the SNAPs and compound muscle action potentials (CMAPs) will be slower. Needle EMG helps to identify the extent of damage to a median nerve, with increased spontaneous activity and fibrillation potentials in the thenar muscles suggesting axonal damage to the median nerve and more severe carpal tunnel syndrome, likely to benefit from surgical treatment [19].

EDX studies are also useful in identifying peripheral polyneuropathies and will often identify the underlying disorder/disease whether it be genetic, disease-related (diabetes, vasculitis, renal disease, viral, autoimmne), paraneoplastic, idiopathic, medication- or alcohol-induced (Table 21.2). For example, EDX is useful for autoimmune disorders such GBS and chronic inflammatory demyelinating polyneuropathy

(CIDP). Typically, progression for GBS lasts up to 4 weeks; while progression to greater than 4 weeks is more indicative of CIDP. Most cases of GBS are characterized by segmental demyelination; however, many patients with typical GBS have evidence of primary axonal degeneration. EMG is useful to help confirm the diagnosis of GBS to allow initiation of early treatment and therefore is performed in the first 1–2 weeks following illness or hospital admission [20].

Imaging

Imaging is integral to evaluation of preganglionic radiculopathy, and/or possible spinal cord compromise. Lumbar root evaluation, cervical and thoracic radiculopathy, and myelopathy are discussed in multiple chapters in this book.

Imaging is being increasingly utilized for evaluation of peripheral nerves, as new techniques and experience with nerve imaging have increased

rapidly in the last decade. As MRI acquisition hardware, and pulse sequences, continue to evolve and improve, MRI is becoming the core study for clinical evaluation of the peripheral nerve. Computed tomography (CT) and CT myelography remain in the nerve-imaging toolbox. Ultrasound, a highly user-skill dependent technique, is used by some for evaluating select peripheral nerves of the extremities (Figure 21.3). Ultrasound of the tibial and radial nerves in patients with chronic diseases, including diabetic neuropathy, is presently the subject of research series. The technique is excellent in showing change in nerve cross-sectional area and echogenicity [21].

Cross-sectional MRI and CT are typically directed at fine anatomic detail, visualizing continuity of nerve, nerve compression or displacement, and variable sensitivity to pathology (e.g. edema, inflammation, neoplastic change). Specialized high-resolution MRI is required, often referred to as MR neurography, due to

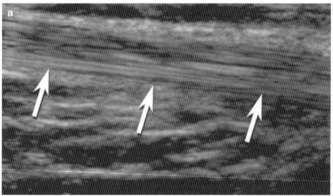

Figure 21.3 Ultrasound image of median nerve at wrist. (a) Longitudinal image of the nerve shows fascicle detail (arrows). (b) Transverse image of the nerve (arrow) shows nodular echogenic pattern reflecting fascicles in cross-section. Note the location between the two flexor tendons of the wrist (T). Although ultrasound can show the delicate structure of nerve fascicles in superficial nerves, the tissue contrast from nerve inflammation or edema, and the spatial relationships to surrounding structures are not as well demonstrated compared with MR neurography (case courtesy of Dr. Sumit Pruthi).

the small size of peripheral nerves, that are typically 1–10 mm in cross-sectional diameter but may be up to 20 mm for the sciatic nerve [22]. For MR neurography, general principles include use of optimized multi-array surface coils tailored to the region of anatomy being imaged. Higher-field-strength magnets help to optimize signal-to-noise ratio and relatively small fields of view are utilized to obtain high resolution in the resulting images. This means that the area of highest interest (area of suspicion) must be determined from the clinical examination to guide the MRI study. It should be emphasized that MR neurography is not a screening study but rather a study targeted to a localized area of suspected nerve dysfunction. Imaging planes are planned for the structures of interest, or, with increasing use of isotropic three-dimensional imaging, are based on volume imaging with postprocessing and multiplanar reformatting to display optimal views of the target nerve(s). This permits visualization of the course of nerves and the relationship and impact of adjacent normal and abnormal structures of interest [23].

MRI protocols typically include T1-weighted series for anatomical definition of fat planes, muscle planes, and the nerve, together with T2-weighted imaging with fat suppression to display the nerve and analyze the T2 signal (normal versus abnormal) within the nerve. T2 weighting is sensitive to the detection of edema and other water-space changes accompanying pathology. Fat suppression is accomplished either through T1 relaxation-based inversion recovery techniques such as short tau inversion recovery (STIR), frequency selective (chemical shift selective) prepulses that saturate out the fat resonance signal, or combined frequency plus chemical-shift selective pulses. Pulse sequence nomenclature and details depend on the specific MR system utilized and its software. Fat-suppression imaging is often challenging due to magnetic-field inhomogeneity (variation across the anatomy of interest) and the magnetic-susceptibility effects at air–tissue interfaces and in the vicinity of metallic implants such as those from orthopedic prosthetic hardware. These artifacts may be particularly troublesome when imaging complex geometric regions such as the brachial plexus or when imaging the upper extremity in large patients when the extremity area of interest lies at the periphery of the magnet-imaging field. Magnetic-field distortion has a variable impact, typically resulting in ineffective fat suppression, but can also cause inadvertent water suppression, which complicates image interpretation

and can result in misdiagnosis. These artifacts can be partially suppressed by techniques that improve magnetic-field homogeneity, for example by placing perfluorocarbon-filled or (less ideally) saline bags along the surfaces of the neck. In addition to fat suppression, contrast enhancement and subacute blood (methemoglobin), which have short T1 relaxation times that may overlap with the short T1 of fat, may also be suppressed with the STIR sequence.

As perineural blood vessels frequently closely parallel the peripheral nerves, these can cause misidentification of blood vessels as possible nerve structures. They can also produce phase-shifted pulsation artifacts (i.e. misregistration of blood-vessel signal outside the vessel lumen), which can interfere with nerve visualization. To counteract these problems strong flow motion suppression techniques are beneficial.

Imaging includes evaluation of muscle groups that may show denervation changes. Such changes are dependent on the stage or chronicity of the denervation process. Thus, recent onset of denervation may show T2-hyperintensity within the involved muscle or muscle group while chronic, longstanding denervation will show fatty infiltration accompanied by muscle atrophy and no hyperintense T2 signal.

The imaging anatomy of the nerve is based on an epineurium confining the nerve fascicles, each fascicle bounded by a perineurial sheath. Within the fascicles, the Schwann cell–axon complex is invested by endoneurium. Nerve pathology is evident by focal or diffuse T2 signal hyperintensity within a nerve, which may be accompanied by enlargement of the nerve. In some cases there may be an altered course of the nerve from extrinsic compression and displacement. The etiology of increased signal intensity on T2-weighted imaging within abnormal nerves is multifactorial. Factors that are likely to contribute include edema in various locations (endoneurial/perineurial, within axons or myelin), disrupted axoplasmic flow, and other axonal pathology (e.g. from demyelination or Wallerian degeneration). Contrast enhancement plays a limited role in nerve imaging for paresthesia although it can be very valuable in the case of tumors or infection. In most cases of entrapment there is no contrast enhancement present. However, homogeneous or heterogeneous contrast enhancement can be seen in cases of tumor, infection, or inflammation, such as Guillian–Barré syndrome.

Relevant to imaging, endothelial tight junctions produce a blood–nerve barrier analogous to the blood–brain barrier and prevent normal contrast enhancement at the level of the perineurium. An exception is the dorsal root ganglion, which does not have a barrier, and can be identified by its normal bright contrast enhancement on T1-weighted post-contrast images. It should be noted that fat-suppressed T1-weighted imaging is essential when evaluating nerves post-gadolinium injection. Contrast-enhancement practices vary. Our approach is to utilize intravenous contrast enhancement for known or suspected neoplasm, inflammation, infection, and for diffuse nerve involvement [22, 23]. Contrast utilization recommendations in the setting of trauma are highly variable. Intravenous contrast may not be required for acute trauma, but may be useful when evaluating for later sequelae, when post-traumatic neuroma formation, and perineural fibrosis may be considerations. As already noted, the use of contrast in cases of entrapment syndrome is not warranted (Figure 21.4).

Specific examples of nerve imaging

Acute peripheral nerve imaging by MR neurography is utilized urgently in some centers for planning microsurgical repair. Another urgent indication may be for diagnosis of rapidly progressive disease, such as GBS, although imaging is only rarely required. GBS has a characteristic appearance including thickening and enhancement of the nerve roots of the cauda equina, predominantly but not exclusively within the anterior

roots, and may involve cranial nerves as well [24] (Figure 21.5). Nerve-root enhancement may occur but is not pathognomonic, and clinical, electrophysiological, and laboratory (including CSF) correlation is critical. Preganglionic nerve-root enhancement is also found in infection, including viral radiculitis (e.g. CMV), Lyme radiculoneuritis, neoplasm (carcinomatosis), and granulomatous disease (e.g. sarcoidosis), among other etiologies.

Less time-critical applications of nerve imaging include elective post-traumatic surgical planning and biopsy planning, in order to enable higher tissue yields by optimizing sampling locations and to improve patient safety.

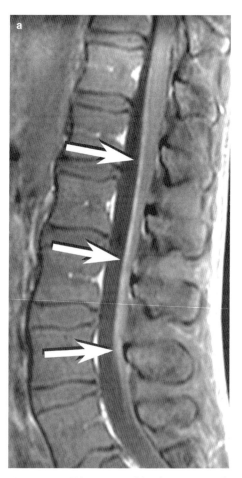

Figure 21.5 GBS. A 23-year-old male patient noted acute onset of numbness and paresthesias of hands and feet followed by rapid onset of gait difficulty and lower extremity weakness over 5 days. Sagittal T1 post-contrast spine image (a) shows enhancement of nerve roots in the cauda equina (arrows). Axial T1 post-gadolinium images (b, c) confirm enhancement of some roots within the cauda equina (arrows). Subsequent work-up confirmed acute inflammatory demyelinating polyneuropathy (GBS).

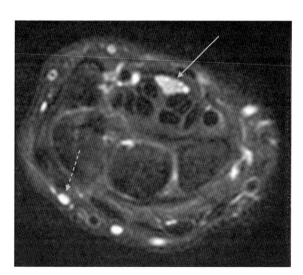

Figure 21.4 Median nerve in patient with carpal tunnel syndrome. Transverse STIR image through carpal tunnel shows flattened, enlarged, and markedly hyperintense nerve (arrow). The fascicular pattern is accentuated. Note signal intensity of nerve approaches that of blood vessels (e.g. dashed arrow).

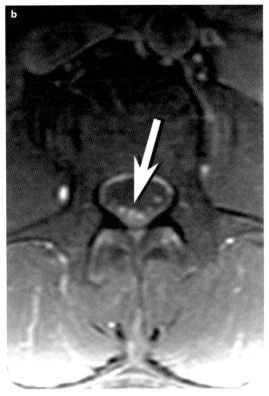

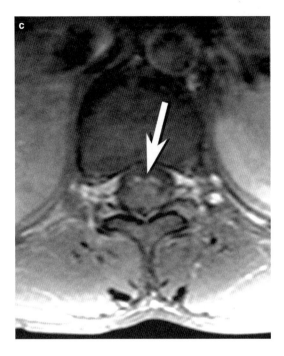

Figure 21.5 (contd.)

Brachial plexus

MRI is the imaging procedure of choice for the detection and elucidation of pathology affecting the brachial plexus (Figure 21.6). There have been dramatic technical improvements recently based on high-resolution, three-dimensional, fat-suppressed imaging with strong fluid weighting and multiplanar reconstruction [25].

Imaging is utilized for stretch injury involving the brachial plexus, which can be seen in neonates with mechanically complicated delivery, and in young and increasingly older (baby boomer) adults from motorcycle accidents (Figure 21.7). Nerve stretching (neuropraxic) and/or frank nerve-avulsion injury may occur in either of these causes. MRI may show nerve root swelling and T2 hyperintensity without nerve discontinuity. Nerve-root avulsion is seen as discontinuity of the nerve and its connection to the spinal cord. The spinal cord may be displaced from the midline toward the contralateral side by tension from the intact nerve roots. A post-traumatic pseudomeningocele may be present with avulsion injury, as well as with intact roots. Although CT myelography was, until recently, the initial imaging test of choice for diagnosis of brachial plexus avulsion injury, since it can provide fine-detail roots within CSF space, more often CT myelography is now used secondarily when high-resolution MRI is inconclusive or provides incomplete information.

In addition to trauma, more typical applications of nerve imaging include differentiation of mechanical and infiltrative patterns of primary nerve (Figure 21.8) or nerve-sheath tumors (Figure 21.9), or adjacent neoplasm reaching the plexus (e.g. Pancoast tumors). Radiation plexopathy (Figure 21.10), which can be acute but is most often delayed by months, typically shows diffuse nerve thickening, loss of fine detail (fascicles) and borders, intrinsic T2 hyperintensity, and may also show mild contrast enhancement [26]. Infectious/inflammatory plexitis may present non-specific patterns. Imaging is not expected to be conclusive for diagnosis in isolation. In hypertrophic neuropathies, such as Charcot–Marie–Tooth disease, the plexus will be thick and T2 hyperintense

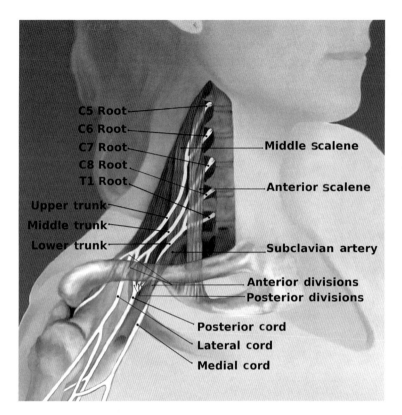

Figure 21.6 Brachial plexus. Schematic diagram of brachial plexus showing major anatomical divisions and several key anatomic relationships. The ventral rami of the nerve roots unite to form the brachial plexus between the anterior and middle scalene muscles. The trunks form within the interscalene triangle, while divisions develop more laterally and cords around the lateral margin of the first rib. Pathology can be described as supra-, retro-, and infraclavicular [25]. The subclavian artery, the floor of the interscalene triangle, provides a convenient landmark for locating and identifying the plexus on sagittal projections.

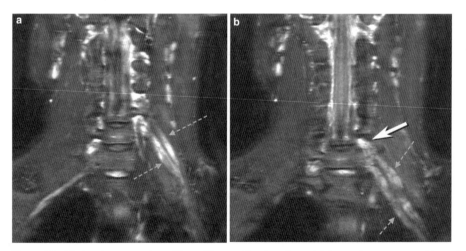

Figure 21.7 Patient in motorcycle accident with a combination of stretch injury and nerve-root avulsions of the left brachial plexus. (a) Hyperintense signal and swollen nerve roots reflecting stretch injuries (dashed arrows). (b) Irregular swelling and T2-hyperintense nerve roots again noted (dashed arrows). Note the pseudomeningocele of C7 root secondary to root avulsion at this level (bold arrow).

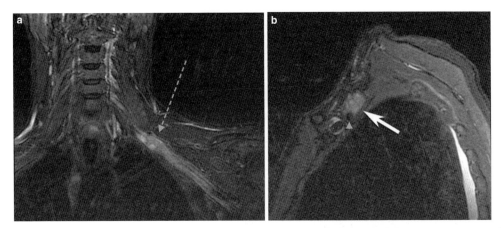

Figure 21.8 Patient with acute myelogenous leukemia. Tumor infiltration of left brachial plexus. (a) Hyperintense T2 infiltrating mass along left brachial plexus divisions and cords (dashed arrow). (b) Sagittal image shows mass indistinguishable from plexus nerves (arrow) and its relation to the subclavian artery, which is seen as a flow void immediately beneath tumor (arrowhead).

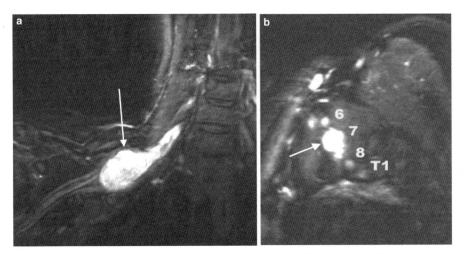

Figure 21.9 Schwannoma of right brachial plexus nerve root is seen with hyperintense T2 signal on this coronal fluid-attenuated inversion recovery (FLAIR) image (a, arrow). (b) Sagittal FLAIR image at the level of the distal roots shows the origin of the tumor (arrow) from the C7 nerve root.

[26, 27]. Similar findings may be seen in CIDP [28] (Figure 21.11).

Lumbosacral plexus and sciatic nerve

Imaging of the lumbosacral plexus and sciatic nerve are utilized when clinical findings or EMG localize to these structures, and/or are not explained by imaging the lumbar spinal canal and neuroforamina. Abnormalities include neoplastic involvement of the plexus or, in inpatients who have had prior surgical or radiation therapy to the pelvis, treatment-related pathology may be seen (scarring, compressive neuropathy from regional deformity, radiation plexopathy). Compressive neuropathy (e.g. piriformis syndrome) and traumatic nerve injury may also be seen [22, 29, 30] (Figure 21.12).

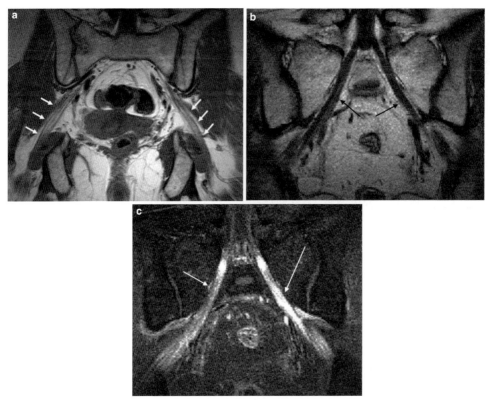

Figure 21.10 (a) Coronal T1 image of normal sacral plexus and sciatic nerves. Note the smooth, delicate "tram-track" appearance of the normal nerve fascicles on each side (arrows). Coronal T1 (b) and STIR (c) images of sacral plexus in patient with bilateral radiation plexitis secondary to radiation treatment for a pelvic malignancy. Note the thickened nerve structures and loss of the normal fascicular pattern in (b) (arrows) and the marked hyperintense T2 signal of the nerves (arrows) in (c).

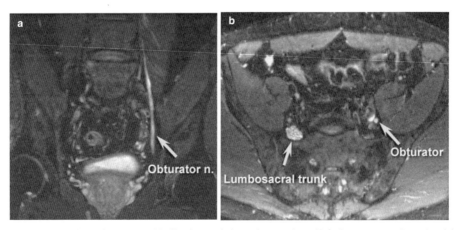

Figure 21.11 Coronal STIR image (a) of lumbosacral plexus shows enlarged left obturator nerve (arrow) with hyperintense T2 signal. Transverse STIR image (b) again shows enlarged, hyperintense T2 signal of the left obturator nerve (labeled arrow) and additionally shows even more marked enlargement and increased T2 signal of the right lumbosacral trunk (labeled arrow) as it passes anterior to the right sacral wing. The patient has CIDP.

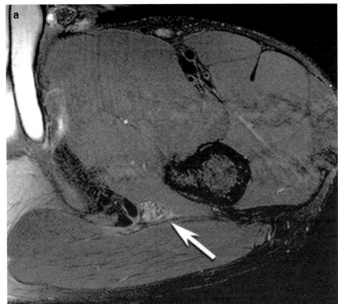

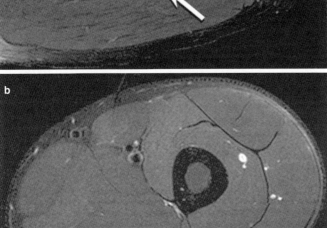

Figure 21.12 Patient suffering GSW to left buttock that passed close to the left sciatic nerve producing severe "shockwave" contusion injury to the nerve but did not transect the nerve. (a) Left sciatic nerve in buttock near the path of bullet (arrow) shows marked swelling and enlargement, inhomogeneous signal of fascicles with some showing increased T2 signal, and others showing decreased signal probably secondary to petechial hemorrhage in the nerve. (b) Axial STIR image of the thigh shows sciatic nerve enlargement to a lesser degree along with homogeneously increased T2 signal (arrow) due to downstream effects of the severe proximal nerve injury.

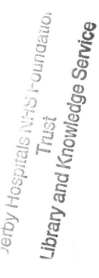

References

1. Asbury AK (1994). Numbness, tingling, and sensory loss. In Isselbacher KJ, Braunwald E, Wilson JD, *et al.*, eds. *Harrison's Principle of Internal Medicine*. 13th edn. New York: McGraw-Hill, pp. 133–136.

2. Dorland WAN (1994). *Dorland's Illustrated Medical Dictionary*. 28th edn. Philadelphia, PA: Saunders.

3. Thompson HG, Rowland LP (1989). Pain and paresthesias. In Rowland LP, ed. *Merritt's Textbook of Neurology*. 8th edn. Philadelphia, PA: Lea and Febiger, pp. 28–31.

4. Goslin KL, Krivickas LS (1999). Proximal neuropathies of the upper extremity. *Neurol Clin* **17**: 525–548.

5. Ferrante MA (2004). Brachial plexopathies: classification, causes, and consequences. *Muscle Nerve* **30**: 547–568.

6. Callaghan BC, Cheng HT, Stables CL, *et al.* (2012). Diabetic neuropathy: clinical manifestations and current treatments. *Lancet Neurol* **11**: 521–534.

7. Hunder GG, Arend WP, Bloch DA, *et al.* (1990). The American College of Rheumatology 1990 criteria for the classification of vasculitis. Introduction. *Arthritis Rheum* **33**: 1065–1067.

8. Windebank AJ (2005). Metal neuropathy. In Dyck PJ, Thomas PK, eds. *Peripheral Neuropathy*, 3rd edn. St. Louis, MO: Elsevier Saunders, pp. 2527–2551.

9. Monforte R, Estruch R, Valls-Solé J, *et al.* (1995). Autonomic and peripheral neuropathies in patients with chronic alcoholism. A dose-related toxic effect of alcohol. *Arch Neurol* **52**: 45–51.

10. Cross NE, Glantz MJ (2003). Neurologic complications of radiation therapy. *Neurol Clin* **21**: 249–277.

11. Krajewski KM, Lewis RA, Fuerst DR, *et al.* (2000). Neurological dysfunction and axonal degeneration in Charcot–Marie–Tooth disease type 1A. *Brain* **123**: 1516–1527.

12. Gomm SA, Thatcher N, Barber PV, Cumming WJ (1990). A clinicopathological study of the paraneoplastic neuromuscular syndromes associated with lung cancer. *Q J Med* **75**: 577–595.

13. Elliott KJ (1994). Other neurological complications of herpes zoster and their management. *Ann Neurol* **35** (suppl): S57.

14. Kumar N (2007). Nutritional neuropathies. *Neurol Clin* **25**: 209–255.

15. Moulin DE, Hagen N, Feasby TE, *et al.* (1997). Pain in Guillain–Barré syndrome. *Neurology* **48**: 328–331.

16. Bates B, Brickley LS, Hoekelman RA (1995). The nervous system: techniques of examination. In Bates B, Brickley LS, Hoekelman RA, eds. *A Guide to Physical Examination and History Taking*, 6th edn. Philadelphia, PA: Lippincott Williams and Wilkins, pp. 505–540.

17. Fisher MA (2002). Electrophysiology of radiculopathies. *Clin Neurophysiol* **113**: 317–335.

18. Preston DC, Shapiro BE (2013). Routine lower extremity nerve conduction techniques. In Preston DC, Shapiro BE, eds. *Electromyography and Neuromuscular Disorders*. Philadelphia, PA: Saunders, pp. 115–124.

19. Preston DC, Shapiro BE (2013). Routine upper extremity, facial and phrenic nerve conduction studies. In Preston DC, Shapiro BE, eds. *Electromyography and Neuromuscular Disorders*. Philadelphia, PA: Saunders, pp. 97–100.

20. Preston DC, Shapiro BE (2013). Electrophysiologic correlations. In Preston DC, Shapiro BE, eds. *Electromyography and Neuromuscular Disorders*. Philadelphia, PA: Saunders, pp. 391–393.

21. Watanabe T, Ito H, Sekine A, *et al.* (2010). Sonographic evaluation of the peripheral nerve in diabetic patients. The relationship between nerve conduction studies, echo intensity, and cross-sectional area. *J Ultrasound Med* **29**: 697–708.

22. Maravilla KR, Bowen BC (1998). Imaging of the peripheral nervous system : evaluation of peripheral neuropathy and plexopathy. *AJNR* **19**: 1011–1023.

23. Chhabra A, Andreisek G, Soldatos T, *et al.* (2011). MR neurography: past, present, and future. *AJR* **197**: 583–591.

24. Zuccoli G, Panigrahy A, Bailey A, Fitz C (2011). Redefining the Guillain–Barré spectrum in children: neuroimaging findings of cranial nerve involvement. *AJNR* **32**: 639–642.

25. Chhabra A, Thawait GK, Soldatos T, *et al.* (2013). High-resolution 3 T MR neurography of the brachial plexus and its branches, with emphasis on 3D imaging. *AJNR* **34**: 486–497.

26. Castillo Castillo M (2005). Imaging the anatomy of the brachial plexus: review and self-assessment module. *AJR* **185** (suppl): S196–204.

27. Thawait SK, Chaudhry V, Thawait GK, *et al.* (2011). High-resolution MR neurography of diffuse peripheral nerve lesions. *AJNR* **32**: 1365–1372.

28. Duggins AJ, McLeod JG, Pollard JD, *et al.* (1999). Spinal root and plexus hypertrophy in chronic inflammatory demyelinating polyneuropathy. *Brain* **122**: 1383–1390.

29. Petchprapa CN, Rosenberg ZS Sconfienza LM, *et al.* (2010). MR imaging of entrapment neuropathies of the lower extremity. Part 1. The pelvis and hip. *Radiographics* **30**: 983–1000.

30. Chhabra A, Chalian M, Soldatos T, *et al.* (2012). 3-T high-resolution MR neurography of sciatic neuropathy. *AJR* **198**: W357–364.

Introduction

Fatigue and weakness are among the most common symptoms observed in a variety of neurological, psychiatric, and medical populations. To manage these symptoms clinically, healthcare providers need accurate and measurable tools and procedures in order to make an appropriate assessment and develop meaningful treatments. As shall be seen in this chapter, neither are clearly available for patient complaints of weakness and especially for fatigue. While thought to represent two distinct symptoms, fatigue and weakness are intricately intertwined, leading to much confusion for the healthcare professionals as well as the patient and family.

Weakness

If a person has lost the ability to exert normal muscular force by moving a limb or the body, we may call this weakness. True weakness, or pathologic loss of muscle strength, may result from disorders of the muscle, neuromuscular junction, nerve, corticospinal tract, spinal cord, brainstem, subcortical white matter, or cortex. Complete loss of muscle contractility is referred to as "plegia": a partial loss of contractility is referred to as "paresis," or the more commonly used term, "paralysis".

Rowland [1] reports that patients who use the term weakness often mean to denote something different from inability to generate muscular force. In fact, people with muscular weakness frequently report that they cannot perform tasks (getting up from a chair, climbing stairs, running) rather than reporting that they are weak. Muscle weakness also does not usually result in a need to lie down after exertion; these symptoms are more common in emotional, psychological, or systemic

disorders causing fatigue (e.g. anemia). Consistent with Rowland's clinical observation, Friedman and Abrantes [2] found that, in Parkinson's disease (PD), self-reported weakness was found to be associated with self-reported fatigue and not with motor symptoms such as tremor, rigidity, bradykinesia, or overall motor severity. Classifying a patient's weakness can proceed most efficiently if the examiner makes a relatively rapid assessment of whether weakness is highly likely, or unlikely, to be pathologic in character based on a brief history of the complaint. Then, the examiner can collect a complete history while the weakness is assessed during the examination, and if unexpected pathologic signs are elicited, additional history can be collected (family history of weakness or neurological disorders, toxin exposures). Important historical features include the parts of the body affected, the period over which the symptoms developed and the rapidity of symptom progression, and associated neurological history, signs, and symptoms. An appropriately directed examination proceeding in this fashion can identify neuromuscular junction disorders (e.g. myasthenia gravis), hemiparesis from stroke or other brain structural disease, and structural disease/stroke in the brainstem or spinal cord. Weakness specific to the neck is almost always a sign of disease of the motor unit [1], and weakness of the facial musculature may be of similar origin, or may be due to cranial neuropathy, pseudobulbar palsy from a brainstem ischemic lesion, or, very rarely, atypical parkinsonism (progressive supranuclear palsy).

Proceeding quickly to the examination is helpful; if a patient is mimicking weakness (conscious malingering or willful factitious disorder) it can uncover inconsistencies in the history and characteristic signs of feigned weakness. These signs can also be present, however, in other somatoform disorders (e.g. hysteria).

A complaint of "fatigue" or "tiredness" is rarely associated with any reflex abnormality or limb weakness, abnormality of muscle tone, or other neuromuscular abnormality on examination. These patients may frequently report aching of the limbs or muscles, but muscle tone and bulk appears normal on examination. The history and physical examination may be highly suggestive of depression in these people, with sighing, and dysthymic affect. These people may also have tight muscles in the neck and shoulders with points of tenderness (trigger points) unaccompanied by redness or swelling, consistent with myofascial pain (more commonly called fibromyalgia). They may also have vague complaints of numbness and tingling, which can migrate and are not consistent with the distribution of a nerve root or sensory nerve.

Fatigue

Despite its high prevalence, fatigue is a non-specific and nebulous construct, which is poorly and inadequately described, understood, defined, assessed, and treated. Despite intensive study, our understanding of fatigue has advanced little over the past 100 years [3]. There are numerous synonyms that have been associated with fatigue, including weakness (Table 22.1). However, as noted above, the extent to which these entities are truly associated with fatigue is questionable. For instance, among the general population and patients seen in general practice, fatigue is twice as common as exhaustion, and up to 10 times more common than weakness or feeling "generally run down" [4]. Several studies of objective measurements of motor fatigue and weakness found little to no relationship between the two. For example, Schwid *et al.* [5] examined objective motor fatigue (loss of maximal capacity to generate force during exercise) and motor weakness (ability to maintain motor output during sustained and repetitive muscle contractions) during 30-second sustained maximal voluntary isometric contractions of the dominant elbow extensors, hand grip, knee extensors, and ankle dorsiflexors in 20 ambulatory multiple sclerosis (MS) patients and 20 age-and sex-matched healthy controls. They found that while fatigue in one muscle tended to correlate with fatigue in other muscles, it was not associated with weakness or ambulatory impairment. This indicates that weakness and fatigue were distinct features of motor dysfunction.

Fatigue is not a unitary construct, but rather multi-dimensional, rendering accurate assessment by practitioners a difficult challenge (Table 22.2). Research for over 100 years has demonstrated that all of the components of fatigue need to be considered in order to fully appreciate the experience of fatigue and its effects. A unified taxonomy of fatigue has recently been suggested [6]. However, to date, research and particularly clinical assessment has focused primarily on only one of these components – the feeling state, that is, the patient's self-report.

For example, the MS council for Clinical Practice Guidelines [7] defines fatigue as "a *subjective* lack of physical and/or mental energy that is *perceived* by the individual or caregiver to interfere with usual and desired activities". Clearly, the focus in clinical practice is on subjective ratings of fatigue only. The rather arbitrary nature of fatigue is further illustrated by the varying definitions of chronic fatigue. The MS Council defines it as "fatigue present for any amount of time on 50% of days for more than *six weeks*, which limits

Table 22.1 Items potentially synonymous with fatigue

Tired, worn out, or run down

Feelings of weakness

Exhaustion

Sleepiness

Lack of energy

Malaise

Effort – in relation to a task

Lack of motivation

Lassitude

Desire for rest

Table 22.2 Components of fatigue

Feeling state	– Self-report of severity, quality, associated symptoms
Behavior	– Decrement in performance, endurance
Affective	– Depression, anxiety, psychosomatic disorders
Mechanism	– Physiology, biochemistry, psychology
Context	– Cultural issues, physical issues (e.g., temperature), social stressors

Adapted from reference [4]

Table 22.3 Chalder fatigue scale. Note the content contamination with questions concerning sleep, depression, cognition, and weakness/strength.

Physical symptoms

Do you have a problem with tiredness?

Do you need rest more?

Do you feel sleepy or drowsy?

Do you have problems starting things?

Do you start things without difficulty but get weak as you go?

Are you lacking in energy?

Do you have less strength in your muscles?

Do you feel weak?

Mental symptoms

Do you have difficulty concentrating?

Do you have problems thinking clearly?

Do you make slips of the tongue when speaking?

Do you find it more difficult to find the correct word?

How is your memory?

Have you lost interest in things you used to do?

functional activities or quality of life". Chronic fatigue in chronic fatigue syndrome (CFS) is defined by such functional limitations over a *6 month* period [8].

Clinical assessment of fatigue is typically measured using one of dozens of self-report instruments available. Self-report instruments typically assess fatigue without defining it, as such fatigue becomes defined *post hoc* based on the questions included in the instrument. In many cases, the questions included may have little or nothing to do with fatigue (Table 22.3). For example, it has not been definitely demonstrated that patients can themselves truly differentiate fatigue from motor impairment, cognitive impairment, sleepiness, depression, or other symptoms in MS. In addition, reports of fatigue are subject to recall bias; for instance, where symptoms may have been present at baseline, but are noted as more serious, or noticed for the first time, only because the patient is now ill [9]. This recall bias thus makes self-reported fatigue scales particularly prone to placebo effects. In one of the first and perhaps most frequently used instrument of self-reported fatigue utilized in persons with MS, the Fatigue Severity Scale (FSS), Krupp *et al.* [10] defined fatigue as "a sense of physical tiredness and lack of energy, distinct from sadness or weakness." While others also defined fatigue as distinct from weakness

or sadness, others include weakness (e.g. Chalder fatigue scale [11]).

This illustrates a key problem and challenge to the use of an interpretation of self-report instruments of fatigue – construct contamination. For example, we now know that sleepiness and fatigue are not the same construct [3]; fatigue does not necessarily lead to cognitive impairment [12]; and, lastly, fatigue is highly correlated with depression [3]. Unfortunately, most self-report instruments include questions which simultaneously assess fatigue, cognitive problems, and depression. Further, such instruments do not differentiate between a host of other factors which may influence the patient's self-assessment, including medication effects, deconditioning, psychiatric factors (e.g. depression), hormonal changes, stress, and sleep patterns.

So what does self-reported fatigue actually tell the clinician? We know a few things from the literature. First, self-reported fatigue does not correlate with objective measures of fatigue (e.g. [5]). This lack of a relationship between self-report and objective performance is the most consistent finding in the literature known for over a century [3]. Second, there is a strong relationship between self-reported fatigue and psychopathology (e.g. depression), although this does not necessarily imply a causal relationship (e.g. [3]). Third, self-reported fatigue is inconsistently related to cognitive impairment. That is, higher self-reported fatigue has been shown to be associated with increased, decreased, and no change in objective cognitive performance (e.g. [12]). Thus, the frequently cited notion that fatigue leads to declines in cognitive performance is highly questionable, not supported by the literature, and likely inaccurate (e.g. [3]). However, self-reported fatigue has also been shown to have some medical predictive value. For example, post-stroke fatigue has been shown to be an independent predictor of death 1 year post stroke [13], is associated with reduced long-term survival [14], and increased risk of "suicidality" [15]. In addition, post-stroke fatigue has also been found to be independently associated with pre-stroke depression, leukoaraiosis, diabetes mellitus, pain, and sleeping disturbances [16]. Self-reported fatigue significantly predicts the development of coronary heart disease, risk of future cardiac events, and even survival following myocardial infarction. These relationships remain even after controlling for the traditional risk factors (e.g. elevated cholesterol, hypertension, smoking, age, etc.) [3]. Importantly, there are conditions where even chronic fatigue is typical and could be considered normal (e.g. pregnancy).

In contrast to self-report, there are many operational definitions of fatigue which mandate a performance-deficit requirement. For example, some state that "fatigue is the decline in performance that occurs in any prolonged or repeated task..." (e.g. Balkin and Westensten [17]). Yet others argue that the overt performance declines are not a necessary consequence of fatigue (e.g. [17]). This is because increased effort can be applied to compensate for declining mental resources. These authors suggested that fatigue should be defined only by its psychological or non-observable aspects. In such cases "subjective" aspects of fatigue can be thought of as "an awareness of the increasing mental effort needed to maintain cognitive performance as cognitive tasks are repeated–performed for extended periods" [17]. It is, lastly, possible that fatigue may represent a perceptual signal – sensed comparison between estimated motor endurance and actual performance, intended to gate or monitor exerted effort [18]. In the chronic fatigue state, like the chronic pain state, underestimated endurance limits a subject's maximal effort without serving its signal value by protecting resources, because resources were actually adequate to performance requirements.

Whether one defines fatigue by self-report or by performance parameters it is clear that singular conceptualizations of fatigue ignore the longstanding understanding that fatigue is multidimensional in nature, and that a broader understanding of fatigue is needed to truly understand this complex phenomenon.

Clinical management of fatigue and weakness

Clinical management of fatigue and weakness is based on management of the underlying disorder. People with subjective fatigue who have parkinsonism are helped by medication adjustment to reduce symptoms, as are people with depression. Disease-modifying therapies as well as targeted medications have been shown to reduce self-reported fatigue in MS, although not consistently. Basic care of pain syndromes, systemic disease, and myasthenia, with their specific targeted interventions, will reduce symptoms and improve fatigue as part of general health.

In motor neuron disease, MS, and other progressive diseases associated with fatigue and weakness, a traditional rehabilitative approach has been to teach the patient energy-conservation techniques: this is an approach directly opposite to exercise recommendations for people with fibromyalgia or deconditioning. However, recent research suggests that therapeutic exercise may be helpful for many chronic and progressive neurological disorders associated with fatigue (e.g. PD [19]). These studies used both resistance (strength building) and endurance (aerobic) approaches in these disorders with some success. Although whether exercise to build endurance and strength is more controversial in diseases of the motor neuron, neuromuscular junction, or muscle, a recent review suggested that adverse effects of exercise are likely to be negligible in these groups, and are "likely to be effective" (level II) to improve health [20]. Lastly, cognitive behavioral therapy has consistently been shown to decrease fatigue in several populations (e.g. DeLuca [3]).

Neuroimaging and weakness

One way in which neuroimaging has been used to study weakness has been through examining structural and functional changes in the brain following injury or disease as well as patterns of recovery (i.e. neuroplasticity and reorganization). In one of the earliest studies of weakness using functional magnetic resonance imaging (fMRI), eight MS patients with mild motor weakness performed a simple finger to thumb opposition movement during scanning [21]. In contrast to healthy controls that showed activation in the contralateral primary motor cortex, MS subjects showed large activation bilaterally in the primary motor cortex, as well as in the contralateral premotor and supplementary motor cortex. Since this work dozens of studies have been published in several clinical populations showing that motor weakness is associated with altered functional cerebral activity (e.g. [22]). Such work has been interpreted as movement-associated cortical reorganization. For instance, weakness in the upper extremities has been associated with an expansion of cortical activation using fMRI in the contralateral hemisphere in relapsing–remitting MS and patients at presentation with clinically isolated syndrome [22]. Patients with more advanced MS tend to show areas extending beyond the classical motor network bilaterally [23]. Mohammadi et al. [24] examined three groups of amyotrophic lateral sclerosis (ALS) patients with: no weakness, mild weakness, or marked weakness of the upper extremity using fMRI during a motor task. All groups showed increased contralateral hemisphere activation relative to healthy controls. However, with increasing weakness, there was a relative decrease in contralateral activation relative to controls. Ipsilateral activation was rare in controls (two of 22 subjects), while in ALS ipsilateral activation increased with increasing weakness.

As would be expected, several studies have shown a relationship between corticospinal tract abnormalities and weakness. Reich *et al.* [25] measured muscle strength in the hips and ankles of 47 persons with MS and examined their relationship with corticospinal-tract abnormalities as measured by various MRI techniques. The MS group was significantly weaker than controls. The magnetization transfer ratio (MTR) in the brainstem was moderately but significantly associated with hip and ankle strength, accounting for 30–45% of the variance. No supratentorial abnormalities were associated with weakness. Brain parenchymal fraction (relative glial and neuronal volume) was not associated with weakness. However, some individuals with profound weakness showed normal corticospinal-tract profiles. This illustrates that weakness may result from a variety of reasons including involvement of regions elsewhere in the brain or in the spinal cord, as well as the degree of volume loss in the brain or spinal cord. This may occur in a number of neurological disorders. For instance, using diffusion tensor imaging (DTI), Yeo *et al.* [26] found that decreased fractional anisotropy (FA) of the corticospinal tract at the midbrain was associated with motor weakness in people with subarachnoid hemorrhage. Several other studies utilized DTI to examine the integrity of the corticospinal tract and motor weakness in various populations including traumatic brain injury (TBI) [27], stroke [28], and brain neoplasms [29]. Other techniques utilized to study motor weakness and cerebral integrity include transcranial magnetic stimulation [30] and a technique called "high-definition fiber tracking (HDFT)," a novel technique to examine axonal loss [31] (Figure 22.1).

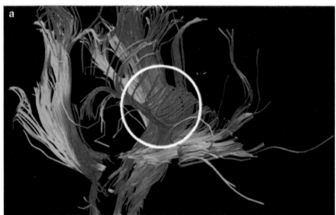

Figure 22.1 DTI fiber tracking (a) and HDFT (b) in a TBI patient at 17 weeks post injury. The DTI fiber tracking shows inaccurate fiber directions and termination points (white circle), whereas the HDFT scan shows accurate details of damaged areas of the right anterior corona radiata without false turns or false continuations. Improved structural accuracy and clinical correlation (motor weakness) was observed with HDFT versus DTI. Reproduced with permission from reference [31].

In coming years, the relationship between these radiological brain biomarkers of motor dysfunction to weakness may help to clarify mechanisms and predictors of weakness in different neurological disorders.

Neuroimaging and fatigue

Structural imaging

Structural imaging studies of fatigue have revealed mixed results depending on the techniques used and the clinical population examined. For instance, most of the early structural imaging studies in MS looking at cerebral abnormalities such as T2- and T1-weighted lesion load or brain parenchymal fraction showed little to no relationship with subjective fatigue (e.g [23]). However, recent studies with more advanced techniques such as voxel-based morphometry and DTI have been generally positive (e.g. [32, 33]), although not always (e.g. [34]). In general, these newer studies, although not all (e.g. [32]), tend to provide support for a model of central fatigue outlined by Chaudhuri and Behan [35], hypothesizing the importance of the non-motor structures of the basal ganglia and its connections (i.e. striatal-thalamic-frontal cortical system). For instance, Calabrese et al. [36] found significant atrophy in the basal ganglia, thalamus, superior frontal gyrus, and inferior parietal gyrus in fatigued versus non-fatigued MS subjects. In fact, numerous studies have now shown the critical role of the basal ganglia (Figure 22.2) and frontal-parietal regions (Figure 22.3) in understanding the neural mechanisms of fatigue [36].

Early structural imaging studies in CFS have also been mixed, with many studies showing increases in white-matter hyperintensities on MRI in these patients versus healthy controls (e.g. [37]), while others have not (e.g. [38]). More recently, studies have shown decreased cerebral volume [39], significantly reduced gray-matter volume, especially in the frontal lobes bilaterally [40], while reduced gray-matter volume in prefrontal cortex in CFS has been shown to be partially reversed with cognitive behavioral therapy [33].

Far fewer structural imaging studies have been conducted in populations other than MS and CFS. Pardini et al. [40] found that subjective fatigue was significantly more severe in persons with penetrating TBI with lesions in the ventromedial prefrontal cortex compared to patients without such lesions, TBI subjects with non-frontal lesions, and healthy controls. An increased load of white-matter hyperintensities was associated with increased subjective fatigue in systemic lupus erythematosus that cannot be explained by depression [41]. In stroke, the early imaging studies examining subjective fatigue have been few and inconclusive (see [42] for a review). However, recent studies in stroke patients found that acute basal ganglia infarcts, particularly in the caudate nucleus significantly predicted post-stroke fatigue [43]. Lastly, Tartaglia et al. [44] showed that increased subjective fatigue was correlated with decreases in the N-acetylaspartate-to-creatine (NAA/CR) ratio using proton magnetic resonance spectroscopy.

It is interesting that the brain regions associated with fatigue in the above studies have also been related to self-rating and self-perception. In a "virtual lesion" paradigm with transcranial magnetic stimulation, Amati et al. [45] demonstrated that dysfunction in medial prefrontal regions may reduce self-estimated abilities. This would be consistent with the idea of a magnitude estimation deficit in this disorder (abnormally decreased estimate of self-performance) separable from poor self-image or dysthymic affect, causing underestimation of self-performance [18].

Taken together, the structural studies overall provide a mixed picture with respect to brain parameters involved in fatigue. However, some limited support for involvement of the basal ganglia and frontal-lobe structures have been reported.

Functional imaging

As with structural imaging, most studies on functional imaging and fatigue come from work in MS and CFS (Figure 22.4).

The most common functional imaging techniques to study fatigue are fMRI and positron emission tomography (PET). For example, Roelcke et al. [46] measured cerebral glucose metabolism in MS patients using ^{18}F-fluorodeoxyglucose (FDG) PET. They found that the fatigued MS group showed significant hypometabolism in the putamen, prefrontal and premotor cortex, and the right supplementary motor area compared to non-fatigued MS. Using specific PET markers, Pavese et al. [47] found that fatigued PD patients had significantly lower serotonin transporter binding in the basal ganglia and thalamus versus non-fatigued patients. These studies suggest that abnormal metabolism in the basal ganglia, prefrontal regions, and thalamus are primary regions associated with fatigue.

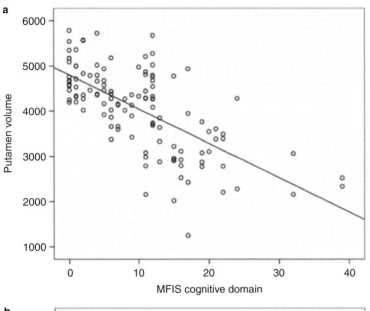

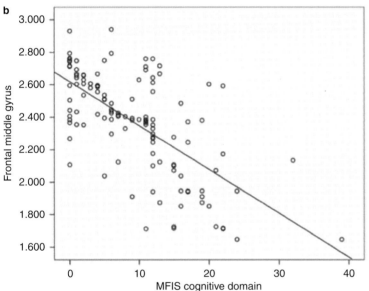

Figure 22.2 Correlations between the modified fatigue impact scale (MFIS) (cognitive domain) and (a) putamen volume (cubic millimeters) and (b) frontal middle gyrus thickness (millimetres). Reproduced with permission from reference [36].

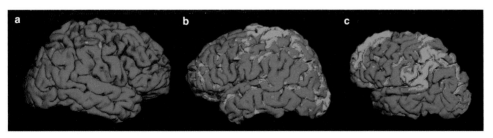

Figure 22.3 Pial surface three-dimensional representation with cortical thickness map overlaid in (a) healthy control, (b) not fatigued relapsing–remitting MS patient, and (c) fatigued relapsing–remitting MS patient. Cortical areas thinner than 2.0 mm are in green while areas greater than 2.0 mm are in red. Reproduced with permission from reference [36].

353

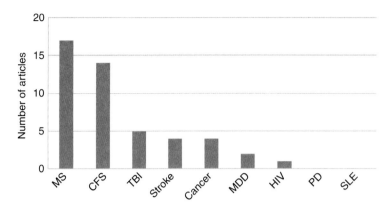

Figure 22.4 Functional neuroimaging articles published by clinical groups. MS = multiple sclerosis; CFS = chronic fatigue syndrome; TBI = traumatic brain injury; MDD = major depressive disorder; HIV = human immunodeficiency virus; PD = Parkinson's disease; SLE = systemic lupus erythematosus. All search terms were limited to English and Human with reviews, case studies, and commentaries excluded. We searched the Pubmed database with terms "("magnetic resonance imaging" OR MRI) OR ("diffusion tensor imaging" OR DTI) OR ("magnetic resonance spectroscopy" OR MRS) OR ("positron emission tomography" OR PET) OR ("single photon emission computerized tomography" OR SPECT) OR ("magnetoencephalography" OR MEG) OR ("magnetic resonance" OR MR) OR ("functional magnetic resonance imaging" OR fMRI) OR neuroimaging". Within those results, we searched "fatigue", "brain" and "functional imaging" and applied these results to each disease type.

Most studies by far have studied fatigue using fMRI. Using fMRI, Filippi *et al.* [23] reported that the fatigued MS group had significantly less functional activation in several regions involved in motor planning and execution compared to the non-fatigued MS group. These authors hypothesized that subjective fatigue was due to disruption of cortical–subcortical functional circuits between the thalamus, basal ganglia, and motor and prefrontal regions of the frontal lobes.

Most functional imaging studies have studied subjective ratings of fatigue. A recent approach is to assess cognitive fatigue objectively by inducing fatigue through task performance during fMRI acquisition, thereby examining brain regions associated with fatigue. DeLuca *et al.* [48] induced and objectively measured cognitive fatigue in MS by administering four trials of a sustained attention task during fMRI acquisition. While there were no group differences in performance accuracy with healthy controls, MS subjects showed a greater increase in brain activity across time relative to controls that showed decreased brain activity over time. Regions increased in MS included the precuneus, superior parietal lobe (BA7), medial/orbital frontal gyrus, inferior parietal lobe, and the caudate in the basal ganglia. A similar finding was observed when the study was conducted in persons with TBI [49] (Figure 22.5). Taken together, these data again support the model of central fatigue outlined by Chaudhuri and Behan [35]. One limitation of both of these studies was that subjective fatigue was not assessed. However, recent preliminary data suggest that subjective fatigue ratings are also strongly correlated with basal ganglia activation [50].

The influence of inducing cognitive fatigue on brain activation during a motor response (finger–thumb opposition task) was examined by Tartaglia *et al.* [51]. During fMRI acquisition, MS subjects first performed the motor task, after which cognitive fatigue was induced by performing a challenging cognitive task (the Paced Serial Addition Test (PASAT)), and then subjects repeated the motor task once again. Compared to the initial motor response, cerebral activation increased significantly on the motor task after fatigue was induced in MS, whereas activation decreased in healthy controls. Increased activation in MS was observed bilaterally in the cingulate gyrus, the postcentral gyrus, and the right prefrontal cortex. Thus, cognitive fatigue could alter the functional response of the brain on motor-task performance.

The relatively few studies examining subjective fatigue and functional imaging in populations other than MS and CFS have yielded generally mixed findings. No relationship was observed between FSS scores and cerebral blood flow in systemic lupus erythemathosus [52], while negative findings were also observed between subjective fatigue and FDG PET abnormalities in HIV-positive patients [53]. Two studies in PD looked at the availability of dopamine in the basal ganglia using single photon emission computed tomography (SPECT) and found no significant relationship with subjective fatigue [54]. In contrast, Abe *et al.* [55] showed reduced frontal lobe perfusion on SPECT and subjective fatigue in PD patients. Fatigue was not associated with depression or degree of disability in this study. Looking at fMRI during the resting state in TBI, Shumskaya *et al.* [56] found

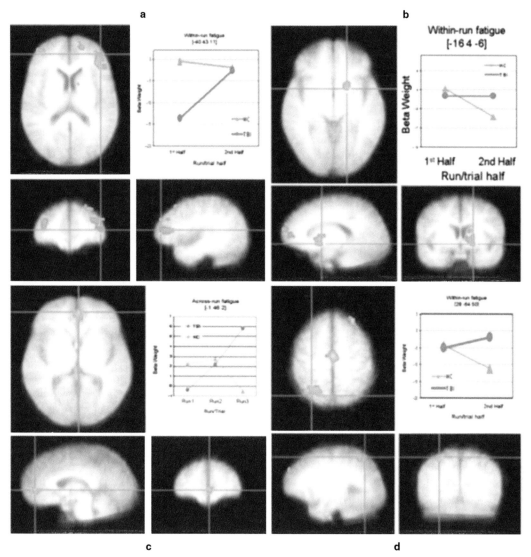

Figure 22.5 Brain activation using fMRI during performance of a fatiguing task in patients with TBI. Axial, corona, and sagittal views for the interaction between group (TBI and healthy) and fatigue (insert graph). Areas of activation include: (a) left frontal middle gyrus; (b) left basal ganglia (caudate/putamen); (c) left anterior cingulate; (d) right superior parietal lobule. Reproduced with permission from reference [49].

abnormal increases in functional connectivity in the right frontoparietal network, and suggested that this abnormal connectivity may be associated with "excessive cognitive fatigue" experienced by persons with TBI.

Conclusions

Although often considered clinically as relatively straightforward with respect to assessment and treatment, it is clear that both weakness and especially fatigue remain nebulous yet ubiquitous constructs.

While highly correlated at clinical presentation, they can be distinguishable with the proper clinical assessment. True muscle weakness must be differentiated from vague complaints of weakness. Self-reported complaints of fatigue are highly correlated with psychopathology; however, they are often separable, and require a keen clinical assessment to disentangle the relationship.

Neuroimaging techniques offer the possibility of improving our assessment of both weakness and fatigue, although neuroimaging requires additional research in order for it to become a mainstream clinical tool for these symptoms. The work with fatigue is particularly promising where there is increasing support and consensus regarding the role of the basal ganglia and its various cerebral connections, which appear to play a pivotal role in our understanding of fatigue. Many neuroimaging studies across several populations tend to support the Chaudhuri and Behan [35] model suggesting that fatigue results from a "failure in the integration of limbic input and motor functions within the basal ganglia affecting the striatal-thalamic-frontal cortical system". Thus, one can at least be hopeful that our increased understanding of the neural underpinnings of the vague concept of fatigue may lead to improved methods for its study and ultimately for its treatment.

References

1. Rowland LP (2010). Syndromes caused by weak muscles. In Rowland LP, Pedley TA, eds. *Merritt's Textbook of Neurology*, 12th edn. Philadelphia, PA: Kluwer, Lippincott Williams and Wilkins, pp. 54–57.

2. Friedman JH, Abrantes A'M. (2012). Self-perceived weakness in Parkinson's disease. *Parkinsonism Related Disord* 18: 887–889.

3. DeLuca J (2005). *Fatigue as a Window to the Brain*. Cambridge, MA: MIT Press.

4. Wessely S, Hotopf M, Sharpe MN (1998). *Chronic Fatigue and its Syndromes*. New York: Oxford University Press.

5. Schwid SR, Thornton CA, Pandya S, *et al.* (1999). Quantitative assessment of motor fatigue and strength in MS. *Neurology* 53: 743–750.

6. Kluger BM, Krupp LB, Enoka RM (2013). Fatigue and fatigability in neurological illness: proposal for a unified taxonomy. *Neurology* 80: 409–416.

7. Multiple Sclerosis Council for Clinical Practice Guidelines (1998). *Fatigue and Multiple Sclerosis: Evidence-Based Management Strategies for Fatigue in Multiple Sclerosis*. Washington, DC: Paralyzed Veterans of America.

8. Fukuda K, Straus SE, Hickie I, *et al.* (1994). The chronic fatigue syndrome: a comprehensive approach to its definition and study. International Chronic Fatigue Syndrome Study Group. *Annals Internal Med* 121: 953–959.

9. Hall GH, Hamilton WT, Round AP (1998). Increased illness experience preceding chronic fatigue syndrome: a case control study. *J Royal Coll Physicians* 32: 274.

10. Krupp LB, LaRocca NG, Muir J, Steinberg AD (1989). The Fatigue Severity Scale. Application to patients with multiple sclerosis and systemic lupus erythematosus. *Arch Neurol* 46: 1121–1123.

11. Chalder T, Berelowitz G, Pawlikowska T *et al.* (1993). Development of a fatigue scale. *J Psychosom. Res* 37: 147–153.

12. Ackerman PL, Kanfer R (2009). Test length and cognitive fatigue: an empirical examination of effects on performance and test-taker reactions. *J Exper Psychol App* 15: 163–181.

13. Stulemeijer M, Fasotti L, Bleijenberg G (2005). Fatigue after stroke. In DeLuca J, ed. *Fatigue as a Window to the Brain*. Cambridge: MIT Press, pp. 73–88.

14. Mead GE, Graham C, Dorman P, *et al.* (2011). Fatigue after stroke: baseline predictors and influence on survival. Analysis of data from UK patients recruited in the International Stroke Trial. *PLoS One* 6: e16988.

15. Tang WK, Lu JY, Mok V, Ungvari GS, Wong KS (2011). Is fatigue associated with suicidality in stroke? *Arch Phys Med Rehabil* 92: 1336–1338.

16. Naess H, Lunde L, Brogger J, Waje-Andreassen U (2012). Fatigue among stroke patients on long-term follow-up. The Bergen Stroke Study. *J Neurological Sci* 312: 138–141.

17. Balkin TJ, Westensten NJ (2011). Differentiation of sleepiness and mental fatigue effects. In Ackerman PL, ed. *Cognitive Fatigue*. Washington, DC: American Psychological Association, pp. 47–66.

18. Heilman KM, Watson RT, Valenstein E (1985). Neglect and related disorders. In Heliman KM, Valenstein E, eds. *Clinical Neuropsychology*, 2nd edn. New York: Oxford University Press.

19. Shulman LM, Katzel LI, Ivey FM, *et al.* (2013). Randomized clinical trial of 3 types of physical exercise for patients with Parkinson disease. *JAMA Neurol* 70: 183–190.

20. Cup EH, Pieterse AJ, Ten Broek-Pastoor JM, *et al.* (2007). Exercise therapy and other types of physical therapy for patients with neuromuscular diseases: a systematic review. *Arch Phys Med Rehabil* 88: 1452–1464.

21. Yousry TA, Berry I, Filippi M (1998). Functional magnetic resonance imaging in multiple sclerosis. *J Neurol Neurosurg Psychiatry* 64 (suppl 1): S85–87.

22. Tomassini V, Matthews PM, Thompson AJ, *et al.* (2012). Neuroplasticity and functional recovery in multiple sclerosis. *Nature Rev Neurol:* 8: 635–646.

23. Filippi M, Rocca MA, Falini A, *et al.* (2002). Correlations between structural CNS damage and functional MRI changes in primary progressive MS. *Neuroimage* 15: 537–546.

24. Mohammadi B, Kollewe K, Samii A, Dengler R, Munte TF (2011). Functional imaging at different disease stages reveals distinct phases of neuroplastic changes in

amyotrophic lateral sclerosis. *Hum Brain Mapp* **32**: 750–758.

25. Reich DS, Zackowskia KM, Gordon-Lipkina EM, *et al.* (2008). Corticospinal tract abnormalities are associated with weakness in multiple sclerosis. *AJNR* **29**: 333–339.

26. Yeo SS, Choi BY, Chang CH, *et al.* (2012). Evidence of corticospinal tract injury at midbrain in patients with subarachnoid hemorrhage. *Stroke* **43**: 2239–2241.

27. Choi GS, Kim OL, Kim SH, *et al.* (2012). Classification of cause of motor weakness in traumatic brain injury using diffusion tensor imaging. *Arch Neurol* **69**: 363–367.

28. Madhavan S, Krishnan C, Jayaraman A, Rymer WZ, Stinear JW (2011). Corticospinal tract integrity correlates with knee extensor weakness in chronic stroke survivors. *Clin Neurophysiol* **122**: 1588–1594.

29. Morita N, Wang S, Kadakia P, *et al.* (2011). Diffusion tensor imaging of the corticospinal tract in patients with brain neoplasm. *Magn Reson Med Sci* **10**: 239–243.

30. Jang SH, Ahn SH, Sakong J, *et al.* (2010). Comparison of TMS and DTT for predicting motor outcome in intracranial hemorrhage. *J Neurological Sci* **15**: 107–111.

31. Shin SS, Verstynen T, Pathak S, *et al.* (2012). High-definition fiber tracking for assessment of neurological deficit in a case of traumatic brain injury: finding, visualization, and interpreting small sites of damage. *J Neurosurg* **116**: 1062–1069.

32. Riccitelli G, Rocca MA, Forn C, *et al.* (2011). Voxelwise assessment of the regional distribution of damage in the brains of patients with multiple sclerosis and fatigue. *AJNR* **32**: 874–879.

33. de Lange F, Koers A, Kalkman J, *et al.* (2008). Increase in prefrontal cortical volume following cognitive behavioural therapy in patients with chronic fatigue syndrome. *Brain* **131**: 2172–2180.

34. Codella M, Rocca M, Colombo B, *et al.* (2002). Cerebral grey matter pathology and fatigue in patients with multiple sclerosis: a preliminary study. *J Neurol Sci* **194**: 71–74.

35. Chaudhuri A, Behan PO (2000). Fatigue and basal ganglia. *J Neurological Sci* **179**: 34–42.

36. Calabrese M, Rinaldi F, Grossi P, *et al.* (2010). Basal ganglia and frontal/parietal cortical atrophy is associated with fatigue in relapsing–remitting multiple sclerosis. *Multiple Sclerosis* **6**: 1220–1228.

37. Lange G, DeLuca J, Maldjian J, *et al.* (1999). Brain MRI abnormalities exist in a subset of patients with chronic fatigue syndrome. *J Neurol Sci* **171**: 3–7.

38. Cope H, Pernet A, Kendall B, David A (1995). Cognitive functioning and magnetic resonance imaging in chronic fatigue. *Br J Psychiatry* **167**: 86–94.

39. Lange G, Holodny A, DeLuca J, *et al.* (2001). Quantitative assessment of cerebral ventricular volumes in chronic fatigue syndrome. *Appl Neuropsychol* **8**: 23–30.

40. Pardini M, Krueger F, Raymont V, Grafman J (2010). Ventromedial prefrontal cortex modulates fatigue after penetrating traumatic brain injury. *Neurology* **74**: 749–754.

41. Harboe E, Greve OJ, Beyer M, *et al.* (2008). Fatigue is associated with cerebral white matter hyperintensities in patients with systemic lupus erythematosus. *JNNP* **79**: 199–201.

42. Kutlubaev MA, Duncan FH, Mead GE (2012). Biological correlates of post-stroke fatigue: a systematic review. *Acta Neurol Scand* **125**: 219–227.

43. Tang WK, Liang, HJ, Chen YK, *et al.* (2012). Poststroke fatigue is associated with caudate infarcts. *J Neurol Sci* **324**: 131–135.

44. Tartaglia M, Narayanan S, Francis S, *et al.* (2004). The relationship between diffuse axonal damage and fatigue in multiple sclerosis. *Arch Neurol* **61**: 201–207.

45. Amati F, Oh H, Kwan VSY, Jordan K, Keenan JP (2010). Overclaiming and the medial prefrontal cortex: a transcranial magnetic stimulation study. *Cogn Neurosci* **1**: 268–276.

46. Roelcke U, Kappos L, Lechner-Scott J, *et al.* (1997). Reduced glucose metabolism in the frontal cortex and basal ganglia of multiple sclerosis patients with fatigue: a ^{18}F-fluorodeoxyglucose positron emission tomography study. *Neurology* **48**: 1566–1571.

47. Pavese N, Metta V, Bose SK, Chaudhuri KR, Brooks DJ (2010). Fatigue in Parkinson's disease is linked to striatal and limbic serotonergic dysfunction. *Brain* **133**: 3434–3443.

48. DeLuca J, Genova H, Hillary F, Wylie G (2008). Neural correlates of cognitive fatigue in multiple sclerosis using functional MRI. *J Neurol Sci* **270**: 28–39.

49. Kohl AD, Wylie GR, Genova HM, Hillary FG, DeLuca J (2009). The neural correlates of cognitive fatigue in traumatic brain injury using functional MRI. *Brain Injury* **23**: 420–432.

50. Wylie GR, Genova H, DeLuca J, Chiaravalloti, N (2012). An investigation of cognitive fatigue in Traumatic Brain Injury using functional magnetic resonance imaging. Presented at the 40th Annual Meeting International Neuropsychological Society, Montreal, QC.

51. Tartaglia M, Narayanan S, Arnold D (2008). Mental fatigue alters the pattern and increases the volume of cerebral activation required for a motor task in multiple

sclerosis patients with fatigue. *Eur J Neurol* **15**: 413–419.

52. Omdal R, Sjöholm H, Koldingsnes W, *et al.* (2005). Fatigue in patients with lupus is not associated with disturbances in cerebral blood flow as detected by SPECT. *J Neurol* **252**: 78–83.

53. Andersen AB, Law I, Ostrowski S, *et al.* (2006). Self-reported fatigue common among optimally treated HIV patients: no correlation with cerebral FDG PET scanning abnormalities. *Neuroimmunomodulation* **13**: 69–75.

54. Schifitto G, Friedman JH, Oakes D, *et al.* (2008). Fatigue in levodopa-naive subjects with Parkinson disease. *Neurology* **71**: 481–485.

55. Abe K, Takanashi M, Yanagihara T (2000). Fatigue in patients with Parkinson's disease. *Behav Neurol* **12**: 103–106.

56. Shumskaya E, Andriessen TM, Norris DG, Vos PE (2012). Abnormal whole-brain functional networks in homogeneous acute mild traumatic brain injury. *Neurology* **79**: 175–182.

Chapter 23

Hearing loss and tinnitus

Mirabelle B. Sajisevi, David M. Kaylie, and Jane L. Weissman

Introduction

Acute hearing loss may be evidence of localized (temporal bone) or systemic disease [1]. Acute tinnitus as an isolated presentation is very rare. However, hearing loss and (non-pulsatile) tinnitus are so closely intertwined that consideration of one merits consideration of the other. In this chapter we will show the intimate relationship between hearing loss, both sensorineural and conductive, with tinnitus.

The presentation of hearing loss and tinnitus is a completely subjective experience. There is often no outward, objective manifestation of inner-ear dysfunction other than patients' reports. For this reason, the acute nature of the start of symptoms is somewhat dependent on patient reporting. This chapter will describe many entities that can lead to hearing loss and/or tinnitus, and we will describe the likelihood of presentation as an acute symptom. Several of these processes are very likely to present immediately with inner-ear symptoms, and others may be less likely to have inner-ear symptoms as the acute presentation; however, they all should remain in the differential diagnosis.

Hearing loss and tinnitus: background

Hearing loss (HL) is either unilateral or bilateral. Bilateral HL may be asymmetric [2]. The division of both acute and chronic HL into sensorineural hearing loss (SNHL) and conductive hearing loss (CHL) focuses the search for an etiology.

Tinnitus is the perception of auditory sensation, often in the absence of external stimuli [3, 4]. Tinnitus is classified as pulsatile (synchronous with heartbeat) and non-pulsatile (continuous), and further classified as subjective (perceived by the patient only) and objective (perceived by the examiner as well as by the patient) [2]. Tinnitus may be unilateral or bilateral.

Tinnitus occurs as a result of hyperactivity in auditory brainstem nuclei. Therefore, it is hypothesized that diseases directly affecting the brainstem can result in tinnitus. Advanced microvascular disease and demyelinating diseases such as multiple sclerosis (MS) affecting the brainstem may cause tinnitus [2]. Chiari I malformation may also result in tinnitus, believed to be due to stretching of the vestibulocochlear nerve [5]. Magnetic resonance imaging (MRI) of the brainstem is the imaging modality of choice [2, 5]. However, except for brainstem infarction and MS, these etiologies are rarely if ever acute.

The most frequent causes of pulsatile tinnitus are vascular tumors (such as glomus tumors and hemangiomas), vascular malformations, and vascular pathology (both arterial and venous) [2, 5–7]. Continuous (non-pulsatile) tinnitus accompanies inner-ear and eighth-cranial-nerve pathology, i.e., often non-pulsatile tinnitus is associated with hearing loss [8]. Continuous tinnitus also accompanies the abnormal muscular contraction of palatal myoclonus and stapedial myoclonus [6, 9].

Tinnitus can be further classified as objective or subjective. Objective tinnitus usually has an identifiable source [1, 6]. A stethoscope can be used to auscultate the eye, preauricular area, parietal or occipital scalp, mastoid, and neck. Subjective tinnitus [2] is the most frequent type of tinnitus but the least likely to have a treatable cause. Non-pulsatile tinnitus is almost always subjective [2].

SNHL (with or without tinnitus)

SNHL is evidence of malfunction of the inner ear, eighth cranial nerve, or brain (including the contralateral and ipsilateral superior olivary complex, lateral lemniscus, inferior colliculus, and finally the medial geniculate nucleus, which is the last auditory nucleus

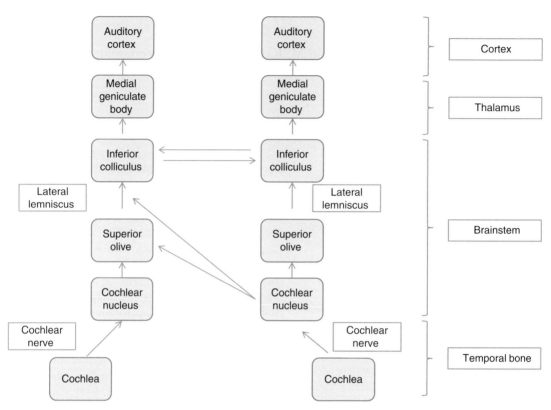

Figure 23.1 The auditory pathway

before the cerebral auditory cortex) [10]. The auditory central nervous system pathways are complex, having both ascending and descending as well as excitatory and inhibitory pathways [10]. Knowledge of the pathways helps guide the central nervous system search for causes of SNHL (Figure 23.1).

Asymmetric SNHL refers to a difference in hearing thresholds or speech discrimination scores between the two ears. There is no uniformly agreed upon definition of asymmetric sensorineural hearing loss. Several have been proposed, and generally a pure-tone threshold difference of 10–15 dB or greater at two contiguous frequencies and/or a speech discrimination difference of greater than 15% between the two ears is considered significant [11].

The most frequent identifiable cause of acute unilateral or asymmetric acute SNHL is a tumor of the cerebellopontine angle (CPA) cistern or internal auditory canal (IAC), and the most frequent of these is a vestibular schwannoma (also known, inaccurately, as acoustic neuroma) [5, 12] (Figure 23.2). Vestibular schwannomas arise from the superior or inferior

division of the vestibular division of the eighth cranial nerve [13]. Other tumors of the IAC and CPA include facial schwannoma, meningioma, and hemangioma [14–16]. Compression of the cochlear nerve or its arterial supply is thought to be the mechanism of sensorineural hearing loss [5]. This is why vestibular schwannomas, though arising from the vestibular nerve, usually present with SNHL. Acute sudden SNHL is frequently the initial presenting symptom of a patient with retrocochlear pathology (i.e. eighth nerve or brain), so therefore it is imperative to image these patients. CPA tumors should remain high in the differential diagnosis of acute SNHL.

In patients with unilateral tinnitus but symmetric hearing loss, the diagnosis of vestibular schwannoma, though less likely, still must be considered. The tumor may be bilateral in the setting of neurofibromatosis type 2. The patient may also have baseline symmetric hearing loss with unilateral tinnitus as the presenting symptom of unilateral acoustic neuroma. Tinnitus as the sole presenting symptom of acoustic neuroma ranges from 2 to 4% [17]. This relatively low percentage makes imaging more debatable in patients with symmetric hearing and unilateral tinnitus. If patients have other associated symptoms or clinical signs, consideration can be given to MRI.

Because schwannomas and meningiomas are usually T2 hypointense, thin-section T2-weighted images

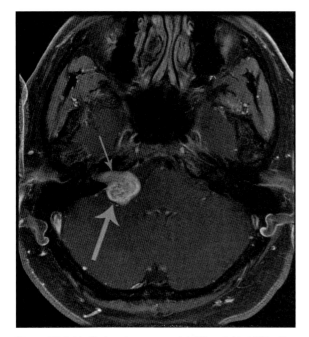

Figure 23.2 Vestibular schwannoma. Axial T1-weighted MRI with gadolinium shows an enhancing mass that fills the right IAC (thin arrow) and extends into the CPA cistern (thick arrow). A meningioma could have the same appearance.

can be used as a screening examination (Figure 23.3a). If the normal IAC contents are not seen well, gadolinium contrast-enhanced T1-weighted images provide additional information (Figure 23.3b).

Large vestibular aqueduct syndrome (LVAS) is the imaging findings of enlarged vestibular aqueduct and other associated inner-ear malformations in the setting of profound SNHL [18, 19]. Computed tomography (CT) shows the enlarged vestibular aqueduct (part of the osseous labyrinth). MRI shows the enlarged endolymphatic duct (part of the membranous labyrinth). Often, the endolymphatic sac is also enlarged: both MRI and CT can detect this. LVAS is one of the most frequent causes of progressive and sudden SNHL in children. In many cases, hearing loss occurs acutely after minor head trauma [18] and in 80% of patients is bilateral [18]. Some authors define a large aqueduct (CT) or duct (MRI) as one with a diameter greater than 1.5 mm [18, 19]. In addition, a larger endolymphatic duct at its origin at the vestibule, compared to size farther out along the duct, correlates with worse hearing [18]. There is a high likelihood that LVAS will present acutely, and, therefore, any child presenting with acute SNHL, with or without tinnitus, should undergo MRI (or CT) to evaluate for LVAS.

Temporal-bone trauma frequently presents with acute SNHL with or without tinnitus. Temporal-bone fractures that violate the inner ear may cause immediate, profound, and often irreversible hearing loss [20] (Figure 23.4). Temporal-bone trauma may cause SNHL loss by direct damage to the cochlear

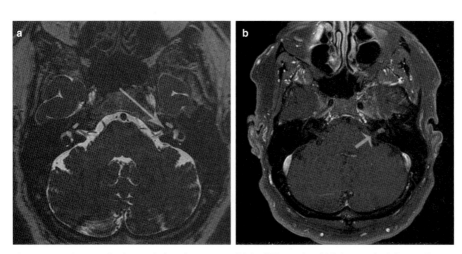

Figure 23.3 Intracanalicular vestibular schwannoma. (a) Axial T2-weighted MR (2-mm slice) shows a hypointense mass (arrow) surrounded by CSF in the fundus (lateral aspect) of the left IAC. (b) Axial T1-weighted image with gadolinium (same patient as in a) shows that the mass (arrow) enhances intensely.

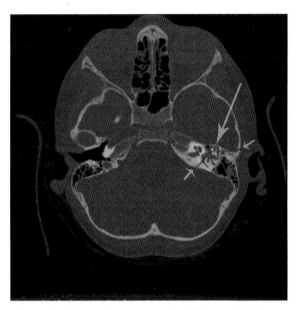

Figure 23.4 Temporal-bone trauma. Axial CT (1-mm thick, bone algorithm) shows an oblique fracture (short arrows) through the left temporal bone, crossing the vestibule. The middle ear is opacified (blood). The "ice cream cone" (ice cream is malleus head, cone is incus body and short process) is slightly malaligned (long arrow), indicating subluxation of the articulation between the two ossicles. The vestibule fracture could cause SNHL. Both the ossicular subluxation and the middle ear blood cause CHL.

nerve, disruption of the membranous labyrinth even without fracture (cochlear concussion), vascular compromise, or hemorrhage into the cochlea [20]. Although SNHL is usually complete and irreversible, some of the damage may be reversible with treatment with a steroid taper [21].

Menière's disease is a clinical [22] (not imaging) diagnosis consisting of episodes of vertigo, SNHL, aural fullness, and tinnitus [23]. The SNHL generally fluctuates with the episodes, affecting one or both ears [11]. One hypothesis is that the tinnitus may be related to endolymphatic hydrops [24]. Imaging in the patient with Menière's disease (generally MRI of the temporal bones and brain) is obtained to exclude other causes of the symptoms and hearing loss [22], and not to make the diagnosis of Menière's disease. The symptoms of Menière's disease can be quite disturbing to patients and it is imperative to rule out severe, acute, potentially treatable pathology, including stroke.

Occupational, environmental, and recreational exposure to noise can result in acute and permanent SHL with associated tinnitus [11, 25]. There are no known imaging findings.

Intracranial hypertension is an important cause of pulsatile tinnitus [6]. This may have an identifiable

cause (e.g. an obstructing mass causing hydrocephalus), or may be so-called idiopathic intracranial hypertension (IIH). IIH (formerly known as pseudotumor cerebri) may present with acute pulsatile tinnitus [2, 26], and with multiple symptoms in addition to the tinnitus, including headache and vision disturbances [2]. Previously, imaging studies in IIH were believed not to show abnormalities [2]. However, it is now known that MRI may show fullness of the optic nerve heads and flattening of the posterior surface of the globes (the MRI correlate of papilledema), cerebrospinal fluid (CSF) distending the optic nerve sheaths, and so-called empty sella (CSF flattening the pituitary along the floor of the sella). IIH rarely presents as acute pulsatile tinnitus, but should be kept in the differential diagnosis.

MRI is the study of choice for patients with unilateral or asymmetric SNHL with or without continuous tinnitus. Because most CPA tumors are hypointense with respect to CSF on T2-weighted sequences, some have advocated "high-resolution" (1-mm slice thickness, or less) T2-weighted MRI for screening of the IAC [27]. If the normal IAC contents are not clearly seen, additional pulse sequences can be obtained after gadolinium administration. If MS or acute ischemia are possible etiologies, brain imaging including diffusion-weighted MRI for acute stroke sensitivity, T2 and fluid-attenuated inversion recovery (FLAIR) and pre- and post-contrast images of the brain should be obtained as well.

Conductive hearing loss (with or without tinnitus)

Conductive hearing loss results from pathology of the middle ear and "outer" ear (including external auditory canal). Non-pulsatile tinnitus can be associated with conductive hearing loss.

Obstruction of the external auditory canal by cerumen, tumors, or stenosis can lead to CHL, and obstruction of the ear canal with foreign bodies or cerumen can cause acute CHL as can acute otitis media. This can be diagnosed with otoscopy and generally does not require imaging. Congenital or acquired cholesteatoma can present with CHL in 60–87% of patients [28], but again this is not acute.

Otosclerosis is an idiopathic osteodystrophy of the temporal bone, and primarily the otic capsule [29]. Overgrowth of abnormal bone at the oval window occurs in stages, starting with a hypervascular

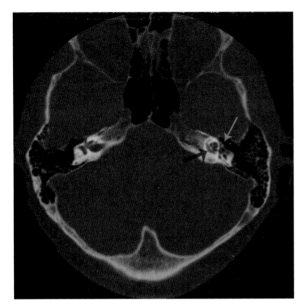

Figure 23.5 Otosclerosis. Axial CT (1-mm slice, bone algorithm) shows overgrowth of abnormally lucent bone anterior to the left oval window in the location of the fissula ante fenestram (fenestral otosclerosis) (white arrow), and a lucent halo around the left cochlea (cochlear or retrofenestral otosclerosis) (black arrow).

otospongiosis stage [29] called fenestral otospongiosis, which on CT appears as abnormal radiolucent bone at the fissula ante fenestram [5] just anterior to the oval window (Figure 23.5). Pulsatile tinnitus often accompanies this phase. The vascular spaces eventually fill in with bone causing stapes fixation and tinnitus which is often non-pulsatile. As the disease progresses, sometimes sclerotic bone overgrowth can be seen at the margin of the oval window [5]. A lucent halo around the cochlea on CT (called retrofenestral or cochlear otosclerosis) is often seen in the presence of mixed hearing loss (SNHL and CHL). Sometimes the abnormal bone of otosclerosis is faintly hyperintense on T2-weighted images. It is very unlikely that a patient with otosclerosis will present acutely with hearing loss and/or tinnitus. These symptoms progress slowly and otosclerosis should remain low on the differential diagnosis of patients with acute hearing loss with or without tinnitus.

Head trauma, including from blast injury, isolated barotrauma, direct penetration of the ear drum, and temporal-bone fracture, may cause CHL [30]. Any trauma causing middle-ear hemorrhage will cause CHL, as blood interferes with normal movement of the ossicles. Additionally, longitudinal temporal-bone fractures displace the posterosuperior wall of the external auditory canal and the tegmen tympani,

creating a shearing effect within the middle ear, tympanic membrane rupture, and disarticulation of the ossicular chain [30] (Figure 23.4). Any patient who experiences head trauma with acute hearing loss with or without tinnitus should be evaluated for temporal-bone fracture and middle-ear injury. Imaging should include high-resolution (e.g. ≤ 1-mm slice thickness) CT imaging with multiplanar reformats.

Tinnitus (additional causes)

Pulsatile tinnitus can arise from turbulent blood flow due to vascular malformations, vascular tumors, heart disease, or vascular occlusion [2, 8]. Arterial dissection (with luminal occlusion or narrowing) is the most likely to be acute [2].

Venous etiologies

Abnormalities of the dural venous sinuses and jugular bulb are not uncommon, but they rarely will present as acute tinnitus. When they do, it is most likely pulsatile in nature. Although acute presentation is rare, it is worth noting the venous etiologies that can be the cause of pulsatile tinnitus.

A dural venous sinus stenosis can result in turbulent flow and pulsatile tinnitus [2]. CT venography (CTV) or MR venography (MRV) are both able to detect this [2]. Sigmoid sinus thrombosis can result in variable clinical presentations including acute pulsatile tinnitus [31, 32]. Both MRI (with MRV) and CT (with CTV) can detect dural venous sinus thrombus [33] (Figure 23.6).

An aberrant sigmoid sinus runs anteromedially from the usual sigmoid sinus course [2]. Venous pulsations can be transmitted into the inner ear through the posterior semicircular canal or endolymphatic sac. MRV can show the aberrant course of the vessel, but CT shows the relationships to various osseous structures to advantage [2]. The dural sinuses are paired, although one side is usually larger [2]. This asymmetry is generally considered a normal variant. However, if there is a focal stenosis of a dural venous sinus, there can be turbulent blood flow causing tinnitus [2, 32, 34, 35].

Auscultation of the distal (low cervical) portion of the internal jugular vein demonstrates a venous hum in approximately half the adult population [2]. Compression of the jugular vein, by a mass for example, may result in turbulent flow resulting in tinnitus [2]. CT of the neck and upper chest can aid in diagnosis [2].

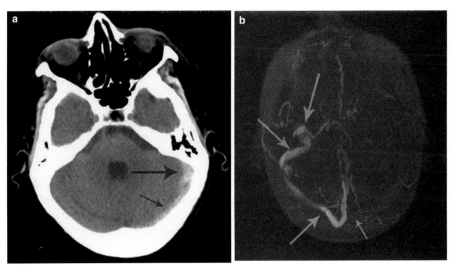

Figure 23.6 Dural venous sinus thrombosis. (a) Axial CT of the brain without intravenous contrast shows abnormal hyperdensity of the thrombus in the left transverse sinus (small arrow) and at the junction of the transverse and sigmoid sinuses (long arrow). (b) Axial view of an MRV of the same patient shows absence of the expected signal in the left transverse sinus (short arrow) and sigmoid sinus and internal jugular vein. The three corresponding structures on the right side have normal hyperintensity (long arrows).

Jugular bulb variants have been reported as causes of pulsatile tinnitus [2]. The jugular bulb is an expansion at the junction of the sigmoid sinus and the internal jugular vein at the skull base [2,5]. If the most cephalad portion of the jugular bulb extends superior to the tympanic annulus (the ring of bone to which the tympanic membrane attaches) it is considered to be a "high riding jugular bulb" [2, 36]. A jugular-bulb diverticulum is defined as a focal polypoid extension of the jugular bulb superiorly between the posterior wall of the IAC and the vestibular aqueduct [7, 32]. Dehiscence of the jugular bulb is another variant in which a superolateral extension of the jugular bulb protrudes into the middle-ear cavity through a dehiscent sigmoid plate [2, 5, 7, 32]. These are seen best on CT of the temporal bone, often in the coronal plane [2]. No intravenous contrast is necessary as it is the osseous anatomy that is important. When these variants are identified it may be important that other causes of pulsatile tinnitus continue to be pursued [37], as it is unclear how or why these variants cause acute tinnitus.

Arterial etiologies

Internal carotid artery (ICA) dissection or stenosis can cause turbulent blood flow and result in pulsatile tinnitus [2, 38, 39]. Acute carotid artery dissection is likely to present with acute pulsatile tinnitus, and it should remain high in the differential diagnosis of acute

pulsatile tinnitus. CT angiography (CTA) and magnetic resonance angiography (MRA) can both identify the intimal flap and narrowed arterial lumen [2, 39]. Fat-suppressed T1-weighted axial MRI shows the intrinsically hyperintense methemoglobin in the false lumen of the arterial dissection [39] (Figure 23.7). Gadolinium administration is not necessary to identify the narrowed ICA lumen or methemoglobin on axial images.

Fibromuscular dysplasia is an idiopathic, non-inflammatory, and non-atherosclerotic disease leading to stenosis of small and medium-sized arteries [40]. When it affects the internal carotid arteries, the most common presentation is intracranial ischemia but tinnitus is the next most common presentation [2]. CTA [39] and MRA are both able to confirm the diagnosis, as is the more invasive catheter angiography. All show the characteristic beaded appearance of the affected artery, caused by multiple focal stenoses and dilations [2]. Angiography is not required for diagnosis but may be used if an interventional procedure is planned [2].

Atherosclerosis of the intracranial (petrous, cavernous) and extracranial (cervical) ICA is very common. Tinnitus can result from stenosis of the artery anywhere along its course, especially at the carotid bifurcation or petrous carotid [2, 6]. Calcified plaques are the hallmark of the disease, which can be precisely characterized on CTA [2] and MRI/MRA. Atherosclerosis is a chronic, slowly progressive problem, which generally does not present with acute pulsatile

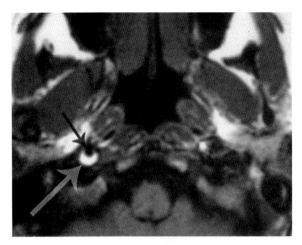

Figure 23.7 Internal carotid artery dissection. Axial T1-weighted MRI (no gadolinium) shows the right ICA lumen (black arrow) partially surrounded and narrowed by a hyperintense crescent (white arrow) that represents methemoglobin in the false lumen of the arterial dissection.

tinnitus. It should remain low on the differential diagnosis of acute pulsatile tinnitus.

An aberrant ICA develops when the ICA fails to develop normally in utero [2, 5, 37]. A collateral vessel, the inferior tympanic artery, undergoes compensatory hypertrophy and anastomosis with the caroticotympanic artery in the middle ear [5]. The enlarged inferior tympanic artery enters the skull through its own foramen, the inferior tympanic canaliculus, and courses through the medial portion of the middle ear, where it may have the CT appearance of a mass, and then joins up with the petrous carotid artery [5]. This is a rare entity and should be low on the list of causes for acute pulsatile tinnitus.

Dehiscence of the ICA canal is more common in the setting of aberrant ICA and usually occurs near the basal turn of the cochlea [5, 7, 26]. The carotid is considered dehiscent if it lacks a boney covering as it courses through the mesotympanum [2]. CT is the imaging modality of choice, with the aberrant ICA appearing as a tubular structure coursing horizontally through the middle ear and there is dehiscence if the latter is present [5]. Dehiscence of the ICA is also unlikely to present as an acute pulsatile tinnitus.

A persistent stapedial artery can occur with a normal ICA or in conjunction with an aberrant carotid artery [6, 41]. The stapedial artery is a fetal artery that normally undergoes regression before birth [5]. A persistent stapedial artery may be seen on CT as an aberrant vessel in the middle ear as it runs across the promontory before coursing along the tympanic portion of the facial nerve to enter into the middle cranial fossa [5].

Additional findings on CT include an absent foramen spinosum, subtle enlargement of the tympanic segment of the ipsilateral facial nerve inferior to the lateral semicircular canal, and a unique relationship of aberrant vessel to the stapes [2, 5]. Persistent stapedial artery is a rare congenital anomaly and is low on the differential diagnosis of acute pulsatile tinnitus.

An aneurysm adjacent to the vestibulocochlear nerve may cause pulsatile tinnitus [2]. CTA and MRA may both be diagnostic. CTA and catheter arteriography have comparable diagnostic accuracy in aneurysms larger than 5 mm [42]. Catheter angiography is indicated if endovascular embolization (treatment) is contemplated.

Vascular malformations

Arteriovenous malformations (AVMs) are abnormal communications between arteries and veins. They can be situated in the dura, brain parenchyma, or extracranial soft tissues [2, 43] (Figure 23.8). Extracranial AVMs are usually clinically evident. Parenchymal AVMs are characterized by a tangle of enlarged or numerous arteries and veins around a central nidus [2]. Dural AVMs, also known as dural arteriovenous fistulas, usually have a direct communication between an artery and a vein without an intervening nidus [5]. The cavernous sinus and transverse sinus are frequently involved [41]. Findings of AVM on MRI include flow-void clusters, an engorged superior ophthalmic vein, white-matter hyperintensities due to gliosis from shunting of blood, intracranial hemorrhages, and vascular enhancement or dilated leptomeningeal medullary vessels [5]. MRA findings may include an identifiable fistula, the presence of venous-flow-related enhancement, and the prominence of extracranial vessels [5, 43]. CTA is also used for the detection of dural arteriovenous fistulae [44, 45], which are often overlooked initially by imaging as the findings can be subtle. However, combined signs of abnormally prominent arterial feeders, "shaggy" tentorium, and asymmetric jugular venous attenuation (evidence of early venous drainage) have an accuracy greater than 90% [44]. Cerebral catheter angiography allows endovascular treatment (embolization) as well as diagnosis [2, 5, 43, 44].

Vascular tumors

Glomus tumors are benign vascular tumors that arise from glomus bodies, structures of neural crest origin. Glomus tympanicum tumors arise along the course of

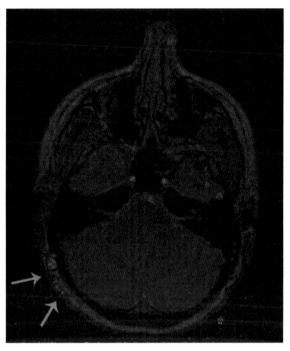

Figure 23.8 Arteriovenous fistula. Axial base image from time-of-flight MRI shows a cluster of abnormal vessels (arrows) in the scalp overlying the right occipital bone.

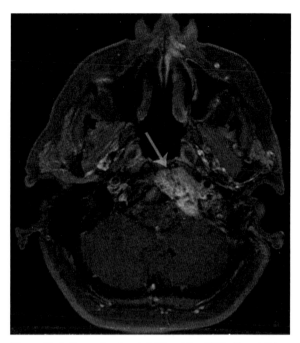

Figure 23.9 Glomus jugulare. Axial T1-weighted MRI with gadolinium and fat suppression shows an intensely but heterogeneously enhancing mass (arrow) extending beyond the left jugular fossa into the clivus. The hypointensities are tumor vessels. The enhancing tumor and the hypointense tumor vessels create the "salt and pepper" MRI appearance characteristic of glomus tumors.

Jacobson's nerve on the medial aspect of the middle ear [2]. They are most frequently located on the cochlear promontory but can arise anywhere in the medial mesotympanum [2]. CT is the imaging modality of choice due to the fact that glomus tympanicum tumors are surrounded by bone and air [2]. When small, the tumor can be seen as a round mass on the cochlear promontory. Glomus tumors show intense enhancement on MRI, but enhancement may be difficult to appreciate on CT, especially in small glomus tympanicum tumors [2]. Cavernous hemangioma of the middle ear can mimic glomus tympanicum clinically, on CT and MRI, and on otoscopy [2].

Glomus jugulare tumors arise in the jugular bulb and can erode the cortex of the jugular fossa and extend into the middle ear [2]. On CT, characteristic erosion of the superior lateral jugular foramen is a diagnostic clue [2]. MRI studies (both T2-weighted images and gadolinium-enhanced T1-weighted images) reveal high-signal-intensity tumor parenchyma interspersed with numerous flow voids, the "salt and pepper" appearance [2] (Figure 23.9). The inferior extent of the tumor may be difficult to identify

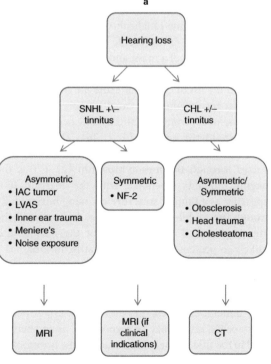

Figure 23.10 Diagnostic algorithms: (a) for hearing loss and (b) for tinnitus

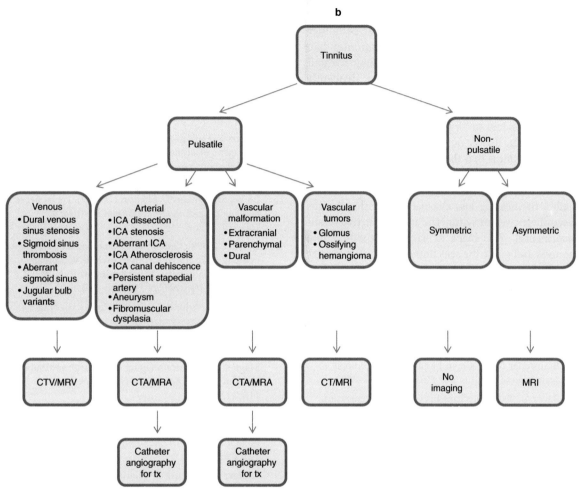

Figure 23.10 (cont.)
Abbreviations: CHL, conductive hearing loss; IAC, internal auditory canal; LVAS, large vestibular aqueduct syndrome NF-2.

on both MRI and CT due to the intense enhancement of both the tumor and the internal jugular vein. MRI with contrast may improve delineating the extent of the mass [5].

Ossifying hemangiomas occur on the facial nerve, most often in one of two characteristic locations, on the geniculate ganglion and within the IAC [46]. When they arise on the geniculate ganglion, facial paralysis is common, and when they arise in the IAC, SNHL is more common [2]. These tumors can be seen on MRI as an enhancing mass along the course of the facial nerve. The appearance is not diagnostic, as a similar appearance occurs with vestibular schwannoma or facial schwannoma [2]. CT will show the stippled calcification pattern characteristic of ossifying hemangioma [2].

Vascular tumors are fairly common; however, they generally will present with slowly progressive pulsatile tinnitus. They should be considered in patients with acute-onset pulsatile tinnitus, but are less likely to be the cause than other etiologies.

Conclusion

In conclusion, SNHL is evidence of pathology of the inner ear (membranous labyrinth), eighth cranial nerve, or brain [47]. CHL is evidence of pathology along the pathway from the external auditory canal, across the tympanic membrane and ossicular chain [47]. Continuous tinnitus often accompanies SNHL. Acute pulsatile tinnitus is rare, but may be seen with many of the entities described in this chapter.

Patients who present with unilateral non-pulsatile tinnitus and asymmetric hearing loss are more likely to have an imaging finding (retrocochlear pathology such as vestibular schwannoma or meningioma) than patients who have eighth-nerve pathology without tinnitus [12]. Hearing loss and tinnitus frequently coexist. Tinnitus can occur with both SNHL and CHL. Patients presenting with acute symptoms of either hearing loss or tinnitus need to be fully evaluated for both. It may not be apparent to the patient with acute tinnitus that they have hearing loss as well. This information is important for deciding the correct imaging work-up. It is important to determine whether the hearing loss associated with the tinnitus is asymmetric versus symmetric and conductive versus sensorineural. This helps to narrow the differential diagnosis and guide the selection of diagnostic studies (Figure 23.10).

References

1. Heller A (2003). Classification and epidemiology of tinnitus. *Otolaryngology Clin N Am* **36**: 239–248.

2. Branstetter B, Weissman J (2006). The radiologic evaluation of tinnitus. *Eur Radiol* **16**: 2792–2802.

3. Bauer C (2004). Mechanisms of tinnitus generation. *Curr Opin Otolaryngol Head Neck Surg* **12**: 413–417.

4. Bauer C, Brozoski T (2011). Effect of tinnitus retraining therapy on the loudness and annoyance of tinnitus: a controlled trial. *Ear Hearing* **32**: 145–155.

5. Vototh S, Shah R, Cure J (2010). A compartment-based approach for the imaging evaluation of tinnitus. *AJNR* **31**: 211–218.

6. Sismanis A (2003). Pulsatile tinnitus. *Otlaryngol Clin N Am* **36**: 389–402.

7. Sonmez G, Basekim C, Ozturk E, Gungo A, Kizilkaya E (2007). Imaging of pulsatile tinnitus; a review of 74 patients. *Clinical Imaging* **31**: 102–108.

8. Saunders J (2007). The role of central nervous system plastiicty in tinnitus. *Science Direct* **40**: 313–334.

9. Han B, Lee H, Kim T, Lim J, Shin K (2009). Tinnitus: characteristics, causes, mechanisms, and treatments. *J Clin Neurol* **5**: 11–19.

10. Mills J, Weber P (2001). Anatomy and physiology of hearing. In Bailey B, ed. *Head and Neck Surgery – Otolaryngology*. Philadelphia, PA: Lippincott Williams and Wilkins, pp. 1621–1640.

11. Chau J, Cho J, Fritz D (2012). Management of adult sensorineural hearing loss. *Otolaryngol Clin N Am* **45**: 941–958.

12. Levy R, Arts H (1996). Predicting neuroradiologic outcome in patients referred for audiovestibular dysfunction. *AJNR* **17**: 1717–1724.

13. Kartush J, Brackmann D (2012). Acoustic neuroma update. *Otolaryngol Clin N Am* **29**: 377–392.

14. De La Cruz A, Teufert K (2009). Transcochlear approach to the cerebellopontine angle and clivus lesions: indications, results and complications. *Otology Neurol* **30**: 373–380.

15. Mowry S, Hansen M, Gantz B (2012). Surgical management of internal auditory canal and cerebellopontine angle facial nerve schwannoma. *Otology Neurol* **33**: 1071–1076.

16. Lo W, Brackmann D, Shelton C (1989). Facial nerve hemangioma. *Annals Otol Rhinol Laryngol* **98**: 160–161.

17. Dawes P (1999). Outcome of using magnetic resonance imaging as an initial screen to exclude vestibular schwannoma in patients presenting with unilateral tinnitus. *J Laryngol Otol* **113**: 118–822.

18. Campbell A, Adunka O, Zhou B, Qaqish B, Buchman C (2011). Large vestibular aqueduct syndrome: anatomic and functional parameters. *Laryngoscope* **121**: 352–357.

19. Hirsch B, Weissman J, Curtin H, Kamerer D (1992). Magnetic resonance imaging of the large vestibular aqueduct. *Arch Otolaryngol Head Neck Surg* **118**: 1124–1127.

20. Lyos A, Marsh M, Jenkins H, Coker N (1995). Progressive hearing loss after transverse temporal bone fracture. *Arch Otolaryngol Head Neck Surg* **121**: 795–799.

21. Kramer M, Shattuck T, Charnock D (1997). Traumatic hearing loss following air-bag inflation. *N Engl J Med* **337**: 574–574.

22. Weissman J, Hirsch B (1997). Review: the imaging of Menière's disease. *Otolaryngol Clin N Am* **30**: 1105–1116.

23. Kaylie D, Jackson C, Gardner E (2005). Surgical management of Menière's disease in the erea of gentamicin. *Otolaryngol Head Neck Surg* **132**: 443–450.

24. Yoshida T, Teranishi M, Kato M, et al. (2012). Endolymphatic hydrops in patients with tinnitus as the major symptom. *Eur Arch Otorhinolaryngol* **270**: 3043–3048.

25. Yankaskas K (2013). Prelude: noise-induced tinnitus and hearing loss in the military. *Hearing Res* **295**: 3–8.

26. Sismanis A (2001). Tinnitus. *Curr Neurol Neurosci Reports* **1**: 492–499.

27. Daniels R, Swallow C, Shelton C, et al. (2000). Causes of unilateral sensorineural hearing loss screened by high-resolution fast spin echo magnetic resonance imaging:

review of 1, 070 consecutive cases. *Am J Otology* **21**: 173–180.

28. Barath K, Huber A, Stampli P, Varga Z, Kollias S (2011). Neuroradiology of cholesteatomas. *AJNR* **32**: 221–229.

29. Goodhill V, Harris I, Canalis R (2000). Otosclerosis In Canalis R, Lambert P, eds. *The Ear*. Philadelphia, PA: Lippincott Williams and Wilkins, pp. 467–487.

30. Conoyer J, Kaylie DM, Jackson CG (2007). Otologic surgery following ear trauma. *Otolaryngol Head Neck Surg* **137**: 757–761.

31. Brors D, Shafers M, Shick B, *et al.* (2001). Sigmoid and transverse sinus thrombosis after closed head injury presenting with unilateral hearing loss. *Neuroradiology* **43**: 144–146.

32. Krishnan A, Mattox D, Fountain A, Hudgins P (2006). CT arteriography and venography in pulsatile tinnitus: preliminary results. *AJNR* **27**: 1635–1638.

33. Stam J (2005). Thrombosis of the cerebral veins and sinuses. *N Engl J Med* **352**: 1791–1798.

34. Dietz R, Davis W, Hamsberger H, Jacobs J, Blatter D (1994). MR imaging and MR angiography in the evaluation of pulsatile tinnitus *AJNR* **15**: 879–889.

35. Russell E, De Michaelis B, Wiet R, Meyer J (1995). Objective pulse-synchronous "essential" tinnitus due to narrowing of the transverse dural venous sinus. *Int J Tinnitus* **1**: 127–137.

36. Remley K, Coit W, Harnsberger H, *et al.* (1990). Pulsatile tinnitus and the vascular tympanic membrane: CT, MR, and angiographic findings. *Head Neck Radiology* **174**: 383–389.

37. Madani G, Conor SEJ (2009). Imaging in pulsatile tinnitus. *Clin Radiol* **64**: 319–328.

38. Elijovich L, Kazmi K, Gauvrit J, Law M (2006). The emerging role of multidetector row CT angiography in the diagnosis of cervical arterial dissection: preliminary study. *Neuroradiology* **48**: 606–612.

39. Vertinsky A, Schwarz N, Fischbein N, *et al.* (2008). Comparison of multidetector CT angiography and MR imaging of cervical artery dissection. *AJNR* **29**: 1753–1760.

40. Plouin P, Perdu J, La Batide-Alanore A, *et al.* (2007). Fibromuscular dysplasia. *Orphanet J Rare Dis* **2**: 28.

41. Kang M, Escott E (2008). Imaging of tinnitus. *Otlaryngol Clin N Am* **41**: 179–193.

42. Ni W, Tian Y, Jiang H *et al.* (2013). Preliminary experience of 256-row multidetector computed tomographic angiography for detecting cerebral aneurysms. *J Comput Assisted Tomogr* **37**: 233–241.

43. Shin E, Lalwani A, Dowd C (2000). Role of angiography in the evaluation of patients with pulsatile tinnitus. *The Laryngoscope* 1916–1920.

44. Narvid J, Do H, Blevins N, Fischbein N (2011). CT angiography as a screening tool for dural arteriovenous fistula in patients with pulsatile tinnitus: feasibility and test characteristics. *AJNR* **32**: 446–453.

45. Willems P, Brouwer P, Barfett J, terBrugge K, Krings T (2011). Detection and classification of cranial dural arteriovenous fistulas using 4D-CT angiography: initial experience. *AJNR* **32**: 49–53.

46. Shelton C, Brackmann D, Lo W, Carbery J (1991). Intratemporal facial nerve hemangiomas. *Otolaryngol Head Neck Surg* **104**: 116–121.

47. Weissman JL (1996). State of the art: hearing loss. *Radiology* **199**: 593–611.

Appendix: Risks associated with imaging procedures in acute neurologic disease

Magnetic resonance imaging (MRI)

The MRI instrument

The MRI environment is associated with multiple major risk factors for patients as well as MRI staff, visiting medical personnel (e.g. emergency room physicians and anesthesiologists), and ancillary emergency personnel (e.g. police and firefighters).

Implanted and indwelling ferrous objects may undergo potentially dangerous translation and rotational motions when subjected to the large static magnetic fields of the MRI instrument when the patient (or staff) are approaching or are within the immediate magnet environment, and again when the patient emerges from that environment. Missile fatalities and all-too-common near-misses have been caused by many objects, including infusion pumps, anesthesia machines, scissors/clamps such as those originally within medical personnel pockets, cleaning tools (metallic buckets), and hardware associated with fire rescue (fire extinguishers) or police (weapons), among others.

Electrical currents can be induced in wire leads as they move through the main magnetic field and from transient magnetic fields associated with the gradient coils that are employed during image acquisition. Implants with potential electric circuits (e.g. leads and wires) and electromechanical devices (e.g. implanted drug infusion pumps and pacemakers) may pose additional risks of burns, damage to device, and device malfunction.

The general approach used by many MRI centers is to utilize multiple tiers of screening for risk (the clinicians requesting a study, the patient, the MRI personnel); metal detectors and physical zones with more restricted entry more proximal to the magnet environment; and frequent reference by MRI personnel to key resources regarding safety of specific (ferrous) devices, at specific magnetic fields, with requirements for strong written documentation regarding the implanted devices.

Most MRI-related burns are first degree (sunburns), usually associated with faulty surface coils or from suboptimal or incorrect positioning of the coil apparatus. Inadvertent electrical circuits and areas of heating may derive from patient sweat, patient position in scanner, and materials or chemicals on the patient's skin including some tattoos. Some medication patches may heat up and produce transient high (dangerous) doses of drug.

Detailed published recommendations for a safe MRI environment have been recently updated by Kanal *et al.* [1].

MRI contrast – nephrogenic systemic fibrosis

Apart from immediate anaphylactic contrast reactions (see below), the main risk of intravenous MRI contrast is nephrogenic systemic fibrosis (NSF). The risk associations for NSF are kidney disease and MRI contrast agents, with stronger associations suggested for more severe kidney disease, dialysis, higher contrast agent doses and possibly specific gadolinium (Gd) chelate formulations. Gd itself is a highly toxic rare-earth metal. The MRI contrast agents all include various formulations of Gd metal ion with a chelating agent to tightly bind the Gd, but there is always some free Gd. There is controversy regarding the exact mechanism and even the agent(s) responsible for NSF [2], but some concern that relative risk may be associated in part with MRI contrast agents with greater free Gd availability.

The most frequent clinical manifestations of NSF, occurring days to months and rarely years after exposure, are in the skin, the extremities more so than trunk, with reddened or darkened papules, patches, plaques, variable degrees of swelling, tightening, and thickening. It is now well recognized that the disorder is systemic, and can result in fibrosis in multiple organs.

Most MRI facilities have implemented restrictive guidelines. These may include a requirement for a serum creatinine screen or estimated glomerular filtration rate (eGFR) measurement, based on the patient's age (e.g. 60 years or above), or when there is an indication of risk for any renal disease. Typically, an MRI center may have specific absolute contraindications for intravenous MRI contrast, with possible exceptions in specific, well-documented emergency settings, and/or may have pre-set dose reduction policies for patients who undergo dialysis or for specific ranges of eGFR. There are already early indications that such strategies are effective [3].

MRI contrast reactions

Life-threatening anaphylactic contrast reactions (e.g. laryngeal edema and bronchospasm with respiratory compromise, and cardiovascular collapse) can and do occur with Gd-based MRI contrast. In one large retrospective review of 158 439 doses of MRI contrast, 0.0404% of the doses had adverse effects [4]. Most were mild (nausea, vomiting, and rash). Of the 64 doses with adverse effects, 11 of these (17.2%) were considered moderate. Moderate reactions included symptomatic urticaria, mild bronchospasm, vaso-vagal reactions, tachycardia, and diffuse erythema. Four of the 64 doses with adverse reactions (6.3%) were associated with major reactions. Major, life-threatening reactions may require treatment with immediate life support, epinephrine, and/or require treatment by emergency physicians, or transfer to an emergency room. Less immediately threatening reactions are often self-limited, and require observation and or treatment with diphenhydramine. Patients considered to be at higher risk for contrast reactions may be pre-treated by protocols that often contain corticosteroids and, depending on the timing relative to the contrast injection study, may include H1 inhibitors [5].

Pregnancy and MRI

MRI employs very strong static magnetic fields, fluctuating magnetic fields, and radiofrequency irradiation, all of which are considered to have small but not-zero influences on biological tissues, with special concerns particularly in the early stages of pregnancy. Guidelines for MRI in pregnant patients are available in the literature [1, 5], and generally include careful review and consideration of the risks and benefits and alternative imaging strategies.

MRI contrast agents are considered to cross the placenta, enter the fetal bloodstream, and their presence in amniotic fluid permits gut entry through swallowing. Although the risk to the fetus is unknown, it is considered potentially harmful; consequently, the use of MRI contrast during pregnancy requires special consideration [1, 5].

X-Rays and other ionizing radiation in diagnostic imaging

Diagnostic X-ray in non-pregnant adults until recently was considered to be relatively non-invasive, but has received considerable attention in both the lay press and professional literature from recognition of adverse events including dramatic skin burns and hair loss associated with perfusion computed tomography (CT), and tissue necrosis during long diagnostic or more often interventional (fluoroscopic) procedures. There are also more theoretical but very concerning risks to the population from ever-increasing exposure to X-ray primarily from the dramatic increase in CT utilization in the past decade [6], and this is especially concerning in children [7].

Specifically, for CT, there is increased risk associated with multiple scans repeated in one imaging session within restricted regions of anatomy. For example, perfusion CT requires time-series (repeat) imaging over the same slices, and there is at least theoretical concern for repeat scans over multiple sessions where cumulative doses may be high. CT (or any imaging study) should always be performed with the lowest possible exposure dose that achieves diagnostic quality.

CT-based screening procedures carry special increased risk of cancer related to dosing large patient populations, potentially multiple times over an individual lifetime. Pediatric imaging in general is considered an important risk that requires thoughtful consideration and planning, and alternative diagnostic imaging strategies (e.g. ultrasound) when feasible and appropriate [7].

X-rays in CT are potentially teratogenic as well as mutagenic. Pregnant and possibly pregnant patients may require special consideration including written consent. Non-contrast MRI rather than CT may be recommended for pregnant/possibly pregnant patients whenever clinically reasonable. Other risks such as cataracts from lens exposure are minimized by use of optimized scan planes.

371

Intravascular (iodinated) contrast

There is an anaphylactic risk associated with intravascular CT contrast, the risk factors and adverse outcomes generally similar to those described above for MRI. Historically, the likelihood of CT contrast reactions exceed those for MRI but, with modern CT contrast (non-ionic formulations), the incidence of life-threatening anaphylactic reactions, as well as more minor reactions (nausea/vomiting), has decreased, but has not been eliminated.

In one large retrospective series, with 298 491 doses of low-osmolar iodinated contrast injections, there were 458 adverse reactions, for an adverse effect rate of 0.153%. Fifteen of the 458 reactions (3.3%) were considered severe; seven required treatment with epinephrine, 10 required transfer to an emergency department [4]. There was one death in a 79-year-old within 20 minutes of injection with cardiovascular collapse while the patient was waiting for transport after the CT.

CT contrast medium is also associated with acute renal failure and worsening of chronic nephropathy. The contribution and risk of specific CT contrast agents to acute renal failure is a controversial topic, in part as the study patients often have multiple, potentially independent risk factors at the time of their CT [8]. CT contrast increases the osmotic load; consequently, patients with significant cardiac disease may be at risk, which may require use of lower osmolality and contrast volumes.

Guidelines for contrast administration in patients considering the various risk factors have been published [5]. Similar to MRI, imaging facilities typically require a recent serum creatinine or eGFR screen [9], or an alternative measure of renal function for patients meeting a predetermined threshold for risk. Patients receiving multiple CT studies within short intervals, and especially those with additional risk factors, require greater scrutiny for renal toxicity from intravenous contrast. Protocols are available for hydration during or before the CT in higher-risk patients [5].

Metformin is frequently used in patients with type 2 diabetes. Concerns for renal impairment and an increased risk of lactic acidosis with renal failure induced by intravascular iodinated contrast have led to policies for withholding doses of metformin prior to contrast-enhanced CT. After holding metformin doses, imaging-center policies also vary for retesting renal function, and establishing normal renal function prior to restarting metformin. Metformin policy is most controversial with regard to patients who have normal baseline renal function, where evidence for risk is currently limited [10].

The American College of Radiology (ACR) Manual on Contrast Media (www.acr.org) provides a detailed and up-to-date discussion of risk factors for contrast reaction, premedication, and other recommendations [5].

Myelographic contrast agents

Myelography is currently performed with non-ionic contrast agents, generally utilizing the lowest total dose and volume required for the specific procedure and anatomy of interest. As for all contrast agents, there is a risk of rare anaphylactic reactions. Hypotensive episodes (vasovagal) during myelography are not uncommon. Consequently, some facilities routinely require placement of an intravascular (venous) access device for rapid therapeutic intervention.

Much more uncommon are procedure-associated life-threatening risk for brain herniation from changes in cerebrospinal fluid (CSF) pressure (large intracerebral mass lesions) and rare but potentially catastrophic injection of contrast directly into the spinal cord (e.g. cervical myelography with C1–C2 puncture). Additional risks include nerve damage from spinal needle trauma, infection (meningitis), induced inflammation, and CSF leak with post-procedure spinal headache, which may be severe and prolonged.

The risk of seizures with modern myelographic contrast agents is low. Surveys suggest that most, but not all, practitioners continue to stop seizure-threshold-lowering drugs ~ 48 hours before and through 24 hours after myelography [11]. The risk of intraspinal bleeding is most often typically assessed with coagulation studies and through the consideration of risk factors, and is minimized by discontinuing antiplatelet agents, aspirin, or non-steroidal anti-inflammatory drugs.

Angiography

Formal catheter angiography includes risks associated with intravascular contrast agents as described above, although intra-arterial injection has typically been associated with lower, but not zero, anaphylactic complications compared to intravenous injection [12]. Additionally, as for other sources of ionizing X-irradiation, there is an important risk of skin injury including burns, hair loss, and tissue necrosis associated with long or repeated procedures. These radiation injuries are often delayed, appearing weeks or months after the procedure [13].

Catheter-associated risks include local bleeding at the puncture site, direct vessel injury, pseudoaneurysm, dissection, occlusion, stroke, and death [12, 14, 15]. The risk is related to the type of procedure, and individual risk factors including age. In one large cerebral angiography series [14] the complication rate was 1.3%, with 0.5% permanent complications. Risk factors included age, cardiovascular disease, and catheter time. Lower complications rates have also been reported [12, 15].

Nuclear medicine

Nuclear medicine procedures are only rarely utilized in acute neurologic presentations, but may be part of an early diagnostic evaluation. Positron emission tomography (PET) is typically now performed as combined PET/CT. The CT provides anatomic correlation, but also allows attenuation correction to lower the PET dose compared to earlier PET techniques. However, the risk of ionizing radiation is from the combined exposure of the positron emitter and the CT exposure. In PET, the radiopharmaceutical, for example ^{18}F-fluorodeoxyglucose, emits a positron that travels only a few millimeters before interacting with an electron; the positron-electron annihilation event results in gamma photons that are detected. Although "low dose" CT is typically utilized in PET/CT, the total ionizing radiation doses of PET/CT are substantial [16].

SPECT/CT also has an ionizing radiation risk, and some risk from more stringent head (therefore neck as well) positioning compared to PET/CT, which should be considered in patients with cervical spine injury.

References

1. Expert Panel on MR Safety, Kanal E, Barkovich AJ, *et al.* (2013). ACR guidance document on MR safe practices: *J Magn Reson Imaging* **37**: 501–530.
2. Idee JM, Port M, Dencausse A, Lancelot E, Corot C (2009). Involvement of gadolinium chelates in the mechanism of nephrogenic systemic fibrosis: an update. *Radiologic Clin N Am* **47**: 855–869.
3. Wang Y, Alkasab TK, Narin O, *et al.* (2011). Incidence of nephrogenic systemic fibrosis after adoption of restrictive gadolinium-based contrast agent guidelines. *Radiology* **260**: 105–111.
4. Hunt CH, Hartman RP, Hesley GK (2009). Frequency and severity of adverse effects of iodinated and gadolinium contrast materials: retrospective review of 456, 930 doses. *AJR* **193**: 1124–1127.
5. ACR Committee on Drugs and Contrast Media (2013). ACR Manual on Contrast Media. Version 9. American College of Radiology. See: www.acr.org.
6. Fazel R, Krumholz HM, Wang Y, *et al.* (2009). Exposure to low-dose ionizing radiation from medical imaging procedures. *N Engl J Med* **361**: 849–857.
7. Miglioretti DL, Johnson E, Williams A, *et al.* (2013). The use of computed tomography in pediatrics and the associated radiation exposure and estimated cancer risk. *JAMA Pediatr* **10**: 1–8.
8. Davenport MS, Khalatbari S, Cohan RH, *et al.* (2013). Contrast material-induced nephrotoxicity and intravenous low-osmolality iodinated contrast material: risk stratification by using estimated glomerular filtration rate. *Radiology* **268**: 719–728.
9. Davenport MS, Khalatbari S, Cohan RH, Ellis JH (2013). Contrast medium-induced nephrotoxicity risk assessment in adult inpatients: a comparison of serum creatinine level- and estimated glomerular filtration rate-based screening methods. *Radiology* **269**: 92–100.
10. Goergen SK, Rumbold G, Compton G, Harris C (2010). Systematic review of current guidelines, and their evidence base, on risk of lactic acidosis after administration of contrast medium for patients receiving metformin. *Radiology* **254**: 261–269.
11. Sandow BA, Donnal JF (2005). Myelography complications and current practice patterns. *AJR* **185**: 768–771.
12. Thiex R, Norbash AM, Frerichs KU (2010). The safety of dedicated-team catheter-based diagnostic cerebral angiography in the era of advanced noninvasive imaging. *AJNR* **31**: 230–234.
13. Koenig TR, Wolff D, Mettler FA, Wagner LK (2001). Skin injuries from fluoroscopically guided procedures: part 1, characteristics of radiation injury. *AJR* **177**: 3–11.
14. Willinsky RA, Taylor SM, TerBrugge K, *et al.* (2003). Neurologic complications of cerebral angiography: prospective analysis of 2,899 procedures and review of the literature. *Radiology* **227**: 522–528.
15. Dawkins AA, Evans AL, Wattam J, *et al.* (2007). Complications of cerebral angiography: a prospective analysis of 2,924 consecutive procedures. *Neuroradiology* **49**: 753–759.
16. Huang B, Law MW, Khong PL (2009). Whole-body PET/CT scanning: estimation of radiation dose and cancer risk. *Radiology* **251**: 166–174.

Index